D0021721

FUNCTIONAL FOODS

HOW TO ORDER THIS BOOK

BY PHONE: 800-233-9936 or 717-291-5609, 8AM–5PM Eastern Time

BY FAX: 717-295-4538

BY MAIL: Order Department
Technomic Publishing Company, Inc.
851 New Holland Avenue, Box 3535
Lancaster, PA 17604, U.S.A.

BY CREDIT CARD: American Express, VISA, MasterCard

BY WWW SITE: http://www.techpub.com

FUNCTIONAL FOODS

Biochemical & Processing Aspects

Edited by

G. Mazza, Ph.D.

Agriculture and Agri-Food Canada

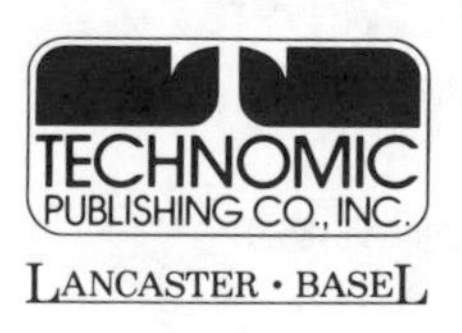

LANCASTER · BASEL

Functional Foods
a **TECHNOMIC**® publication

Technomic Publishing Company, Inc.
851 New Holland Avenue, Box 3535
Lancaster, Pennsylvania 17604 U.S.A.

Printed in the United States of America

10 9 8 7 6 5 4 3 2 1

Main entry under title:
Functional Foods: Biochemical and Processing Aspects

A Technomic Publishing Company book
Bibliography: p.
Includes index p. 439

Library of Congress Catalog Card No. 98-85171
ISBN No. 1-56676-487-4

To my wife Rachel, my daughter Victoria, and my sons Michael and Joseph who received less of my attention while this book was being written/edited.

Table of Contents

Foreword

FUNCTIONAL foods, designer foods and nutraceuticals—terms used interchangeably to refer to foods or isolated food ingredients that deliver specific nonnutritive physiological benefits that may enhance health—have clearly emerged as major food industry buzzwords of the late 1990s. Initially viewed as a passing fad, the concept of formulating foods for their ancillary health benefits is a trend that is quickly moving into the corporate mainstream [1,2]. The topic of functional foods has been the focus of numerous international meetings [3] and one of the leading topics of interest within the field of food technology in 1997 [4]. With a current (1997) U.S. market value estimated at $86 billion and a growth rate of +7.5% [5], the functional food/nutraceutical trend is clearly one that will continue to grow as we enter the next millennium.

A significant driving force in the functional foods marketplace is consumer demand—the quest by consumers to optimize their health through food. The "health race for health-promoting ingredients" was identified as the fourth most important trend in the food industry in 1996 [6], while the most recently released HealthFocus Trend Report [7] found that the percentage of today's shoppers who believe that certain foods can help to reduce their reliance on drugs and medical therapies increased significantly in just 2 years—from 42% to 52%. Finally, in a recent R&D Magazine survey (in *Food Processing*) of the top 100 food companies, functional foods/nutraceuticals were identified as the single most important consumer trend impacting new food product development [8]. Increasing consumer demand for healthier foods or food ingredients is not likely to dwindle as baby boomers attempt to stave off the chronic health problems associated with aging and realize that dietary intervention can be a safe and cost-effective alternative to drugs or other more traditional therapies.

Research and development activity in the functional foods arena is no longer relegated to companies "on the fringe," since a number of industry conglomerates have recently made substantial commitments of resources to the development of such products. Having broken new ground in 1984 by utilizing an unapproved health claim on its All Bran® cereal to raise consumer awareness about the importance of fiber in colon cancer prevention, Kellogg's has once again established itself as an innovator by being the first major food conglomerate to formally establish a Functional Foods Division [9]. In April of 1997, Kellogg's petitioned the U.S. Food and Drug Administration under the Nutrition Labeling and Education Act (NLEA) of 1990 for a health claim on the role of dietary fiber from wheat bran in reducing the risk of colon cancer [10]. This petition follows on the success of the first food-specific health claim, awarded in January of 1997 to the Quaker Oats Company, for the association between the consumption of soluble fiber from whole oat products and a reduced risk of coronary heart disease [11]. Another large company that has made a commitment to the development of functional foods is the Campbell Soup Company, which introduced its Intelligent Quisine home-delivered meal program in 1996 [12]. Developed in consultation with the American Heart Association and the American Diabetes Association, Intelligent Quisine is specifically formulated for individuals with elevated blood cholesterol, diabetes, and high blood pressure. Five clinical trials conducted at eight universities (involving 1,200 subjects) have demonstrated that, after following this meal plan for 10 weeks, 73% of the participants reduced their blood cholesterol, 75% reduced their blood pressure, and 62% reduced their blood sugar. Clearly, food companies are beginning to respond to leading consumer health concerns.

Nonfood companies are also venturing into the functional food/nutraceutical arena. For example, Johnson & Johnson's McNeil Consumer Products division recently announced that it has acquired the U.S. marketing rights for the cholesterol-lowering margarine Benecol [13], a functional food whose sales have reached $17 million annually in Finland, a country with a population of only 3 million adults. DuPont has recently acquired Protein Technologies International [14], the leading manufacturer of soy protein isolate, a functional ingredient that has been the focus of intense research efforts because of its ability to lower cholesterol [15] and possibly reduce the risk of cancer [16], osteoporosis [17], and symptoms associated with menopausal transition [18].

Market activity for functional foods increases significantly in response to a more flexible regulatory environment. For example, in Japan, which is the first and only country to have established a specific approval process for functional foods—Foods for Specified Health Use (FOSHU)—80 approved FOSHU products have been developed in less than 5 years [19].

A critical issue in the regulation of functional foods, particularly if any claims are to be made in the labeling of these products, is the identification of the active component responsible for the purported health benefits. As Dr. Alison Stephen astutely points out in Chapter 14, Regulatory Aspects of Functional Products, "It is unacceptable anywhere to be told that a product of any kind has a particular action if it is uncertain whether or not it contains the right components to bring about that action." Thus, companies that wish to utilize the oat/coronary heart disease health claim on a product, for example, must be able to demonstrate that the product bearing the claim contains 0.75 grams of β-glucan—the physiological component responsible for the cholesterol-lowering effect—per reference amount customarily consumed (RACC). This level is based on a total daily intake of 3 grams (the effective dose) of β-glucan per day, consumed over four eating occasions.

Although several recent books have emerged on the topic of functional or designer foods [20–22], none has addressed the issue of processing, which can profoundly affect the health-enhancing potential of a functional food. Processing of a functional food may have profound effects on the specific health benefits it claims to deliver. If, for example, the physiological effect of β-glucan were altered significantly during processing, it is conceivable that the lipid-lowering properties associated with it could be lost, a result that is obviously undesirable. Conversely, certain processing techniques may *enhance* the health benefits of a functional food. A good example of this can be seen with flax, an oilseed that, because of its significant α-linolenic acid content, is highly susceptible to oxidation. As illustrated in Chapter 4 by Oomah and Mazza, microencapsulation of flaxseed oil produces a product with very high oxidative stability, which has many applications for new, health-enhancing products.

Foods are composed of a myriad biologically active constituents that may contribute to health enhancement [23]. *Functional Foods: Biochemical and Processing Aspects,* in addition to providing a comprehensive overview of an array of these biologically active compounds from both plant and animal sources, is unique in its ability to shed light on how the processing of these phytochemicals and zoochemicals may impact the health benefits of functional foods. The information in this book will thus be of value to anyone interested in this tremendously exciting and rapidly growing area in the food and nutrition sciences, and I am grateful to G. (Joe) Mazza for giving me the opportunity to review the information herein and provide these comments.

REFERENCES

1. Best, D. 1997. "All Natural and Nutraceutical," Prep. Foods 166(6):32–38.
2. Hollingsworth, P. 1997. "Mainstreaming Healthy Foods," Food Technol. 51(3): 55–58.

3. First International Conference on East-West Perspectives on Functional Foods. 1996. Nutr. Rev. 54(11):S1–S202.
4. Neff, J. and J. R. Holman. 1997. "How the Latest Products Toe the Fine Line Between Food and Drugs," Food Proc. 58(4):23–26.
5. Anon. 1997. "Nutraceuticals Trend Takes Root Despite Definitional Challenges," Nutr. Bus. J. 11(8):1–3, 15.
6. Sloan, E. 1996. "The Top 10 Trends to Watch and Work on," Food Technol. 50(7):55--71.
7. Gilbert, L. 1996. "HealthFocus Trend Report," HealthFocus, Des Moines, IA.
8. Kevin, K. 1997. "The 1997 Top 100® R&D Survey," Food Proc. 58(6):65–70.
9. VanValkenburgh, J. 1996. "Kellogg Co. Adds New Anti-Disease-Oriented Food Division," Commercial Appeal, Oct. 29.
10. Anon. 1997. "FDA Reviewing Petition for Wheat Bran Fiber/Colon Cancer Health Claim," Food Label. Nutr. News 5(35):17–18.
11. Food and Drug Administration. 1997. "Food Labeling: Health Claims; Oats and Coronary Heart Disease; Final Rule," Department of Health and Human Services, Part III, 21 CFR, Part 101, January 23.
12. O'Donnell, C. D. 1997. "Campbell's R&D Cozies Up to the Consumer," Prep. Foods 166(10):26–30.
13. Neff, J. 1997. "Foods of Tomorrow. Big Companies Take Nutraceuticals to Heart," Food Proc. 58(10):37–42.
14. Ricciuto, M. 1997. "DuPont to Acquire Protein Technologies International from Ralston Purina," Press Release, DuPont, Wilmington, DE.
15. Anderson, J. W., B. M. Johnstone, M. E. Cook-Newell. 1995. "Meta-Analysis of the Effects of Soy Protein Intake on Serum Lipids," N. Engl. J. Med. 333:276–282.
16. Messina, M. and S. Barnes. 1991. "The Role of Soy Products in Reducing Risk of Cancer," J. Natl. Cancer Inst. 83(8):541–546.
17. Arjmandi, B. H., L. Alekel, B. W. Hollis, D. Amin, P. Guo, M. Stacewicz-Sapuntzakis and S. Kukreja. 1996. "Dietary Soybean Protein Prevents Bone Loss in an Ovariectomized Rat Model of Osteoporosis," J. Nutr. 126:161-167.
18. Albertazzi, P., F. Pansini, G. Bonaccorsi, L. Zanotti, E. Forini and D. De Aloysio. 1997. "The Effect of Dietary Soy Supplementation on Hot Flushes," Obstet. Gynecol. 91:6–11.
19. Bailey, R. 1997. "The Status of Foods for Specified Health Use (FOSHU) in Japan," Presented at NUTRACON '97, Las Vegas, NV, July 18, 1997.
20. Goldberg, I., ed., 1994. Functional Foods, Designer Foods, Pharmafoods, and Nutraceuticals, New York, Chapman & Hall.
21. Finley, J. W., D. J. Armstrong, S. Nagy and S. F. Robinson, eds. 1996. Hypernutritious Foods, Auburndale, FL, Agscience, Inc.
22. LaChance, P. A., ed. 1997. Nutraceuticals: Designer Foods III. Garlic, Soy and Licorice, Trumbull, CT, Food & Nutrition Press, Inc.
23. Steinmetz, K. A. and J. D. Potter. 1991. "Vegetables, Fruit, and Cancer. II. Mechanisms," Cancer Causes Control 2:427–442.

CLARE M. HASLER
Urbana, Illinois

Preface

THIS book provides a comprehensive treatment of the physiological effects of foods and food components capable of promoting good health and preventing or alleviating diseases. Our objective was to assemble in one volume the large amount of information that has been published in recent years on the nature and physiological effects of biologically active components of major plant foods (cereals, oilseeds, fruits, and vegetables), dairy and fish products. Opportunities for the application of existing and novel food processing methods to the manufacturing of food products with health-enhancing effects are also discussed in various chapters.

Entire chapters are devoted to functional food products from oats, wheat, rice, flaxseed, mustard, fruits, vegetables, fish and dairy products. The chapter on designer vegetable oils covers all the recent developments in vegetable oils, including genetically modified oils and engineering and production of structured lipids. Functional products from quinoa, amaranth, beans, ginseng, echinacea, and other botanicals are covered in separate chapters. The book ends with an authoritative chapter on the present regulatory status of functional foods in the United States, Japan, Canada, and the European Union. This chapter also discusses assessment of natural products for use in promoting human health and as medicinal agents. The issue of where the burden of proof to show an effect of a food product on a physiological or biochemical process lies and costs of making health claims are also considered.

With over 1,800 literature references, this book is expected to benefit food scientists and technologists, food process engineers, biochemists, nutritionists, public health professionals, as well as entrepreneurs, who are designing, processing, and marketing new functional food products. Everyone who believes in the need for foods that combine nutritional and medical benefits, and believe that such foods can be produced, will find this book invaluable.

As editor, I wish to express my sincere appreciation to the 26 contributors who, by giving freely of their expertise, have made the book possible. Many thanks are also due to Paul Ferguson and Linda Kerr, who helped with the preparation of portions of the book. My gratitude is also extended to several of my colleagues at Agriculture and Agri-Food Canada and elsewhere who read and commented on the drafts of various chapters; in particular, I thank Clare Hasler, Carrie Thomson, Robert Ackman, and the staff and management of Technomic Publishing Co., Inc., especially Eleanor Riemer.

I shall be very obliged to readers who would call my attention to aspects that have been neglected and to errors or omissions that might appear in this book.

G. MAZZA

List of Contributors

BEER, Michael U.
Department of Food Science
Swiss Federal Institute of Technology
CH-8092 Zurich, Switzerland

BLACK, Richard
Nestlé Canada Inc.
Sheppard Avenue West
Toronto, ON M2N 6S8 Canada

CHAMPAGNE, Elaine T.
USDA ARS Southern Regional
Research Center
P.O. Box 19687
New Orleans, LA 70179 USA

CHAO, Eunice
Kellogg Canada Inc.
6700 Finch Avenue West
Etobicoke, ON M9W 5P2 Canada

CUI, Wuwei
Food Processing and Quality
Improvement Program
Agriculture and Agri-Food Canada
Guelph, ON Canada

DELAQUIS, Pascal
Food Research Program
Agriculture and Agri-Food Canada
Pacific Agri-Food Research Centre
Summerland, BC V0H 1Z0 Canada

ESKIN, N. A. Michael
Department of Food & Nutrition
University of Manitoba
Winnipeg, MB R3T 2N2 Canada

FITZPATRICK, Kelley
Plant Biotechnology Institute
National Research Council of Canada
110 Gymnasium Place
Saskatoon, SK S7N 0W9 Canada

GIRARD, Benoit
Food Research Program
Agriculture and Agri-Food Canada
Pacific Agri-Food Research Centre
Summerland, BC V0H 1Z0 Canada

GURAYA, Harmeet
USDA ARS Southern Regional
Research Center
P.O. Box 19687
New Orleans, LA 70179 USA

GUZMÁN-MOLDONADÓ, S. H.
Depto. de Biotecnología
y Bioquímica
Centre de Investigación y de Estudios
Avanzados del IPN
Apdo. Postal 629, 36500 Irapuato,
GTO México

HASLER, Clare M.
The Functional Foods for Health
Program
Department of Food Science and
Human Nutrition
University of Illinois at
Urbana-Champaign
103 Agricultural Bioprocess Lab,
M/C 640
1302 West Pennsylvania Avenue
Urbana, IL 61801 USA

JELEN, Pavel
Department of Agricultural,
Food and Nutritional Science
University of Alberta
Agriculture-Forestry Centre Building
Edmonton, AB T6G 2P5 Canada

LI, Thomas S. C.
Food Research Program
Agriculture and Agri-Food Canada
Pacific Agri-Food Research Centre
Summerland, BC V0H 1Z0 Canada

LUTZ, Susan
Food Processing Development
Alberta Agriculture, Food and Rural
Development
Leduc, AB T9E 6M2 Canada

MAZZA, G. (Joe)
Food Research Program
Agriculture and Agri-Food Canada
Pacific Agri-Food Research Centre
Summerland, BC V0H 1Z0 Canada

McCASKILL, Don R.
Riceland Foods Inc.
P.O. Box 927
Stuttgart, AR 72160 USA

McDONALD, Bruce E.
Department of Foods and Nutrition
University of Manitoba
Winnipeg, MB R3T 2N2 Canada

MOLDENHAUER, Karen A.
Rice Research & Extension Center
University of Arkansas
P.O. Box 351
Stuttgart, AR 72160 USA

OOMAH, B. Dave
Food Research Program
Agriculture and Agri-Food Canada
Pacific Agri-Food Research Centre
Summerland, BC V0H 1Z0 Canada

PAREDES-LÓPEZ, Octavio
Depto. de Biotecnología
y Bioquímica
Centro de Investigación y de Estudios
Avanzados del IPN
Apdo. Postal 629, 36500 Irapuato,
GTO México

SHAHIDI, Fereidoon
Department of Biochemistry
Memorial University of
Newfoundland
St. John's, NF A1B 3X9 Canada

SIMMONS, Curt
Kellogg Company
Science and Technology Center
235 Porter Street, P.O. Box 3423
Battle Creek, MI 49016-3423 USA

STEPHEN, Alison
College of Pharmacy and Nutrition
University of Saskatchewan
110 Science Place
Sakatoon, SK S7N 5T9 Canada

WANG, Larry
Biological Sciences
University of Alberta
Edmonton, AB T6G 2E9 Canada

WOOD, Peter
Centre for Food and Animal Research
K.W. Neatby Building
Agriculture and Agri-Food Canada
Central Experimental Farm
Ottawa, ON K1A 0C6 Canada

CHAPTER 1

Functional Oat Products

P. J. WOOD[1]
M. U. BEER[1]

1. INTRODUCTION

THE Food and Drug Administration (FDA) of the USA has recently allowed a health claim for an association between consumption of diets high in oatmeal, oat bran, or oat flour and reduced risk of coronary heart disease. This represents the first health claim for a specific food under the Nutrition Labeling and Education Act (1990) and follows on a long history of investigation and controversy. The claim is based on the many clinical studies that concluded that oat products may reduce serum cholesterol levels, a risk factor for coronary heart disease, but the magnitude and the significance of the reduction have been variable and sources of argument. The FDA analysis separated studies into those done with subjects having normal or elevated cholesterol levels, and those done with subjects who were on a fat-reduced (<30% of calories) diet, or the more normal North American levels of fat intake. Many other variables make comparison of studies difficult, such as nature of product and daily dose; type of control diet or baseline cholesterol level from which change is determined; management, if any, of nutrient intake; recording of diet; changes in subject weight; sex and age of subjects; and study duration and design. Nevertheless, the overall conclusion from the FDA review was that oats could indeed lower serum cholesterol levels, specifically low-density lipoprotein (LDL) cholesterol, without change in the high-density lipoprotein (HDL) fraction; on this basis a health claim for reduced heart disease risk was allowed. The FDA has allowed that the

[1]Centre for Food and Animal Research, Agriculture and Agri-Food Canada, Ottawa, ON, Canada.

main active ingredient, in this respect, is the soluble fibre $(1 \rightarrow 3)(1 \rightarrow 4)$-$\beta$-D-glucan, or β-glucan.

Uncertainties remain as does a need for further research. There is no consensus on mechanism of action, and although a daily intake of 3 g β-glucan per day is suggested as a minimum, better dose response information (which may vary with population group), and elucidation of physicochemical characteristics needed for physiological response is needed. β-Glucan was accepted as the main active ingredient, but this does not imply that any source of β-glucan is allowed; the health claim is specifically for oat bran, rolled oats (oatmeal), and oat flour. However, the ruling does open the way for new claims such as for novel oat products or barley, if sufficient supporting evidence is provided.

This chapter will review the nature of oats as related to properties that might alleviate, or reduce, the risk of chronic disease, such as diabetes and heart disease. Since β-glucan and viscosity appear to be important for modifying blood lipids and attenuating blood glucose and insulin responses, the focus will be on this component and its properties. Where appropriate, β-glucan of other cereals, particularly barley, will be referred to for comparison. There is good reason to suppose that barley may similarly reduce serum cholesterol levels [1].

There are in oats a multitude of components with the potential for modifying blood lipids [2] or conferring other physiological benefits; in horses, for example, oats are believed to contribute to friskiness, a psychological modification with mixed blessings in humans. The outer layers of oats are similar to those of other cereals in being a good source of insoluble dietary fibre with the attendant capacity to improve colonic function and possibly reduce the risk of colon cancer. Many other functionally distinct components such as waxes, lignin, phytate, vitamins, minerals, and phenolics concentrate in these layers [3]. Some of these compounds are powerful antioxidants and may possess potent pharmacological properties. Oats are a whole-grain food capable of providing nutritious sustenance in a more general sense, that is to say, it provides protein, energy, vitamins, minerals, and a good amino acid balance [4]. Thus, oats fulfill admirably the description of a functional food, as one that, in addition to providing all normal attributes of a food—basic sustenance, pleasing taste and texture—also confers a specific health benefit.

2. NATURE OF OAT PRODUCTS

2.1. WHOLE OATS

The common cultivated food and feed oat is the species *Avena sativa*. Two excellent books review the chemistry, technology, production, utilization, and nutritional value of oats [5,6].

Figure 1.1 shows an outstanding line drawing of an oat seed, based on de-

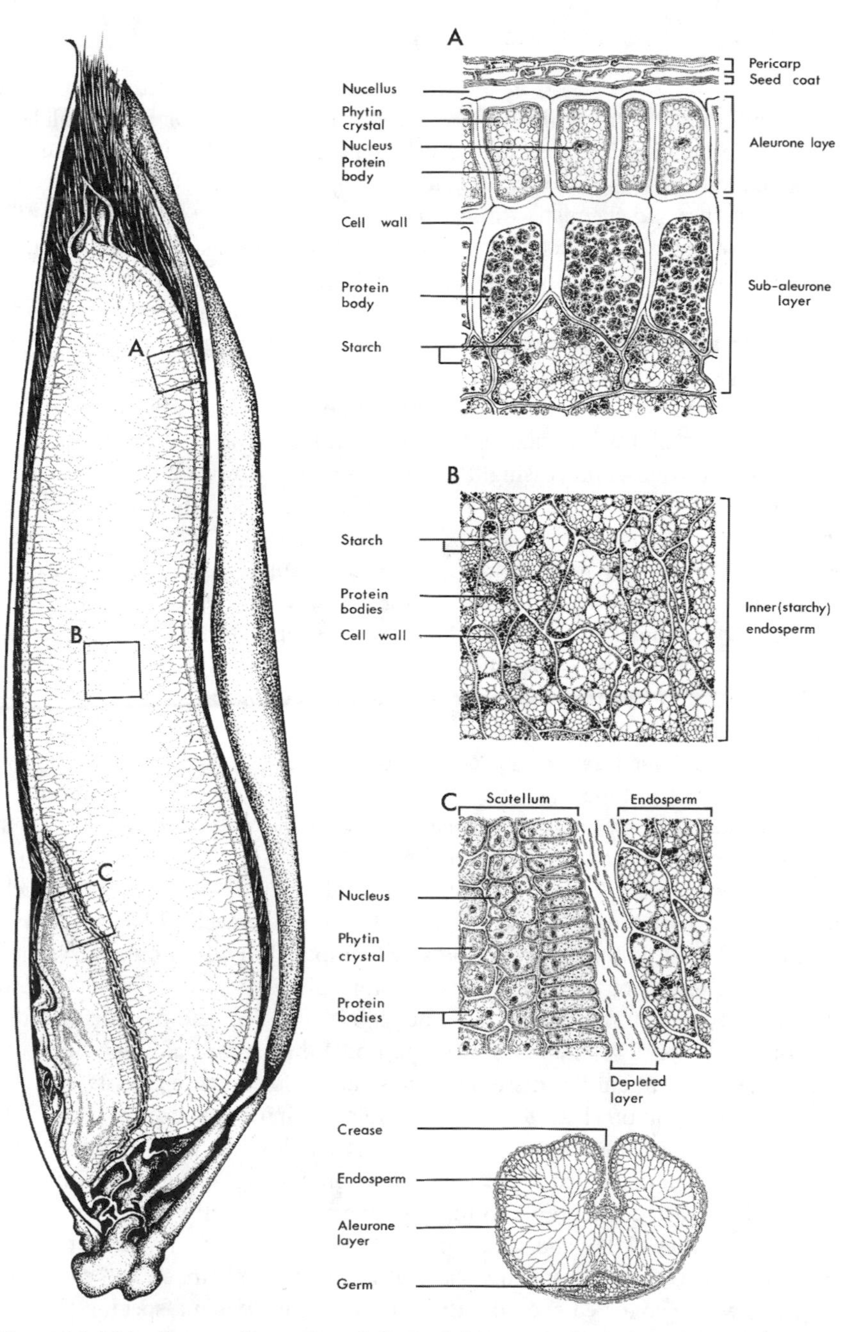

Figure 1.1 Major features of an oat kernel. On the left is a seed with the hull, showing the major structural characteristics. At the bottom right is a cross-sectional area showing a portion of the germ. A, B, and C are magnifications of the portions of the bran, inner starchy endosperm, and germ as indicated, detailing the different tissues and microstructures. (Reprinted from Reference [14], with permission.)

tailed micrographs drawn by F. Wong under the direction of R. G. Fulcher. This representation has been extensively reproduced in the literature, and is included again here since it serves as a succinct reminder of the diversity of microstructure and chemistry throughout the seed. It is easy to see that significant variations in these details, such as cell wall thickness, may occur in different cultivars. These characteristics of oats, and their potential variations, in effect control the manner in which oats are processed and utilized as food.

As harvested, oats (except for some naked or hull-less types) retain their hull (husk), which accounts for about 25–30% of the seed, oats for food use are first "de-hulled" (sometimes termed "hulled). While readily digested by ruminants, the highly lignified and fibrous covering is not suitable for human consumption without processing. Properly processed however, it makes a useful fibre ingredient for the food industry. Unprocessed hulls contain silicate particles, sometimes called spicules, which have a barbed nature and can irritate the mouth, esophagus, and possibly the gastrointestinal tract. These are removed for food products. Phenolics (lignin) may also be removed to give a white product known as oat fibre—this is almost entirely insoluble dietary fibre, and should not be confused with oat bran. In a study with oat fibre involving type II diabetic subjects, a transitory lowering of fasting blood glucose and LDL-cholesterol levels was observed (during hospitalization phase), but was not retained during the "ambulatory" phase [7]. Stool weight was increased but transit time was unchanged and the fibre was resistant to fermentation. Thus, oat fibre may provide stool bulking and reduce constipation, but potential benefits from fermentation are absent [8].

Details of further processing to primary food products and ingredients such as rolled oats, oatmeal, flour, and bran have been reviewed [9,10,11]. An essential difficulty in the milling of oats, as compared to wheat or corn, relates to the soft nature of the kernel and the lipid distribution throughout. These features make both removal of the outer lignified layers and particle classifications (and hence separation of a white flour) difficult. In addition, the moment the groat structure is disrupted, lipase and lipoxygenase activity, and atmospheric oxidation, lead to fatty acid release and formation of oxidized, products with an unpleasant flavor. To prevent this, the oats or groats are given a high-moisture heat treatment before processing. Given these difficulties and the fact that there is no readily identifiable functional utility or end product, such as gluten and break-making for wheat, starch for corn, or malt for barley, it is hardly surprising that oat has been the "cinderella" crop, despite its well recognized overall nutritional value. Now that a specific physiological function—cholesterol lowering—has been identified, it is likely that new processes and ingredients will appear with oat bran representing the first generation.

Selective dye-binding characteristics allow detection of β-glucan [12] and microscopic evaluation of distribution, either visually or by microspectrofluorometric mapping (Figure 1.2 [13]). Oat β-glucan was shown to be distrib-

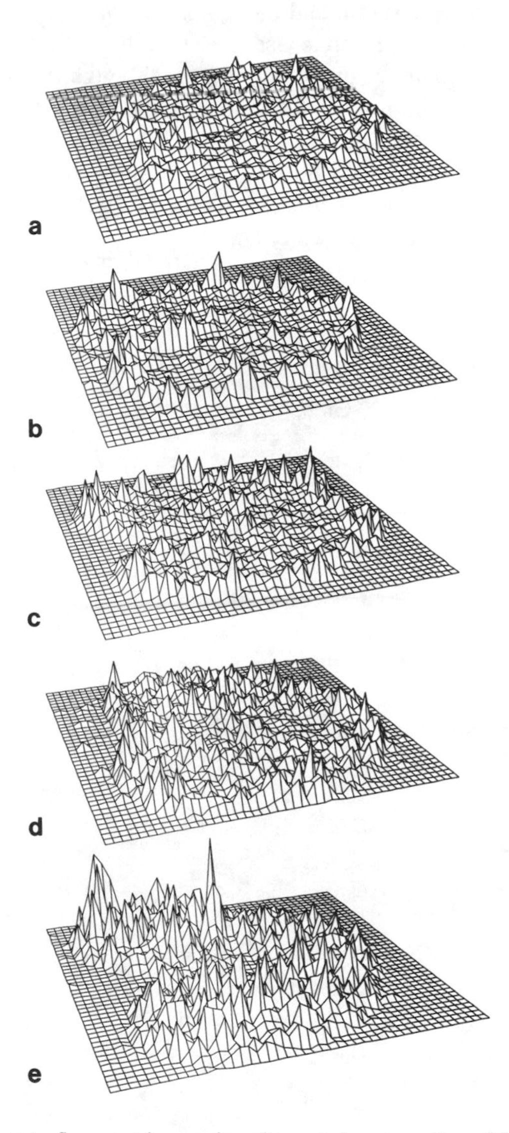

Figure 1.2 Microspectrofluorometric mapping of a central cross section of five oat cultivars (% β-glucan in parenthesis) showing the relative fluorescence intensity of bound calcofluor indicative of β-glucan distribution: (a) Donald, (3.7%); (b) OA516-2, (4.0%); (c) Tibor, (4.6%); (d) Woodstock, (5.1%); (e) Marion, (6.4%). (Reprinted from Reference [13], with permission.)

uted throughout the endosperm and located in the endosperm cell walls. Microscopy indicates that β-glucan is also present in the aleurone walls [14], apparently in lesser amounts than the endosperm although the possibility of interference with dye-binding or fluorescence intensity makes quantitation uncertain. Chemical analysis showed that β-glucan constitutes about 75% of the endosperm cell walls [15]. $(1 \rightarrow 3)(1 \rightarrow 4)$-$\beta$-D-Glucan has only been confirmed in the Graminae, or grasses, although a structurally very similar polysaccharide is present in some lichens [16]. The largest (seed) amounts of β-glucan are found in barley (3–11%) and oats (3–7%), with lesser amounts

TABLE 1.1. β-Glucan Content of Oat Groats.

Reference	Source of Variation	Country	Range of β-Glucan (% dwb)
Åman & Graham [18]	C[1], E[2]	Sweden	2.2–4.2[4]
Åman [19]	C, E	Sweden	2.7–3.6[4]
Asp et al. [20]	C, E	Sweden	3.5–5.7
Autio et al. [21]	C	Finland	3.0–5.3
Bauer & Geisler [22]	C, E	Germany	3.2–6.1
Bhatty [23]	C, E	Canada	1.8–6.1
Brunner & Freed [24]	C, E	USA	3.7–6.6
Cho & White [25]	C, E	USA	3.0–6.4
Ganßmann [26]	C, E	Germany	3.3–5.9
Henry [27]	C	Australia	3.8–4.0[5]
Holthaus et al. [28]	C	USA	3.7–6.1
Hymphreys et al. [29]	C, E	Canada	3.5–6.9
Jackson et al. [30]	C, E	USA	3.7–5.1[4]
Lim et al. [31]	C, E	USA	3.0–6.5
Miller et al. [32]	C, E, S[3]	Canada	1.8–5.5
Miller et al. [33]	C, E	Canada	3.9–6.0
Peterson [34]	C, E	USA	4.6–7.5
Peterson et al. [35]	C, E	USA	3.1–7.3
Saastamoinen [36]	C, E	Finland, Sweden	1.9–5.1[6]
Saastamoinen et al. [37]	C, E	Finland	3.9–6.3
Welch & Lloyd [38]	C	UK	3.2–6.3
Wood et al. [39]	C	Canada	3.9–6.8

[1]C = cultivars and lines.
[2]E = environmental effects (year, location).
[3]S = species.
[4]Not dehulled.
[5]Not clear if dehulled.
[6]Groat loss during dehulling.

reported in rye (1–2%) and wheat (<1%). Only trace amounts have been reported in corn, sorghum, rice and other cereals of importance as food [17].

There is a wide range of β-glucan content in the oat groat (Table 1.1), although the range is somewhat less than in barley. Environment as well as genotype affect levels. Care must be taken when comparing literature values that the same base for measurement has been used, which for food uses should be the groat (the hulls contain no β-glucan).

2.2 OAT BRAN

The microstructural characteristics of oat bran have been described in a recent review [40]. In anatomical terms, cereal bran is considered to be the outer layers of the kernel, which include a number of morphologically distinct layers ending in going from the outside into the kernel, with the aleurone cells (Figure 1.1). In practice, milling processes do not yield such a well-defined selection of tissue, even for wheat, which presents less problems to the miller than oats, and for which a variety of advanced milling methods have been developed over the years. These milling methods are sufficiently established for wheat so that a reasonable consistency can be expected from commercial products. That is not the case for oat bran, which led to the American Association of Cereal Chemists (AACC) adopting the following as a definition [41]:

> Oat bran is the food which is produced by grinding clean oat groats or rolled oats and separating the resulting oat flour by sieving, bolting and/or other suitable means into fractions such that the oat bran fraction is not more than 50% of the starting material, and has a total β-glucan content of at least 5.5% (dry weight basis) and a total dietary fibre content of at least 16.0% (dry weight basis), and such that at least one-third of the total dietary fibre is soluble fibre.

This definition was also accepted by the FDA for the health claim ruling.

The definition is not highly demanding of β-glucan level. Indeed, some cultivars significantly exceed 5.5% without processing (Table 1.1). The definition does make a requirement for some fractionation, however. The outer layers of the groat and other cell walls, especially from the aleurone and (in many cultivars) thick-walled sub-aleurone endosperm, are resistant to attrition and these materials (the main source of insoluble dietary fibre) tend to predominate in the coarse fraction, which the definition identifies as the bran. Since β-glucan is the major component of the endosperm cell walls, the thick sub-aleurone walls represent a particularly rich source and contribute to the higher β-glucan content of bran. As a consequence of these microstructural details, it is possible that an anatomically "pure" oat bran might be depleted rather than enriched in β-glucan. The endosperm is essential for β-glucan-rich material and in some cultivars in particular, at least as determined by calcofluor staining and microspectrofluorometric mapping ([13], Figure 1.2), the β-glucan is rather evenly distributed throughout the endosperm.

Although 5.5% β-glucan is the suggested minimum level, quality commercial brans might reasonably be expected to contain 7% or more. Table 1.2 summarizes reported data on β-glucan levels possible in bran from different milling methods. Since it is possible to obtain fractions considerably enriched in β-glucan, but in low yield, the recovery of the β-glucan, as a percentage of the total in the groat, is important. Cultivar and environment not only influence β-glucan content, but also the enrichment possible in processing to bran (Table 1.2 [21,26,39]). The composition of oat brans has been reviewed in detail [44].

Commercial methods for oat bran production have been reviewed [10,11]. Without defatting, or use of liquid processing, it is difficult to achieve brans that are highly enriched in β-glucan. To obtain brans with β-glucan content >10% for subsequent extraction of oat gum and for clinical trials, Wood et al. [45] used defatted oats and air classification similar to the process patented by Hohner and Hyldon [46]. Additional processes, in which full fat flours were first dry sieved then sieved in aqueous ethanol, were also developed. A number of processes are described in the patent literature [47,48] which apply the principle of fractionation in organic solvent and aqueous alcohols. One, based on a preliminary aqueous steeping step, is presently used for the production of oat fractions for the cosmetic industry (see Table 1.2 [49,50]).

2.3. β-GLUCAN ISOLATES

At present no purified oat β-glucan products are commercially available for the food industry. Fine chemical-grade material (Megazyme International Ireland Ltd. Co., Wicklow) is available as is material for the cosmetic industry (Canamino Inc., Saskatoon, SK, Canada). Methods for production at pilot plant scale (>1 kg), used to obtain material for clinical studies have been reported [45,51].

An interesting new product, known as Oatrim, was developed by Inglett [52] and is presently marketed by Quaker Oats–Rhône Poulenc and by ConAgra–Mountain Lake Manufacturing. Oatrim is prepared by extraction of oats or oat bran with hot water containing a heat-stable α-amylase to give a low dextrose-equivalent maltodextrin containing from 1–10% by weight of β-glucan. Like other maltodextrins, Oatrim may act as a fat replacer, allowing manufacture of fat-reduced products, and may incorporate, in addition, the benefits possible from viscous soluble fibre.

TABLE 1.2. β-Glucan Enrichment in Bran by Laboratory-Scale Milling Processes.

Reference	Process	Groat β-Glucan (% dwb)	Flour β-Glucan (% dwb)	Bran β-Glucan (% dwb)	Bran Yield (% of whole)	EF[1]
Autio et al. [21]	EtOH sieve	3.0–5.3	—	11.8–18.3	—	3.2–5.1
Ganßmann [26]	Dry sieve	4.4–5.4	1.4–1.9	7.8–10.6	37–40	1.9–2.1
Knuckles et al. [42]	Defatted, roller mill, sieve	4.7	0.6	21.2	18	4.5
Paton et al. [unpub.]	Steep, EtOH sieve	3.9–6.8	—	14.7–19.1	13–23	2.8–3.5
Wood et al. [39]	Falling number mill, sieve	3.9–6.8	1.6–2.3	5.8–8.9	48–58	1.3–1.6
Wood et al. [43]	Dry sieve, EtOH sieve	4.2–6.7	—	10.8–13.4	26–34	1.6–3.2

[1]EF = Enrichment factor (β-glucan in bran/β-glucan in original seed).

3. NATURE AND ANALYSIS OF OAT β-GLUCAN

3.1. ANALYSIS

It is important from the regulatory point of view, and also for research and development, that components believed to have physiological benefit in a functional food can be specifically analyzed. β-Glucan can be analyzed as dietary fibre, but unlike for other dietary fibres, more specific and well-accepted methods are available. This makes β-glucan a particularly useful model fibre for study. Identification can be achieved specifically, among other components of food or digesta [53], as described above by use of microscopy and dye-binding. Dye-binding can also be used to sensitively and specifically analyze β-glucan in solution [54]. Enzyme methods for analysis are also available. The method of Åman and Graham [18] uses a β-glucanase enzyme to quantitatively convert β-glucan to glucose, which is then determined using glucose oxidase. This method depends on first removing all starch by use of α-amylase, which must be β-glucanase free. A method developed by McCleary and Glennie-Holmes [55] uses a specific $(1 \rightarrow 3)$ $(1 \rightarrow 4)$-β-D-glucan-4-glucanohydrolase to solubilize and quantitatively extract the β-glucan as oligosaccharides, which are then converted to glucose using a specific β-glucosidase. The necessary highly specific enzymes are available commercially as a kit and the method, supported by collaborative studies by both the Association of Official Analytical Chemists and AACC, has been accepted as the analysis of choice by the FDA in the oat health claim [56].

3.2 STRUCTURE

Purified oat β-glucan is a linear, unbranched polysaccharide composed of 4-*O*-linked β-D-glucopyranosyl units (≈70%) and 3-*O*-linked β-D-glucopyranosyl units (≈30%) [57]. The $(1 \rightarrow 3)$ linkages occur singly, and most of the $(1 \rightarrow 4)$ linkages occur in groups of two or three [43,57,58], leading predominantly to a structure of β-$(1 \rightarrow 3)$-linked cellotriosyl and cellotetraosyl units. On the basis of linkage analysis, or ^{13}C-NMR spectra [43,58], oat and barley β-glucan and the noncereal β-glucan, lichenan, appear almost structurally identical, but analysis of oligosaccharide fragments released by enzymes reveal differences [43,59]. The relative amounts of the oligosaccharides produced by the action of lichenase, a highly specific $(1 \rightarrow 3)(1 \rightarrow 4)$-β-D-glucan-4-glucanohydrolase (EC 3.2.1.73) [59], constitute a fingerprint of structure. The oligosaccharides are conveniently and rapidly analyzed by high-performance anion-exchange chromatography (HPAEC, Figure 1.3). Since no purifications or sample clean-up are needed, it is possible to do structural analysis of all β-glucan in a flour or product rather than a purified portion not necessarily representative of the whole.

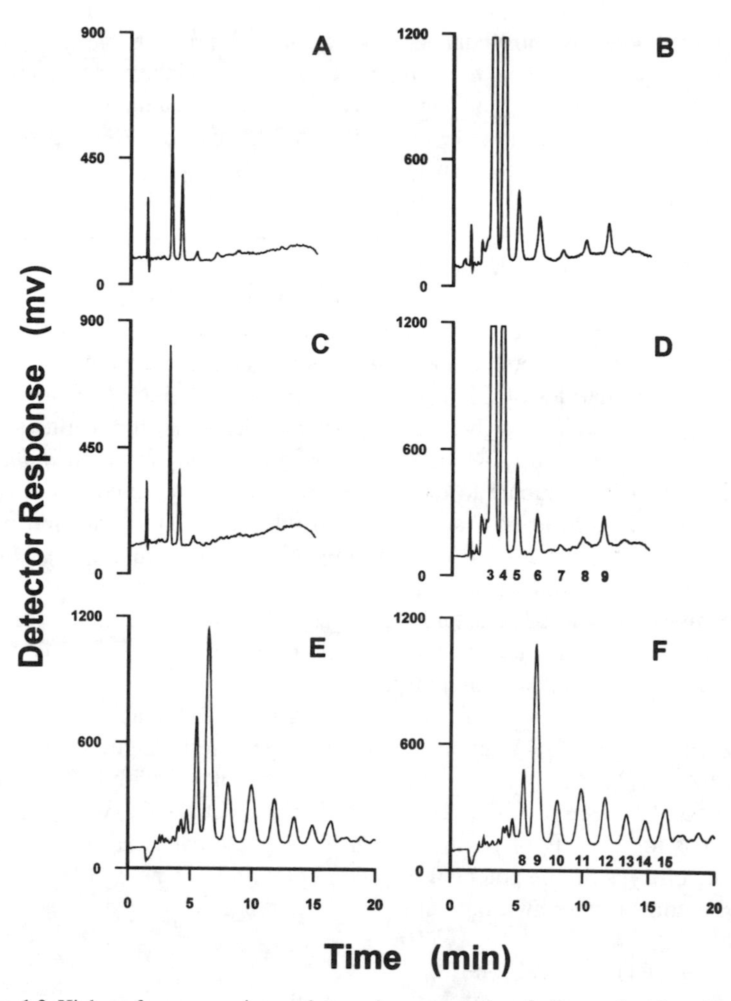

Figure 1.3 High-performance anion exchange chromatography of oligosaccharides released by lichenase from oat (A, B, E) and barley (C, D, F) β-glucan. (A–D) show soluble oligosaccharides, (B) and (D) are at high concentration to detect DP 5-9. (E) and (F) show water-insoluble oligosaccharides (solubilized in methyl sulfoxide before chromatography).

The molar ratio of $(1 \rightarrow 3)$-linked cellotriosyl to $(1 \rightarrow 3)$-linked cellotetraosyl units, which constituted 85–90% by weight of the polysaccharides was lower for oats (2.1–2.4) than it was for barley (2.8–3.3), rye (3.0–3.2), or wheat (3.0–3.8) [16,59].

In addition to 3-*O*-β-cellobiosyl- and cellotriosyl-D-glucose, a number of higher DP oligosaccharides and an insoluble precipitate are formed by the action of lichenase (Figure 1.3). Because the enzyme is specific for β-$(1 \rightarrow 4)$-linked

3-substituted glucopyranosyl units, these additional products must represent oligosaccharides containing more than two β-(1 $\rightarrow$ 4)-linked glucopyranosyl units and terminated at the reducing end by a β-(1 $\rightarrow$ 3)-linked glucose (i.e., cellodextrins terminated at the reducing end by a 3-linked unit). These structures were confirmed by methylation analysis and ^{13}C-NMR [16,59].

Both the total (7–9%) and relative amounts of lichenase-solubilized oligosaccharides of DP > 4 from β-glucan from different cultivars of oat (and barley) are conserved [59]. The increased proportion of DP 9, relative to 7 and 8, material in the water-soluble fraction presumably reflects slight solubility of the DP 9 oligosaccharide found in the mostly water-insoluble product ($\approx$3–5% yield). In both oat and barley, the water-insoluble material contained oligosaccharides of DP 7-15, but the largest fraction ($\approx$40%) was of DP 9 (Figure 1.3). These higher DP oligosaccharides arise from cellulose-like portions of the molecule, which must have functional importance for the plant, and which contribute to molecular extension (and hence viscosity) in solution [60]. It is believed (barley β-glucan) that the major structural building blocks are distributed randomly throughout the molecules [61], but the distribution of the cellulose-like regions is unknown.

The above review of structure deals with the major identified features; some minor variations may exist. Although not detected in recent analysis, it was widely believed that consecutive β-(1 $\rightarrow$ 3) linkages occurred [16]; this feature may be present, as might alternating (1 $\rightarrow$ 3) linkages and (1 $\rightarrow$ 4) linkages in minor (<1%) amounts. Protein or peptide linkage has also been suggested [62], and MW and viscosity loss on incubation with a β-glucanase free trypsin has been reported [21,63], but Johansen et al. [64] were unable to detect loss in viscosity of β-glucan isolates or crude oat bran extracts in the presence of trypsin. The potential for bound protein influencing MW and viscosity requires further investigation.

3.3. MOLECULAR WEIGHT

Despite the considerable interest in the problems caused in the brewing and feed industry by the viscosity of barley β-glucan, studies of molecular weight (MW) of cereal β-glucans have been rare. This probably reflects the difficulty in obtaining reliable data [65]. Earlier studies reported values as low as 2.7×10^4 (oats [66]) or as high as 40×10^6 (barley [67]). The high value of the latter study was attributed to a protein association. The most detailed, rigorous study of the MW of oat β-glucan has been that of Vårum and colleagues [62,68,69], but these studies were restricted to samples that had been depolymerized by sonication. For these low MW samples, the Mark-Houwink equation was determined as:

$$[\eta]\ (\text{mL/g}) = 6.7 \times 10^{-2}\ M_n^{0.75}$$

[62,69]. Vårum et al. [68] reported an aggregation phenomenon, which may be related to unusual rheology reported for depolymerized oat β-glucan [70].

Size exclusion chromatography potentially provides a simple method for determining MW and MW distribution. Without MW-sensitive detectors, standards of established MW are required; for this, the commercially available dextran and pullulan have often been used. Because of the differences in molecular conformation (shape) between the α-linked glucan standards and β-glucan [69], the values for β-glucan may be significantly overestimated. MW values should then be reported as dextran or pullulan equivalents [63] or a process known as universal calibration applied [67,69].

Recently, chromatography systems using light-scattering detectors in combination with refractive index detectors have become commercially available. These detectors deal with different polymer conformations by using low-angle laser light scattering (LALLS), multi-angle laser light scattering (MALLS), or right-angle laser light scattering (RALLS) in combination with viscometric detection. In crude extracts of oats, the use of these nonspecific detectors to evaluate β-glucan is not possible, because of unknown contributions from co-extracted substances (starch, proteins). This problem may be overcome by addition of a fluorescence detector exploiting the specific dye-binding of Calcofluor by β-glucan [71]. This system may also be used to quantitate the β-glucan [71,72].

Using high-performance-size exclusion chromatography with calcofluor detection, and oat β-glucan standards evaluated by LALLS, Wood et al. [71] reported MW of β-glucan in crude extracts from several oat, barley and rye cultivars. The MW of oat β-glucan ($\approx 3 \times 10^6$) was greater than that from barley ($2–2.5 \times 10^6$) or rye (1×10^6). Bhatty [73] suggested MW of $>2 \times 10^6$ for oat and barley β-glucan, again oat > barley. Mälkki et al. [63] reported lower values (1.5×10^6) for β-glucan from oat bran concentrates, examining differences in MW of β-glucan related to processing. Using columns calibrated with β-glucan standards whose MW was established using RALLS and viscometry, Beer et al. [74] reported somewhat lower MWs of β-glucan in extracts from various oat and barley cultivars than Wood et al. [71], but confirmed a significant difference between oats and barley. Autio et al. [22] reported cultivar variations in MW with a highest value of 1.5×10^6. These data are summarized in Table 1.3. Discrepancies can be attributed both to the measuring system and extraction and isolation methods. It is unlikely that a "true" MW or MW distribution of oat β-glucan as it exists in the cell wall is measurable. It is, however, possible to aim for determining the maximum possible MW that can be extracted.

Sample pretreatment prior to extraction is important. Clearly, if β-glucanases are present, they must be inactivated, or it must be recognized that any sample isolated without this step may have been depolymerized. The impact that this may have can perhaps be appreciated by realizing that the cleavage of one bond

TABLE 1.3. Molecular Weight of β-Glucan in Oat Bran and Oat Flour.

Reference	Source	PT[1]	Solvent	Temperature (°C)	Duration (min)	Detection[2]	MW (10^{-6})
Autio et al. [21]	Oat Bran	1	H_20	70	60	A	1.5
Beer et al. [51]	Oat Bran	2	Na_2CO_3	40	30	C	1.1
Beer et al. [74]	Oat Flour	2	H_20	90	120	B	2.0–2.5
Beer et al. [75]	Oat Bran	1	Na_2HPO_4	37	135	B	1.1–1.9
Mälkki et al. [63]	Oat Bran	1	Na_2CO_3	70	120	A	0.4–1.5
Sundberg et al. [76]	Oat Bran	2	Na_2CO_3	60	120	B	2.7
Wood et al. [71]	Oat Flour	2	Na_2CO_3	60	120	B	3.0
	Oat Bran	2	Na_2CO_3	60	120	B	3.1

[1]Sample pre-treatment: 1 = no pretreatment; 2 = Sample ethanol treated prior to extraction.
[2]Detection Method: A = multiangle laser light scattering detection; B = calcofluor post-column detection with β-glucan standards; C = refractive index detection with pullulan standards.

in 12,000 can halve the MW of a high-MW β-glucan. Although more external cleavage locations are less drastic, it does not require a high level of enzyme activity for a potentially devastating effect on viscosity, as the formula in the section on viscosity shows. Wood et al. [71] reported that without inactivation of β-glucanases, β-glucan extracted from commercial oats prior to steam-heat treatment and flaking was of lower MW than β-glucan from oats pretreated with ethanol (2 h at 85°C, 70% ethanol), and was unstable compared to that from steam-heat treated rolled oat. This effect may be from β-glucanases released from contaminating microorganisms in the kernel; we have generally observed that, without heat treatment, extracts are of lower MW and may be unstable. If microorganisms are the source of the hydrolases, it is to be expected that this phenomenon will be variable.

Measurement of MW requires material in solution, and decisions need to be made whether to use mild conditions and get less extraction or use more vigorous reagents and risk degradation. Using hot water or carbonate buffer (pH 10) as extraction media [71,74], only 50–70% of total β-glucan was solubilized, leaving over 30% of the total β-glucan insoluble and of unknown MW. Sodium hydroxide gives total extraction [77], but the work of Beer et al. [74] showed that MW of β-glucan was significantly decreased by NaOH.

McCleary [78] reported that increasing temperature of extraction leads to increase in MW of barley β-glucan as determined by intrinsic viscosity of extracts. Similarly, we have found [unpublished data] that the MW of oat β-glucan extracted at 90°C is up to 30% higher than that of β-glucan extracted at 37°C.

3.4. SOLUBILITY

The term *solubility* is perhaps a misnomer where dietary fibre and specifically oat (or barley) β-glucan are concerned. Solubility refers to extractability under certain specified conditions of sample preparation, solvent, temperature, time, liquid: solids ratio. Comparison of data from several studies dealing with the extraction or solubility of β-glucan from oat and barley [e.g., 51,71,78,79,80] is difficult because of the many variables involved. As with MW determination, endogenous enzymes, whether originating from the cereal itself or from contaminating microorganisms, may be important; amounts of β-glucan extracted from untreated flour are higher than from ethanol-treated samples [71]. However, the solubilizing effect of depolymerization might be offset by changes in the cell walls on drying leading to lower extractability [67].

Extraction of cereal β-glucan with mild reagents and conditions is incomplete. There are as yet no fully satisfactory molecular or microstructural explanations for this resistance to, and sample differences in, solubilization [16], although it is evident that MW may play a role [78]. Also, thicker cell walls, such as the sub-aleurone endosperm of many cultivars, show a greater resistance to extraction [81]. However, wheat β-glucan, despite thin endosperm cell walls, is extremely resistant to extraction [82]. McCleary [78] reported that ≈90% of the total barley β-glucan was extracted in successive treatments with water at 40, 65, and 95°C, whereas Wood et al. [71] found ≈45% of barley and 70% of oat β-glucan extracted by carbonate (pH 10) at 60°C. Beer et al. [74] found ≈65% of the total β-glucan in oats and waxy barley and ≈50% in non-waxy barley was extracted by hot water (90°C) containing a thermostable, β-glucanase free, α-amylase. Additional hot water extractions and a final DMSO extraction increased the total β-glucan solubilized to ≈80%; total extraction was achieved using sodium hydroxide. Both alkali (NaOH) [77] and acid (dilute perchloric or sulphuric acid) [54,83] have been used for complete extraction, necessary for analysis, but both lead to depolymerization.

In the framework of evaluating the nutritional and physiological aspects of cereal β-glucan, an *in vitro* extraction system that mimics human digestion is perhaps more appropriate. Such a system was developed to evaluate the effects of process and cooking on β-glucan [75], and is reported below.

3.5. RHEOLOGY

Oat β-glucan is a linear, high molecular-weight polysaccharide, which, in the absence of chain ordering and association and above a certain minimum (entanglement) concentration, gives highly viscous, shear thinning solutions. The viscosity (η) is highly concentration dependent, which, combined with shear (S) dependency, means comparison of data must be at the same shear rate and concentration. A power law,

$$\eta = KS^{n-1}$$

may be used to assist in comparison but such comparisons need to be made over a similar range of shear rates since the relationship does not hold over a wide range. On this basis, Wood [16] reported that oat gum (≈80% β-glucan) prepared in the laboratory had higher K (theoretical viscosity at the shear rate of 1 s^{-1}) and n (flow behavior index, a measure of shear thinning behavior) than pilot plant-prepared oat gum, which was used in clinical studies. An oat gum prepared by Autio et al. [84] had similar properties to the laboratory-prepared gum of Wood. Two samples prepared by alkaline extraction [73] had significantly higher n values than those reported by Wood [16] and Autio et al. [84]. A survey by Autio et al. [21] indicated that different cultivars yield β-glucans of widely different values of n (0.48–0.93), for 18.6–463 s^{-1} indicating that a wide range of MW distributions is possible. These measurements were done at concentrations (≈0.3%) rather close to the dilute region where less molecular entanglement leads to more Newtonian behavior (e.g., $n = 0.93$). Measurements by Wikström et al. [85] were also at low concentrations, but over a much wider shear rate range they found n values (≈ 0.45) indicative of much greater shear thinning. This illustrates the difficulty of making useful comparisons between data obtained in different laboratories. These difficulties were further illustrated by Wood et al. [86] where, depending on concentration and shear rate used for comparison, one oat gum preparation might appear from 1.5 to 16 times "more viscous" than another.

More generally valid treatments of shear rate dependency of random coil polymers in solution than the simple power law have been described, which allow for low shear rate Newtonian behavior [87]. That proposed by Morris [88] relates the viscosity (at any shear rate) to zero shear (low shear rate plateau) viscosity (η_0), shear rate and the rate, $S_{1/2}$, at which viscosity reduces to half that of the zero shear value. For the β-glucan used in clinical trials [89] at 1% w/v, a value for η_0 of 2.0 Pa · s and 32 s^{-1} for $S_{1/2}$ was found (Wood, unpublished data).

Doublier and Wood [70] showed that for an oat gum containing 80% β-glucan,

$$\eta_{sp0} \propto (c[\eta])^{3.9}$$

where η_{sp0} is zero shear specific viscosity, c is concentration and $[\eta]$ intrinsic viscosity, holds for oat gum, above about 0.3% concentration, as expected from random coil behavior in solution similar to, for example, guar gum. From this it can be seen that above 0.3% viscosity is highly concentration dependent; a doubling of concentration could produce a 15-fold increase in viscosity. Since

$$[\eta] = K(\mathrm{MW})^{\alpha}$$

and $\alpha = 0.72{-}0.75$ for oat β-glucan [69, Beer et al. unpublished data], viscosity is also highly sensitive to MW.

Doublier and Wood [70] used flow and dynamic (oscillatory) viscosity measurements to evaluate pilot plant-prepared oat gum and two samples depolymerized by partial acid hydrolysis for use in clinical studies [89]. The unhydrolyzed sample showed expected flow and dynamic viscosity behavior. The zero shear rate Newtonian plateau was evident ($\eta_0 = 1.2$ Pa · s for a 0.78% w/v concentration on a β-glucan basis). G'' was greater than G' at low frequencies and G' increased more rapidly with frequency. Hydrolysis reduced the MW of the samples from about 1 million to 360,000 and 100,000. As expected, the lower the MW, the lower the viscosity at all shear rates, but unexpectedly there was evidence of weak gel characteristics in the partially hydrolyzed samples. In both these samples, at low frequency in the mechanical spectra, the storage modulus G' was greater than the loss modulus G'', and a zero shear Newtonian plateau was not evident in flow measurements.

The oscillatory measurements of Autio [90] were similar to those of Doublier and Wood [70] for unhydrolyzed oat gum (G'' was greater than G' at low frequencies) typical of entangled random coil polymers. Wikström et al. [85], on the other hand, observed a low-frequency area in which G' was greater than G'', indicating the weak gel characteristic reported by Doublier and Wood [70] for partially hydrolyzed β-glucan. The rheology of β-glucans of different MW distributions requires further examination.

4. PHYSIOLOGICAL EFFECTS OF OAT β-GLUCAN IN HUMANS

Although this review deals mainly with human clinical trials, many useful animal studies have been done, and these may be particularly helpful in determining mechanism.

4.1. CARBOHYDRATE METABOLISM

Beneficial effects of oats in the treatment of diabetes were reported as long ago as 1913 [91]. Attenuation of postprandial blood glucose and insulin response is believed to be of benefit in both healthy and diabetic people; response to a food may be estimated by the glycemic index, a comparison of the food with a white bread control. Rolled oats and commercial oat bran only moderately lower glycemic index [92]. Although many factors in a food influence glycemic index, in pioneering studies, Jenkins et al. [93] showed that soluble fibres, but not insoluble fibre, attenuated postprandial blood glucose and insulin levels and that the effect was viscosity dependent.

Braaten et al. [94] compared the effectiveness of oat and guar gum in lowering blood glucose and insulin levels after an oral glucose load in healthy subjects. Both gums significantly and identically lowered postprandial blood glucose and insulin levels compared with the control of glucose alone.

An experimental high β-glucan ($\approx 15\%$) oat bran was compared with cream of wheat (wheat farina) to which an approximately equivalent amount of β-glucan was added. The meals, which included white bread, were designed to be similarly textured hot cereal types [95]. The oat bran and cream of wheat plus oat gum meals reduced the postprandial plasma glucose and insulin levels compared with the control wheat farina in both healthy and Type 2 diabetic subjects. The study showed that both the native cell wall fibre of oat bran and an isolated oat gum incorporated into a meal act similarly to lower postprandial plasma glucose and insulin levels.

Wood et al. [89] showed that increasing the dose of oat gum successively reduced the plasma glucose and insulin response to an oral glucose load relative to control without gum. Further, reduction of the viscosity of the oat gum by acid hydrolysis reduced or eliminated the capacity to decrease postprandial glucose and insulin levels.

When all the data from oat and guar gum experiments were combined, a highly significant linear relationship was found between log (viscosity) of the mixtures consumed and the glucose and insulin response (Figure 1.4). The re-

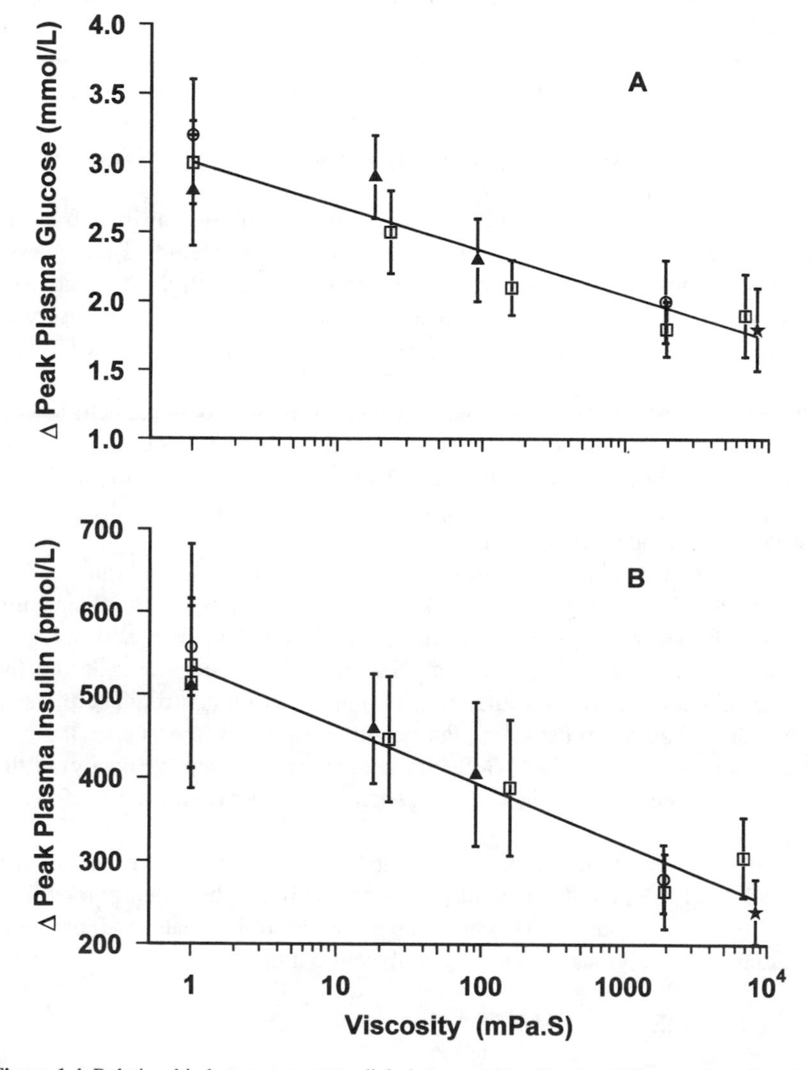

Figure 1.4 Relationship between postprandial glucose and insulin rise (difference from baseline) in response to a 50-g oral load, and logarithm viscosity (at 30 s^{-1}), of different gum drinks. Different doses, unhydrolyzed oat gum, □; acid hydrolyzed oat gum, ▲; "instantized oat gum," ○; guar gum, ★. Bars show between subject standard errors. (Reprinted from References [89], with permission from the Nutrition Society.)

lationship showed that 79–96% of the changes in plasma glucose and insulin were attributable to viscosity, and that changes occur at relatively low doses or viscosity. While individual comparisons did not detect significant differences from control (because of insufficient subject sample size), the combined regression demonstrated that low doses, such as might be obtained from a single serving of rolled oats, could be effective. The data also demonstrated that equivalence of materials, such as guar and oat gum [94], might simply reflect measurement at levels where major differences in viscosity led to statistically undetectable differences in response. Thus, reduction of the mean peak blood glucose increment from 2.1 to 2.0 mmol/L (less than standard error) would require a doubling of viscosity from 1.0 to 2.0 Pa · s (at a shear rate of 30 s^{-1}).

Hallfrisch et al. [96] fed β-glucan isolate in the form of Oatrim extracts to mildly hypercholesterolemic subjects over a 5-week period. There was a lower postprandial insulin and glucose responses with both the 1% and 10% β-glucan product, but a clear dose response to β-glucan was not observed. The doses used in the tolerance test (based on body weight) were low to moderate (average for men ≈0.5 and 3 g).

Incorporation of a high β-glucan (≈19%) oat bran into a spaghetti to provide 5.2 g of β-glucan did not affect postprandial blood glucose in 10 healthy subjects, but did decrease insulin response [97]. On the basis of the liquid model of Wood et al. [89], this dose would have been expected to significantly lower blood glucose response.

Tappy et al. [98] studied the effect of a similar high β-glucan bran (≈15%) incorporated into an extruded breakfast cereal. Subjects with noninsulin-dependent diabetes mellitus consumed meals with 4 g, 6 g, and 8.4 g of β-glucan, and all three breakfasts significantly decreased the peak and the average glucose and insulin increments compared to a control. There was a significant relationship between plasma glucose peak or area under the glucose curve and the amount of β-glucan in the cereals or log (viscosity) of the suspended cereals. These data are in general agreement with those of Wood et al. [89].

In general, depending on dose, viscosity and food form, oat products may have a low glycemic index and may confer this effect when incorporated into meals or other products. However, commercial rolled oats and oat bran should not be viewed as markedly low glycemic index foods.

4.2. LIPID METABOLISM

The study of de Groot et al. [99], who observed that feeding 140 g of rolled oats to healthy young men lowered serum cholesterol by 11% in three weeks, appears to be the first report of the effect of oats on serum lipids. The studies of Anderson and colleagues [100–105] perhaps did most to bring the potential cholesterol-lowering effect of oats to public attention, showing that oat bran might reduce total serum cholesterol in hypercholesterolemic subjects by as much as 20% with no change in high-density lipoprotein (HDL) cholesterol.

There have been over 50 studies on the effect of oat products on serum cholesterol levels in humans [106,107]. These generally indicate that oat products may lower serum cholesterol levels, although there are studies in which no effect was observed and for which there are no rigorously established explanations [108–110]. There are, however, reasonable explanations for the "negative" paper of Swain et al. [111], which attracted much public attention in January 1990. This paper compared cream of wheat with oat bran without controlling the fat intake of subjects (who, inappropriately, were mainly young females with normal cholesterol levels and who were already consuming relatively high-fibre diets). Both products apparently displaced fat from the diet, which the authors said accounted for all of the 7.2% reduction of serum cholesterol levels observed with both cereals. In fact, the fat intake during the oat phase was higher than during the wheat phase. Despite a design that clearly would make detection of a specific oat effect difficult, there was a statistically significant improvement in the LDL/HDL-cholesterol ratio during the oat phase.

There are many useful reviews of the effect of oats on blood lipids; especially useful critical reviews are those of Anderson et al. [112], the *Federal Register* [56,107] and Welch [4]. This review will, be restricted to aspects dealing specifically with the active component, β-glucan, and dose response to this polysaccharide.

The ability of viscous polysaccharides to lower serum cholesterol levels is well known [112], and most studies have supposed that β-glucan is the active component of oats [113]. The FDA oat claim has determined that an effective daily intake of β-glucan is 3 g, but few attempts have been made to establish a dose response that may differ between different subject groups and depend upon baseline level. Davidson et al. [114] examined the effect of oatmeal and oat bran on serum cholesterol levels in hypercholesterolemic subjects in a dose response study. Subjects were randomly assigned to three oatmeal and three oat bran doses with wheat bran as control. At Week 6 of treatment, compared to the control, significant reductions in both total and LDL-cholesterol levels were obtained in the treatment groups who were receiving 88 g of oatmeal, 56 g of oat bran, and 84 g of oat bran, corresponding to 3.6 g, 4.0 g, and 6.0 g of β-glucan, respectively. The authors reported an inverse correlation between serum cholesterol levels and β-glucan intake but did not report statistics—a significant regression would mean all levels studied were significant, although in the individual comparisons only three treatments showed significant effects.

In another dose response study [109] no significant effects were observed, but the products used (from New Zealand) had low β-glucan levels

(3.7–4.2%). Nevertheless, the daily intake of β-glucan at the highest dose of bran consumed was probably similar to the FDA suggested minimum of 3 g.. Although much has been made [12] of the low β-glucan levels of New Zealand oat brans, no detailed analyses of these brans have been published.

Ripsin et al. [115] used strict criteria to select a number of oat bran studies for a meta-analysis, from which it was concluded, *inter alia,* that daily doses of β-glucan >3 g were needed for good effect.

There have been only three studies with isolated β-glucan extracts. Wood and co-workers prepared oat gum, about 80% β-glucan, on a large scale [46], which enabled the first clinical trials of isolated oat β-glucan. The product was well characterized [40,44,60,71,86,89]. In a placebo-controlled cross-over design, 19 hypercholesterolemic subjects were fed 7.2 g of oat gum daily. Weekly blood lipid measurements enabled setting a baseline level from which the LDL- and total cholesterol levels were reduced by 10.0% and 9.2%, respectively, in 4 weeks (Figure 1.5). There was no change in HDL-cholesterol. Of the 19 subjects, there were five whose LDL-cholesterol at Week 4 of the oat gum phase did not change from their baseline values beyond their individual 95% confidence interval. These are "statistical" nonresponders and it is not known whether there is a biochemical basis for the difference. The LDL-cholesterol lowering of the remaining 14 subjects was 13%.

Beer et al. [116] have also reported clinical trials using well-characterized [51] oat β-glucan extracts. While Beer et al. observed an increase in HDL-cholesterol, no changes in total or LDL-cholesterol levels were found; possible explanations were that the subjects were normocholesterolemic, feeding was for just 2 weeks and the product had a low solubility.

Behall et al. [117] used a 1 and 10% β-glucan level of Oatrim and found significant lowering of total and LDL-cholesterol but the data were confounded somewhat by the weight losses of the subjects. Most cholesterol lowering (9%) took place while establishing subjects on a maintenance diet, which contained 1.3 g per day of soluble β-glucan. A further 8% reduction occurred on increasing soluble β-glucan intake to 2.1 g per day with Oatrim, and an additional 5% reduction was achieved with the much larger increase in intake to 8.7 g per day. There was a decrease in fat consumption in going from the maintenance diet to Oatrim, possibly contributing to the cholesterol lowing, and it is possible that the effects of establishing the subjects on a controlled diet may have continued into the Oatrim phase. Nevertheless, the data suggest that the optimum daily intake of β-glucan might be quite modest (ca. 6 g). Overall, the subjects achieved an average reduction in serum cholesterol of 22%, and lost weight.

It is surprising that in the many oat bran studies, very few reported the β-glucan content of the product used. The β-glucan content of oat bran or whole oat samples may differ greatly (Tables 1.1 and 1.2) and furthermore, processing and storage may influence solubility and MW. Using an *in vitro* system

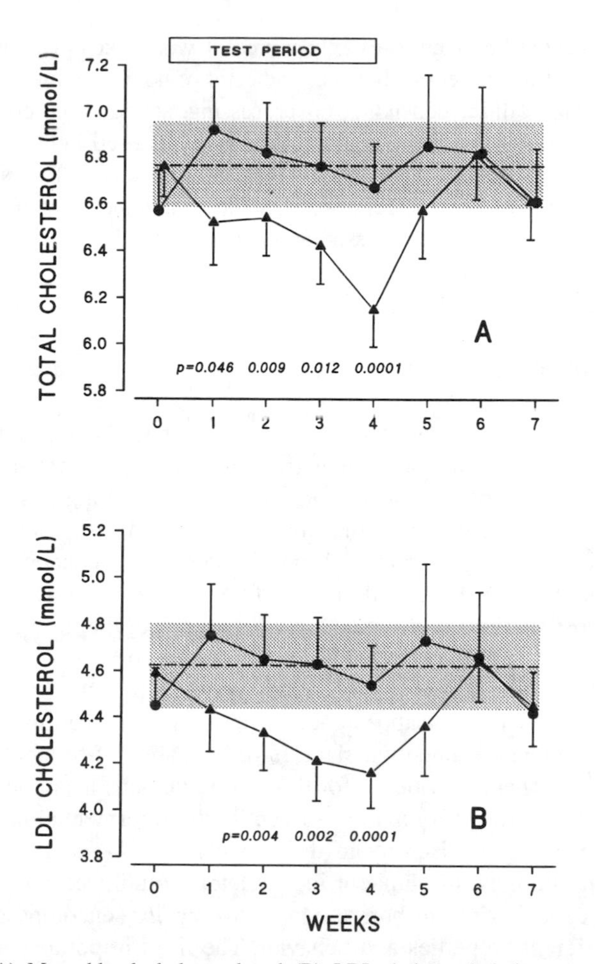

Figure 1.5 (A) Mean blood cholesterol and (B) LDL-cholesterol during oat gum (▲) and placebo (●) phases (0–4 weeks) of study. Period from 4–7 weeks is washout between phases or poststudy when oat gum was given last. Dotted line is baseline, and shading represents the 95% confidence interval about the mean. Error bars are SEM. (Reprinted from Reference [113], with permission.)

simulating the human digestion, Beer et al. [75] showed differences in extractability and MW of β-glucan in oat brans and muffins. Three oat bran samples showed differences in extractability and MW of β-glucan; baking of muffins increased extractability but decreased MW. A major difference in extractability between muffins from different recipes was also detected.

This could translate into significant differences in physiological effect if levels are not in the area of plateau response. Although simulating human digestion, the method cannot be taken to exactly represent what takes place in the upper gastrointestinal tract of people, but is an indicator of how solubilization and MW of products might differ depending on processing, storage, and cooking methods. It would be worthwhile to evaluate any products used in clinical trials for their relative capacities to increase gastrointestinal viscosity. Certainly, studies on the cholesterol-lowering effect of oats should be conducted with well-characterized products, and better dose response data established.

4.3 MODE OF ACTION OF β-GLUCAN

4.3.1 Glycemic Response

Dietary fibres are not digested by human enzymes. They provide a solids content in the upper gastrointestinal tract, modifying the physical environment with potential physiological consequences. Following passage through the upper gastrointestinal tract, the fibre is fermented in the lower gastrointestinal tract, again with potential physiological consequences. Although these characteristics are generally true of fibres, there are considerable variations, the most significant of which are whether or not the fibre is solubilized during digestion and, once in solution, the degree to which it modifies the rheology of the lumen. The classifications may not be entirely distinct. Animal studies have shown disappearance of fibre and β-glucan in the small intestine and β-glucan is depolymerized [53], indicative of fermentation in the small intestine. There is evidence for this also in humans in studies of ileostomates [76]. Fibres also vary in their susceptibility to fermentation. Solubilization of fibre increases viscosity in the lumen in a MW- and concentration-dependent fashion, but insoluble or incompletely solubilized fibres also modify rheological behavior. In short, the term *dietary fibre* encompasses material of many different properties and behavior. The most important properties of oat β-glucan are likely to be its ability to increase solution viscosity and a likely rapid fermentation in the large intestine.

In animal studies, oat β-glucan delayed gastric emptying, increased gastrointestinal transit time, increased luminal viscosity, and increased the thickness of the so-called unstirred layer [118–120]. These characteristics, typical of viscous fibres such as the more extensively studied guar gum, are associated with slowed nutrient absorption, reduced blood glucose and insulin levels, and other changes. In the model used by Wood et al. [89], the biochemical manifestations of oat β-glucan consumption (blood glucose and insulin levels) were $\approx$90% viscosity dependent. The greatest effect probably arises simply from the increased luminal viscosity modifying convective mixing and transport to the gut wall [93,121,122]. Short chain fatty acids (acetate, propionate, and butyrate) produced by fermentation in the colon may also influence the production of glucose and its utilization by peripheral tissues [123].

4.3.2 Serum Lipids

Although most evidence indicates that only soluble fibres lower serum cholesterol levels, the mechanisms by which these do so are uncertain; unlike glycemic response, a role for viscosity is not well established in clinical studies, but has been demonstrated in a hamster model [124]. In humans, a low-viscosity gum (acacia) did not lower serum cholesterol levels while a mixture of high-viscosity gums did, but this experimental design was also comparing chemical structure [125]. In other experiments, much higher doses of gum acacia (arabic) did lower serum cholesterol levels [126], but this comparison does not distinguish specifically between dose and viscosity, which requires examination of differing molecular weights of the same gum. Recently, a partially depolymerized guar gum was shown to lower serum cholesterol levels [127], but this product was of relatively high MW (similar to the MW of oat β-glucan used by Braaten et al. [113]). Partially depolymerized gums, or naturally occurring low-viscosity gums, such as gum arabic, may develop adequate viscosity at sufficiently high concentration. Dose and extent of depolymerization must be considered in evaluating whether viscosity has a role in serum cholesterol reduction.

Although most investigations measure the medium or long-term effect of the fibre on fasting serum lipoproteins, recent studies have examined postprandial lipid responses [128,129]. The effects of soluble fibres on postprandial events, such as the way in which absorption of nutrients occurs, may be significant. Certainly, viscous polysaccharides known to have these postprandial effects also lower serum cholesterol levels over the longer term. Psyllium significantly lowered serum cholesterol levels when consumed with breakfast, but not when consumed between meals [130].

The following have been proposed as possible mechanisms for cholesterol reduction.

(1) Cholesterol and bile acid excretion: There is increased excretion of bile acids and cholesterol with increased intake of soluble fibre [131,132], but cholesterol lowering and sterol excretion are not always related [103]. Changes in absorption and re-absorption may be caused by binding to fibre, although recent data could not detect binding of glycocholic acid to β-glucan [133]. Mixing and diffusion changes caused by increased viscosity [134–136], and changes in emulsification, could also influence absorption and re-absorption [137].

(2) Insulin secretion: Insulin plays a role in lipid metabolism and may stimulate cholesterol synthesis [138] and hepatic synthesis and secretion of very-low-density lipoproteins [139]. Soluble fibres reduce the rise in blood glucose and insulin [100,122,140–142] and the lower insulin may lead to lower serum cholesterol levels. This mechanism is supported by

the fact that other means of achieving lower insulin, such as slowed absorption by a nibbling diet (17 meals per day compared to 3), have also led to lowered serum cholesterol levels [143].

(3) Short-chain fatty acids (SCFA): Acetic, propionic and butyric acids are produced by fermentation in the colon and may modify cholesterol synthesis [144–146]. Propionate inhibited cholesterol synthesis in isolated rat hepatocytes [147] and lowered serum cholesterol levels in rats and pigs [148]. However, other data do not support a major role for SCFA in lowering serum cholesterol. At physiological concentrations (1 mmol/L) propionate did not affect cholesterol synthesis in perfused liver [148]. Perfusing propionate into the colon of humans did not lower serum cholesterol [149]. Finally, in hypercholesterolemic subjects with ileostomy, with a virtually suppressed fermentation process, oat bran produced a significant reduction of serum total and LDL-cholesterol comparable to that measured in human subjects with a functional colon [150]. However, SCFA reaching the liver have the capacity to modulate lipid and carbohydrate synthesis and secretion [151] and much remains to be learned about the physiological effects of SCFA.

(4) Rate of fat absorption: The absorption step necessitates an appropriate dispersion of lipid molecules in the aqueous phase and a proper interaction with the intestinal mucosa. As discussed above, increasing the viscosity of the intestinal contents decreases luminal mixing by increasing resistance to the convective effects of intestinal contractions [152]. In addition, viscous fibres including oat gum have been shown to increase the thickness of the so-called unstirred layer adjacent to the mucosa [118], and cholesterol uptake by everted rat jejunal sacs was inhibited by oat gum.

(5) Lipase activity: Dietary fibre may bind or inactive pancreatic lipase. In *in vitro* conditions there was marked inhibition of pancreatic lipase in the presence of wheat bran, oat bran, sugar-beet fibre, and psyllium, with triglycerides as substrate [153,154]. In gastric conditions, soluble fibres of sufficiently high viscosity significantly lowered the extent of lipid emulsification and, accordingly, slightly reduced the extent of triglyceride hydrolysis catalyzed by gastric lipase [155].

4.3.3. Cell Proliferation and Interaction with Carcinogens

The production of SCFA from fermentation is associated with a stimulation of colonic cell proliferation, which has been associated with enhanced tumorigenesis [156]. This finding has raised the suggestion that some soluble fibre rather than acting to protect against colon cancer, like insoluble fibres such as wheat bran, might instead enhance tumor development. These data on cell proliferation have been related to studies showing promotion of 1,2-

dimethylhydrazine (DMH) induced cancers in rats by soluble fibres [157]. In other studies of chemically induced cancer in rats [158], butyrate, which slows growth of cancer cells *in vitro,* was associated with inhibition of tumor development, but the location of butyrate production must be the distal colon for it to be effective in reducing the incidence of tumor initiation in response to DMH. Thus, wheat bran was an effective inhibitor while rapidly fermentable fibres sources (guar and oat bran) were not.

Other behavior that might promote, rather than inhibit, tumor development has been shown by *in vitro* studies that demonstrated that soluble fibres, including barley β-glucan [159], help maintain hydrophobic carcinogens in solution. This could diminish the protective effect believed to be exerted by insoluble fibre.

5. CONCLUSIONS

It is now well established that oat β-glucan, like many other viscous polysaccharides, may reduce serum cholesterol levels in hypercholesterolemic subjects, thereby reducing risk of heart disease. Rolled oats, oat bran, and other products including barley have sufficient β-glucan to be food sources capable of providing this health benefit. Whether or not these foods elicit the desired physiological effect, however, depends on many factors, some of which are only poorly understood. Viscosity appears to be important and though not necessarily causal, it has been well established for attenuation of blood glucose and insulin response. Accordingly, factors controlling viscosity are important. These factors include amount of β-glucan, solubility, molecular weight, and structure. For most products, the amount of β-glucan is readily determined or well known, but the effects of processing and cooking on solubility and molecular weight are less well understood. It is not yet established that viscosity is required for cholesterol lowering, and testing this hypothesis should be a priority for clinical research. Uncertainty about the mechanisms of action inevitably leads to uncertainty about benefits and potential for disagreement and controversy. Further clinical studies to establish barley as capable of lowering serum cholesterol may be needed, although the high number of studies done for oats should hardly be necessary. A clear understanding of β-glucan properties and mechanism of action would be preferable to accumulating clinical data that are inherently variable.

Much progress has been made in the characterization of cereal β-glucan but many knowledge gaps remain. We do not know the basis for solubility differences and additional study of solution behavior, such as rheological evaluation of different molecular weight distributions, is needed. In particular, the basis for development of gel-like characteristics is unknown. There remains disagreement on molecular weight, and suggestions that peptides or protein are involved in the structure leading to high molecular weight need further study.

More detailed information on the influences of soluble fibres on events throughout the gastrointestinal tract is needed and β-glucan may have particular advantages for such studies. The effects of SCFA, including proportions and site of production, would seem to have importance in this respect. The ability of β-glucans to bind metabolites, nutrients or carcinogens, or their interference with such binding, clearly could have great physiological significance and certainly any mechanism that has the potential to promote rather than prevent carcinogenesis merits close study.

6. REFERENCES

1. McIntosh, G. H., J. Whyte, R. McArthur and P. J. Nestel. 1991. "Barley and wheat foods: influence on plasma cholesterol concentrations in hypercholesterolemic men," Am. J. Clin. Nutr. 53:1205–1209.
2. Qureshi, N. and A. A. Qureshi. 1993. "Tocotrienols: Novel hypocholesterolemic agents with antioxidant properties," Vitamin E in Health and Disease, L. Packer and J. Fuchs, New York, NY: Marcel Decker Inc. pp. 247–267.
3. Collins F. W. 1986. "Oat Phenolics: Structure, Occurrence and Function," Oats: Chemistry and Technology, F. H. Webster, St. Paul, MN: Amer. Assoc. Cereal Chem. pp. 227–295.
4. Welch, R. W. 1995. "Oats in human nutrition and health," The Oat Crop, R. W. Welch, London, New York: Chapman and Hall. pp. 433–479.
5. Webster, F. H. 1986. Oats: Chemistry and Technology, St. Paul, MN: Amer. Assoc. Cereal Chem.
6. Welch, R. W. 1995. The Oat Crop. London, New York, NY: Chapman and Hall.
7. Anderson, J. W., C. C. Hamilton, J. L. Horn, D. B. Spencer, D. W. Dillon and J. A. Zeigler. 1991. "Metabolic effects of insoluble oat fibre on lean men with type II diabetes," Cereal Chem. 68:291–295.
8. Stephen, A. M., W. J. Dahl, D. M. Johns and H. N. Englyst. 1997. "Effect of oat hull fibre on human colonic function and serum lipids," Cereal Chem. 74: 379–383.
9. Deane, D. and E. Comers. 1986. "Oat cleaning and processing," Oats: Chemistry and Technology, Webster, F. H., St. Paul, MN: Amer. Assoc. Cereal Chem. pp. 371–412.
10. Paton, D. and M. K. Lenz. 1993. "Processing: Current practice and novel processes," Oat Bran, P. J. Wood, St. Paul, MN: Amer. Assoc. Cereal Chem. pp. 83–112.
11. Ganßmann, W. and K. Vorwerk. 1995. "Oat milling, processing and storage," The Oat Crop, R. W. Welch, London, New York, NY: Chapman and Hall. pp. 369–408.
12. Wood, P. J., R. G. Fulcher and B. A. Stone. 1983. "Studies on the specificity of interaction of cereal cell wall components with Congo red and Calcofluor. Specific detection and histochemistry of $(1 \rightarrow 3)(1 \rightarrow 4)$-$\beta$-D-glucan," J. Cereal Sci. 1:95–110.

13. Miller, S. M. and R. G. Fulcher. 1994. "Distribution of $(1 \rightarrow 3)(1 \rightarrow 4)$-$\beta$-D-glucan in kernels of oats and barley using microspectrofluorimetry," Cereal Chem. 71:64–68.
14. Fulcher, R. G. 1986. "Morphological and chemical organization of the oat kernel," Oats: Chemistry and Technology, F. H. Webster, St. Paul, MN: Amer. Assoc. Cereal Chem. pp. 47–74.
15. Miller, S. M., R. G. Fulcher, A. Sen and J. T. Arnason. 1995. "Oat endosperm cell walls: I. Isolation, composition and comparison with other tissues," Cereal Chem. 72:421–427.
16. Wood, P. J. 1993. "Physiochemical characteristics and physiological properties of oat $(1 \rightarrow 3)(1 \rightarrow 4)$-$\beta$-D-glucan," Oat bran, P. J. Wood, St. Paul, MN: Amer. Assoc. Cereal Chem. pp. 83–112.
17. Wood, P. J. 1992. "Aspects of the chemistry and nutritional effects of non-starch polysaccharides of cereal," Developments in Carbohydrate Chemistry, R. J. Alexander and H. F. Zobel, St. Paul, MN: Amer. Assoc. Cereal Chem. pp. 293–314.
18. Åman, P. and H. Graham. 1987. "Analysis of total and insoluble mixed-linked $(1 \rightarrow 3)(1 \rightarrow 4)$-$\beta$-D-glucans in barley and oats," J. Agric. Food. Chem. 35: 704–709.
19. Åman, P. 1987. "The variation in chemical composition of Swedish oats," Acta. Agric. Scand. 37:347–352.
20. Asp, N.-G., B. Mattsson and G. Önning. 1992. "Variation in dietary fibre, β-glucan, starch, protein, fat and hull content of oats grown in Sweden 1987–1989," Euro. J. Clin. Nutr. 46:31–37.
21. Autio, K., O. Myllymäki, T. Suortti, M. Saastamoinen and K. Poutanen. 1992. "Physical properties of $(1 \rightarrow 3)(1 \rightarrow 4)$-$\beta$-D-glucan preparates isolated from Finnish oat varieties," Food Hydrocolloids 5:513–522.
22. Bauer, S. K. and G. Geisler. 1996. "Variabilität im β-Glucangehlat der Haferkaryopse von 132 Kulturhafer- und 39 Wildhafergenotypen," J. Agro. Crop Sc. 176:151–157.
23. Bhatty, R. S. 1992. "β-Glucan content and viscosities of barleys and their roller-milled flour and bran products," Cereal Chem. 69:469–471.
24. Brunner, B. R. and R. D. Freed. 1994. "Oat grain β-glucan content affected by nitrogen level, location, and year," Crop. Sci. 34:473–476.
25. Cho, K. C. and P. J. White. 1993. "Enzymatic analysis of β-glucan content in different oat genotypes," Cereal Chem. 70:539–542.
26. Ganßmann, W. 1994. "β-Glucangehalte in deutschen Hafersorten und Laborversuche zur Anreicherung von β-Glucan und Gesamtballastoffen," Getreide Mehl und Brot 6:45–49.
27. Henry, R. J. 1987. "Pentosan and $(1 \rightarrow 3)(1 \rightarrow 4)$-$\beta$-D-glucan concentrations in endosperm and whole grain of wheat, barley, oats and rye," J. Cereal Sci. 6:253–258.
28. Holthaus, J. F., J. B. Holland, P. J. White and K. J. Frey. 1996. "Inheritance of β-glucan content in oat grain," Crop Sci. 36:567–572.
29. Humphreys, D. G., D. L. Smith and D. E. Mather. 1994. "Nitrogen fertilizer and seeding date induced changes in protein, oil and β-glucan contents of four oat cultivars," J. Cereal Sci. 20:283–290.
30. Jackson, G. D., R. K. Berg, G. D. Kushnak, T. K. Blake and G. I. Yarrow. 1994.

"Nitrogen effects on yield, beta-glucan content, and other quality factors of oat and waxy hulless barley," Commun. Soil Sci. Plant Anal. 25:3047–3055.

31. Lim, H. S., P. J. White and K. J. Frey. 1992. "Genotypic effects on β-glucan content of oat lines grown in two consecutive years," Cereal Chem. 69:262–265.
32. Miller, S. S., P. J. Wood, L. N. Pietrzak and R. G. Fulcher. 1993. "Mixed linkage β-glucan, protein content, and kernel weight in *avena* species," Cereal Chem. 70:231–233.
33. Miller, S. S., D. J. Vincent, J. Weisz and R. G. Fulcher. 1993. "Oat β-glucan: an evaluation of eastern Canadian cultivars and unregistered lines," Can. J. Plant Sci. 73:429–436.
34. Peterson, D. M. 1991. "Genotype and environment effects on oat beta-glucan concentration," Crop Sci. 31:1517–1520.
35. Peterson, D. M., D. M. Wesenberg and D. E. Burrup. 1995. "β-Glucan content and its relationship to agronomic characteristics in elite oat germplasm," Crop. Sci. 35:965–970.
36. Saastamoinen, M., S. Plaami and J. Kumpalainen. 1992. "β-Glucan and phytic acid content of oats cultivated in Finland," Acta Agric. Scand. 42:6–11.
37. Saastamoinen, M., S. Plaami and J. Kumpalainen. 1992. "Genetic and environmental variation in β-glucan content of oats cultivated or tested in Finland," J. Cereal Sci. 16:279–290.
38. Welch, R. W. and J. D. Lloyd. 1989. "Kernel (1 → 3)(1 → 4)-β-D-glucan content of oat genotype," J. Cereal Sci. 9:35–40.
39. Wood, P. J., J. Weisz and P. Fedec. 1991. "Potential for β-glucan enrichment in brans derived from oat (*Avena sativa* L.) cultivars of different (1 → 3)(1 → 4)-β-D-glucan concentration," Cereal Chem. 68:48–51.
40. Fulcher, R. G. and S. S. Miller. 1993. "Structure of oat bran and distribution of dietary fibre components," Oat Bran, P. J. Wood, St. Paul, MN: Amer. Assoc. Cereal Chem. pp. 1–24.
41. Anonymous 1989. "AACC committee adopts oat bran definition," Cereal Foods World 34:1033.
42. Knuckles, B. E., M. M. Chiu and A. A. Betschart. 1992. "β-Glucan-enriched fractions from laboratory-scale dry milling and sieving of barley and oats," Cereal Chem. 198–202.
43. Wood, P. J., J. Weisz and B. Blackwell. 1991. "Molecular characterization of cereal β-glucans. Structural analysis of oat β-D-glucan and rapid structural evaluation of β-D-glucans from different sources by high-performance liquid chromatography of oligosaccharides released by lichenase," Cereal. Chem. 68: 31–39.
44. Marlett, J. A. 1993. "Comparisons of dietary fibre and selected nutrient compositions of oat and other grain fractions," Oat Bran, P. J. Wood, St. Paul, MN: Amer. Assoc. Cereal Chem. pp. 49–82.
45. Wood, P. J., J. Weisz, P. Fedec and V. B. Burrows. 1989. "Large-scale preparation and properties of oat fractions enriched in (1 → 3)(1 → 4)-β-D-glucan," Cereal Chem. 66:97–103.
46. Hohner, G. A. and R. G. Hyldon. 1977. "Oat groat fractionation process," U.S. Patent 4,028,468.
47. Myllymäki, O., Y. Mälkki and K. Autio. 1994. "Process for fractionating crop into industrial raw material," U.S. Patent 5,312,636.

48. Oughton, R. W. 1980. "Process for the treatment of comminuted oats," U.S. Patent 4,211,695.
49. Burrows, V. D., R. G. Fulcher and D. Paton. 1984. "Processing aqueous treated cereals," U.S. Patent 4,435,429.
50. Collins, F. W. and D. Paton. 1992. "Method of producing stable bran and flour products from cereal grains," U.S. Patent 5,169,660.
51. Beer, M.U., E. Arrigoni and R. Amadò. 1996. "Extraction of oat gum from oat bran: Effects of process on yield, molecular weight distribution, viscosity and $(1 \rightarrow 3)(1 \rightarrow 4)$-$\beta$-D-glucan content of the gum," Cereal Chem. 73:58–62.
52. Inglett, G. E. 1991. "Method for making a soluble dietary fibre composition from oats," U.S. Patent 4,996,063.
53. Johansen, H. N., K. E. Bach-Knudsen, P. J. Wood and R. G. Fulcher. 1997. "Physicochemical properties and the degradation of oat bran polysaccharides in the gut of pigs," J. Sci. Food Agric. 73:81–82.
54. Jørgensen, K. G. 1988. "Quantification of high molecular weight $(1 \rightarrow 3)(1 \rightarrow 4)$-$\beta$-D-glucan using calcofluor complex formation and flow injection analysis. I. Analytical principal and its standardization," Carlsberg Res. Commun. 53:277–285.
55. McCleary, B. V. and M. Glennie-Holmes. 1985. "Enzymic quantification of $(1 \rightarrow 3)(1 \rightarrow 4)$-$\beta$-D-glucan in barley and malt," J. Inst. Brew. 91:285–295.
56. Anonymous 1997. "Food labeling: Health claims; oats and coronary heart disease," Federal Register 62:3584–3601.
57. Parrish, F. W., A. S. Perlin and E. T. Reese. 1960. "Selective enzymolysis of poly-β-D-glucans, and structure of the polymers," Can. J. Chem. 38:2094–2104.
58. Dais, P. and A. S. Perlin. 1982. "High field, 13C-NMR spectroscopy of β-D-glucans, amylopectin and glycogen," Carbohydr. Res. 100:103–116.
59. Wood, P. J., J. Weisz and B. A. Blackwell. 1994. "Structural studies of $(1 \rightarrow 3)(1 \rightarrow 4)$-$\beta$-D-glucans by ^{13}C-NMR and by rapid analysis of cellulose-like regions using high-performance anion-exchange chromatography of oligosaccharides released by lichenase," Cereal. Chem. 71:301–307.
60. Buliga, G. S., D. A. Brant and G. B. Fincher. 1986. "The sequence statistics and solution conformation of a barley $(1 \rightarrow 3)(1 \rightarrow 4)$-$\beta$-D-glucan," Carbohydr. Res. 157:139–156.
61. Staudte, R. G., J. R. Woodward, G. B. Fincher and B. A. Stone. 1983. "Water soluble $(1 \rightarrow 3)(1 \rightarrow 4)$-$\beta$-D-glucans from barley (*hordeum vulgare*) endosperm. III. Distribution of cellotriosyl and cellotetraosyl residues," Carbohydr. Polym. 3:299–312.
62. Vårum, K. M. and O. Smidsrød. 1988. "Partial chemical and physical characterization of $(1 \rightarrow 3)(1 \rightarrow 4)$-$\beta$-D-glucans from oat (*Avena sativa* L.) aleurone," Carbohydr. Polym. 9:103–117.
63. Mälkki, Y., K. Autio, O. Hänninen, O. Myllimäki, K. Pelkonen, T. Suortti and R. Törrönen, R. 1992. "Oat bran concentrates: physical properties of β-glucan and hypocholesterolemic effects in rats," Cereal Chem. 69:647–653.
64. Johansen, H. N., P. J. Wood and K. E. Bach-Knudsen. 1993. "Molecular weight changes in the $(1 \rightarrow 3)(1 \rightarrow 4)$-$\beta$-D-glucan of oats incurred by the digestive processes in the upper gastrointestinal tract of pigs," J. Agric. Food Chem. 41: 2347–2353.
65. Harding, S. E., K. M. Vårum, B. T. Stokke and O. Smidsrød. 1991. "Molecular

weight determination of polysaccharides," Advances in Carbohydr. Anal. 1: 63–144.

66. Acker, L., W. Diemar and E. Samhammer. 1955. "The lichenin of oats. I. Properties, preparation and composition of the muciparous polysaccharides," Z. Lebensm. Unters. Forsch. 102:225–231.
67. Forrest, I. S. and T. Wainwright. 1977. "The mode of binding of β-glucans and pentosans in barley endosperm cell walls," J. Inst. Brew. 139:535–545.
68. Vårum K. M., O. Smidsrød and D. Brant. 1992. "Light scattering reveals micelle-like aggregation in the (1 → 3)(1 → 4)-β-D-glucans from the oat aleurone," Food Hydrocolloids 4:497–511.
69. Vårum, K. M., A. Martinsen and O. Smidsrød. 1991. "Fractionation and viscometric characterization of a (1 → 3)(1 → 4)-β-D-glucan from oat, and universal calibration of a high-performance size exclusion chromatographic system by the use of fractionated β-glucans, alginates and pullulans," Food Hydrocolloids 5:363–373.
70. Doubler, J. L. and P. J. Wood. 1995. "Rheological properties of aqueous solutions of (1 → 3)(1 → 4)-β-D-glucan from oats (*Avena sativa* L.)," Cereal Chem. 72:335–340.
71. Wood, P. J., J. Weisz and W. Mahn. 1991. "Molecular characterization of cereal β-glucans. II. Size-exclusion chromatography for comparison of molecular weight," Cereal. Chem. 68:530–536.
72. Suortti, T. 1993. "Size exclusion chromatographic determination of β-glucan with postcolumn reaction detection," J. Chromatogr. 632:105–110.
73. Bhatty, R. S. 1995. "Laboratory and pilot plant extraction and purification of β-glucans from hull-less barley and oat brans," J. Cereal Sci. 22:163–170.
74. Beer, M. U., P. J. Wood and J. Weisz. 1997. "Molecular weight distribution and (1 → 3)(1 → 4)-β-D-glucan content of consecutive extracts of various oat and barley cultivars," Cereal Chem. (in press).
75. Beer, M. U., P. J. Wood, J. Weisz and N. Fillion. 1997. "Effect of cooking and storage on the amount and molecular weight of (1 → 3)(1 →)-β-D-glucan extracted from oat products by an *in vitro* digestion system," Cereal Chem. (submitted).
76. Sundberg, B., P. J. Wood, A. Lia, H. Andersson, A.-S. Sandberg, G. Hallmans and P. Åman. 1996. "Mixed-linked β-glucan from breads of different cereals is partly degraded in the human ileostomy model," Am. J. Clin. Nutr. 64:878–885.
77. Carr, J. M., J. L. Glatter, J. L. Jeraci and B. A. Lewis. 1990. "Enzymic determination of β-glucan in cereal-based food products," Cereal Chem. 67:226–229.
78. McCleary, B. V. 1988. "Purification of (1 → 3)(1 → 4)-β-D-glucan from barley flour," Methods in Enzymology, W. A. Wood and S. T. Kellogg, San Diego, CA: Academic Press. pp. 511–514.
79. Åman, P., H. Graham and A.-C. Tilly. 1989. "Content and solubility of mixed-linked (1 → 3)(1 → 4)-β-D-glucan in barley and oats during kernel development and storage," J. Cereal Sci. 10:45–50.
80. Anderson, M. A., J. A. Cook and B. A. Stone. 1978. "Enzymatic determination of (1 → 3)(1 → 4)-β-D-glucans in barley grain and other cereals," J. Inst. Brew. 84:233–239.
81. Wood, P. J. and R. G. Fulcher. 1978. "Interaction of some dyes with cereal β-glucans," Cereal Chem. 55:952–966.

82. Beresford G. and B. A. Stone. 1983. "(1 → 3)(1 → 4)-β-D-Glucan content of triticum grains," J. Cereal Sci. 1:111–114.
83. Ahluwahlia, B. and E. E. Ellis. 1984. "A rapid and simple method for the determination of starch and β-glucan in barley and malt," J. Inst. Brew. 90:254–259.
84. Autio, K., Myllymäki and Y. Mälkki. 1987. "Flow properties of solutions of oat β-glucans," J. Food Sci. 52:1364–1366.
85. Wikström, K., L. Lindahl, R. Andersson and E. Westerlund. 1994. "Rheological studies of water-soluble (1 → 3)(1 → 4)-β-D-glucans from milling fractions of oat," J. Food Sci. 59:1077–1080.
86. Wood, P. J., J. T. Braaten, F. W. Scott, D. Riedel and L. M. Poste. 1990. "Comparison of viscous properties of oat and guar gum and the effects of these and oat bran on glycemic index," J. Agric. Food Chem. 38:753–757.
87. Morris, E. R., A. N. Cutler, S. B. Ross-Murphy and D. A. Rees. 1981. "Concentration and shear rate dependence of viscosity in random coil polysaccharide solutions," Carbohydr. Polym. 1:5–21.
88. Morris, E. R. 1990. "Shear-thinning of 'random coil' polysaccharides: characterization by two parameters from a simple linear plot," Carbohydr. Polym. 13:85–96.
89. Wood, P. J., J. T. Braaten, F. W. Scott, K. D. Riedel, M. S. Wolynetz and M. W. Collins. 1994. "Effect of dose and modification of viscous properties of oat gum on plasma glucose and insulin following an oral glucose load," Brit. J. Nutr. 72: 731–743.
90. Autio, K. 1988. "Rheological properties of solutions of oat β-glucans," Gums and Stabilizers for the Food Industry 4, G. O. Phillips, D. J. Wedlock and P. A. Williams, Oxford: IRL Press.
91. Allen, F. M. 1913. Studies Concerning Glycosuria and Diabetes, W. M. Leonard, Boston.
92. Foster-Powell, K. and J. B. Miller. 1995. "International tables of glycemic index," Am. J. Clin. Nutr. 62:871S–890S.
93. Jenkins, D. J. A., T. M. S. Wolever, A. R. Leeds, M. A. Gassull, J. B. Dilawari, D. V. Goff, G. L. Metz and K. G. M. Alberti. 1978. "Dietary fibres, fibre analogues and glucose tolerance: importance of viscosity," Brit. Med. J. 1:1392–1394.
94. Braaten, J. T., P. J. Wood, F. W. Scott, K. D. Riedel, L. M. Poste and M. W. Collins. 1991. "Oat gum, a soluble fibre which lowers glucose and insulin in normal individuals after an oral glucose load: comparison with guar gum," Am. J. Clin. Nutr. 53:1425–1430.
95. Braaten, J. T., F. W. Scott, P. J. Wood, K. D. Riedel, M. S. Wolynetz, D. Brulé and M. W. Collins. 1994. "High β-glucan oat bran and oat gum reduce postprandial blood glucose and insulin in subjects with and without type 2 diabetes," Diabetes Med. 11:312–318.
96. Hallfrisch, J., D. J. Schofield and K. M. Behall. 1995. "Diets containing soluble oat extracts improve glucose and insulin response of moderately hypercholesterolemic men and women," Am. J. Clin. Nutr. 61:379–384.
97. Holm J., B. Koellreutter and P. Würsch. 1992. "Influence of sterilization, drying and oat bran enrichment of pasta on glucose and insulin responses in health subjects and on the rate and extent of in vitro starch digestion," Eur. J. Clin. Nutr. 46:629–640.
98. Tappy, L., E. Gügolz and P. Würsch. 1996. "Effects of breakfast cereals containing various amounts of β-glucan fibres on plasma glucose and insulin responses in NIDDM subjects," Diabetes Care 19:831–834.

99. De Groot, A. P., R. Luyken and N. A. Pikaar. 1963. "Cholesterol-lowering effect of rolled oats," Lancet 2:303–304.
100. Anderson, J. W. 1980. "Dietary fibre and diabetes," Medical Aspects of Dietary Fibre, G. A. Spiller and R. M. Kay, New York, NY: Plenum Medical Book Co. pp. 193–221.
101. Anderson, J. W., L. Story, B. Sieling, W. L. Chen, M. S. Petro and J. Story, 1984. "Hypocholesterolemic effects of oat bran or bean intake for hypercholesterolemic men," Am. J. Clin. Nutr. 40:1146–1155.
102. Anderson, J. W. 1985. "Physiological and metabolic effects of dietary fibre," Fed. Proc. 44:2902–1906.
103. Anderson, J. W. and N. J. Gustafson. 1988. "Hypocholesterolemic effects of oat and bean products," Am. J. Clin. Nutr. 48:749–753.
104. Anderson, J. W., D. Spencer, C. Hamilton, S. Smith, J. Tietyen, C. Bryant and P. Oeltgen. 1990. "Oat-bran cereal lowers serum total and LDL-cholesterol in hypercholesterolemic men," Am. J. Clin. Nutr. 52:495–499.
105. Anderson, J. W., H. G. Norman, D. A. Deakins, S. F. Smith, D. S. O'Neal, D. W. Dillon and P. R. Oeltgen. 1991. "Lipid response of hypercholesterolemic men to oat-bran and wheat-bran intake," Am. J. Clin. Nutr. 54:678–683.
106. Anderson, J. W. and S. R. Bridges. 1993. "Hypocholesterolemic effects of oat bran in humans," Oat Bran, P. J. Wood, St. Paul, MN: Amer. Assoc. Cereal Chem. pp. 139–157.
107. Anonymous 1996. "Food labeling: Health claims; oats and coronary heart disease," Federal Register 61:296–313.
108. Mackay, S. and M. J. Ball. 1992. "Do beans and oat bran add to the effectiveness of a low fat diet?" Eur. J. Clin. Nutr. 46:641–648.
109. Leadbetter J., M. J. Ball and J. I. Mann. 1991. "Effects of increasing quantities of oat bran in hypercholesterolemic people," Am. J. Clin. Nutr. 54:841–845.
110. Törrönen, R., L. Kansanen, M. Uusitupa, O. Hänninen, O. Myllymäki, H. Härkönen and Y. Mälkki. 1992. "Effects of oat bran concentrate on serum lipids in free-living men with mild to moderate hypercholesterolaemia," Europ. J. Clin. Nutr. 46: 621–627.
111. Swain, J. F., I. L. Rouse, C. B. Curley and F. M. Sacks. 1990. "Comparison of the effects of oat bran and low-fibre wheat on serum lipoprotein levels and blood pressure," New. Engl. J. Med. 322:147–152.
112. Anderson, J. W., D. A. Deakins, T. L. Floore, B. M. Smith and S. E. Whitis. 1990. "Dietary fiber and coronary heart disease," Critical Rev. in Food Sci. and Nutr. 29:95–147.
113. Braaten, J. T., P. J. Wood, F. W. Scott, M. S. Wolynetz, M. D. Lowe, P. Bradley-White and M. W. Collins. 1994. "Oat β-glucan reduces serum cholesterol concentration in hypercholesterolemic subjects," Europ. J. Clin. Nutr. 48:465–474.
114. Davidson, M. H., L. D. Dugan, J. H. Burns, J. Bova, K. Story and K. B. Drennan. 1991. "The hypocholesterolemic effects of β-glucan in oatmeal and oat bran," JAMA 265:1833–1839.
115. Ripsin, C. M., J. M. Keenan, D. R. Jacobs, P. J. Elmer, R. R. Welch, L. Van Horn, K. Liu, W. H. Turnbull, F. W. Thye, M. Kestin, M. Hegsted, M. H. Davidson, L. D. Dugan, W. Dehmark-Wahnefried and S. Beling. 1992. "Oat products and lipid lowering—a meta analysis," J. Am. Med. Assoc. 267:3317–3325.

116. Beer, M. U., E. Arrigoni and R. Amadò. 1995. "Effects of oat gum on blood cholesterol levels in healthy young men," Eur. J. Clin. Nutr. 49:517–522.

117. Behall, K. M., D. J. Schofield and J. Hallfrisch. 1997. "Effect of beta glucan level in oat fibre extracts on blood lipids in men and women," J. Am. Col. Nutr. 16:46–51.

118. Lund, E. K., J. M. Gee, J. C. Brown, P. J. Wood and I. T. Johnson. 1989. "The effect of oat gum on the physical properties of the gastrointestinal contents and the uptake of D-galactose and cholesterol by rat small intestine *in vitro,*" Brit. J. Nutr. 62:91–101.

119. Vachon C., J. D. Jones, P. J. Wood and L. Savoie. 1988. "Concentration effect of soluble dietary fibres on postprandial glucose and insulin in the rat," Can. J. Physiol. Pharmacol. 66:801–806.

120. Bégin, F., C. Vachon, J. D. Jones, P. J. Wood and L. Savoie. 1989. "Effect of dietary fibres on glycemia and insulinemia and on gastrointestinal function in rats," Can. J. Physiol. Pharmacol. 67:1265–1271.

121. Edwards, C. A., N. A. Blackburn, L. Craigen, P. Davison, J. Tomlin, K. Sugden, I. T. Johnson and N. W. Read. 1987. "Viscosity of food gums determined in vitro related to their hypoglycemic actions," Am. J. Clin. Nutr. 46:72–77.

122. Jenkins, D. J. A. 1980. "Dietary fibre and carbohydrate metabolism," Medical Aspects of Dietary Fiber, Spiller, G. A. and R. M. Kay, New York, NY: Plenum Medical. pp. 175–192.

123. Jenkins, D. J. A., A. L. Jenkins, T. M. S. Wolever, V. Vuksan, A. V. Rao, L. U. Thompson and R. G. Josse. 1995. "Dietary fibre, carbohydrate metabolism and diabetes," Dietary Fiber in Health and Disease, D. Kritchevsky and C. Bonfield, St. Paul, MN: Eagan Press. pp. 137–145.

124. Gallaher, D. D., C. A. Hassel and K.-J. Lee. 1993. "Relationship between viscosity of hydroxypropyl methylcellulose and plasma cholesterol in hamsters," J. Nutr. 123:1732–1738.

125. Jensen, C. D., G. A. Spiller, J. E. Gates, A. F. Miller and J. H. Whittam. 1993. "The effect of Acacia gum and a water soluble dietary fibre mixture on blood lipids in humans," J. Am. College Nutr. 12:147–154.

126. McClean Ross, A. H., M. A. Eastwood, W. G. Brydon, J. R. Anderson and D. M. W. Anderson. 1983. "A study of the effects of dietary gum arabic in humans," Am. J. Clin. Nutr. 37:368–375.

127. Blake, D. E., C. J. Hamblett, P. G. Frost, P. A. Judd and P. R. Ellis. 1997. "Wheat bread supplemented with depolymerized guar gum reduces the plasma cholesterol concentration in hypercholesterolemic human subjects," Am. J. Clin. Nutr. 65:107–113.

128. Cara, L., C. Dubois, P. Borel, M. Armand, M. Senft, H. Portugal, A.-M. Pauli, P.-M. Bernard and D. Lairon. 1992. "Effects of oat bran, rice bran, wheat fibre, and wheat germ on postprandial lipemia in health adults," Am. J. Clin. Nutr. 55:81–88.

129. Dubois, C., M. Armand, M. Senft, H. Portugal, A.-M. Pauli, P.-M. Renard, H. Lafont and D. Lairon. 1995. "Chronic oat bran intake alters postprandial lipemia and lipoproteins in healthy adults," Am. J. Clin. Nutr. 61:325–333.

130. Wolever, T. M. S., D. J. A. Jenkins, S. Mueller, D. L. Boctor, T. P. Ransom, R. Patten, E. S. Chao, K. McMillan and V. Fulgoni. 1994. "Method of administration influences the serum cholesterol-lowering effect of psyllium," Am. J. Clin. Nutr. 59:1055–1099.

131. Judd, P. A. and A. S. Truswell. 1981. "The effects of rolled oats on blood lipids and fecal steroid excretion in man," Am. J. Clin. Nutr. 34:2061–2067.

132. Kirby, R., J. W. Anderson, B. Sieling, E. Rees, W. Chen, R. Miller and R. Kay. 1981. "Oat-bran selectively lowers serum low-density lipoprotein cholesterol concentrations of hypercholesterolemic men," Am. J. Clin. Nutr. 34:824–829.

133. Bowels, K. R., K. R. Morgan, R. H. Furneaux and G. D. Coles. 1996. "^{13}C CP/MAS NMR study of the interaction of bile acids with barley β-D-glucan," Carbohydr. Polym. 29:7–10.

134. Kritchevsky, D., S. A. Tepper, G. T. Goodman, M. M. Weber and D. M. Klurfeld. 1984. "Influence of oat and wheat bran on cholesterolemia in rats," Nutr. Rep. Int. 29:1353–1359.

135. Story, J. A. and D. Kritchevsky. 1976. "Comparison of the binding of various bile acids and bile salts in vitro by several types of fibre," J. Nutr. 106:1292–1294.

136. Vahouny, G. V., R. Tombes, M. M. Cassady, D. Kritchevsky and L. Gallo. 1980. "Dietary fibres: V. Binding of bile salts, phospholipids and cholesterol from mixed micelles by bile acid sequestrants and dietary fibres," Lipids 15:1012–1018.

137. Blackburn, N. A., J. S. Redfern, H. Jarjis, A. M. Holgate, I. Hanning, J. H. B. Scarpello, I. T. Johnson, and N. W. Read. 1984. "The mechanism of action of guar gum in improving glucose tolerance in man," Clin. Sci. 66:329–336.

138. Bhathena, S. J., J. Avigan and M. E. Schreiner. 1974. "Effect of insulin on sterol and fatty acid synthesis and hydroxymethylglutaryl CoA reductase activity in mammalian cells grown in culture," Proc. Natl. Acad. Sci. USA 71:2174–2178.

139. Reaven, G. M. and R. M. Bernstein. 1978. "Effect of obesity on the relationship between very low density lipoprotein production rate and plasma triglyceride concentration in normal and hypertriglyceridemic subjects," Metabolism 27: 1047–1054.

140. Jenkins, D. J. A., T. M. S. Wolever, A. L. Jenkins and R. H. Taylor. 1978. "Dietary fibre, carbohydrate metabolism and diabetes," Mol. Aspects. Med. 9:97–112.

141. Jenkins, D. J. A. 1991. "Dietary fibre and other antinutrients: metabolic effects and therapeutic implications," Current Topics in Nutrition and Disease. Nutritional Pharmacology, G. A. Spiller, New York, NY: Alan R Liss Inc. pp. 117–145.

142. Dreher, M. L. 1987. "Dietary fibre and its physiological effects," Handbook of Dietary Fibre. An Applied Approach, M. L. Dreher, New York, NY: Marcel Dekker Inc. pp. 199–279.

143. Jenkins, D. J. A., T. M. S. Wolever, V. Vuksan, F. Brighenti, S. Cunnane, R. Venketeshwer, A. L. Jenkins, G. Buckley, R. Patten, W. Singer, P. Corey and R. G. Josse. 1989. "Nibbling versus gorging: metabolic advantages of increased meal frequency," New Engl. J. Med. 321:929–934.

144. Bridges, S. R., J. W. Anderson, D. A. Deakins, D. W. Dillon and C. L. Wood. 1992. "Oat bran increases serum acetate of hypercholesterolemic men," Am. J. Clin. Nutr. 56:455–459.

145. Chen, W.-J. L., J. W. Anderson and D. Jennings. 1984. "Propionate may mediate the hypercholesterolemic effects of certain soluble plant fibres in cholesterol-fed rats," Proc. Soc. Exp. Biol. Med. 175:215–218.

146. Cummings, J. H., E. W. Pomare, W. J. Branch, C. P. E. Naylor and G. T. MacFarlane. 1987. "Short chain fatty acids in human large intestine, portal, hepatic, and venous blood," Gut 28:1221–1227.

147. Wright, R. S., J. W. Anderson and S. Bridges. 1990. "Propionate inhibits hepatocyte lipid synthesis," Proc. Soc. Expt. Biol. Med. 195:26–29.
148. Topping, D. L. 1995. "Propionate as a mediator of the effects of dietary fibre," Dietary Fibre in Health and Disease, D. Krichevsky and C. Bonfield, St. Paul, MN: Eagan Press. pp. 340–345.
149. Wolever, T. M. S., P. Spadafora and H. Eshuis. 1991. "Interaction between colonic acetate and propionate in man," Am. J. Clin. Nutr. 53:681–687.
150. Zhang, J. X., G. Hallmans, H. Andersson, I. Bosaeus, P. Åman, P. Tidehag, R. Stenling, E. Lundin and S. Dahlgren. 1992. "Effect of oat bran on plasma cholesterol and bile acid excretion in nine subjects with ileostomies," Am. J. Clin. Nutr. 56:99–105.
151. Remesy, C., C. Demigne and C. Morand. 1992. "Metabolism and utilization of short chain fatty acids produced by colonic fermentation," Dietary Fibre—A Component of Food, T. F. Schweizer and C. A. Edwards, London, UK: Springer. pp. 137–150.
152. Eastwood, M. 1995. "Physicochemical properties of dietary fibre in the foregut," Mechanism of Action in Human Physiology and Metabolism, C. Cherbut, J. L. Barry, D. Lairon and M. Durand, Paris, France: John Libbey Eurotext. pp. 17–28.
153. Lairon, D., H. Lafont, J. L. Vigne, G. Nalbone, J. Leonardi and J. C. Hauton. 1985. "Effects of dietary fibres and cholestyramine on the activity of pancreatic lipase *in vitro,*" Am. J. Clin. Nutr. 42:629–638.
154. Hendrick, J. A., T. Tadokoro, C. Emenhiser, U. Nienaber and O. R. Fennema. 1992. "Various dietary fibres have different effects on lipase-catalyzed hydrolysis of tributyrin *in vitro,*" J. Nutr. 122:269–277.
155. Pasquier, B., M. Armand, F. Guyon, C. Castellain and D. Lairon. 1994. "Soluble fibres alter emulsification of dietary fat in vitro," Proceedings of the European workshop on Mechanisms of Action of Dietary Fibre on Lipid and Cholesterol Metabolism, D. Lairon, Luxembourg: Commission of the European Communities. pp. 45–47.
156. Zhang, J. and J. R. Lupton. 1994. "Dietary fibres stimulate colonic cell proliferation by different mechanisms at different sites," Nutr. Cancer 22:267–276.
157. Bauer, H. G., N.-G. Asp, A. Dahlquist, P. E. Fredlund, M. Nyman and R. Öste. 1981. "Effect of two kinds of pectin and guar gum on 1,2-dimethylhydrazine initiation of colon tumors and on fecal β-glucuronidase activity in the rat," Cancer Res. 41:2518–2523.
158. McIntyre, A, P. R. Gibson and G. P. Young, 1993. "Butyrate production from dietary fibre and protection against large bowel cancer in a rat model," Gut 34:386–391.
159. Harris, P. J., A. M. Robertson, M. E. Watson, C. M. Triggs and L. R. Ferguson. 1993. "The effects of soluble-fibre polysaccharides on the adsorption of a hydrophobic carcinogen to an insoluble fibre," Nutr. Cancer. 19:43–45.

CHAPTER 2

Physiologically Functional Wheat Bran

E. CHAO[1]
C. SIMMONS[2]
R. BLACK[3]

1. INTRODUCTION

HUMAN health is inextricably linked with diet, and within the last 10 years, research teams combining epidemiologists, nutritionists, oncologists, biochemists and microbiologists have been able to demonstrate the potent health effects of many of the foods that are a part of the traditional diet. In North America, the food industry plays a pivotal role in shaping that diet. The food industry is also in a unique position to translate the benefits of research in nutrition and food science into commercially viable foods for the "human diet" (and so human health). Thus, in recent years there has been an explosion of research geared towards developing a better understanding of precisely *how* diet can affect health and general body physiology. In the United States, the use of "health claims" is another effort to encourage the general public to select foods as part of a diet that may directly promote health. Health claim, as authorized through the enactment of the Nutrition Labeling and Education Act of 1990 (NLEA) in the United States, is any claim made in the label of a food that expressly, or by implication, characterizes the relationship of that food or one or more of its components to a disease- or health-related condition. While it is still too early to tell if there has been a significant impact on dietary patterns in the U.S. population

[1]Kellogg Canada Inc., Etobicoke, Ontario, Canada.
[2]Kellogg Company, Battle Creek, Michigan, USA.
[3]Nestlé Canada Inc. and Department of Nutritional Sciences, Faculty of Medicine, University of Toronto, Toronto, ON, Canada.

as a result of this effort, the NLEA has spurred research in this area, both within North America and around the world, in an effort to better understand and quantify the effects of diet on health and human physiology.

Currently in the United States, a health claim for a food or food component is based on "significant scientific agreement" on the totality of the publicly available evidence, something that has been exceedingly difficult to define. However, it has been acknowledged that some specific issues must be addressed by the science: (1) identifying the public health benefit that will derive from the use of the claim; (2) the safe and optimum level of the substance to be consumed; (3) the potential of the claim to actively influence consumption patterns of the food; (4) the prevalence of the disease- or health-related condition in the population; and (5) the relevance of the claim in the context of the total diet.

Much of the research in this area has focused on specific nutrients or components of specific foods. Wheat and wheat bran provide an excellent example of this research process, as our understanding of the physiologic effects of dietary fiber has progressed from simply alleviating constipation to actively reducing the risk of some types of chronic diseases.

The role of cereal grains in gastrointestinal health has long been recognized. As early as the fifth century B.C., Hippocrates, the Father of Medicine, recommended eating wholemeal bread "for its salutary effect upon the bowel" [1]. In this century, the work of physicians such as Burkitt, Painter, Trowell and Walker has renewed interest in the potential benefits of dietary fiber in the prevention of several chronic diseases. Dietary fiber, resistant to digestion by human digestive enzymes, is concentrated in the bran fraction of whole grains. More recently, in the last decade, other components present in whole grains, though nonessential as nutrients, have also been associated with certain health benefits. These substances include phenolic compounds (such as lignans and phytoestrogens), tocotrienols and phytic acid.

Wheat is one of the major grains in the diet of a vast number of the world's population and, therefore, can play an important role in the nutritional quality of the diet and human health. Wheat bran in particular, widely available as a food ingredient, is probably the most studied fraction of the grain. This chapter will focus on the physiological functions of wheat bran, related to its role in enhancing health and the management and risk reduction of some chronic diseases. The health-related effects of other associated wheat components will also be discussed in brief. An outline of the chemistry and processing of wheat will be introduced as background information.

2. STRUCTURE AND COMPOSITION OF WHEAT KERNELS

Like other typical cereal grains, wheat kernels (caryopses) contain three main anatomical parts: an embryo (germ), an endosperm, and a pericarp (fruit coat, containing layers making up the bran) that covers the endosperm (Figure 2.1).

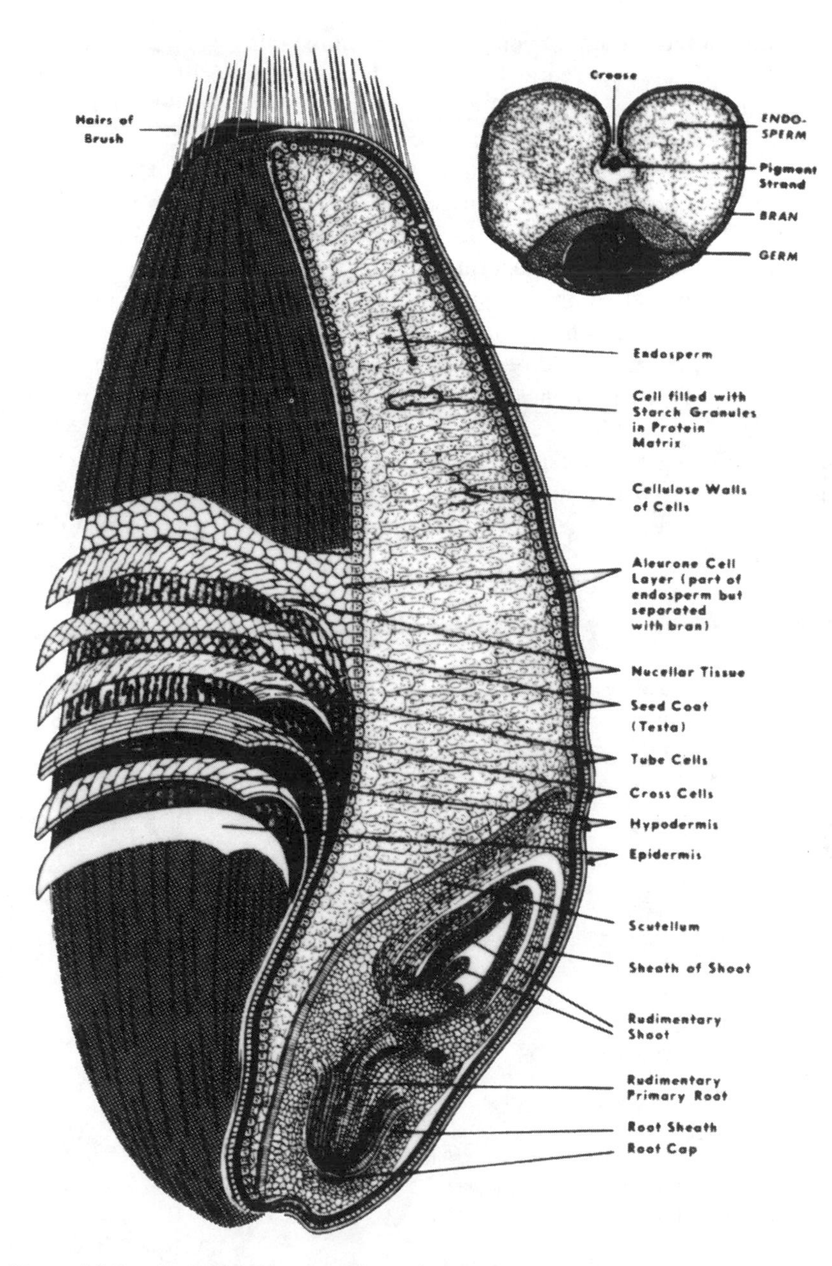

Figure 2.1 Longitudinal and cross sections of a wheat kernel. (Reprinted from Reference [2], with permission from American Association of Cereal Chemists, Inc.)

The structural relationships among these parts in the intact grain and the major milled fractions are depicted in Table 2.1. Although variation exists across and within wheat varieties, typical kernels are about 8 mm in length and 4 mm in width at their midpoint, weighing about 35 mg.

The outermost bran layers are fiber rich. Starch and protein are concentrated in the endosperm, while the germ is high in fat. The bran and germ fractions are also high in vitamins and minerals. Commercial bran fractions always have some endosperm material associated with them, to varying degrees, depending on mill practice. The germ is typically removed in the milling process as a final product. Actual amounts of various biochemical constituents within kernels vary across varieties. Even more pronounced than in the past, these varietal differences are due not only to soil and environmental influences, but are also impacted by genetic manipulation within and across wheat types and classes. Generalizations about anything other than gross composition can be misleading. Much of the general composition data published, particularly in texts, reflect varieties no longer commercially available.

TABLE 2.1. Ideal Relationship Between Botanical Constituents and Major Mill Fractions.

Grain Component		Mill Factions
Grain (caryopsis)		
1. Pericarp (fruit coat)		
a. Outer pericarp		
Outer epidermis (epicarp)	Beeswing	
Hypodermis		
Thin-walled cells—remnants over most of grain, but cell walls remain in crease and attachment region; includes vascular tissue in crease		
b. Inner pericarp		
Intermediate cells		
Cross cells		Bran
Tube cells (inner epidermis)		
2. Seed		
a. Seed coat (testa) and pigment strand		
b. Nucellar epidermis (hyaline layer)		
c. Endosperm		
Aleurone layer		
Starchy endosperm		White flour
d. Embryo		
Embryonic axis		
Scutellum		Germ

Source: Adapted from Reference [3].

3. MILLING

Milling of grains typically falls into one of two categories: wet milling or dry milling. Specialized milling technology has developed recently to allow fractionation of grains to meet very specific needs. However, wheat is typically dry milled. The purpose of dry milling is to separate the main anatomical parts of the grain (bran, endosperm and germ) as efficiently as possible. A simplified mill flow process is depicted in Figure 2.2.

Wheat milling is accomplished through a series of paired rolls and sifters that serve to facilitate separation of the major components of the grain — with flour, bran and germ as primary products. Many nonuniversal terms are used for various milled bran fractions, including "heavy bran," "light bran," "fine bran," "coarse bran" and "ground bran." It is critical to understand the identity of the bran fraction of interest, regardless of the semantics used to describe it. To simplify matters, we compare in Table 2.2 whole wheat, high-density (higher content of starchy endosperm material)

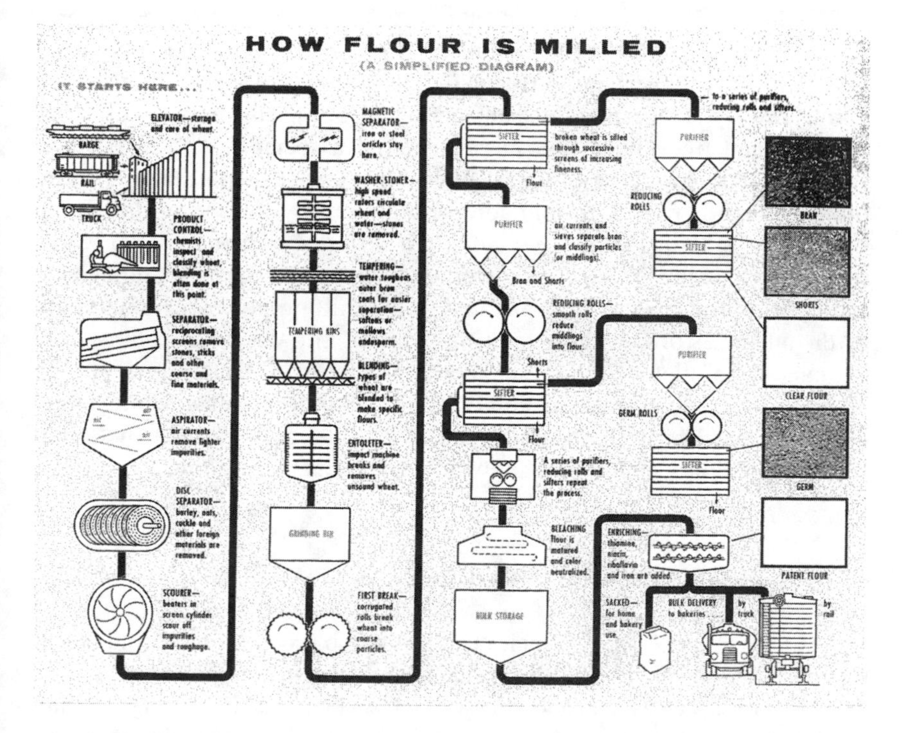

Figure 2.2 Flour milling. (Reprinted from Reference [4], copyright © 1987; by permission of VCH Publishers, a subsidiary of John Wiley & Sons, Inc.)

TABLE 2.2. Composition of Whole Wheat and Representative Bran Fractions.

Material[1]	Size[2]	Protein (%)	Fat (%)	Starch (%)	Dietary Fibre (%)
Whole wheat	2000	10.2	1.5	65.0	12.0
High density bran	2200	12.5	1.7	61.1	13.0
Low density bran	1400	15.5	3.1	21.1	37.0

[1]All materials were analyzed and results reported on an "as is" moisture basis, 14.5%, 13.1%, and 11.7% for whole wheat, high-density bran, and low-density bran, respectively.
[2]Size is mean particle (or kernel) size, reported in microns.
Source: Kellogg Company Laboratory values.

bran and low-density (lower content of starchy endosperm material) bran. These bran fractions vary in where they come off the milling process, as described below, and vary physically in particle size. Bran containing approximately 35–40% dietary fiber (low density as described in Table 2.2) is a common milled product used as a raw material in breakfast cereal production. It is produced in the "break" section of the mill (containing a series of break rolls) where corrugated rolls allow gross separation of the fibrous branny layers from the endosperm and germ. This bran material has adhering and free floury endosperm material associated with it, but is a very concentrated source of wheat fiber. Floury endosperm material sifted from the bran is processed into commercial flour by further milling in the "reduction" side of the mill (containing a series of reduction rolls) where striated rolls reduce the size of materials further. A variety of intermediate and hybrid products can be generated in the milling process, limited only by the attributes of the wheat entering the mill, mill design, capability, and the overall abilities of the miller. For example, high-density bran can be produced at the first break section of a mill, and represents a whole kernel of wheat that has been sheared open, with little loss of bran, but from which some floury endosperm and whole germ can be sifted out.

4. BREAKFAST CEREAL PROCESSING

A variety of process technologies can be used to produce hot or cold breakfast cereals from grain-based ingredients, including whole grains as well as their fractions, such as bran and flour. Breakfast cereal manufacturing typically involves these basic steps, their sequence depending on the specific processing

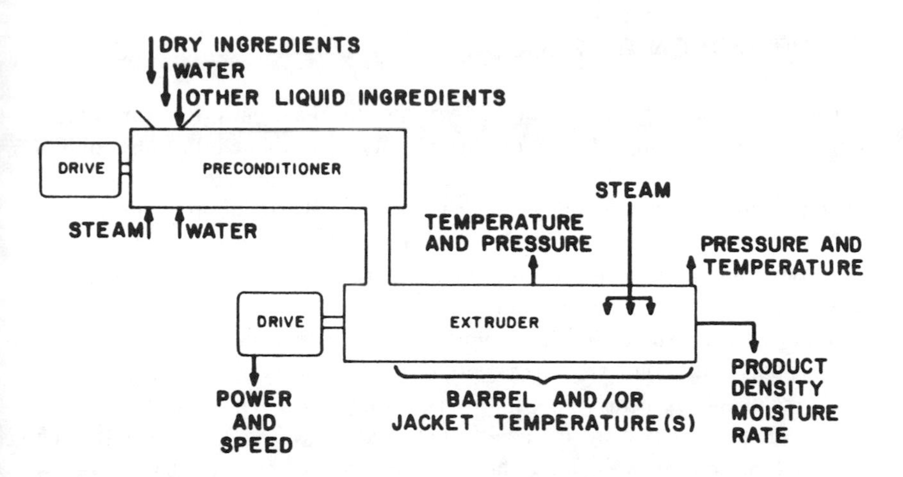

Figure 2.3 Diagram of an extruder indicating process variables requiring monitoring. (Reprinted from Reference [5], with permission from American Association of Cereal Chemists, Inc.)

methods: addition of flavoring, conditioning or tempering, cooking, drying, shaping/forming (e.g., flaking, shredding), toasting, vitamin spray/coating (optional), and packaging. One widely practiced technique for cooking cereals involves continuous processing in an extruder (Figure 2.3). Formulated ingredients that can be preconditioned to facilitate cooking are exposed to heat, moisture, pressure and shear in this operation. Once cooked, materials are typically dried to remove moisture that aids in subsequent processing.

Many technologies are utilized to process preconditioned or cooked grain materials, including: flaking grains or grain pieces by roller milling, puffing, which involves pressure differentials as the basis for expansion, shredding of cooked grains and the formation of "mats" from shreds in various orientations, blending of grains and slurry components (consisting of a syrup mixture which binds ingredients together) for granola-type products, and drum drying of cooked flours to produce farinas and typical baby cereals.

5. HEALTH BENEFITS OF WHEAT BRAN FIBER

The useful role of wheat bran in promoting regularity and preventing constipation is generally accepted. In addition, growing research has focused on its protective effect against colon and breast cancers. The following is a review of the evidence supporting these major physiological benefits of wheat bran.

5.1. PROMOTION OF REGULARITY

Not only does the amount of fiber in the diet have an effect on colonic function, the type of fiber and its digestibility or fermentability also play a significant role. Both soluble and insoluble fibers have value in promoting regularity in colonic function, as measured by stool weight and transit time, but they promote regularity via different mechanisms. Insoluble fibers, such as those from wheat bran, are resistant to fermentation by colonic bacteria and increase fecal bulk by retaining water [6,7].

Soluble fibers, such as those from vegetables and fruits and some grains such as oats and barley, are extensively broken down by bacteria and provide readily available substrate for colonic bacterial growth. These fibers increase fecal weight primarily by increasing bacterial mass and gases, one of the principal end products of fermentation [7,8]. This decrease in density or increase in volume of fecal mass causes threshold volume in the rectum to be reached rapidly, thereby triggering the mechanisms of defecation. Since fecal bulk and transit time are inversely correlated, fibers that increase fecal weight also reduce transit time [9,10]. Shortened transit time limits the opportunity for re-absorption and hardening of the intestinal contents, thus preventing impaction and constipation. Although fecal volume is responsible for triggering bowel movement, this important parameter is not often measured because of technical problems [11,12].

Among the different sources of dietary fiber as fecal bulking agents, wheat bran is probably the most studied and among the most effective. In fact, wheat bran is often used as a standard against which the laxative effects of novel fiber sources are compared [13,14]. Among the different fiber sources compared by Cummings (1993), wheat bran ranked among the highest in fecal bulking, exceeding fibers from fruit and vegetables, gums and mucilages, cellulose, oats, corn, legumes and pectin [3] (Table 2.3).

5.1.1. Chemical Composition and Structure of Wheat Bran

The digestibility and fermentability of fiber are dependent on both its chemical composition and structure, which in turn also determines its physicochemical characteristics [15]. Cellulose (typically 15–24% of dietary fiber in wheat bran) and lignin, a major component of cell walls (5–10% of wheat bran fiber) [16,17], were components of wheat bran that survived the digestive process essentially unaltered in a fiber balance study [18]. The cellular structure of bran, well retained under different methods of fiber preparation [19], is another key factor contributing to its resistance to digestion and fermentation. In the human, wheat bran fiber is only 36% digested [7]. Scanning electron microscope studies of bran before and after passage through the gut provide further evidence that the cellular structure is retained virtually intact [20].

TABLE 2.3. Average Increase in Fecal Output per Gram Fiber Fed.

Source	Increase in Fecal Bulk/Fiber (g/g ± SEM)	Number of Studies	Comments
Wheat	5.4 ± 0.7	41	Mainly wheat bran
Fruit and vegetables	4.7 ± 0.7	28	Carrots, peas, cabbage, apple, potato, banana, prunes, mixed sources
Gums and mucilages	3.7 ± 0.5	27	Psyllium/ispaghula, tragacanth, xanthan, sterculia, bassara, xylan, agar, gum arabic
Cellulose	3.5 ± 0.8	7	Also carboxymethyl-methylcellulose cellulose
Oats	3.4 ± 1.1	4	Oat bran or oats
Corn	3.3 ± 0.3	5	Corn meal or bran
Legumes	2.2 ± 0.3	17	Soya products
Pectin	1.2 ± 0.3	11	Degree of methoxylation unimportant

Average increase in fecal output per gram fiber fed.
Reprinted with permission from Reference [8]. Copyright CRC Press, Boca Raton, Florida. © 1993.

The fiber structure is also a major factor in the water-holding capacity of wheat bran. It is believed that bound (as opposed to trapped) water which remains associated with the fiber contributes to fecal bulking in individuals with normal bowel function [7,9]. Bound water was estimated to be the main component (48%) of the increase in fecal weight among subjects consuming a high-fiber diet enriched with wheat bran for three weeks (+18 g dietary fiber from wheat bran compared to a control diet with 22 g dietary fiber). The remaining proportions of the increased fecal weight were attributed to free water (22%), water associated with bacteria and fiber from the controlled diet (20%), and extra bacteria excreted (10%) [7]. These studies together would suggest that wheat bran, being resistant to digestion and fermentation in the intestine, increases fecal mass primarily by retaining water associated with the fiber structure and colonic microflora, thus contributing to its laxative effects.

5.1.2. Physical Form

Several studies have shown that the fecal bulking effect of wheat bran is reduced as particle size decreases [21,22]. Particle size of bran above 500 μm appears to be of critical importance in increasing fecal output [23]. There has been concern that particle size below 200 μm may actually contribute to constipation [23]. However, data on the laxative effect of wheat bran in this lower-particle size range are limited.

Particle size of bran is apparently not affected by mastication and digestion in the small intestine [17]. Particle size can affect the fecal bulking effect of wheat bran by altering water-holding capacity, resistance to colonic bacterial fermentation, and entrapment of finely dispersed gas produced by colonic bacteria [21]. Larger particle size has been associated with higher *in-vitro* water-holding capacity [21,24] and higher moisture content in the feces [22]. The greater resistance to digestibility of cellulose in coarse bran compared to fine bran may also contribute to the difference in fecal bulking effect between the two bran types [22]. Further, the large wheat bran particles take a curly shape on fermentation, providing a physical resistance to the removal of interstitial water and dispersed gases, thus counterbalancing the absorptive capacity of the colon [12].

From a food processing perspective, the range of particle size in commercially available wheat bran offers many functional benefits. While fiber particle size may affect its colonic effects, the range of particle size typically found in commercially available wheat bran (coarse bran $>$1400 μm to very finely ground bran $<$500 μm) is well within that reported to be associated with fecal bulking effects.

5.1.3. Effect of Processing

The biological effect of cooking on cereal fiber has not been clearly defined although some studies suggest that cooked bran has less effect on fecal bulking than a comparable dose of raw bran. In an experimental study in which the colonic effects of raw and cooked wheat bran (in the form of breakfast cereal) were compared directly at two doses (12, 20 g/d for raw bran, 13.2 and 22 g/d for cooked bran), significant reduction in transit time was achieved with the higher dose of raw bran but not with either dose of the cooked bran [11]. Comparing fecal wet weight at the lower dose, the increase was higher with raw bran; at the higher dose, the difference between bran types was insignificant. The lack of dose response with raw bran was an unexpected finding in this study. In a review of the literature, Cummings reported significantly higher average increase in fecal output for raw bran (7.2 g/g fiber) than cooked bran (4.9 g/g fiber) [8]. It is possible that some form of processing may modify the fiber structure and, thus, the digestibility and water-holding capacity of wheat bran. This in turn could alter its fecal bulking property. However, the practical significance of this is probably limited as wheat bran in different processed forms continues to show efficacy in promoting regularity [25].

5.1.4. Dose Response

The dose response relationship between wheat bran fiber and fecal output was studied in a group of healthy volunteers who consumed wheat fiber cereals in amounts that provided 0.3, 5.6, 9.5, 11.2, 19.0 and 28.4 g dietary fiber per day for 14 days. A linear dose response (2.7 g increase in fecal weight per g increase in wheat fiber) was observed across the six levels of fiber intake. The increase in fecal weight was independent of the initial daily fecal weight of the volunteers [25]. Dose response relationship between wheat fiber and increase in stool weight was also observed in the study of Stephen et al. in which healthy subjects consumed one of four different amounts of bran-enriched wholemeal bread (30, 60, 110, 170 g/d) in addition to white bread [26]. These data support a dose-dependent effect of wheat bran fiber on fecal bulking and its use in graded amounts in the management of constipation.

5.2. MANAGEMENT OF SOME COMMON GASTROINTESTINAL DISORDERS

5.2.1. Constipation

Most definitions of constipation include infrequent bowel action—twice a week or less [27]. Since constipation is perceived in various ways, many different symptoms are associated with it. Often people complain of constipation if their stools are too hard or too small, if they strain or experience pain in defecation, have infrequent bowel movements or have the feeling of incomplete defecation. Certainly, low fiber intake is one factor in the development of constipation.

There have been few controlled studies on the effectiveness of fiber and wheat bran in relieving constipation [28]. Review of available data suggests that constipated patients had lower stool output and slower transit time with or without bran supplementation, and responded less well to similar doses of bran than control subjects [29]. The author suspected that the constipated patients in some studies were particularly selected and might not be representative of all constipated patients. Also, since constipation is an ill-defined symptom, differences in the degree of constipation between studies may also complicate the assessment of wheat bran efficacy in constipation management. It is possible that a motility disorder of the colon, which is either primary or secondary to an underlying disease or an altered lifestyle, is responsible for constipation. In some instances, complete reversal or relief of constipation may not be achieved with dietary fiber supplementation alone. However, *preventing* constipation with supplemental fiber intake from wheat bran has been shown to be an effective strategy in up to 60% of elderly patients and in children [12].

5.2.1.1. Effects of Gender and Age

Constipation is more common in women than men [27]. Some research suggests that women may need more fiber for normal laxation compared to men. On average, women had smaller stools and slower transit time than men despite similar intakes of dietary fiber [26,30]. A higher proportion of women (17%) than men (1%) passed less than 50 g of stools per day [31]. Men, with higher average basal fecal outputs, also had greater response for a given increase in fiber intake [25]. The effect of gender on stool weight may be explained entirely by differences in transit [26]. In addition, more women may experience constipation because of hormonal changes. For example, it has been suggested that slower transit due to altered hormone levels underlies the constipation associated with pregnancy [32].

It is well recognized that the elderly are more prone to developing constipation than younger age groups. However, age was not found to be correlated with fecal output in one study in which age ranged from 17–62 years [26]. Several factors can contribute to decreased regularity in large bowel function in the elderly: decreased colonic muscular tone and motility; low fluid intake due to decreased sensitivity to thirst; intolerance to high-fiber foods due to denture problems; reduced food intake; physical inactivity; and medications including habitual laxative use [33,34].

Constipation is also a common clinical problem in childhood but its manifestation is different from that in adults [35]. Most children are reported to pass stools of an extremely large size, suggesting colonic overdistension and insensitivity. Other problems may also develop as a result of constipation. Encopresis (chronic overflow diarrhea or fecal soiling) may result when the internal rectal sphincter is chronically distended [35]. Fecal soiling may also occur as the internal rectal sphincter is chronically held open.

Management in childhood should aim at preventing constipation by establishing normal colonic muscular tone and ensuring adequate intake of fiber and fluid, which together promote regular passage of softer stools and slowly allowing the return of normal rectal function and tone [36]. A recent recommendation from the American Health Foundation proposes that a reasonable goal for dietary fiber intake during childhood and adolescence may be approximately equivalent to the age of the child plus 5 g per day [36]. Based on this "Age + 5" formula, minimal dietary fiber intake would range from 8 g/d at age 3, to 25 g/d by age 20. This can be contrasted with recommendations for adults, which generally range from 25 to 35 g/d.

5.2.2. Diverticulosis

Diverticulosis refers to abnormalities of the colon characterized by the presence of sacs protruding through the colonic wall. The treatment of uncomplicated diverticulosis aims to relieve symptoms and to prevent or postpone its complications. The best results have been achieved with unprocessed, coarse wheat bran in maximum amounts tolerated or at least 10–25 g/d in divided portions added to foods [37]. Similar fiber intake can also be achieved by whole wheat bread, high-fiber breakfast cereals or biscuits. Recommended amounts are usually reached by gradually increasing over 4 to 6 weeks. Patients' bloating and discomfort may increase before improvement is obtained. It appears that patients with diverticular disease exhibit only about 50% of the response to bran seen in healthy individuals [8]. The mechanism for the role of dietary fiber in the prevention or management of diverticulosis is unclear. The hypothesis of Painter that diverticular disease being a result of colonic underfilling would suggest that correcting this condition by maintaining certain fecal mass with high-fiber diet could potentially reduce the risk of developing diverticulosis [38].

5.2.3. Irritable Bowel Syndrome

Irritable bowel syndrome (IBS) is characterized by progressive large bowel irregularity with altering constipation and diarrhea, is often accompanied by pain. While the genesis of IBS is not known, many think that it is caused by colonic or intestinal spasm. Treatment aims at control or relief of symptoms, although usually not completely or permanently.

High-fiber diets are widely used in treating IBS, especially for patients with constipation [39]. Often divided doses of unprocessed wheat bran (up to 12–16 grams administered four times daily) are prescribed, which is gradually reduced to the optimally effective tolerable dose. Alternately, the patient may start with smaller doses and gradually increase until the desired effect is achieved. However, there are no hard data documenting the effectiveness of fiber or bran in IBS [39,40,41]. As high as 55% of the patients in one study of 100 IBS cases complained about aggravated symptoms [41]. Common complaints include bloating and distension, which are not uncommon with sudden increase in fiber intake. These undesirable effects may disappear spontaneously within a few weeks but may necessitate decreasing fiber quantity or eliminating fiber completely in patients who remain intolerant [39]. In some patients with IBS, intolerance to wheat products has been implicated [41].

5.3. COLON CANCER RISK REDUCTION

Colon cancer, the second leading cause of cancer death in North America, has been associated with dietary risk factors that may be controlled. Since there has been little change in the efficacy of treatment for colon cancer (as measured by 5-year survival rates), prevention will likely prove to be the most powerful tool in reducing the mortality of the disease [42]. The benefit of a diet characterized by high-fiber foods in colon cancer risk reduction has been well recognized although the dietary components involved have not been clearly defined [12,43]. Greenwald et al. reviewed 40 epidemiologic studies that probed for an association between dietary fiber and colon cancer incidence [44]. In 95% of these studies, there was a significant inverse relationship between measures of fiber intake and colon cancer risk. A protective effect linked to the fiber content of diet is further supported by a combined analysis of 13 case-control studies by Howe et al. [45]. Growing evidence suggests that not all fibers are equal in their protective effect against colon cancer. Among the different sources of fiber that have been studied, wheat bran appears to have the most consistent inhibiting effect on colon cancer development.

5.3.1. Controlled Clinical Trials

There are four major reports of randomized, double-blind, placebo-controlled clinical trials of wheat bran in patients with resected adenomatous colon polyps. Three studies demonstrated a protective effect of wheat bran. Surrogate endpoints or biomarkers for cancer (e.g., the number of adenomatous polyps, levels of fecal bile acids) were used in these studies. In the first study of wheat bran in colon neoplasia, 58 patients with familial adenomatous polyposis were followed for 4 years [46]. Subjects were assigned into one of three diet groups: low-fiber control diet, low-fiber diet supplemented with ascorbic acid and α-tocopherol, or high-fiber diet supplemented with wheat bran cereal (22.5 g dietary fiber/day) plus ascorbic acid and α-tocopherol. Among compliant patients who consumed at least 11 g/d of fiber from the wheat bran supplement, polyp number decreased proportionately with the amount of fiber ingested even after adjustment for vitamins.

In the Australian Polyp Prevention Trial, 24 patients were randomized into one of eight treatment groups using a partially blind, placebo-controlled factorial design [47]. Subjects received low-fat (20–30% energy) high-fiber (25 g fine raw bran diet) and 20 mg beta-carotene, alone or in combination. A total of 306 subjects had completed the study at the end of the 4 years. Although no single intervention had a protective effect on total adenomas, the combination of low-fat and high-fiber significantly reduced the incidence of large adenomas at 24 and 48 months, suggesting that these interventions may reduce tumor growth.

The randomized, double-blind study of Alberts et al. reported a statistically significant association between wheat bran fiber in the form of a breakfast cereal (13.5 g fiber/d) and reduction in fecal bile acid (both primary and secondary) concentrations and excretion rates in 50 patients with resected colon adenomas at 9 months [48].

The Canadian Intervention Trial reported by McKeown-Eyssen et al. failed to show a protective effect of a low-fat, high-fiber diet including a wheat bran snack product in 165 patients after 2 years [49]. However, the nonsignificant fiber effects observed in this study cannot be attributed entirely to wheat fiber as the actual consumption of the wheat bran snack product or total wheat fiber intake in the treatment and control groups was not reported.

5.3.2. Other Epidemiological Studies

Epidemiological research on colon cancer risk with estimates of fiber intake from cereal grains including wheat bran or whole wheat has reported significant protective effects of cereal fiber in several ecological studies [50–54]. A slightly reduced risk of colon or rectal cancer was observed in two case-control studies but not at levels that reached statistical significance [55,56]. At least one prospective cohort study supports an inverse relation between colorectal adenomas and fiber intake from specific sources including cereal grains [57]. A retrospective cohort study of Nordic males suggests that a higher fiber intake is associated with a lower incidence of colon cancer [58]. In a review of over 55 studies on the link between fiber and colon cancer, Hill concluded that cereals are strongly protective [59]. This protective benefit was most pronounced with high-fiber cereals, particularly those containing wheat bran.

5.3.3. Animal Studies

Certainly animal studies support a unique role for wheat bran, as it has been shown to significantly affect biomarkers of colon cancer. In rat models of colon cancer induced by a carcinogen (e.g., 1,2 dimethyhydrazine or DMH), wheat bran is considered to be the type of fiber that most consistently inhibits the development and growth of colon cancer [60]. Reviewing the animal literature on wheat bran and tumor incidence, McIntyre and colleagues concluded that in the overwhelming majority of studies, wheat bran given throughout the study period was protective, even when feeding was initiated during the post-initiation or promotion phase of cancer development [61]. The presence of sufficient levels of micronutrients may also be important in supporting the protective effect of wheat bran [61].

In an examination of the dose effect of wheat bran on colon cancer, Alabaster et al. fed rats a high fat (20% w/w), low-calcium (0.18% w/w) diet supplemented with 1%, 4% or 8% dietary fiber from wheat bran for 2 weeks prior, 1 week during and 22 weeks after injection with the carcinogen azoxymethane

(2 injections of 15 mg/kg body weight, separated by 7 days) [62]. At the completion of the study, there was significantly lower tumor incidence and tumor multiplicity as a function of increased dietary fiber (Figure 2.4). Alabaster and his research team went on to examine the effect of processed wheat bran by incorporating wheat bran into one of two different forms of breakfast cereal: a flake or an extruded product [63]. No significant difference in the efficacy between processed and raw wheat bran was found (Figure 2.5). Further, using foci of aberrant crypts/cm^2 of colon as a biomarker, the researchers noted reduction

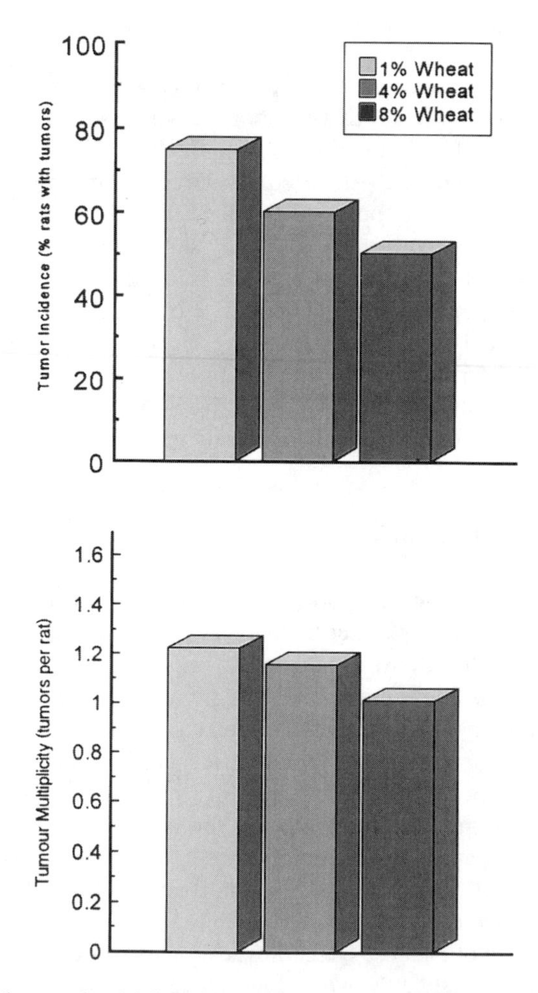

Figure 2.4. Incidence and multiplicity of colon tumors in rats. Diets were high-fat, low-calcium, with 1%, 4%, or 8% fiber from wheat bran. Cancer was induced following 2 s.c. injections of azoxymethane, separated by 7 days. (Adapted from Reference [62]. Reprinted from Reference [89] with permission of The American Institute for Cancer Research.

in colon cancer risk as cereal intake was increased. This type of research is a key step in determining the possible public health benefits of food products that are available in the market place and enjoy wide acceptance. If an ingredient or a food in the processed form, relative to its raw, unprocessed counterpart, shows no beneficial effects, or perhaps even worse, shows a beneficial effect but is unacceptable to the consumer, then there is little chance of success for public health improvements. In translating research results into tangible benefits, the food scientist must work closely with medical and nutrition experts to develop foods that can have positive impact on health, be cost effective, and be acceptable to the public.

5.3.4. Proposed Mechanisms

Several mechanisms have been proposed for the protective effect of dietary fiber in colon carcinogenesis [64]. For wheat bran fiber in particular, the bile acid mechanism has been studied most extensively with human data available, while the other proposed mechanisms require further development.

5.3.4.1. Bile Acid Excretion

Bile acids, and secondary bile acids in particular, have been shown to be tumor promoters and associated with colorectal cancer risks in animals and

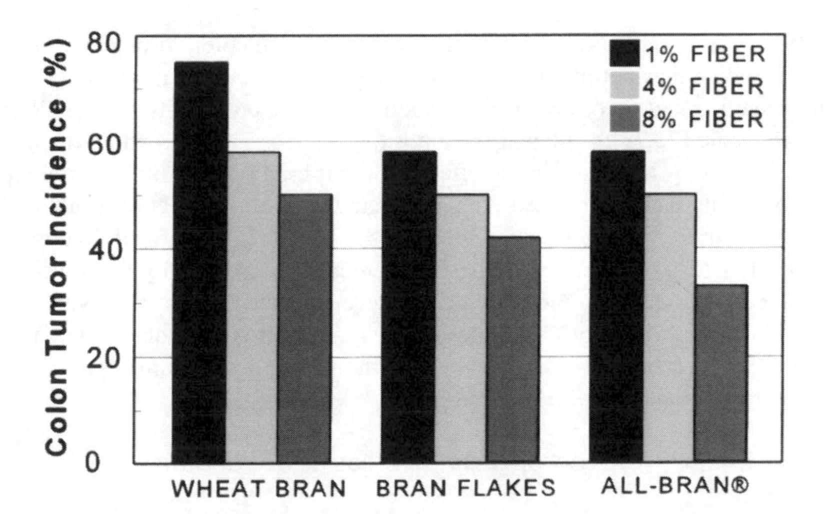

Figure 2.5. Effects of wheat bran cereals on colon tumor incidence in rats (% rats with tumors). Diets were high-fat, low-calcium, with 1%, 4%, or 8% fiber from wheat bran, Kellogg's® Complete® Bran Flakes, or Kellogg's® All-Bran® cereals. Cancer was induced following 2 s.c. injections of azoxymethane at 1 week intervals. (Adapted from Reference [63].) ®Kellogg Company

humans [48,65]. As indicated earlier, because of its fecal bulking effect, wheat bran fiber also shortens transit time and reduces exposure of colonic cells to bile acids [65,66]. Its bulking property in turn has a dilution effect on the fecal concentrations of bile acids, which may also contribute to its protective effects [48,67]. In addition, wheat bran is thought to bind bile acids and increase their excretion and elimination [65,66,68].

5.3.4.2. Effects on SCFAs, Butyrate and Mucosal Cell Proliferation

Another emerging hypothesis suggests that colonic fermentation products such as short-chain fatty acids (SCFAs), and butyrate in particular, may modulate carcinogenesis. Wheat bran, though generally considered a slow fermentable fiber, has been shown in the rat model to be positively associated with high butyrate concentrations in the distal colon, and with reduced tumor mass [69]. In humans, increased concentrations of SCFAs and butyrate in fecal samples of subjects fed 5 g of wheat bran daily for four weeks has also been observed [70]. Data on [^{3}H]thymidine rectal mucosa cell labelling index in a pilot study suggested that wheat bran supplementation (13.5 g/d for 2 months) inhibits DNA synthesis and rectal mucosa cell proliferation in patients with familial polyposis [71]. This in turn would suggest a reduced risk of colon cancer.

5.3.4.3. Effects on Colonic Microflora

Wheat bran may also have an indirect effect on the colon through its influence on colonic microflora by: (1) reducing microflora enzyme activity and the rate of formation of bacterial metabolites that are potentially mutagenic or carcinogenic [72,73]; (2) favouring a positive balance in the growth of beneficial bacteria [74]. Results in the effect of wheat bran on colonic bacterial enzyme activity have been mixed, in part due to the diluting effect of fecal bulking and differences in feeding duration. In the human study of Reddy in which 13–15 g of wheat bran fiber supplement was taken daily for 8 weeks, significant decreases in the activities of several bacterial enzymes were observed, notably those of β-glucuronidase, 7α-dehydroxylase and nitroreductase [72]. These enzymes are involved in the production of tumor promoters and in the metabolism of procarcinogens.

5.3.5. Unique Physicochemical Properties of Wheat Bran

Compared to fiber from other cereal grains such as corn and oat bran, wheat bran appears to have the greatest effect in reducing fecal mutagenicity, secondary bile acid concentrations, bacterial enzyme activities and tumor mass [69,75–77]. These differences may in part be due to differences in the fermentability of the fibers. Although fermentable soluble fibers, such as those from vegetables and fruits and some grains such as oats and barley, also increase fecal weight by increasing bacterial mass and gases [7,8], they do not have the same effect as wheat bran fiber on inhibiting tumor development in the colon [78].

Wheat bran components such as cellulose, lignin, and its cellular structure (key factors contributing to its slow fermentability and water-holding capacity) are believed to play a major role in its colon cancer-protective effects. Another important physicochemical property of wheat bran is its ability to bind cytotoxic substances such as bile acids and food mutagens, making them less likely to be re-absorbed in the colon [48,79–80]. Induction of cytochrome P-450 dependent enzymes in the small intestine has also been suggested as a possible mechanism [81]. Nonfiber components of wheat bran including phenolic compounds and phytic acid may also contribute to its anti-carcinogenic effects (see Section 6).

In summary, evidence available to date from a broad range of animal and epidemiological studies, including controlled clinical trials, provides strong support for a protective role of wheat bran in reducing the risk of colon cancer development. Emphasizing cereal and grain products as part of a low-fat, high-fiber diet is consistent with current diet recommendations in many developed countries.

5.4. BREAST CANCER RISK REDUCTION

Exciting data linking fiber intake to a reduction in breast cancer risk are beginning to emerge. While the epidemiological association between increased dietary fiber and a reduced risk of breast cancer [82,83] is confounded by the fact that high-fiber diets are typically low in fat and high in fruit and/or vegetable consumption, more rigidly controlled experimental studies have provided additional support for the role of dietary fiber in the prevention of breast cancer.

5.4.1. Epidemiological Studies

Elevations in bioavailable estrogen have been linked to an increased risk of developing breast cancer [84–86], and estrogens are acknowledged as a necessary factor in the genesis of breast cancer (if not the growth) [87]. Recent data do show that women with breast cancer have higher levels of circulating estrogens, and higher levels of bioavailable estrogens, than do women who are breast cancer free [88] (Table 2.4). Furthermore, risk of breast cancer increases as bioavailable estrogen increases (Table 2.5). Thus, the implication is that if it is possible to reduce the levels of circulating estrogens, and particularly, the amount of circulating *bio-available* estrogen, it may be possible to reduce the risk of developing breast cancer [84,86].

TABLE 2.4. Mean Levels of Estrone, Total Estradiol, Bioavailable (Free) Estradiol, and Bound Estradiol in Women with Breast Cancer (Case) and Breast Cancer Free (Control).

Estrone and Estradiol	Case	Control	% Difference
Estrone (pg/ml)	14.0[2]	11.4	18.5%
Total estradiol (pg/ml)	33.6[1]	27.7	17.6%
Free estradiol (pg/ml)	0.47[1]	0.36	23.4%
Albumin-bound estradiol (pg/ml)	19.4[1]	14.7	24.2%
SHBG-bound estradiol (pg/ml)	12.8	11.9	7.0%
Free estradiol (%)	1.42[1]	1.34	5.6%
Albumin-bound estradiol (%)	58.9[1]	54.1	8.1%
SHBG-bound estradiol (%)	39.7[1]	44.6	11.0%

[1] $p < 0.001$, paired *t* test; [2] $p < 0.01$, paired *t* test.
Reprinted from Reference [89] with permission of the American Institute for Cancer Research.

That diet may play a role in altering estrogen metabolism appears to be supported by comparisons between vegetarian and omnivorous women. In the study of Goldin and Gorbach of pre- and post-menopausal women, estradiol and estriol fecal excretions were higher in vegetarians (who consumed a high-fiber diet) than omnivores (consuming a low-fiber diet) [90]. As expected, vegetarians had lower plasma estradiol levels than omnivores. However, other

TABLE 2.5. Adjusted (for Quetlet Index) Odds Ratios for Breast Cancer for Quartiles of Various Measures of Estrone and Estradiol: Total, Bioavailable (Free), and Bound.

	Quartile				
Estrone and Estradiol	I	II	III	IV	*p*
Estrone (pg/ml)	1.0	2.2	3.7	2.5	<0.10
Total estradiol (pg/ml)	1.0	0.9	1.8	1.8	<0.10
Free estradiol (pg/ml)	1.0	1.4	3.0	2.9	<0.01
Albumin-bound estradiol (pg/ml)	1.0	1.1	2.7	2.2	<0.01
SHBG-bound estradiol (pg/ml)	1.0	1.0	1.1	1.3	ns
Free estradiol (%)	1.0	1.7	1.9	2.0	ns
Albumin-bound estradiol (%)	1.0	1.3	2.1	3.3	<0.001
SHBG-bound estradiol (%)	1.0	0.70	0.40	0.32	<0.01

Reprinted with permission from Reference [89] with permission of the American Institute for Cancer Research.

dietary or lifestyle factors could also contribute to these reported differences in estrogen metabolism between the two groups.

5.4.2. Controlled Clinical Trials

Once again, as with colon cancer, some researchers have ascribed a unique role in estrogen metabolism to the consumption of wheat products as compared to other common grains. In a study of 62 pre-menopausal women, Rose and colleagues [91] reported that wheat bran (but not corn or oat bran) significantly reduced the amount of circulating estrogens in the plasma, specifically serum estrone and estradiol levels [91]. This was accomplished by supplementing the diet with an average of 15 to 30 g/d of wheat bran, representing 6 to 12 g/d of dietary fiber. Furthermore, these changes were accomplished without any attempt to reduce dietary fat intake. Others have made similar observations [92,93,94, see 95 for review]. The unique property of wheat bran fiber may help explain why some epidemiological studies fail to report a protective effect of dietary fiber on breast cancer risk. Negative findings in these studies may be due in part to low intake of wheat bran or total fiber or to a limited range of fiber intakes among study participants.

Wheat bran in the form of ready-to-eat breakfast cereals also favourably influenced breast cancer risk in a study that examined the effects of three levels of wheat bran supplementation in the form of Kellogg's® All-Bran® cereal in amounts that provided 5, 10 or 20 g dietary fiber/day (equivalent to ¼ to 1 cup cereal/day) for 2 months. Changes in the major serum estrogens during both the luteal and follicular phases of the menstrual cycle were monitored. Increasing the level of wheat bran, particularly in the luteal phase, produced a significant reduction (10–20%) in the serum estrogen levels [96].

5.4.3. Animal Studies

Similarly, in animal models of breast cancer, Cohen et al. have documented a 30% decrease in tumor incidence in rats fed a diet containing 10% wheat bran compared to rats receiving no supplemental wheat bran [97]. In another study, Arts et al. reported that while tumor incidence did not decrease with increased fiber from wheat bran, tumor weights and multiplicity were significantly reduced in the high-fiber diet group [98]. Taken together, these studies provide encouraging data and support linking increased wheat bran fiber with reduced breast cancer risk.

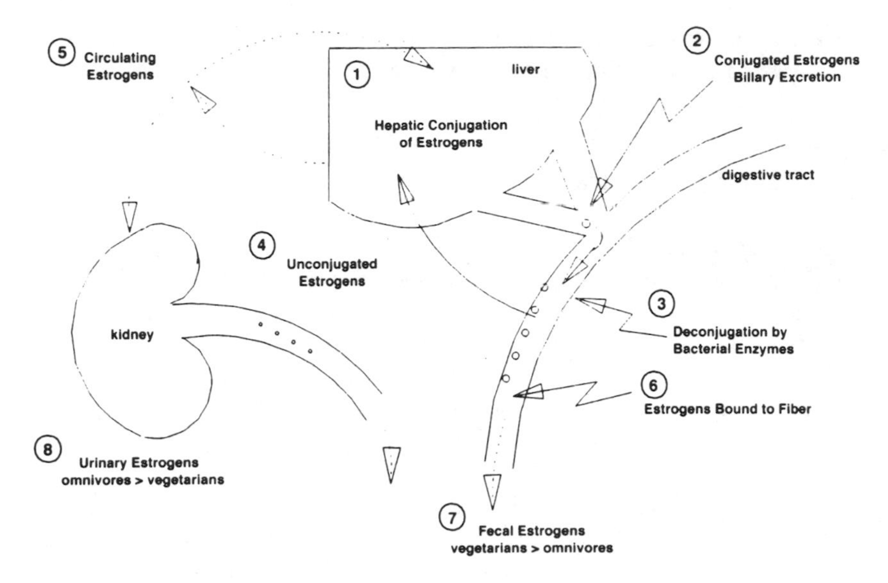

Figure 2.6. Enterohepatic circulation of estrogens. ① Estrogens are conjugated in the liver. ② The conjugated estrogens are excreted in the bile as part of the digestive process. ③ In the lumen, β-glucoronidase enzymes act to deconjugate the estrogens, which permits ④ the re-uptake of free estrogens into the hepatic circulation and ⑤ general circulation. ⑥ However, wheat bran fiber (1) may act to inhibit the action of the β-glucoronidase enzymes; (2) may bind and prevent the enzymes from accessing the conjugated estrogens; or (3) may bind the free estrogens following deconjugation, all of which prevent or inhibit re-uptake. ⑦ Thus, vegetarians with high-fiber diets excrete more estrogens in the feces, compared to omnivores (low fiber diets), ⑧ with the result that urinary excretion of estrogens is somewhat reduced in vegetarians (total estrogen excretion, fecal and urinary combined, is greater in vegetarians). (Adapted from Reference [95].)

5.4.4. Proposed Mechanisms

The mechanism for these effects may be a result of an alteration in the enterohepatic cycling of estrogens [93,99] (Figure 2.6). When conjugated estrogens are secreted in the bile, wheat bran minimizes deconjugation by β-glucoronidase enzymes, an otherwise essential digestive process in the re-absorption of the estrogens from the lumen into the hepatic circulation. It may be that wheat bran renders much of the conjugated estrogens inaccessible to the enzymes by binding the estrogens in some manner [100]. Alternatively, wheat bran may directly inhibit the activity of the enzymes themselves, perhaps through a subtle alteration of the intestinal environment rendering conditions less than optimal for the β-glucoronidase enzymes. It is even possible that the enzymes successfully cleave the conjugated estrogens, but the wheat bran subsequently binds the "free" estrogen and prevents re-uptake. In any case, the result is an increased excretion of estrogens in the feces, and a reduction in circulating levels.

5.5. RISK REDUCTION IN CORONARY HEART DISEASE AND DIABETES MELLITUS

While the beneficial effects of soluble fiber on lipid and carbohydrate metabolism are well accepted [23], only recently has the role of insoluble fiber received increased attention. The Nurses Study and the Health Professionals Study suggest that habitual insoluble fiber (cereal fiber) intake is associated with a reduced risk of developing type II diabetes and coronary heart disease (CHD) [101,102]. Other inverse associations between cereal fiber intake and non-lipid risk factors for CHD such as blood pressure and fibrinogen have also been suggested in cross-sectional studies [103]. Also of interest are the differences in effects among cereal grains on hepatic lipogenesis in animal models [104,105]. Postulates of responsible agents range from the type of carbohydrate to the presence of specific cholesterol inhibitors (such as tocotrienols and tocopherols in wheat germ). Given the preliminary nature of these results, their significance in relation to human health remains to be established.

6. HEALTH BENEFITS OF OTHER WHEAT COMPONENTS

Several phytochemicals present in whole wheat may also have health benefits. These are relatively new areas of investigation in the nutrition field and limited data are available on the role these compounds play in health promotion. Phytic acid (inositol-phosphate), a component of wheat bran (4.8%, [106]), more commonly known for its inhibitive effect on mineral bioavailability, has recently received attention for its anti-cancer effect. Phytic acid is a natural plant antioxidant and its ability to suppress iron-catalyzed oxidative reactions provides one plausible mechanism, among others, for its protective role in carcinogenesis observed in animal models [106,107]. The inhibitory effect of phytic acid on oxidative reactions may also be related to its binding or mineral chelating potential [108,109]. Phytic acid is strongly negatively charged at pH normally encountered in foods, thus making it very reactive with other positively charged groups such as cations and proteins [110]. Up to 4 g of phytic acid in foods can survive the small intestines and enter the colon, an amount that may be sufficient to influence colonic health [107]. Phytic acid has also been suggested to reduce the risk for mammary tumors, particularly when the level of dietary minerals such as calcium and iron is high [107]. While observations from studies of phytic acid in pure or various salt forms appear encouraging, the role of phytic acid in wheat bran requires further study [111].

Phenolic compounds in plant components, such as lignan, have also received a high level of research interest in the last decade for their potential role in the prevention of sex hormone-related cancer [112]. While present in cereal grains such as wheat, these products are not a concentrated source of lignan compared to other plant sources such as flaxseed. Other phenolic compounds, such as phenolic acid, are abundant in whole grains, particularly in the bran layer, with ferulic acid in the largest concentration in wheat bran (764 mg/100 g, [107]). These compounds may be beneficial to health because of their antioxidant property [107].

7. DIETARY RECOMMENDATIONS AND WHEAT BRAN CONSUMPTION

While research to date supporting the beneficial health effects of wheat bran fiber is strong, public awareness of its important role in the human diet appears to be low apart from its function in maintaining regularity. There is no recommendation at present about how much fiber should come from specific sources. However, a target for cereal fiber consumption may be made based on available data. In clinical trials that show wheat bran to be beneficial in risk reduction of colon cancer, fiber intake from this source in the range of 10–15 g/d [in addition to the basal fiber level (15–20 g/d)] would be a reasonable guide. This level of intake is also consistent with the effect of wheat bran on fecal output and bile acid excretion in dose response studies [25,67].

While the evidence linking the preotective effect of wheat bran in breast cancer may be limited, some researchers have made practical recommendations about its consumption as part of a healthy diet and lifestyle. For example, advising on protection against breast cancer, Weisburger and Kroes [83] concluded, "The most appropriate preventive mesures are a limited fat intake, daily vegetable and fruit intake, and wheat bran fiber, the avoidance of obestity and regular exercise." Following an assessment of diet and breast cancer risk in Australia, which uncovered an inverse relationship between fiber intake and breast cancer risk, Baghurst and Rohan [113] recommended that, "increased use of breakfast cereals (especially those with a bran base), peas, beans (including soya beans), dried fruits and nuts can significantly elevate an individual's daily fiber intake." These guidelines are consistent with current diet recommendations in many western countries aimed at reducing chronic disease risks in the general public and in promoting dietary fiber intake from a variety of food sources, to reach a target range of 20–35 g/day.

8. CONCLUSIONS

Increasingly, the issue for the food industry becomes one of understanding the health benefits of food and diet and of targeting research towards elucidating the physiologically active components and their mechanisms of action. Many of these physiologically active compounds are found in well-known food sources, in addition to those less recognized. Wheat, as well as soya, and perhaps onion and garlic, many fruits and vegetables, are just a few among a wide variety of foods with potential health benefits. Research designed to understand and *enhance* these benefits is critically important. Clearly, such a targeted approach could lead to the development of "functional foods." However, it is difficult at this stage to precisely determine (1) the impact of such foods on the health of the general public (depending upon acceptance of the food by the public); or (2) the food industry's desire to become involved in this type of research (given the high cost of investment, well in excess of $2 million to pursue a health claim in the United States). Because of the potential health benefits, we are already witnessing a rapid increase of research in this area, and of subsequent translation of these findings from the lab bench to the kitchen table.

Many foods currently available in our diet have demonstrated physiologic effects inasmuch as health risk is concerned. Investment in research to advance our understanding of these foods should take on higher priority as many of these foods are widely accepted by consumers and have great potential from both health and economic perspectives. There is also the need to advance our understanding of how to communicate a health/diet message to the public. Partnerships between those in industry, government, non-profit organizations, and academia should facilitate the development of scientific consensus on these issues in order that truthful, useful, health/diet messages can be communicated and acted upon.

9. REFERENCES

1. Dreher, M. L. 1987. Handbook of Dietary Fiber—An Applied Approach, New York: Marcel Dekker. p. 5.
2. Hoseney, R. C. 1986. "Structure of cereals," Principles of Cereal Science and Technology, St. Paul, MN: American Association of Cereal Chemists, Inc. p. 3.
3. Evers, A. D., D. B. Bechtel. 1988. "Microscopic structure of the wheat grain," Wheat Chemistry and Technology, Vol. 1, Y. Pomeranz, St. Paul, MN: American Association of Cereal Chemists, Inc. p. 54.
4. Pomeranz, Y. 1988. "Wheat-processing, milling," Modern Cereal Science and Technology. New York, NY: VCH Publishers, Inc. p. 153.
5. Harper, J. M. 1989. "Instrumentation for extrusion processes," Extrusion Cooking, C. Mercier, P. Linko, J. M. Harper, St. Paul, MN: American Association of Cereal Chemists, Inc. p. 40.
6. Cummings, J. H., M. J. Hill, D. J. A. Jenkins, J. R. Pearson, H. S. Wiggins. 1976. "Changes in fecal composition and colonic function due to cereal fiber," Am. J. Clin. Nutr. 29:1468–1473.
7. Stephen, A. M., J. H. Cummings. 1980. "Mechanism of action of dietary fibre in the human colon," Nature 284:283–284.
8. Cummings, J. H. 1993. "The effect of dietary fiber on fecal weight and composition," Handbook of Dietary Fiber in Human Nutrition (2nd edition), G. A. Spiller, Boca Raton, FL: CRC Press, Inc. pp. 263–349.
9. Findlay, J. M., A. N. Smith, W. D. Mitchell, A. J. B. Anderson. 1974. "Effects of

unprocessed bran on colon function in normal subjects and in diverticular disease," Lancet i:146–149 (Feb 2).

10. Stephen, A. M., H. S. Wiggins, J. H. Cummings. 1987. "Effect of changing transit time on colonic microbial metabolism in man," Gut 28:601–609.
11. Wyman, J. B., K. W. Heaton, A. P. Manning, A. C. B. Wicks. 1976. "The effect on intestinal transit and the feces of raw and cooked bran in different doses," Am. J. Clin. Nutr. 29:1474–1479.
12. Health and Welfare Canada, 1990. Nutrition Recommendations—The Report of the Scientific Review Committee, Ottawa: Canadian Government Publishing Centre, pp. 34–39.
13. Health Canada, Health Protection Branch, Food Directorate. June 1994. "Guideline for planning and statistical review of clinical laxation studies for dietary fibre," Appendix 2, Guideline Concerning the Safety and Physiological Effects of Novel Fibre Sources and Food Products Containing Them, Guideline No. 9, revised, November, 1994.
14. Lampe, J. W., R. F. Wetsch, W. O. Thompson, J. L. Slavin. 1993. "Gastrointestinal effects of sugarbeet fiber and wheat bran in healthy men," Eur. J. Clin. Nutr. 47:543–548.
15. Robertson, J. A. 1988. "Physicochemical characteristics of food and the digestion of starch and dietary fibre during gut transit," Proc. Nutr. Soc. 47:143–152.
16. Rasper, V. F. 1979. "Chemical and physical properties of dietary cereal fiber," Food Technology 3:40–44.
17. Holland, B., I. D. Unwin, D. H. Buss. 1988. Cereals and Cereal Products. The Third Supplement of McCance & Widdowson's The Composition of Foods (4th edition), Herts: The Royal Society of Chemistry. p. 9.
18. Dintzis, F. R., J. B. McBrien, F. L. Baker, G. E. Inglett. 1979. "Some effects of baking and human gastrointestinal action upon a hard red wheat bran," Dietary Fibers: Chemistry and Nutrition, GE Inglett and SI Falkehag, New York: Academic Press. pp. 157–171.
19. Robertson, J. A., M. A. Eastwood. 1981. "An examination of factors which may affect the water holding capacity of dietary fibre," Br. J. Nutr. 45:83–96.
20. Williams, A. E., M. A. Eastwood, R. Cregeen. 1978. "SEM and light microscope study of the matrix structure of human feces," Scanning Electron Microscopy 11:707–712.
21. Brodribb, A. J. M., C. Groves. 1978. "Effect of bran particle size on stool weight," Gut 19:60–63.
22. Heller, S. N., L. R. Hackler, J. M. Rivers, P. J. Van Soest, D. A. Roe, B. A. Lewis, J. Robertson. 1980. "Dietary fibre: the effect of particle size of wheat bran on colonic function in young adult men," Am. J. Clin. Nutr. 39:1734–44.
23. Health and Welfare Canada, 1985. Report of the Expert Advisory Committee on Dietary Fibre to the Health Protection Branch, Ottawa.
24. Mongeau, R., R. Brassard. 1982. "Insoluble fiber from breakfast cereals and brans: bile salt binding and water-holding capacity in relation to particle size," Cereal Chem. 59:413–417.
25. Jenkins, D.J.A., R.D. Peterson, M.J. Thome, P.W. Ferguson. 1987. "Wheat fiber and laxation: dose response and equilibration time," Am. J. Gastroenterol. 82(12): 1259–1263.
26. Stephen, A. M., H. S. Wiggins, H. N. Englyst, T. J. Cole, B. J. Wayman,

J. H. Cummings. 1986. "The effect of age, sex and level of intake of dietary fibre from wheat on large-bowel function in thirty healthy subjects," Br. J. Nutr. 56:349–361.

27. Taylor, R. 1990. "Management of constipation," Br. Med. J. 300:1063–1064.
28. Badiali, D., E. Corazziari, F. I. Habib, E. Tomei, G. Bausano, P. Magrini, F. Anzini, A. Torsoli. 1995. "Effect of wheat bran in treatment of chronic nonorganic constipation: a double-blind controlled trial," Dig. Dis. Sci. 40:349–356.
29. Muller-Lissner, S. A. 1988. "Effect of wheat bran on weight of stool and gastrointestinal transit time: a meta analysis," Br. Med. J. 296:615–617.
30. Lampe, J. W., S. B. Fredstrom, J. L. Slavin, J. D. Potter. 1993. "Sex differences in colonic function: a randomised trial," Gut 34:531–536.
31. Cummings, J. H., S. A. Bingham, K. W. Heaton, M. A. Eastwood. 1992. "Fecal weight, colon cancer risk and dietary intake of nonstarch polysaccharides (dietary fiber)," Gastroenterol. 103:1783–1789.
32. Lawson, K., F. Kern, G. T. Everson. 1985. "Gastrointestinal transit time in human pregnancy: prolongation in the second and third trimester followed by postpartum normalization," Gastroenterol. 89:996–999.
33. Institute of Food Technologists. Nutrition and the Elderly, 1986. "A scientific status summary by the Institute of Food Technologists' Expert Panel on food safety & nutrition," Food Technol. 40:81–88.
34. American Dietetic Association. Position of the American Dietetic Association, 1987. "Nutrition, aging and the continuum of health care," Technical Support Paper. J. Am. Diet. Assoc. 87:344–347.
35. McClung, H. J., L. Boyne, L. Heitlinger. 1995. "Constipation and dietary fiber intake in children," Pediatrics 96(Suppl—Part 2):999–1000.
36. Williams, C. L., M. Bollella, E. L. Wynder. 1995. "A new recommendation for dietary fiber in childhood," Pediatrics 96(Suppl—Part 2):985–988.
37. Naitove, A., T. P. Almy. 1993. "Diverticular disease of the colon," Gastrointestinal Disease—Pathophysiology, Diagnosis, Management, M. H. Sleisenger, J. S. Fordtran, Philadelphia: Saunders. pp. 1423–1424.
38. Painter, N. S. 1967. "Diverticulosis of the colon," Am. J. Dig. Dis. 12(2):222–227.
39. Schuster, M. M. 1993. "Irritable bowel syndrome," Gastrointestinal Disease—Pathophysiology, Diagnosis, Management, M.H., Sleisenger, J.S. Fordtran, Philadelphia: Saunders. pp. 1414–1415.
40. Snook, J., H. A. Shepherd. 1994. "Bran supplementation in the treatment of irritable bowel syndrome," Aliment. Pharmacol. Ther. 8:511–514.
41. Francis, C. Y., P. J. Whorwell. 1994. "Bran and irritable bowel syndrome: time for reappraisal," Lancet 344(8914):39–40.
42. Vargas, P. A., D. S. Alberts. 1992. "Primary prevention of colorectal cancer through dietary modification," Cancer 70:1229–1235.
43. National Research Council, 1989. Diet and Health. Implications for Reducing Chronic Disease Risk, Washington, DC: National Academy Press. pp. 291–309.
44. Greenwald, P., E. Lanza, G. A. Eddy. 1987. "Dietary fiber in the reduction of colon cancer risk," J. Am. Diet. Assoc. 87:1178–1188.
45. Howe, G. R., E. Benito, R. Castelleto, J. Cornée, J. Estève, R. P. Gallagher, J. M. Isovich, J. Deng-ao, R. Kaaks, G. A. Kune, S. Kune, K. A. L'Abbé, H. P. Lee, M. Lee, A. B. Miller, R. K. Peters, J. D. Potter, E. Riboli, M. L. Slattery, D. Trichopoulos, A. Tuyns, A. Tzonov, A. S. Whittemore, A. H.

Wu-Williams, Z. Shu. 1992. "Dietary intake of fiber and decreased risk of cancers of the colon and rectum: evidence from the combined analysis of 13 case-control studies," J. Natl. Cancer Inst. 84(24):1887–96.

46. DeCosse, J. J., H. H. Miller, M. L. Lesser. 1989. "Effect of wheat fiber and vitamins C and E on rectal polyps in patients with familial adenomatous polyposis," J. Natl. Cancer Inst. 81(17):1290–97.
47. R. MacLennan, F. Macrea, C. Bain, D. Battistutta, P. Chapuis, H. Gratten, J. Lambert, R. C. Newland, M. Ngu, A. Russell, M. Ward, M. L. Wahlqvist and the Australian Polyp Prevention Project. 1995. "Randomized trial of intake of fat, fiber, and beta carotene to prevent colorectal adenomas," J. Natl. Cancer Inst. 87:1760–66.
48. Alberts, D. S., C. Ritenbaugh, J. A. Story, M. Aickin, S. Rees-McGee, M. K. Buller, J. Atwood, J. Phelps, P. S. Ramanujam, S. Bellapravalu, J. Patel, L. Bettinger, L. Clark. 1996. "Randomized, double-blinded, placebo-controlled study of effect of wheat bran fiber and calcium on fecal bile acids in patients with resected adenomatous colon polyps," J. Natl. Cancer Inst. 88(2):81–92.
49. McKeown-Eyssen, G. E., E. Bright-See, W. R. Bruce, V. Jazmaji and the Toronto Polyp Prevention Group. 1994. "A randomized trial of a low fat high fibre diet in the recurrence of colorectal polyps," J. Clin. Epidemiol. 47(5):525–36.
50. Englyst, H. N., S. A. Bingham, H. S. Wiggins, D. A. T. Southgate, R. Seppänen, P. Helms, V. Anderson, K. C. Day, R. Choolun, E. Collinson, J. H. Cummings. 1982. "Nonstarch polysaccharide consumption in four Scandinavian populations," Nutr. Cancer 4(1):50–60.
51. McKeown-Eyssen, G. E., E. Bright-See. 1985. "Dietary factors in colon cancer: international relationships. An update," Nutr. Cancer 7(4):251–53.
52. McKeown-Eyssen, G. E., E. Bright-See. 1984. "Dietary factors in colon cancer: international relationships," Nutr. Cancer 6(3):160–70.
53. Maisto, O.E., C.G. Bremner. 1981. "Cancer and the colon and rectum in the coloured population of Johannesburg: relationship to diet and bowel habits," S. Afr. Med. J. 60:571–73.
54. Powles, J. W., D. R. R. Williams. 1984. "Trends in bowel cancer in selected countries in relation to wartime changes in flour milling," Nutr. Cancer 6(1): 40–48.
55. Pickle, L. W., M. H. Greene, R. G. Ziegler, A. Toledo, R. Hoover, H. T. Lynch, J. F. Fraumeni. 1984. "Colorectal cancer in rural Nebraska," Cancer Res. 44(1): 363–69.
56. Randall, E., J. R. Marshall, J. Brasure, S. Graham. 1992. "Dietary patterns and colon cancer in western New York," Nutr. Cancer 18(3):265–76.
57. Giovannucci, E., M. J. Stampfer, G. Colditz, E. B. Rimm, W. C. Willett. 1992. "Relationship of diet to risk of colorectal adenoma in men," J. Natl. Cancer Inst. 84(2):91–98.
58. Jensen, O. M., R. MacLennan. 1979. "Dietary factors and colorectal cancer in Scandinavia," Israel J. Med. Sci. 15(4):329–34.
59. Hill, M. 1997. "Cereals, cereal fibre and colorectal cancer risk: a review of the epidemiological literature," Eur. J. Cancer Prev. 6:219–225.
60. Reddy, B. S. 1995. "Nutritional factors and colon cancer," Crit. Rev. Food. Sci. Nutr. 35(3):175–90.
61. McIntyre, A., G. P. Young, T. Taranto, P. R. Gibson, P. B. Ward. 1991. "Different

fibers have different regional effects on luminal contents of rat colon," Gastroenterol. 101(5):1274–81.

62. Alabaster, O., Z. C. Tang, A. Frost, N. Shivapurkar. 1993. "Potential synergism between wheat bran and psyllium: enhanced inhibition of colon cancer," Cancer Letters 75:53–58.
63. Alabaster, O., Z. Tang, N. Shivapurkar. 1997. "Inhibition by wheat bran cereals of the development of aberrant crypt foci and colon tumours," Food and Chemical Toxicology 35(5):517–522.
64. Ausman, L. M. 1993. "Fiber and colon cancer: does the current evidence justify a preventive policy," Nutr. Rev. 51(2):57–63.
65. Hill, M. J. 1991. "Bile acids and colorectal cancer: hypothesis," Eur. J. Cancer Prev. 1(Suppl. 2):69–74.
66. Reddy, B. S., K. Watanabe, J. H. Weisburger, E. L. Wynder. 1977. "Promoting effect of bile acids in colon carcinogenesis in germ-free and conventional F344 rats," Cancer Res. 37(9):3238–42.
67. Lampe, J. W., J. L. Slavin, E. A. Melcher, J. D. Potter. 1992. "Effects of cereal and vegetable fiber feeding on potential risk factors for colon cancer," Cancer 1(3):207–11.
68. Jacobs, L. R. 1988. "Fiber and colon cancer," Gastroenterol. Clin. North Am. 17:747–60.
69. McIntyre, A., P. R. Gibson, G. P. Young. 1993. "Butyrate production from dietary fibre and protection against large bowel cancer in a rat model," Gut 34: 386–91.
70. Treem, W., N. Ahsan, G. Kastoff, M. Shoup, T. Lerer, C. Justinich, J. Hyams. 1995. "Effects of wheat bran and pectin on the production of fecal short-chain fatty acids," Gastroenterol. 108(4):A700 [Abstract].
71. Alberts, D. S., J. Einspahr, S. Rees-McGee, P. Ramanujam, M. K. Buller, L. Clark, C. Ritenbaugh, J. Atwood, P. Pethigal, D. Earnest, H. Villar, J. Phelps, M. Lipkin, M. Wargovich, F. L. Meyskens, Jr. 1990. "Effects of dietary wheat bran fiber on rectal epithelial cell proliferation in patients with resection for colorectal cancers," J. Natl. Cancer Inst. 82(15):1280–85.
72. Reddy, B. S. 1990. "Effect of types of dietary fiber on fecal mutagens and bacterial enzymes in relation to colon cancer," New Developments in Dietary Fibre. I. Furda, C. J. Brine, New York: Plenum Press, 270:159–167.
73. Zakhary, N. I., A. A. El-Aaser, A. A. Abdelhady, S. A. Fathey, F. Aboul-Ela. 1994. "Effect of vicia faba and bran feeding on nitrosamine carcinogenesis and formation," Nutr. Cancer 21(1):59–69.
74. Cheng, B. Q., R. P. Trimble, R. J. Illman, B. A. Stone, D. L. Topping. 1987. "Comparative effects of dietary wheat bran and its morphological components (aleurone and pericarp-seed coat) on volatile fatty acid concentrations in the rat," Br. J. Nutr. 57:69–76.
75. Reddy, B. S., A. Engle, S. Katsifis, B. Simi, H.-P. Bartram, P. Perrino, C. Mahan. 1989. "Biochemical epidemiology of colon cancer: effect of types of dietary fiber on fecal mutagens, acid and neutral sterols in healthy subjects," Cancer Res. 49(16):4629–35.
76. Reddy, B. S., B. Simi, A. Engle. 1994. "Biochemical epidemiology of colon cancer: effect of types of dietary fiber on colonic diacylglycerols in women," Gastroenterol. 106(4):883–89.

77. Reddy, B. S., A. Engle, B. Simi, M. Goldman. 1992. "Effect of dietary fiber on colonic bacterial enzymes and bile acids in relation to colon cancer," Gastroenterol. 102(5):1475–82.
78. Jacobs, L. R. 1987. "Effect of dietary fiber on colonic cell proliferation and its relationship to colon carcinogenesis," Prev. Med. 16(4):566–71.
79. Camire, M. E., J. Zhao, M. P. Dougherty, R. J. Bushway. 1995. "In vitro binding of benzo(a)pyrene by ready-to-eat breakfast cereals," Cereal Foods World 40: 447–50.
80. Ferguson, L. R., P. J. Harris. 1996. "Studies on the role of specific dietary fibres in protection against colorectal cancer," Mutation Res. 350(1):173–84.
81. Lindeskog, P., E. Övervik, T. Hansson, J-Å. Gustafsson. 1986. "Influence of dietary fibre on hepatic and intestinal metabolism in rat," Mutation Res. 204: 553–63.
82. Rose, D. P. 1986. "Dietary factors and breast cancer," Cancer Surv. 5:671–87.
83. Weisburger, J. H., R. Kroes. 1994. "Mechanisms in nutrition and cancer," Eur. J. Cancer Prevent. 3:293–298.
84. Jones, L. A., D. M. Ota, G. A. Jackson, P. M. Jackson, K. Kemp, D. E. Anderson, S. K. McCamant, D. H. Bauman. 1987. "Bioavailability of estradiol as a marker for breast cancer risk assessment," Cancer Res. 47:5224–5229.
85. Langley, M. S., G. L. Hammon, A. Bardsley, R. A. Sellwood, D. C. Anderson. 1985. "Serum steroid binding proteins and the bioavailability of estradiol in relation to breast diseases," J. Natl. Cancer Inst. 75:823–829.
86. Ota, D. M., L. A. Jones, G. L. Jackson, P. M. Jackson, K. Kemp, D. Bauman. 1986. "Obesity, non-protein-bound estradiol levels, and distribution of estradiol in the sera of breast cancer patients," Cancer 57:558–62.
87. Nandi, S., R. C. Guzman, J. Yang. 1995. "Hormones and mammary carcinogenesis in mice, rats, and humans: a unifying hypothesis," Proc. Natl. Acad. Sci. USA, 92:3650–3657.
88. Toniolo, P. G., M. Levitz, A. Zeleniuch-Jacquotte, S. Banerjee, K. L. Koenig, R. E. Shore, P. Strax, B. S. Pasternack. 1995. "A prospective study of endogenous estrogens and breast cancer in postmenopausal women," J. Natl. Cancer Inst. 87:190–197.
89. Black, R. 1996. "Wheat bran, colon cancer and breast cancer: what do we have? what do we need?" Dietary Phytochemicals in Cancer Prevention and Treatment, AICR, New York, NY: Prenum Press. pp. 223, 226–227.
90. Goldin, B. R., S. L. Gorbach. 1988. "Effect of diet on the plasma levels, metabolism, and excretion of estrogens," Am. J. Clin. Nutr. 48:787–790.
91. Rose, D. P., M. Goldman, J. M. Connolly, L. E. Strong. 1991. "High-fiber diet reduces serum estrogen concentrations in premenopausal women," Am. J. Clin. Nutr. 54:520–525.
92. Goldin, B. R., M. N. Woods, D. L. Spiegelman, C. Longcope, A. Morrill-LaBrode, J. T. Dwyer, L. J. Gualtieri, E. Hertzmark, S. L. Gorbach. 1994. "The effect of dietary fat and fiber on serum estrogen concentrations in premenopausal women under controlled dietary conditions," Cancer 74:1125–1131.
93. Gorbach, S. L., B. R. Golden. 1987. "Diet and the excretion and enterohepatic cycling of estrogens," Preventive Medicine 16:525–531.

94. Heber, D., J. M. Ashley, D. A. Leaf, R. J. Barnard. 1991. "Reduction of serum estradiol in postmenopausal women given free access to low-fat high-carbohydrate diet," Nutrition 7:137–140.
95. Rose, D.P. 1992. "Dietary fiber, phytoestrogens, and breast cancer," Nutrition 8: 47–51.
96. Rose, D., M. Lubin, J. Connolly. 1997. "Effect of diet supplementation with wheat bran on serum estrogen levels in the follicular and luteal phase of the menstrual cycle," Nutrition 13(6):535–539.
97. Cohen, L. A., M. E. Kendall, E. Zang, C. Meschter, D. P. Rose. 1991. "Modulation of N-nitrosomethylurea-induced mammary tumor promotion by dietary fiber and fat," J. Natl. Cancer Inst. 83:496–501.
98. Arts, C. J. M., T. H. Albert, H. J. De Bie, H. Van Den Berg, P. Van't Veer, G. S. J. Bunnik, J. S. H. Thijssen. 1991. "Influence of wheat bran on nmu-induced mammary tumor development, plasma estrogen levels and estrogen excretion in female rats," J. Steroid Biochem. Molec. Biol. 39:193–202.
99. Gorbach, S. L. 1984. "Estrogens, breast cancer, and intestinal flora," Rev. Infect. Dis. 6:S85–90.
100. Arts, C. J. M., C. A. R. L. Govers, H. Van Den Berg, M. G. E. Wolters, P. Van Leeuwen, J. H. H. Thussen. 1991. "*In vitro* binding of estrogens by dietary fiber and the *in vivo* apparent digestibility tested in pigs," J. Steroid Biochem. Molec. Biol. 38:621–628.
101. Freskens, E. J., S. M. Virtanen, L. Rasanen, J. Tuomilehto, J. Stengard, J. Pekkanen, A. Nissinen, T. D. Kromhout. 1985. "Dietary factors determining diabetes and impaired glucose tolerance: a 20-year follow-up of the Finnish and Dutch cohorts of the seven countries study," Diabetes Care 18:1104–12.
102. Rimm, E. B., A. Ascherio, E. Giovannucci, D. Spiegelman, M. J. Stampfer, W. C. Willett. 1996. "Vegetable, fruit and cereal fibre intake and risk of coronary heart disease among men," J. Am. Med. Assoc. 275:447–451.
103. Fehily, A. M., J. E. Milbank, J. W. Yarnell, T. M. Hayes, A. J. Kubiki, R. D. Eastham. 1982. "Dietary determinants of lipoproteins, total cholesterol, viscosity, fibrinogen and blood pressure," Am. J. Clin. Nutr. 36:890–896.
104. Maurice, D. V., L. S. Jensen. 1979. "Hepatic lipid metabolism in domestic fowl as influenced by dietary cereal," J. Nutr. 109:872–882.
105. Qureshi, A. A., V. Chaudhary, F. E. Weber, E. Chicoye, N. Qureshi. 1991. "Effects of brewer's grain and other cereals on lipid metabolism," Nutr. Res. 11: 159–168.
106. Graf, E., J. W. Eaton. 1990. "Antioxidant functions of phytic acid," Free Radical Biol. & Med. 8:61–69.
107. Thompson, L. U. 1994. "Antioxidants and hormone-mediated health benefits of whole grains," Crit. Rev. Food Sci. Nutr. 34(5&6):473–497.
108. Graf, E., J. W. Eaton. 1993. "Suppression of colonic cancer by dietary phytic acid," Nutr. Cancer 19(1):11–19.
109. Alabaster, O., Z. Tang, N. Shivapurkar. 1996. "Dietary fiber and the chemopreventive modelation of colon carcinogenesis," Mutat. Res. 350(1):185–97.
110. Thompson, L. U. 1989. "Nutritional and physiological effects of phytic acid," Food Proteins, J. Kinsella, W. Soucie, Champaign, IL: A.O.C.S. pp. 410–431.
111. Jenab, M., L. U. Thompson. 1997. "The role of phytic acid in wheat bran on

colon carcinogenesis," 16th International Congress of Nutrition, July 27–August 1, 1997, Montreal, Canada. p. 270 [Abstract PT 526].

112. Thompson, L. U. 1993. "Potential health benefits and problems associated with antinutrients in foods," Food Res. Intl. 26:131–149.

113. Baghurst, P. A., T. E. Rohan. 1994. "High-fiber diets and reduced risk of breast cancer," Int. J. Cancer 56:173–176.

CHAPTER 3

Functional Products From Rice

K.A. MOLDENHAUER[1]
E.T. CHAMPAGNE[2]
D.R. McCASKILL[3]
H. GURAYA[2]

RICE (*Oryza sativa* L.), a major cereal crop, is the staple food source for half of the world population. Rice is an excellent source of calories, in the form of starch, and has the added benefit of providing protein with higher nutritional quality than that in other cereal grains. It is hypoallergenic, easily digested, and has versatile functional properties. Improving and increasing the world's supply will depend on the development of improved varieties, improved production practices, and new products that capitalize on rice's unique components and functional properties.

1. COMPOSITION OF RICE KERNELS

The rice kernel is composed of a hull, consisting of the lemma, palea, sterile lemmas and rudimentary glumes, the caryopsis or brown rice, and an embryo (Figure 3.1). A cross-section of the kernel further characterizes the components of the brown rice and embryo (Figure 3.2). The bran consists of several cell layers, including the pericarp, tegmen and aleurone. It is usually removed with much of the embryo during commercial milling operations. The hull comprises approximately 20% of the rice kernel, the bran and embryo about 8–12%, and the endosperm or milled rice 70–72% on an average.

[1]University of Arkansas, Rice Research and Extension Center, P.O Box 351 Stuttgart, AR 72160, USA
[2]USDA ARS Southern Regional Research Center, P.O. Box 19687, New Orleans, LA 70179, USA
[3]Riceland Foods, Inc. P.O. Box 927, Stuttgart, AR 72160, USA

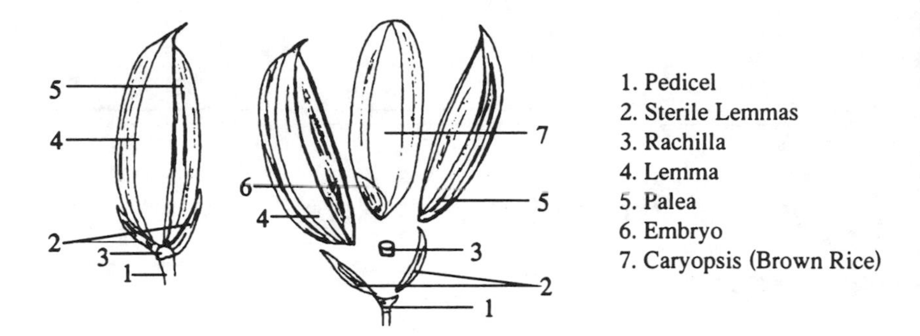

Figure 3.1 Structure of a rice grain. (Adapted from K. Hoshikawa. 1989. "The Growing Rice Plant and Anatomical Monograph." Nobunkyo, Tokyo, p. 10)

From a marketing standpoint there are three forms of rice: rough, brown, and milled. Rough rice, or paddy, is the harvested unshelled rice as it comes from the field. Brown rice, also referred to as shelled rice, husked rice, cargo rice or loozian, is rice from which the hull has been removed by shelling or hulling. Finally, milled rice, sometimes referred to as white rice, is rice in which all or most of the bran has been removed by some operation of milling called scouring or whitening (Figure 3.3). Usually this milling is followed by the operation of polishing in which the remaining traces of bran are removed from the kernel leaving a smooth, white surface.

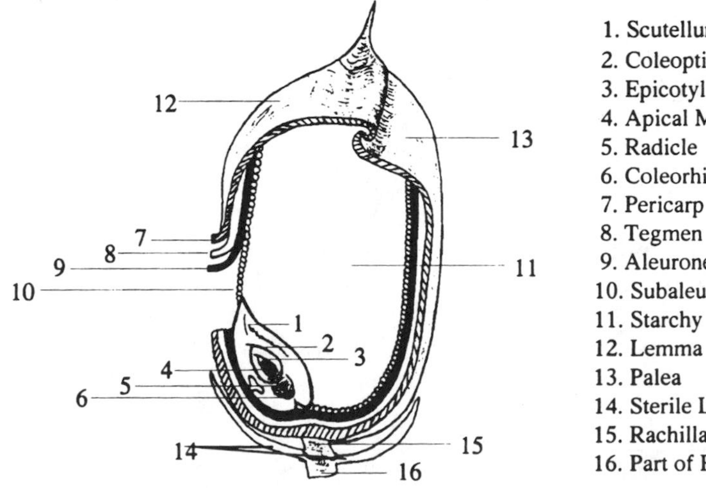

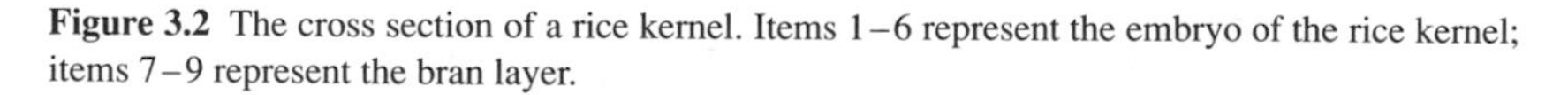
Figure 3.2 The cross section of a rice kernel. Items 1–6 represent the embryo of the rice kernel; items 7–9 represent the bran layer.

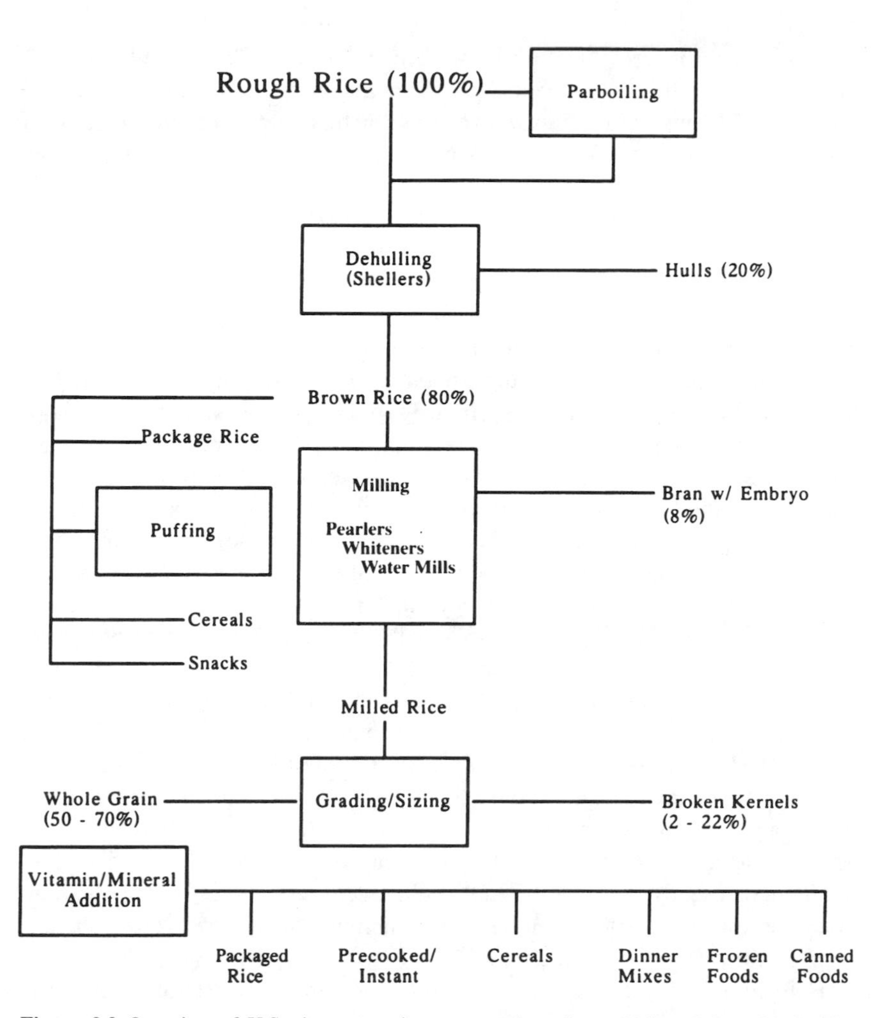

Figure 3.3 Overview of U.S. rice processing steps and products. (Adapted from McCaskill, D.R., and Orthoefer, F.T. 1993. Proceedings of Rice Utilization Workshop "Developing Innovative, Non-Conventional Uses for Rice." August 5–6, 1993, New Orleans, LA, pp. 58–67.)

2. RICE BRAN

Rice bran is one of the most abundant, underutilized co-products produced in the U.S. rice milling industry. In 1995, about 173 million hundredweights of rice were produced in the U.S., resulting in 13.9 million hundredweights of rice bran [1]. Historically, this bran has been used in an unstabilized form as an animal feed ingredient. With improvements in methods of rice bran stabilization during the past 20 years, there are currently many arenas for using rice bran. Many new and innovative uses for this co-product in the form of value-added food and nonfood products are currently being investigated by the industry.

Bran layers of the rice kernel contain the highest concentration of nutrients. Rice bran is extracted for oil and is a potential source for protein and other nutrients. Commercial rice bran contains 11.5–17.2% protein, 12.8–29.6% fat, 6.2–31.5% fiber (with soluble dietary fiber accounting for 1.9–2.4%), and 8.0–17.7% ash, depending on the processing conditions [2–4]. The amount of starch in the bran ranges from 10–55%, depending upon the degree of milling [4]. Phosphorus, primarily in the form of phytates, is a major mineral constituent of rice bran. Potassium, magnesium and silicon are also present at high levels; levels of sodium and calcium are low [4]. The bran is abundant in the B-vitamins and tocopherols but low in Vitamins A and C [4].

Rice bran contains primarily insoluble fiber (cellulose) and soluble fiber (hemicellulose). Insoluble fiber adds bulk to the gastrointestinal (GI) tract in humans causing more frequent stools that pass through the system more quickly, requiring less pressure to expel, and absorbing more bile acids thereby preventing their reentry into circulation [5]. This lowers the amount of bile absorption/reabsorption of dietary and or endogenous lipid by the lower intestinal tract and promotes the synthesis of more bile acids from available cholesterol [3,6]. Lowering serum cholesterol levels in the blood, specifically the low-density lipoprotein (LDL) fraction, aids in cardiovascular health and tends to lessen gallstone formation [6]. Animal and human studies show cholesterol lowering from a hypercholesterolemic status with rice bran. Reductions usually occur in the LDL (atherogenic) fraction [4]. Specific bran fractions that show hypocholesterolemic activity include rice bran oil, unsaponifiable matter, and protein [3].

Hemicellulose, unlike other forms of dietary fiber, consists of several carbohydrate components, including hexoses, pentoses, hexuronic acids, plus amino acids [5] in various combinations and quantities that influence its functional properties. The quantities of the sugars (arabinose, glucose, galactose, xylose, etc.) in rice hemicellulose vary by the rice cultivar tested and the environment in which the rice is grown. Differences of quantities of these sugars varied from 7.1% to 13.7% for xylose in the cultivar Starbonnet grown in Louisiana and Arkansas, respectively [5]. The amount of the protein/amino acids associated with hemicellulose also varied widely from 9.6% for Louisiana-grown Starbonnet, a long-grain cultivar, to 26.4% for California-grown Calrose, a medium-grain type [7]. Therefore, the potential exists for plant breeders to increase the soluble fiber content in rice bran through the selection process. Studies comparing the bile acid-binding ability of the hemicellulose in the bran from Starbonnet and Calrose with wheat bran [5] have shown cultivar differences. The hemicellulose in the medium-grain Calrose demonstrated greater binding capacity than that in either the long-grain rice or wheat bran. Hemicellulose in Calrose bound 25.7, 40.3, 21.9, and 28.4%, respectively, of the four bile acids cholate, glycocholate, taurocholate, and glycotaurocholate, while that in Starbonnet and wheat bran bound only from 10.7 to 21.1% of the bile acids [5]. Further testing is required to discover whether the increase in bile-binding capacity is inherently greater in the medium-grain rices than long-grain rices or whether the individual cultivars or the California environment causes the greater binding capacity. If variability exists among cultivars, then it could be beneficial to select cultivars with these characteristics for future use.

Rice bran is potentially a valuable source of natural antioxidants such as tocopherols, tocotrienols, and oryzanols [8]. Increased concern over the safety of synthetic antioxidants like butylated hydroxyanisole (BHA) and butylated hydroxytoluene (BHT) has increased the interest in finding effective and economical natural antioxidants. Antioxidants extracted from rice bran potentially could satisfy this demand. Results from studies [9] have shown that rice antioxidants at 500 ppm (level not restricted by FDA) provide the same level of antioxidant activity as a mixture of BHA/BHT at 200 ppm (FDA maximum).

An overview of both commercial and theoretical rice bran processing and utilization is shown in Figure 3.4. Utilization of rice bran for human consumption has been limited in the past due to the tendency towards rapid development of rancidity and because of the microbial activity generally associated with raw rice bran [10–12]. The process of milling abrades the external cell layers (bran) down to the endosperm, thoroughly mixing the bran material. Native lipase enzymes, which are located in the testa cells, come in contact with the oil in the aleurone and sub-aleurone layers, causing rapid hydrolysis of the oil fraction within raw bran, resulting in a rapid increase in free fatty acids and glycerol [13,14]. This enzymatic deterioration, or lipolysis, within the rice bran, is a process known as hydrolytic degradation [3,4,15]. Heating bran in the presence of moisture permanently denatures lipolytic enzymes [16] and destroys lipolytic microbes. As long as the bran remains sterile, the enzyme activity will not increase [17].

Stabilization processes preserving rice bran from hydrolytic degradation have been accomplished through three general processes, including retained-moisture heating, added-moisture heating, and dry heating at atmospheric pressure [18]. Enzyme inactivation by heat using low-cost extrusion equipment has proven to be the most efficient and controllable method for stabilization [12]. Saunders and coworkers at the USDA-ARS Western Regional Research Center in Albany, California, developed an extrusion process that stabilizes bran through use of a screw-type cooker extruder to generate heat by compression and friction as bran is forced through a constriction orifice [4,

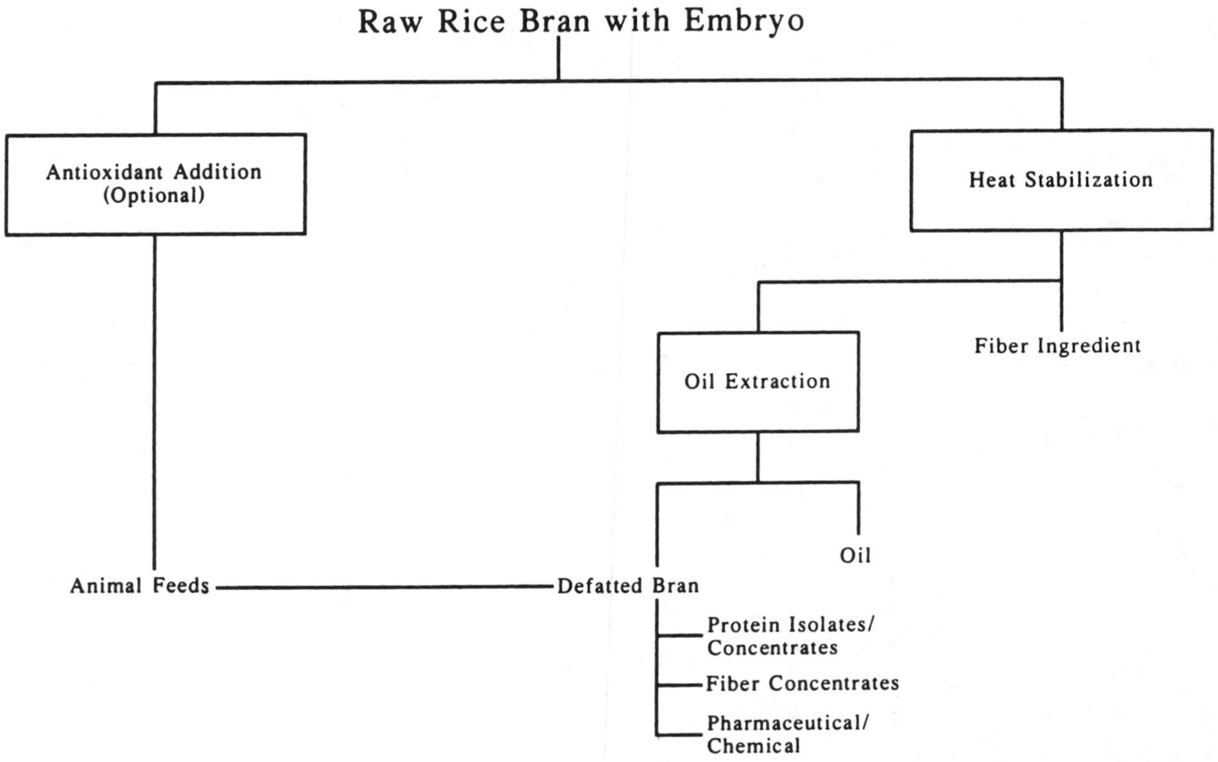

Figure 3.4 Processing and utilization of rice bran. (Adapted from McCaskill, D.R., and Orthoefer, F.T. 1993. Proceedings of Rice Utilization Workshop "Developing Innovative, Non-Conventional Uses for Rice." August 5–6, 1993, New Orleans, LA. pp. 58–67.)

6,18]. The extrusion method is a retained-moisture heating process that not only inactivates the native rice bran lipases, but also greatly reduces the microbial load and destroys insects [6,18]. Further drying and storage of the rice bran at or below 12% moisture ensures maximum benefit from the heat sterilization [4,6,18]. Variations of this method are commonly used to commercially stabilize rice bran in both small and large volumes. Extrusion cookers do not require added water, injected steam, or a source of external heat, but instead cook by converting the mechanical energy of the drive screw into heat through friction and shear as granular material is compressed, worked and forced through an orifice [18].

Nutritional qualities of rice bran may be improved by heat treatment [13] involved in the stabilization of the bran. Low levels of trypsin inhibitors and hemagglutinin from the germ are present in raw rice bran, and are destroyed under conditions that denature lipolytic enzymes [14]. Full-fat stabilized rice bran is used in specialty baked products, muffins, multigrain breads and related health or natural foods to increase fiber and protein content. Stabilized rice bran can also be shipped to an extraction plant to recover and refine high-quality rice oil. Again, the crude oil fraction of rice bran is a source of commercially valuable antioxidants and cholesterol-lowering agents [4].

Defatted rice bran contains an increased percentage of fiber ranging from 35–48% [6], and can be used in speciality high-fiber products and baked goods. Rice bran fractions also possess emulsifying [19] and foaming properties for baked products [20,21], meringues and whipped toppings. These fractions reportedly provide other benefits, such as leavening and texturization. Defatted rice bran contains about 15–20% protein [22] that can be extracted with dilute alkali to produce a bran protein concentrate that is 50–60% protein [19]. Bran protein has good nutritional quality for human consumption. In contrast to most other cereal protein, rice bran protein has a high lysine content [23]. Rice bran has been reported to have a PER (protein efficiency ratio) of 1.6–1.9 and a digestibility of 70–75% [19]. The protein concentrate has reportedly an even higher PER of 2.0–2.5 and digestibility of 90% due to the removal of fiber and phytic acid. Thus, rice bran protein concentrates would make excellent nutritional additives for food products. With the added benefit of low allergenicity, it is well suited for infant formulations [24], for example. Potential nonfood uses for rice bran proteins include biodegradable films and adhesives for the paperboard industry [25,26].

3. RICE BRAN OIL

Rice bran oil is another co-product of the rice milling industry. The rice bran (with germ) fraction contains the majority of the oil in the rice kernel. The oil content of clean rice bran is 20–22%, which is similar to that of soybeans and cottonseed [27,28]. However, dilution of the bran with hulls or with rice starch from overmilling the endosperm may reduce the oil content to 15–20% [22]. Only about 40% of the world rice crop is milled in two-stage rice mills, which allow removal of the hulls from the bran and yield clean rice bran [28]. Once milled, rice bran oil is exposed to lipases in the bran, which result in its rapid breakdown to free fatty acids at an initial rate of 5–7% by weight of the oil per day [29]. Duc to the rapid increase in free fatty acids, either refining of the edible oil or rice bran stabilization by enzyme inactivation must occur as soon as possible after milling to prevent excessive oil refining losses. Stabilization of the bran allows storage for future use and is addressed in Section 2.

The yield of refined rice bran oil depends on the age and storage conditions of the rice, milling practices, bran stabilization, conditions used for extraction, and the method of refining the oil. Extraction can occur either at high or low temperatures. Many organic solvents can be used for rice bran oil extraction, with the most popular being *n*-hexane [30]. Hexane extraction at about 60°C results in the inclusion of most of the gums and waxes in the micella, which yields a greater quantity of crude oil (95–99%), but only an 80% yield of refined oil [15,30]. The gums and waxes are then removed [31,32]. Conversely, low-temperature extraction at about 18°C removes neutral oil, with minimal quantities of gums and waxes, and may yield 98% refined oil [15]. Two major types of refining used with rice bran oil are alkali and physical. Alkali refining works well with oils that contain relatively high amounts of free fatty acids, but results in a greater loss of neutral oil [15,28]. Physical refining, on the other hand, depends on molecular distillation from a thin film, and refining losses can approach the actual free fatty acid content [15,28]. Physical refining is usually followed by a light alkali refining to remove the last traces of free fatty acids. Discoloration, high levels of free fatty acids, and wax are the problems most often encountered in refining rice bran oil. Timely bran stabilization and careful control of temperatures during extraction and refining can greatly reduce these problems [28,30]. Refined oil can be bleached with activated bleaching clay just as any other vegetable oil.

Rice bran oil is excellent for frying foods giving low peroxide, foam, free fatty acid and polymer formation [30,33]. It is more stable under frying conditions than many of the other common vegetable oils because of the more even balance between linoleic and oleic acid, the very low level of linolenic acid, and the high level of powerful antioxidants [15,28]. Palmitic, oleic, and linoleic acids represent 95% of the fatty acids in rice bran oil [15]. These can be isolated by acidulation of the soap stock and separated by fractional crystallization to give a variety of melting point ranges [28]. Potential applications include paints, resins, soaps, cosmetics, and pharmaceuticals.

High-temperature hexane extraction may result in 3–4% wax in the crude oil. These waxes can be isolated and purified by crystallizing and precipitating at low temperature [30]. They may be centrifuged or filtered off and then washed with acetone or ethanol to remove residual oil. Rice bran wax is composed of esters of long-chain fatty acids, C^{16}—C^{26}, and fatty alcohols, C^{22}—C^{30} in length [15,28]. It is FDA-approved as a coating for fresh fruits and vegetables to prevent moisture loss and as a release agent for plastic packaging materials intended for food contact. It is also used in confectioneries, lipstick, and other cosmetics [30]. Rice bran wax is similar in characteristics to carnauba wax, and is potentially more plentiful than carnauba wax [15,23,30].

Fats are an integral part of human diets supplying calories and essential fatty acids. The quantity and quality of the fat utilized in U.S. diets have been demonstrated to play an important role in obesity, coronary heart disease, and cancer. High cholesterol levels have been associated with an increased risk of heart disease. Studies have shown this risk is associated with high levels of LDL cholesterol and correspondingly low levels of high-density lipoprotein (HDL) cholesterol [34]. LDL cholesterol is raised when diets are high in saturated fats compared to polyunsaturated fats [35]. Hegsted et al. [36] and Keys et al. [37] demonstrated with their predictive equations that gram for gram, saturated fats elevated serum cholesterol levels twice as fast as polyunsaturated fats lowered them. Monounsaturated fatty acids were neutral according to these equations, and dietary cholesterol had only a moderate cholesterol-elevating effect. More recent studies in humans have shown that replacement of dietary saturated fatty acid by monounsaturated fatty acids resulted in reductions of LDL cholesterol that were either equal to [38,40], less than [41], or greater than polyunsaturated fatty acids [42].

Rice bran oil has been reported to have the beneficial effect of lowering serum cholesterol [35,43–48]. A rice bran oil diet reduces total serum cholesterol and LDL cholesterol, and Apo B compared to other fat sources [43], and has had no effect on triglycerides, HDL cholesterol and serum Apo A levels [43]. Even though the fatty acid profile of rice oil can be quite different from other hypocholesterolemic vegetable oils with 20% saturated fatty acids and about equal amounts of polyunsaturated and monounsaturated fatty acids at about 40% each, rice bran oil still has the effect of lowering serum cholesterol [35,49]. Many studies have drawn the conclusion that it is the unsaponifiable fraction of the rice oil that helps to lower cholesterol levels [43,50–52]. Rice bran oil contains an unusually high level of unsaponifiable matter (up to 4.4%), several times greater than that in most other vegetable oils [15,35,51]. The unsaponifiable matter is a mixture of 43% plant sterols (campersterol, stigmasterol, B-sitosterol, and others), 28% triterpene alcohols (24-methylene cycloartanol and cycloartenol), 10% 4-methyl sterols and 19% less polar compounds such as aliphatic alcohols and other hydrocarbons [53]. Many of the unsaponifiable component parts of rice bran oil have hypocholesterolemic action due to various mechanisms. Unsaponifiable sterols such as phytosterols and triterpene alcohols can have a significant effect on LDL cholesterol level at relatively low intake by inhibiting dietary cholesterol absorption and enhancing fecal sterol and bile secretions [35,50]. Oryzanol was a name given to a mixture of ferulic acid esters of the triterpenoid alcohol by Kaneko and Tsuchiya [54]. Components of γ-oryzanol have been identified as ferulate esters of cycloartenol, 24-methylene cycloartanol, campersterol, B-sitosterol and other sterols [55]. It comprises 20–30% of the unsponifiable matter of 1.1–2.6% of the oil [46,55], and has been reported to have hypolipidemic activity [43]. The high content of tocotrienols, which are members of the vitamin E family, in rice bran oil may inhibit cholesterol synthesis [35,55]. Qureshi et al. [56–58] suggested that tocotrienol, an unsaponifiable component of palm oil and rice oil, can inhibit cholesterol synthesis and lower serum cholesterol levels in various animal models. Either one of these mechanisms could result in the upregulation of LDL receptor sites and thereby increase the liver uptake of circulating LDL cholesterol and decrease the serum levels of LDL cholesterol [43].

The oryzanols and tocotrienols are two co-products from rice bran oil which by themselves may be of value. The tocotrienols are members of the vitamin E family and possess antioxidant activity. Other physiological actions attributed to the tocotrienols include decreasing serum cholesterol, decreasing hepatic cholesterol synthesis by suppression of hydroxy methyl glutaryl coenzyme A reductase, and antitumor activity [55]. There has been interest in the compound oryzanol for pharmacological uses like growth-accelerating action in animals, regulation of estrous cycle, and the ability to promote skin-capillary circulation [54].

As rice co-products like oil become more important to the rice industry, rice lines that have higher oil contents may be selected and released as speciality lines for production. Recently, equations have been derived for use with NIR technology to predict chemical constituents such as amylose, fat (oil), protein, and water in rice lines [59]. With the advent of these equations, utilization of NIR technology to evaluate rice breeding lines is possible. In the future as NIR becomes a selection tool utilized by rice breeding programs, rice lines with higher oil contents will be able to be selected.

4. RICE STARCH

White rice resulting from milling of brown rice is the endosperm of the kernel and is composed primarily of starch (90%, d.b.). Rice starch, as with other starches, consists of two polymeric forms of glucose, amylose and amylopectin (Figure 3.5). Amylose primarily has linear chains with only 3–4 branched chains on average [60–62] and comprises 0–33% of the rice starch content [63]. Amylopectin is a highly branched polymer having on the average 96% alpha-1,4 bonds and 4% alpha-1,6 bonds. These two molecules are organized into a radially anisotropic, semi-crystalline structure in the starch granule [64–65].

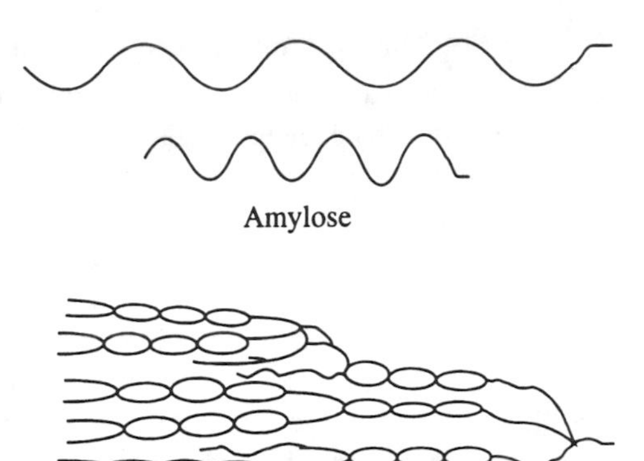

Figure 3.5 Diagram showing fragments of an amylose molecule, a linear starch molecule, and an amylopectin molecule, a branched starch molecule.

Rice starch granules are very small compared to those in other cereal grains, ranging in size from 3 to 5 microns. Twenty to 60 of these small polyhedral granules develop in an amyloplast forming a spherical to ellipsoidal compound granule, varying from 7 to 39 microns in diameter [66–67].

Isolated, native rice starch is a very fine, very white powder that provides applications as a cosmetic dusting powder, laundry-stiffening agent, paper and photographic paper powder, sugar coating in confectionery, and excipient for pharmaceutical tablets. Gelatinized rice starch has a bland taste and is smooth, creamy and spreadable, making it a good custard starch. Rice starch granules are about the same size as homogenized fat globules, thus providing similar texture perception. Waxy rice starch, which has excellent freeze-thaw stability, has found applications as a fat replacer in frozen desserts and in gravies in frozen dinners. Waxy rice starch also shows resistance to high-temperature (sterilization, UHT, microwave) treatments. Rice maltodextrins are commercially produced by partially hydrolyzing starch at high temperature or with enzymes to dextrose equivalents up to 20. Being bland and soluble in cold or hot water, they serve as carriers for flavor and provide bulk in products such as frostings, soups, sauces, and salad dressings.

Rice starch provides functional and neutraceutical roles when isolated and *in situ*. *In situ* starch determines the eating and processing qualities of the grain. Amylose content is considered the most contributory factor [68]. In general, rice with low amylose content cooks moist, soft and clingy, whereas rice with high amylose content cooks dry, fluffy, and firm. Waxy rice tends to lose its shape when cooked and is very sticky. In the U. S., rice is classified into three grain types: long, medium, and short, depending on length/width ratios (Table 3.1). U.S. long-grain rice cultivars typically have intermediate to high amylose contents and are marketed primarily as milled rice, parboiled rice, quick-cooking rice, and in packaged rice mixes. In contrast, the medium-and short-grain cultivars have low amylose contents. They are preferred for ready-to-eat (RTE) breakfast cereals, baby foods, and brewing. There are also special-purpose rices. Newrex and Rexmont are extra-high amylose cultivars (greater than 24%) with improved processibility for manufacturing into canned soups, quick-cook, and frozen rice products [69].

Rice appears to be quickly and completely digested, which results in a high glycemic response [70] and low colonic fermentation [71]. The composition and structure of the rice starch *in situ* affects the digestibility of rice. It is believed that starch digestibility is mainly determined by amylose content. In general, rice with high amylose content has a lower glycemic index (digests at a slower rate). However, amylose alone is not a good predictor of rice digestibility. Rice varieties with similar amylose contents have shown lower [72–73], higher [74], or similar [75] *in vitro* starch digestibilities. Structural differences in amylose in different varieties or complexing of amylose with lipid may affect digestibility. Goddard et al. [72] proposed that in high-amylose rice, amylose-lipid complexes could delay starch hydrolysis, thus eliciting flatter glucose and insulin responses.

Cooking procedure [76] and time [75] could also affect digestibility of rice. A two-step domestic cooking procedure consisting of boiling and baking polished rice can limit *in vitro* digestibility rates [76]. Panlasigui et al. [75] found that rice varieties with similar amylose content that were cooked for the minimum cooking time (when 90% of granules are gelatinized or no longer

TABLE 3.1. Official U.S. Length/Width Ratios Used to Determine Grain Type.

Grain Type	Grain Form	Length/Width Ratio	Apparent Amylose Content (%)
Long	Rough (paddy) kernel	3.4:1 and greater	
Long	Brown kernel	3.1:1 and greater	
Long	Milled kernel	3.0:1 and greater	21–23
Medium	Rough kernel	2.3:1–3.3:1	
Medium	Brown kernel	2.1:1–3.0:1	
Medium	Milled kernel	2.0:1–2.9:1	15–20
Short	Rough kernel	2.2:1 and less	
Short	Brown kernel	2.0:1 and less	
Short	Milled kernel	1.9:1 and less	15–20

Adapted from the United States Standards for Rice USDA (1989) and personal communication with B. D. Webb.

opaque) had the same degree of gelatinization, and their starch digestion rates and glycemic responses were similar. But when all rice cultivars were cooked for the same time, the digestibility varied due to differences in gelatinization properties.

Processing of rice is another factor affecting the digestibility of rice. Processing can affect compexation of lipid with starch and the degree of gelatinization, which in turn affect digestibility. Technologies such as extrusion cooking, explosion puffing and instantization improve rice starch digestibility, yielding products with glycemic indices higher than those of conventionally cooked white rice. Several studies [77–79] on insulin-dependent diabetics, noninsulin-dependent diabetics and healthy subjects have shown that parboiling and quick-cooking parboiling treatments markedly reduce the glycemic response to rice. Casiraghi et al. [79] found *in vitro* starch digestibility decreased in the following order: polished rice > quick-cooking parboiled rice > parboiled rice. Parboiled rice is hardened by a special steam-pressure process before milling which gelatinizes some of the starch in the grain, seals in nutrients, and makes the grain resistant to overcooking [80]. It is done to reduce stickiness and increase the milling yield. Gelatinized starch can reassociate later during storage [81]. Some doubt exists regarding the nature of the associative bonding in parboiled rice starch. Parboiling treatments induce a change in x-ray diffraction pattern from A-type pattern for raw starch to V-type pattern for amylose-lipid complexes, with no evidence of starch retrogradation, characterized by B-type of pattern [81]. The authors suggested that low enzymatic availability of parboiled rice can be an effect of starch-lipid interaction. However, Hibi et al. [82], working on cooked white rice, demonstrated that starch-lipid complexes are metastable and during storage changed to a more stable structure partly characterized by B-type pattern via an amorphous state.

Ito et al. [83] studied changes of fine structures of rice grain and found that rice digestibility is directly related to the gap volume in grains, constituted of micro and macro pores. The micro pores are an index of the degree of starch gelatinization while macro pores are an index of starch availability to α-mylase. Casiraghi et al. [79] also suggested that lower *in vitro* digestibility and flattened glycemic response of parboiled and quick-cooking parboiled rices without any increase in the amount of unabsorbed starch could be due to higher cohesiveness of the grain or different pore-size distribution in rice grain.

For nutritional purposes, starch has been classified into three types based on its digestibility: rapidly digestible starch, slowly digestible starch, and resistant starch [84]. The formation of starch resistant to digestion *in vivo* during high-moisture thermal treatment was found to be limited, and parboiled (0.8%) and quick-cooking parboiled rices (0.8%) had levels slightly higher than untreated rice (0.4%) [79]. Ortuno et al. [85] also found brown short-grain and parboiled long-grain rices had the higher contents of slowly digestible and resistant starch compared to white rices.

The extent to which rice is chewed before swallowing will affect its digestibility. It is very important when comparing the results of studies to see if the samples were macerated or intact. How accessible the starch is to the hydrolysis enzyme will affect measured digestibility. In the Ortuno et al. study [85], the samples were not ground before or macerated after cooking. The whole rice grains gave higher percentage of slowly digestible and resistant starch than was observed in the Casiraghi et al. study [79] in which the samples were macerated. Recently, Guraya and James [86] determined that the rate of digestion for whole kernels decreased in the order: untreated polished > parboiled > tempered parboiled. However, the rates of digestibility were the same for the three samples when the kernels were macerated and were significantly lower than those of the whole kernels. O'Dea et al. [87], comparing ground and unground rices, also demonstrated the importance of the surface area/starch ratio in determining the rate of *in vivo* and *in vitro* hydrolysis.

Opportunities abound for rice starch in isolated and *in situ* forms in functional/neutraceutical foods. As mentioned earlier, the small granule size of rice starch lends to applications as a fat replacer. Current applications use waxy rice starch because of its innate heat and freeze-thaw stability. The development of stable fat replacers using nonwaxy rice starch would be desirable. More desirable from an economic and availability viewpoint would be to develop fat replacers using nonwaxy rice flours. Development of rice starch-based foods with low glycemic index would be beneficial to diabetics and athletes. A starch-based sports beverage or food bar that slowly digests would be beneficial in maintaining blood glucose concentration and carbohydrate oxidation during the latter stage of exercise for the athlete. Rice, with its bland flavor and nutritionally valuable protein, would serve well as the starting material for such food products.

5. REFERENCES

1. Arkansas Agricultural Statistics for 1995. 1996 Arkansas Agricultural Experiment Station Report Series 334.
2. Kahlon, T.S., R.M. Saunders, F.I. Chow, M.M. Chiu and A.A. Betschart. 1990. "Influence of rice bran, oat bran and wheat bran on cholesterol and triglycerides in hamsters," Cereal Chem. 67:439–443.
3. Kahlon, T.S., F.I. Chow and R.N. Sayre. 1994. "Cholesterol-lowering properties of rice bran," Cereal Foods World 39:99–103.
4. Wells, J.H. 1993. "Utilization of rice bran and oil in human diets," Louisiana Agriculture 36(3):5–8.
5. Normand, F.L., R.L. Ory and R.R. Mod. 1987. "Binding of bile acids and trace minerals by soluble hemicelluloses of rice," Food Technol. 41:86–99.

6. Babcock, D. 1987. "Rice bran as a source of dietary fiber," Cereal Foods World 32:538–539.
7. Mod, R.R., E.J. Conkerton, R.L. Ory and F.L. Normand. 1978. "Hemicellulose composition of dietary fiber of milled rice and rice bran," J. Agric. Food Chem. 26:1031–1035.
8. Godber, J.S. and J.H. Wells. 1994. "Rice bran: as a viable source of high value chemicals," Louisiana Agriculture 37(2):13.
9. Hettiarachchy, N., P.S. Landers, K. Griffin and U. Kalapathy. 1994. "Utilization of rice bran proteins in food," Arkansas Rice Research Studies 1993, Wells, B.R., ed. Fayetteville, AR: Arkansas Agricultural Experiment Station Research Series 439. pp. 205–211.
10. Godber, J.S., D. Martin, T.S. Shin, G. Setlhako, C. Tricon and M. Gervais. 1993. "Quality parameters important in rice bran for human consumption," Louisiana Agriculture 36(3):9–12.
11. Martin, D., J.S. Godber, G. Setlhako, L. Verma and J.H. Wells. 1993. "Optimizing rice bran stabilization by extrusion cooking," Louisiana Agriculture 36(3):13–15.
12. McCaskill, D.R. and F.T Orthoefer. 1993. Proceedings of Rice Utilization Workshop Developing Innovative, Non-Conventional Uses for Rice. August 5–6, 1993, New Orleans, LA. pp. 58–67.
13. Barber, S. and C. Benedito de Barber. 1980. "Rice bran: chemistry and technology," Rice: Production and Utilization, Luh, B.S., ed. Westport, CT: AVI Publishing Co., Inc. pp. 790–862.
14. Luh, B.S., S. Barber and C. Benedito de Barber. 1991. Rice Utilization Vol. II., Luh, B.S., ed. New York, NY: AVI Book Published by Van Nostrand Reinhold. pp. 313–362.
15. Sayre, R.N. 1988. "Rice bran as a source of edible oil and higher value chemicals," presented at the American Association of Cereal Chemists 73rd. Annual Meeting, October 12, 1988. San Diego, California. pp. 1–11.
16. Barber, S., J.M. Camacho, R. Cerni, E. Tortosa and E. Primo. 1977. "Process for the stabilization of rice bran, I. Basic research studies," Proceedings of Rice By-Products Utilization International Conference Vol II. Rice By-Product Preservation, Barber, S. and E. Tortosa, ed. Valencia: Institute for Agriculture Chemistry and Food Technology. Valencia, Spain, 1974. pp. 49–62.
17. Loeb, J.R. and R.Y. Mayne. 1952. "Effect of moisture on the microflora and formation of free fatty acids in rice bran," Cereal Chem. 29:163–175.
18. Sayre, R.N., R.M. Saunders, R.V. Enochian, W.G. Schlutz and E.C. Beagle. 1982. "Review of rice bran stabilization systems with emphasis on extrusion cooking," Cereal Foods World 27:317–322.
19. Marshall, W.E. 1993. "Utilization of rice bran/hulls in value-added products," Proceedings of Rice Utilization Workshop Developing Innovative, Non-Conventional Uses for Rice. August 5–6, 1993, New Orleans, LA. pp. 68–76.
20. James, C. and S. Sloan. 1984. "Functional properties of edible rice bran in model systems," J. Food Sci. 49:310–311.
21. Hettiarachchy, N.S., U. Kalapathy and K. Griffin. 1994. "Natural antioxidants from fenugreek and rice bran," Arkansas Rice Research Studies 1993. Wells, B.R., ed. Fayetteville, AR: Arkansas Agricultural Experiment Station Research Series 439. pp. 218–221.
22. Randall, J.M., R.N. Sayre, W.G. Schultz, R.Y. Fong, A.P. Mossman, R.E. Tribel-

horn and R.M. Saunders. 1985. "Rice bran stabilization by extension cooking for extraction of edible oil," J. Food Sci. 50:361–368.

23. Juliano, B.O. 1985. "Rice bran," Rice: Chemistry and Technology, Juliano, B.O., ed. St. Paul, MN: American Association of Cereal Chemistry. pp. 647–687.
24. Landers, P.S., B.R. Hamaker and N.S. Hettiarachchy. 1993. "Utilization of rice bran proteins in food," Arkansas Rice Research Studies 1992, Wells, B.R., ed. Fayetteville, AR: Arkansas Agricultural Experiment Station Research Series 431. pp. 198–203.
25. Hettiarachchy, N.S. and R. Gnanasambandam. 1995. "Simple methods to determine rice quality and investigations of novel, value-added uses of rice bran: Part B," Arkansas Rice Research Studies 1994, Wells, B.R., ed. Fayetteville, AR: Arkansas Agricultural Experiment Station Research Series 446. pp. 239–247.
26. Hettiarachchy, N.S. and R. Gnanasambandam. 1996. "Protein-based biodegradable films from rice bran: preparation and properties," Arkansas Rice Research Studies 1995, Norman, R.J. and B.R. Wells, ed. Fayetteville, AR: Arkansas Agricultural Experiment Station Research Series 453. pp. 287–295.
27. Enochian, R.V., R.M. Saunders, W.G. Shultz, E.C. Beagle and P.R. Crowley. 1981. "Stabilization of rice bran with extrusion cookers and recovery of edible oil: A preliminary analysis of operations and financial feasibility," Marketing Research Report 1120, USDA–ARS, Washington, D.C. p. 18.
28. Sayre, R.N. and R.M. Saunders. 1990. "Rice bran and rice bran oil," Lipid Technology 2(3):72–76.
29. Desikachar, H.S.R. 1977. "Status report: preservation of by-products of rice milling," Proceedings of Rice By-Products Utilization International Conference Vol II. Rice By-Product Preservation, S. Barber and E. Tortosa ed. Valencia, Spain 1974. pp. 1–32. Valencia: Institute for Agriculture Chemistry and Food Technology.
30. Kao, C. and B.S. Luh. 1991. "Rice oil," Rice Utilization Vol. II, B.S. Luh, ed. New York, NY: AVI Book Published by Van Nostrand Reinhold. pp. 295–311.
31. Bhattacharyya, A.C. and D.K. Bhattacharyya. 1983. "Refining of high FFA rice bran oil by alcohol extraction and alkali neutralization," J. Oil Technol. Assoc. India 15(2):36–38.
32. Sayre, R.N., D.K. Nayyar and R.M. Saunders. 1985. "Extraction and refining of edible oil from extrusion-stabilized rice bran," JAOCS 62(6):1040–1043.
33. Lynn, L., B.J. Steen and R.M. Anderson. 1968. "New rice oil," Food Technol. 22:1250–1252.
34. Hegsted, M. and M.M. Windhauser. 1993. "Reducing human heart disease risk with rice bran," Louisiana Agriculture 36(3):22–24.
35. Nicolosi, R. 1990. "Unsaponifiables in rice bran oil under study," INFORM 1(9): 831–835.
36. Hegsted, D.M., R.D.B. McGandy, M.L. Myers and R.J. Atare. 1965. "Quantitative effects of dietary fat on serum cholesterol in man," Am. J. Clin. Nutr. 17:281–295.
37. Keys, A., J.T. Anderson and R. Grande. 1957. "Prediction of serum-cholesterol responses of man to changes in fats in the diet," Lancet 2:959–966.
38. Mattson, F.H. and S.M. Grundy. 1985. "Comparison of effects of dietary saturated, mono-unsaturated, and polyunsaturated fatty acids on plasma lipids and lipoproteins in man," J. Lipid Res. 26:194–202.

39. McDonald, B.E., J.M. Gerrard, V.M. Bruce and E.J. Corner. 1989. "Comparison of the effect of canola oil and sunflower oil on plasma lipids and lipoproteins on in vivo thromboxane A_2 and prostacyclin production in healthy young men," Am. J. Clin. Nutr. 50:1382–1388.
40. Dreon, D.M., K.M. Varnizan, R.M. Drauss, M.A. Austin and P.D. Wood. 1990. "The effects of polyunsaturated fat vs. monounsaturated fat on plasma lipoproteins," J. Am. Medical Assoc. 263:2462–2466.
41. Sirtori, C.R., E. Tremoli, E. Gatti, G. Montanari, M. Sirtori, S. Colli, G. Gianfranceschi, P. Maderna, C.Z. Dentone, G. Testolin and C. Galli. 1986. "Controlled evaluation of fat intake in the Mediterranean diet: Comparative activities of olive oil and corn oil on plasma lipids and platelets in high risk patients," Am. J. Clin. Nutr. 44:635–642.
42. Mensink, R.P. and M.S. Katan. 1989. "Effect of a diet enriched with monounsaturated or polyunsaturated fatty acids on levels of low-density and high-density lipoproteins cholesterol in healthy women and men," New Eng. J. Med. 321:436-441.
43. Nicolosi, R.J., L.M. Ausman and D.M. Hegsted. 1991. "Rice bran oil lowers serum total and low density lipoprotein cholesterol and apoB levels in nonhuman primates," Atherosclerosis 88:133–142.
44. Nicolosi, R.J. 1993. "Nutritional aspects of rice oil," Proceedings of Rice Utilization Workshop—Developing Innovative, Non-Conventional Uses For Rice, August 5–6, 1993, New Orleans, LA. pp. 87–91.
45. Rukmini, C. and C.T. Raghuram. 1991. "Nutritional and biochemical aspects of the hypolipidemic action of rice bran oil: A review," J. Am. College Nutr. 10:3661–3669.
46. Hegsted M. and C.S. Kousik. 1994. "Rice bran and rice bran oil may lower heart disease risk by decreasing cholesterol synthesis in the body," Louisiana Agriculture 37(2):16–17.
47. Lichtenstein, A.H., L.M. Ausman, W. Carrasco, L.J. Gualtieri, J.L. Jenner, J.M. Ordovas, R.J. Nicolosi, B.R. Glodin and E.J. Shaefer. 1994. "Rice bran oil consumption and plasma lipid levels in moderately hypercholesterolemic humans," Arteriosclerosis and Thrombosis 14(4):549–556.
48. Sharma, R.D., and C. Rukmini. 1986. "Rice bran oil and hypocholesterolemia in rats," Lipids 21:715–717.
49. Raghuram, T.C., B.U. Rao and C. Rukmini. 1989. "Studies on hypolipidemic effects of dietary rice bran oil in human subjects," Nutr. Rep. Intl. 39:889–895.
50. Lees, A.M., H.Y.I. Mok, R.S. Lees and M.A. McCluskey. 1977. "Plant sterols as cholesterol-lowering agents: Clinical trials in patients with hypercholesterolemia and studies of sterol balance," Artheroscerosis 28:325–338.
51. Kahlon, T.S., F.I. Chow and R.N. Sayre. 1994. "Cholesterol-lowering properties of rice bran," Cereal Foods World 39(2):99–103.
52. Sharm, R.D. and C. Rukmini. 1987. "Hypocholesterolemic activity of unsaponifiable matter of rice bran oil," J. Med. Res. 85:278–281.
53. Itho, T., T. Tamura and T. Matsumoto. 1973. "Sterol composition of 19 vegetable oils," JAOCS 50:122–125.
54. Seetharamaiah, G.S. and J.V. Prabhakar. 1986. "Oryzanol content of Indian rice bran oil and its extraction from soap stock," J. Food Sci. Technol. 23:270–273.
55. Rogers, E.J., S.M. Rice, R.J. Nicolosi, D.R. Carpenter, C.A. McClelland and L.J.

Romanczyk. 1993. "Identification and quantitation of γ-oryzanol components and simultaneous assessment of tocols in rice bran oil," JAOCS 70:301–307.
56. Quershi, A.A., N. Prentice, Z.Z. Din, W.C. Burger, C.E. Elson and M.L. Sunde. 1984. "Influence of cultural filtrate of trichoderma viride and barley on lipid metabolism of laying hens," Lipids 19:250–257.
57. Qureshi, A.A., W.C. Burger, C.E. Elson and D.M. Peterson. 1986. "The structure of an inhibitor of cholesterol biosynthesis isolated from barley," J. Biol. Chem. 261:10544–10550.
58. Qureshi, A.A., T.D. Crenshaw, N. Abuirmeileh, D.M. Peterson and C.E. Elson. 1987. "Impact of minor plant constituents on porcine hepatic lipid metabolism. Impact on serum lipids," Atherosclerosis 64:109–114.
59. Bean, M.M., R.E. Miller and M.M. Chiu. 1994. "NIR and DSC—New tools for rice quality evaluations," Proceedings of the Twenty-Fifth Rice Technical Working Group New Orleans, Lousiana: March 5-9, 1994. Texas Agricultural Experiment Station, Texas A&M University, College Station, TX. p. 129.
60. Takeda, Y., N. Maruta, S. Hizukuri and B.O. Juliano. 1989. "Structures of indica rice starches (IR48 and IR64) having intermediate affinities for iodine," Carbohydr. Res. 187:287–294.
61. Takeda, Y., Hizukuri, S. and B.O. Juliano. 1986. "Purification and structure of amylose from rice starch," Carbohydr. Res. 148:299–308.
62. Hizukuri, S., Y. Takeda, N. Maruta and B.O. Juliano. 1989. "Molecular structures of rice starch," Carbohydr. Res. 189:227–235.
63. Juliano, B.O. 1992. "Structure, chemistry, and function of the rice grain and its fractions," Cereal Foods World 37:772–774, 776–779.
64. Nikuni, Z. 1978. "Studies on starch granules," Starch/Staerke 30:105–111.
65. Lineback, D.R. 1984. "The starch granule: Organization and properties," Bakers Digest 58:16, 18–21.
66. Hoshikawa, K. 1968. "Studies on the development of endosperm in rice. II. Development of starch granules in endosperm tissue," Nippon Sakumotsu Gakkai Kiji 37:207.
67. Hayakawa, T., S.W. Seo and I. Igaue. 1980. "Electron microscopic observation of rice grain. I. Morphology of rice starch," J. Jpn. Soc. Starch Sci. 27:173.
68. Webb, B.D. U.S. 1985. "Criteria of quality," Rice Chemistry and Technology. Juliano, B.O., ed. St. Paul, MN: American Association of Cereal Chemists. pp. 425–427.
69. Webb, B.D. 1991. "Rice quality and grades," Rice Utilization Vol. II. Luh, B.S., ed. New York, NY: AVI Book Published by Van Nostrand Reinhold. pp. 89–119.
70. Wolever, T.M.S., D.J.A. Jenkins, V.R.G. Vuksan, G.S. Wong and A.L. Jenkins. 1990. "Glycemic index of foods in individual subjects," Diabetes Care 13:126–132.
71. Kerlin, P., L. Wong, B. Harris and S. Capra. 1984. "Rice flour, breath hydrogen, and malabsorption," Gastroenterology 87:578–585.
72. Goddard, M.S., G. Young and R. Marcus. 1984. "The effect of amylose content on insulin and glucose responses to ingested rice," Am. J. Clin. Nutr. 39:388–392.
73. Juliano, B.O. 1993. "Improving food quality of rice," International Crop Sci. I. 677–681.

74. Rao, P.S.J. 1971. "Studies on the nature of carbohydrate moiety in high yielding varieties of rice," Nutr. 101:879–884.
75. Panlasigui, L.N., L.U. Thompson, B.O. Juliano, C.M. Perez, S.H. Yiu and G. Greenberg. 1991. "Rice varieties with similar amylose content differ in starch digestibility and glycemic response in humans," Am. J. Clin. Nutr. 54:871–877.
76. Gatti, E., G. Testolin and D. Noe. 1987. "Plasma glucose and insulin responses to carbohydrate food (rice) with different thermal processing," Ann. Nutr. Metab. 31:296–303.
77. Wolever, T.M.S., D.J.A. Jenkins and J. Kalmusky. 1986. "Comparison of regular and parboiled rices: explanation of discrepancies between reported glycemic responses to rice," Nutr. Res. 6:349–357.
78. Ramussen, O. and S. Gregersen. 1992. "Influence on the amount of starch on the glycaemic index to rice in non-insulin-dependent diabetic subjects," Br. J. Nutr. 67:371–377.
79. Casiraghi, M.C., F. Brighenti, N. Pellegrini, E. Leopardi and G. Testolin. 1993. "Effect of processing on rice starch digestibility evaluated by in vivo and in vitro methods," J. Cereal Sci. 17:147–156.
80. Dziezak, Z.D. 1991. "Romancing the kernel: A salute to rice varieties," Food Tech. 6:74–80.
81. Bhattacharya, K.R. 1985. "Parboiling of rice," Rice: Chemistry and Technology. Juliano, B.O., ed. St. Paul, MN: American Association of Cereal Chemists. pp. 289–348.
82. Hibi, Y., S. Kitamura and T. Kuge. 1990. "Effect of lipids on the retrogradation of cooked rice," Cereal Chem. 67:7–10.
83. Ito, K., K. Yoshida, N. Okazaki and S. Kobayashi. 1988. "Effect of processing on the pore size distribution and digestibility of rice grain," Agric. Biol. Chem. 52:3001–3007.
84. Englyst, H.N., S.M. Kingman and J.H. Cummings. 1992. "Classification and measurement of nutritionally important starch fractions," Eur. J. Clin. Nutr. 46:S33–S50.
85. Ortuno, J., G. Ros, M.J. Periago, C. Martinez and G. Lopez. 1996. "Cooking water uptake and starch digestible value of selected Spanish rices," J. Food Qual. 19:78–79.
86. Guraya, H. and C. James. 1996. Unpublished data.
87. O'Dea, K., P. Snow and P. Nestel. 1981. "Role of starch hydrolysis in vitro as a predictor of metabolic responses to complex carbohydrates in vivo," Am. J. Clin. Nutr. 34:1991–1993.

CHAPTER 4

Flaxseed Products for Disease Prevention

B. D. OOMAH[1]
G. MAZZA[1]

1. INTRODUCTION

FLAX (*Linum usitatissimum*) is an economically important oilseed crop in Canada. Global production for crop year 1995–1996 was 2.27 million metric tons (MT), with Canada contributing a major share (≈40%) of the production at 0.84 million MT. Canada is the only significant exporter of flaxseed to the European Union, the United States, and Japan, with 0.56 million MT exported in 1996.

Besides being rich in α-linolenic acid oil and good quality protein, flaxseed has potential as a natural source of phytochemicals such as flavonoids, lignans and phenolic acids. The demonstration of clinical activity associated with the consumption of flaxseed has led the U.S. National Cancer Institute (NCI) to target flax as one of the six plant materials for study as cancer-preventive foods [1]. Flax also has a relatively small genome with 15 pairs of small chromosomes of approximately equal size [2], which makes it fairly easy to genetically engineer traits of importance for the production of nutrient-tailored foods or ingredients that provide health benefits, including prevention and treatment of disease. Flaxseed has been consumed in various forms for over 5,000 years as a food ingredient and for its medicinal properties, which are mentioned in the Pen-T's A_0, the great Chinese Pharmacopeia [3].

Flaxseeds are flat, oval, and pointed at one end. The seed contains a seed coat, an embryo consisting of two large, flattened cotyledons, a short

[1]Agriculture and Agri-Food Canada, Pacific Agri-Food Research Centre, Summerland, BC, Canada.

hypocotyl and a radicle [4]. The seed coat in flaxseed is formed from the ovule and consists of five distinct layers, two of which are most important: the epidermal layer, commonly called the mucilage layer, and the testa consisting of pigmented cells which determine the colour of the seed. The structural features of the seed have been well described [4] and are illustrated in Figure 4.1. Cotyledon forms 55%, the seed coat and the endosperm 36%, and the embryo axis 4%, respectively, of the total weight of hand-dissected flaxseed [5]. The seed coat, which makes up most of the hull, can be removed by abrasive dehulling [6]. The hull obtained mechanically comprises approximately 22% of the seed [6].

From the handling, registration and marketing standpoint, there are two types of commercially produced oilseed flax, traditional flax or linseed, and the newly developed solin. The Canadian Grain Commission has established official grades for solin that differ from those of flax. Specifically, Canadian Grain Commission standards specify that solin oil contain less than 5% linolenic acid compared to more than 50% in flaxseed oil, producing an oil of light color suitable for cooking and that solin cultivars have a yellow seedcoat for visual distinguishability [7]. The characteristics of flax and solin cultivars commonly grown on the Canadian prairies are well documented [7–9].

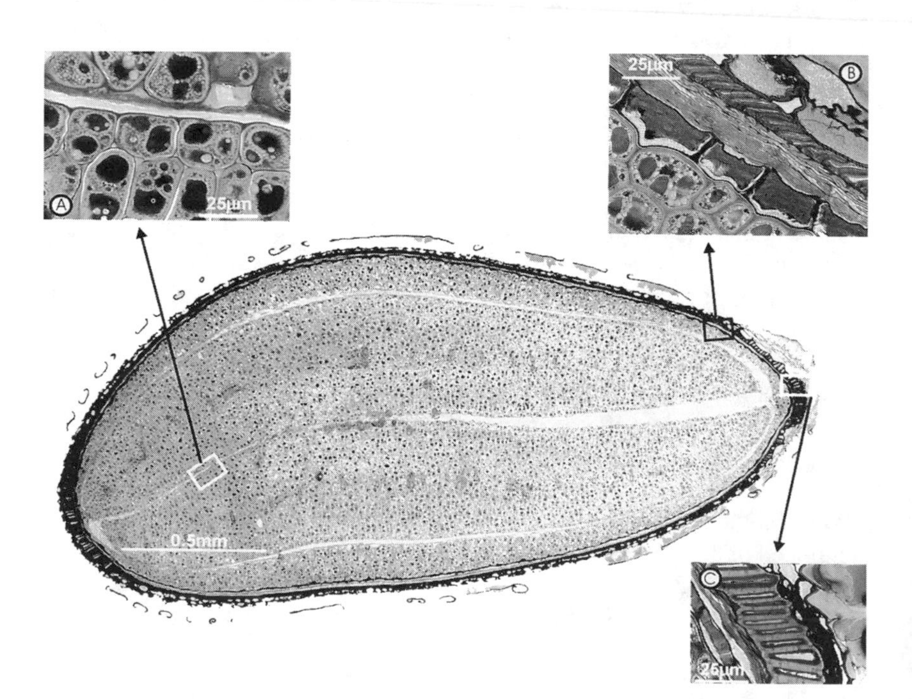

Figure 4.1 Structure of flaxseed cv. NorMan (A) cotyledon, (B) seed coat, (C) mucilage.

2. BIOLOGICALLY ACTIVE COMPONENTS

2.1. LIPIDS

In 1996, flaxseed grown in the Canadian prairie provinces, the major flaxseed-growing area of Canada, contained 5% palmitic acid (16:0); 3% stearic acid (18:0); 17% oleic acid (18:1n–9); 15% linoleic acid (18:2n–6); and 59% α-linolenic acid (ALA; 18:3n–3) based on analyses of 495 samples (Table 4.1) [10–12]. Oil content and quality are highly heritable traits in flaxseed. A wide inter- and intracultivar variation in oil content and quality in a diverse collection of 214 *L. usitatissimum* accessions was reported by Australian workers [13]. In the samples, oleic acid and ALA varied between 13–25% and 46–64%, respectively, and were negatively correlated within and between varieties. Flaxseed varieties from the world collection grown in Morden, Manitoba, Canada, in one year to reduce environmental variation revealed a range of 46–71% ALA. Single seeds from these varieties showed even greater variability in fatty acid composition: oleic acid, 14–60%; linoleic acid 3–21%; and ALA from 31–72% [14]. Environmental factors, such as temperature, particularly after flowering, soil conditions, cultural practices and the presence of disease are known to affect oil content and quality [15,16].

Although flaxseed oil has been consumed for centuries in India, China, and Europe [17], it is traditionally considered a nonedible oil in many western countries due to its rapid oxidation and polymerization, and it does not have GRAS (Generally Recognized as Safe) status [18]. Thus, modification of flaxseed oil to improve its stability and competitiveness as a salad or cooking oil by reducing ALA to <3% was first started in Australia [19,20] and Canada [21,22]. The successful modification of flaxseed oil led to the introduction of solin type varieties with low (<3%) ALA, and concomitant increases in linoleic acids, while having stable concentrations of other fatty acids (Table 4.1). Linola is a trademarked brand of solin. The only registered varieties of solin in Canada are Linola 947 and Linola 989. Reduction in ALA synthesis and the degree of oil unsaturation is due to the inhibition of linoleic acid desaturase enzyme system. These successes have provided impetus to further alter the fatty acid composition of flaxseed, such as the development of flaxseed cultivars rich in oleic acid [23], or palmitic and palmitoleic acids [24]. The high palmitic/low linolenic germplasm provides the opportunity to produce a cocoa-butter replacement oil [25]. Anti-sense RNA technology anticipated to be used to suppress the stearoyl ACP desaturase activity will lead to increases in stearic and oleic acid contents so that the palmitic, stearic and oleic acid levels are of near equal concentration. Such a linseed oil would represent a major new source of SUS (Saturated-Unsaturated-Saturated) triglycerides and should find application in the

TABLE 4.1. Oil, Fatty Acid, and Protein Composition of Flaxseed.

Reference	Oil (%)	Palmitic	Stearic	Oleic	Linoleic	α-Linolenic	Protein (%) ($N \times 6.25$)
DeClercq [10][a]	44.3	5.4	3.3	17.6	14.7	58.7	21.9
DeClercq [11][b]	43.8	5.1	3.1	19.1	14.9	56.8	23.7
Anonymous [12][c]	45.6	5.2	3.5	18.4	15.3	57.2	34.8
Anonymous [12][d] Solin	46.6	5.9	3.4	16.8	71.5	2.3	35.5

[a]Mean of 324 samples of No. 1 Canada Western flaxseed, from 1996 harvest survey, protein, and oil moisture free base.
[b]Ten-year mean data (1986–1995) of No. 1 Canada Western flaxseed (commercial samples).
[c]Three-year average data (1994–1996) of Canadian flaxseed varieties grown in research plots over western Canada ($n = 41$).
[d]1996 data for solin-type flax grown in western Canada.

candy industry. A domestic source of a vegetable oil high in palmitic acid for the manufacture of highly acceptable margarines has great attraction in Canada [25].

The reported biological properties of ALA (Table 4.2) demonstrate a broad spectrum of potential health benefits associated with the consumption of this fatty acid. Studies with deuterated ALA suggest that humans are capable of desaturating and chain elongating it to eicosapentaenoic acid (EPA; 20:5n−3) and decosahexaenoic acid (DHA; 22:6n−3) [26]. Like other n−3 polyunsaturates, ALA inhibits the metabolism of linolenic acid through the desaturation-elongation pathway, resulting in lower plasma and tissue levels of arachidonic acid (AA; 20:4n−6) in various animal models [27–32]. Like EPA, ALA may be an important physiological modulator in the synthesis and metabolism of eicosanoids derived from AA [33]. ALA has inhibitory effects on basal and stimulated production of eicosanoids derived from AA, including thromboxane A_2, leukotrienes B_4 and C, and 12-hydroxyeicosatetraenoic acid [34–36]. Alpha-linolenic acid also alters the *in vitro* production of several prostanoids, including PGE_2, PGF, PGI_2, TxB_2, and leukotriene E_5 [37–41]. Animal studies suggest that ALA can be actively recycled, due to β-oxidation, into other lipids, particularly in the developing brain [42,43]. Clinical ALA deficiency reported in 1982 [44] showed that ALA supplementation

TABLE 4.2. Reported Biological Effects of α-Linolenic Acid.

Biological Effect	Reference
Modulate synthesis and metabolism of eicosenoids derived from arachidonic acid	33
Reduce production of "4 series" leukotrienes	34–36
Contribute to the total pool of lipogenic precursors for brain lipid synthesis	42, 43
Alleviate clinical neurological symptoms, including numbness, visual blurring and paresthesil	44
Protect against cardiovascular disease and myocardial infarction	45, 46
Reduce high blood pressure in hypertensives and lower plasma triglyceride and cholesterol levels	47, 48
Reduce mortality due to cancer	51
Potential antithrombogenic and antiarrhythmic effects	49
Inhibit lymphocyte proliferation with benefits to individuals with immune disorders	50
Retard tumour growth	51
Antiparasitic and antimalarial activities	52
Essential for optimal neurological development in humans	33

(about 1.6 g per day) resolved the clinical neurological symptoms, including numbness, visual blurring, and paresthesia over 3 months. When ALA intake increased threefold in the Lyon "Mediterranean Diet" heart study, a 76% reduction in cardiovascular death was observed [45]. Significantly higher intake of ALA was the main feature of the intervention diet considered responsible for reducing deaths. Recently, an ALA-rich Mediterranean diet was shown to result in a 70% reduction in cardiovascular mortality over a 2-year observation period compared to a control [45]. ALA has been shown to reduce blood pressure in hypertensives [46] and to lower triglycerides and cholesterol [47,48]. The potential antithrombogenic effect of dietary ALA, possibly via EPA formation and/or damping the formation of AA-derived eicosanoids, was suggested by de Lorgeril et al. [45], but reduced mortality could also have been mediated via an antiarrhythmic effect as suggested previously from the DART trial [49]. Diets containing ALA inhibit lymphocyte proliferation in animals and immune response in healthy humans, which led Kelly [50] to conclude that a high intake of ALA may be beneficial to individuals with autoimmune disorders. In addition to the evidence that dietary ALA may retard tumour growth, a number of reports indicate that it may also have a role in metastasis [51]. Flaxseed oil possesses strong antimalarial properties and has a substantial inhibitory effect on the parasites, probably due to the metabolic effect of the hydroperoxides of the highly unsaturated fatty acids [52]. It has been suggested that ALA is dietarily essential for optimal neurological development in humans, especially during fetal and early postnatal life [33].

Flaxseed also contains phospholipids from which 2.9% of sterol glycosides can be extracted [53]. The sterols can be further fractionated into cholesterol (2% of sterol fraction), campesterol (26%), stigmasterol (7%), sitosterol (41%), Δ^5-avenasterol (13%), cycloartenol (9%), and 24-methylenecycloartanol (2%) [54].

2.2. PROTEINS

Flaxseed as a source of vegetable protein is commercially available in the form of seed, full-fat flour (i.e., milled flaxseed), and meal. Flaxseed and flour are the least refined form of flax protein ingredients. Prime-quality flaxseed meal must contain no less than 30% protein. There are two commercial grades of flaxseed meal. The most common grade available contains 30–32% protein, while the second most common is rated at 40% protein.

The literature on the composition, functionality and uses of flaxseed proteins has been reviewed recently [55,56]. Variability in the protein content of flaxseed has been attributed to genetic and environmental factors. Cool growing conditions usually results in lower protein but higher oil content [57]. However, genetic variation for protein content in flax cultivars is limited [14], since a survey of 400 entries from the world collection showed a range of 39–45% protein content in oil free meal. Flaxseed grown in nine countries with greatly varying environment showed little difference (23.3–24.7%) in protein content [58]. As in other oilseeds, a strong negative correlation is observed between the oil and protein content of the seed [59,60]. Higher seed protein levels can be achieved by crop management such as increased application of nitrogen (N) and phosphorus (P) fertilizers [61].

The protein fraction contains a favourable ratio of amino acids (Table 4.3) with lysine, threonine and tyrosine as the limiting amino acids. It is a good source of the sulfur amino acids methionine and cystine. Flaxseed meal has an essential amino acid index of 69 compared with 79 and 75 for soybean and canola meals, respectively. Similarly, the protein score, based on most limiting amino acid, relative to FAO (Food and Agriculture Organization) nutri-

TABLE 4.3. Amino Acid Composition of Flaxseed, Flaxseed Meal, and Protein Isolate (g/100 g protein).

Amino Acids	Flaxseed cv. NorLin[a]	Commercial Flaxseed Meal[b]	Protein Isolate from Flaxseed[c]
Alanine	4.4	5.5	5.1
Arginine	9.2	11.1	10.4
Aspartic acid	9.3	12.4	11.0
Cystine	1.1	4.3	NR
Glutamic acid	19.6	26.4	24.6
Glycine	5.8	7.1	4.9
Histidine	2.2	3.1	5.7
Isoleucine[d]	4.0	5.0	5.2
Leucine[d]	4.0	7.1	6.5
Lysine[d]	4.0	4.3	5.3
Methioine	1.5	2.5	3.2
Phenylalanine[d]	4.6	5.3	7.3
Proline	3.5	5.5	7.5
Serine	4.5	5.9	4.9
Threonine	3.6	5.1	3.6
Tryptophan[d]	NR	1.7	NR
Tyrosine	2.3	3.1	3.0
Valine[d]	4.6	5.6	5.6

[a]Data from Reference [55].
[b]Data from Reference [9].
[c]Data from Reference [63].
[d]Essential amino acid.
NR = not reported.

tional requirements, is 82 for flaxseed meal and 67 for soybean meal [62]. The nutritional value of flaxseed meal is comparable to that of soybean meal. Net protein utilization and protein efficiency ratios are slightly lower, while protein scores are higher than those of soybean meal (Table 4.4).

The flax products commonly available for use in food formulation are the whole flaxseed, stabilized flaxseed (i.e., flaxseed that has gone through a defined heat treatment) and flaxseed meal. Defatted flaxseed meal, flaxseed protein concentrate and isolate have been obtained in the laboratory but are not yet commercially available. These products differ widely in their composition and functional characteristics. The compositions of these products are given in Table 4.5. The isolated flaxseed protein has the highest level of protein (87%) with only trace amounts of lipids. Therefore, this product may provide minimal effects of lipids on flavour and acceptability. The protein isolate was tested in fish sauce, meat emulsion, and ice cream [73]. However, in fish sauce, large quantities of the preparation had to be used in order to stabilize the product. In ice cream, it yielded products of lower quality than those produced with gelatin, and the preparation was unsuitable for a meat emulsion due to its insufficient gelling properties. Flaxseed protein concentrate contains 66% protein with some lipids. Commercial flaxseed meal contains only 39% protein and up to 14% lipids, which reduces its value as a protein source and as a functional ingredient. Whole flaxseed contains only 24% protein with 44% lipid and 10% carbohydrates. The high lipid content adds to the caloric contribution of this product. The high polyunsaturated fat content can stimulate increased oxidation.

The solubilities of flaxseed proteins in the Osborne series of solvents are unique relative to other oilseeds but comparable to those of sunflower [74]. About 25% of the seed nitrogen is soluble in distilled water, about 30% is solubilized by 1 M NaCl, and the major fraction (42%) can be extracted with 0.1 N NaOH. Only 4% of the residue is soluble in 70% ethanol. Globulins constitutes 70–85% of flaxseed proteins of which two-

TABLE 4.4. Comparison of Nutritional Value for Flaxseed and Soybean Meals.

	Flaxseed	Soybean
Biological value	61.6–77.4	72.8
Net protein utilization	57.8	61.4
Digestibility	72.9–91.6	90.5
Protein efficiency ratio	0.79–1.76	2.32
Protein score	56.5–82	47.0

Data from References [62, 64–69 (for flaxseed), 70 (for soybean)].

TABLE 4.5. Composition of Flaxseed Protein Products.

Flaxseed Protein Product	Protein (N × 6.25)	Lipid	Carbohydrate	Ash
Isolated flaxseed protein[a]	86.6	Trace	NR	NR
Flaxseed protein concentrate[a]	65.5	0.8	NR	NR
Commercial flaxseed meal[b]	39.2	13.6	NR	5.58
Defatted flaxseed meal[b]	42.2	0.6	17.8	7.42
Whole flaxseed[b]	23.5	43.8	9.9	4.81

[a]Data from Reference [71].
[b]Data from Reference [72].
NR = not reported.

thirds has a molecular weight of 250,000 and the remainder is of low molecular weight [75].

The poor water solubility of flaxseed proteins is confirmed in the nitrogen extractability curve, flaxseed meal proteins being only 20–24% soluble between pH 2 and 6 [71,76,77]. Flaxseed protein isolate prepared by an alkali extraction-acid precipitation method showed a greater acid and alkali solubility than soy protein isolate [71], and moderate to high solubility in low and high concentrations of sodium chloride. In the presence of NaCl, the solubility minimals are shifted to lower pH values. The buffer capacity of flaxseed protein is maximal at an acid pH below the isoelectric region and minimal in the alkaline region.

Flaxseed products generally exhibit favorable water absorption, oil absorption, emulsifying activity and emulsion stability compared with the corresponding soybean products [76]. However, the alkali-extracted, acid-precipitated flaxseed protein isolate has higher water absorption properties and binds four times more oil than soybean isolate. The emulsifying properties of flaxseed proteins are pH-dependent and are adversely influenced by NaCl. Flaxseed proteins also show high foaming characteristics. Incorporation of sodium chloride enormously increases the foam stability of flaxseed protein from a half life of 22 minutes to over 600 minutes.

Flaxseed proteins are structurally more lipophilic than soybean proteins. Their hydrophilic properties are influenced by the presence of polysaccharide gums in flaxseed protein preparations [56,76]. The gum in flaxseed has been implicated in enhancing viscosity, water-binding, emulsifying and foaming properties of linseed protein products [76,78]. Modification of flaxseed proteins by heat treatment effectively improves water absorption, but reduces fat absorption, nitrogen solubility, foaming and emulsion characteristics [79].

Trypsin-inhibitor activity (TIA) has been reported in a sample of flaxseed meal [75]. Bhatty [80] recently compared the trypsin-inhibitor activity of flaxseed meal with those of raw soybean and rapeseed meal. Flaxseed meal contained only about one-half of the TIA (42–51 TIA units) of rapeseed meal (99 TIA units) and much less than the soybean meal (1650 units). Trypsin-inhibitor activity of raw flaxseed meal was reduced by 50–70% in commercial samples of flaxseed. Amylase-inhibitor and haemagglutinating activities have not been detected in flaxseed.

Another class of native seed proteins called "oleosins," or oil-body proteins, are structural proteins found in the seeds. They are highly lipophilic with a unique secondary structure, which permits their central core to be embedded in oil bodies, while the more hydrophilic *N*- and *C*-termini reside on the cytoplasmic site [81]. Oleosin from flaxseed has proven highly beneficial in the production and purification of recombinant proteins in plants for industrial and pharmaceutical applications. Flaxseed has a number of advantages in this system that are based on using the oil as part of the purification process [82,83].

2.3. POLYSACCHARIDES

The high dietary fiber of flaxseed is well known [9,78,84]. Flaxseed polysaccharide gum or mucilage may have nutritional value as a dietary fiber, which appears to play a role in reducing diabetes and coronary heart disease risk, preventing colon and rectal cancer, and reducing the incidence of obesity [84,85].

Flaxseed hydrocolloidal gum, also referred to as mucilage, comprises about 8% of the seed weight [9,78]; however, its yield is dependent on extraction regimes and can range from 3.5 to 9.4% [78,86–88]. An experiment with 10 commercial cultivars from Canada showed genotypic and seasonal differences in hydrocolloid gum content of flaxseed with location having no influence on this trait. However, the gum content in flaxseed, determined as sedimentation value, showed cultivar differences ranging from 48–90 ml and regional differences ranging from 48–71 ml [89]. The yellow seed coat seems to be linked to a low gum content [59,90]. Gums extracted from yellow flaxseeds exhibit stronger rheological properties than those from brown seeds due to their significantly lower acidic fraction and higher amounts of neutral polysaccharides [90].

Fiber content has also been associated with seed coat color. Meal from yellow-seeded flax contains less crude fiber (8.7 vs. 11.7%) and less neutral detergent fiber (24 vs. 29%) than meal from brown-seeded flax [66]. A significant negative correlation exists between fiber and oil content of flaxseed [59]. Fiber content also exhibits positive heterosis, indicating a significant scope for improvement in flax breeding [91].

There appears to be some genetic variation in the water-soluble carbohydrate content in existing flax cultivars. Oomah et al. [92] observed a range of 3.6–8.0% in water-soluble carbohydrate content of 109 entries from the world collection. The ratio of rhamnose to xylose, an indicator of the viscous behavior of flaxseed gum, varies considerably among flaxseed cultivars (from 0.3–2.2). The proportion of uronic acid and xylose also differs considerably among cultivars [90,93], while other saccharides are independent of genotype.

Flaxseed mucilage behaves like a typical viscuous fiber in its ability to reduce postprandial blood glucose responses [94]. Preliminary studies showed that adding 25 g flaxseed mucilage to a 400 ml solution containing 50 g glucose reduced the area under the blood response curve by 27% compared to oral glucose alone [95]. Soluble fiber is believed to reduce glycemic responses by increasing the viscosity of the small intestinal contents and delaying the digestion and absorption of carbohydrates [96–98].

Studies with flaxseed meal and flaxseed oil demonstrate a complementary action of several lipid-lowering modalities [99]. The studies of Bierenbaum et al. [100] and Cunnane et al. [101,102] both agree that flaxseed-supplemented diets reduce total serum cholesterol and LDL-cholesterol significantly. High-density lipoprotein cholesterol levels either rise slightly or remain constant. However, the supposition here is that some aspect of the dietary fiber of flaxseed produced the effect rather than the whole flaxseed oil or the ALA in that oil. Flaxseed incorporated into the diet, either raw or in baked products, also improves glucose tolerance. Again the improvement in glucose tolerance may be an effect of the dietary fiber and not related to the flaxseed oil.

2.4. LIGNANS

Lignans are phenolic compounds formed by the union of two cinnamic acid residues and comprised of a 2,3-dibenzylbutane nucleus (Figure 4.2) [103]. Plant lignans possess multiple oxygenated substituents in the aromatic rings and notably in the *para*-position that make them different in structure from mammalian lignans. Although the biological role of lignans in plants is unclear, the antifungal and insecticidal properties of these compounds indicate a possible role in plant host-defence systems, while in some plants they may function as growth regulators [104]. Lignans also possess antimitotic and antioxidative activities, and may play a role as anticancer agents in humans [103–105].

When flaxseed was fed to rats [106], monkeys and humans [107] phenomenal increases in the urinary excretion of enterolactone and enterodiol were demonstrated. Secoisolariciresinol diglycoside (SDG) was subsequently isolated from flaxseed and shown to be the precursor of enterodiol and enterolactone [106]. Flaxseed was found to be the champion plant species for lignan production when fed to rats (Figure 4.3). The relative abundance of precursors to enterolactone and enterodiol was quantified by expressing urinary lignan excretion per gram of dietary components fed to rats.

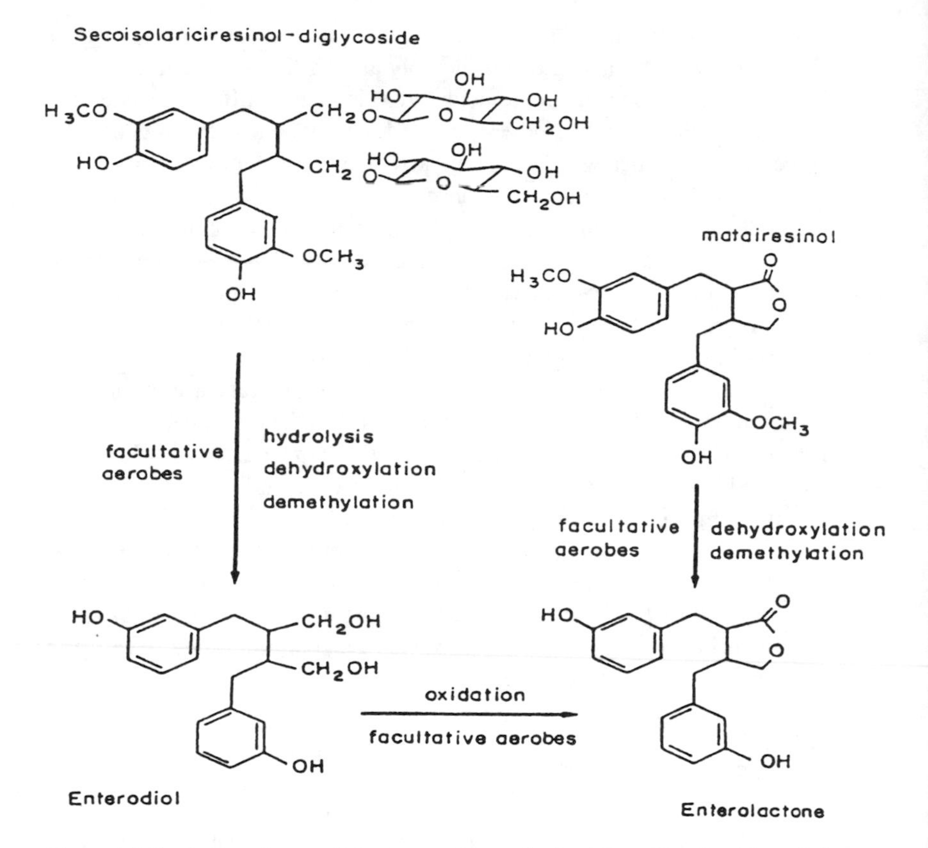

Figure 4.2 Production of enterodiol and enterolactone by fecal flora. (Reprinted from Reference [103], with permission from AOCS Press.)

Following synthesis by intestinal bacteria, lignans are absorbed from the intestine, transported to the liver, and secreted in bile [108]. Although the exact site of absorption is uncertain, recent studies suggest that the colon is the major site for metabolism and absorption [103].

A limited description of the isolation of lignan glycosides appeared as early as 1956 [109] and more information has been forthcoming recently [106–108,110]. The interest in flax lignans has generated several methods for their determination, especially by HPLC [111], ionspray mass spectrometry [112], liquid chromatography-mass spectrometry [113], and most recently, isotope dilution gas chromatographic-mass spectrometric method [114]. The pharmaceutical industry's interest in lignans as a chemical class relates mainly to their antimitotic activity [104]. The antimitotic activity of several lignans resembling enterolactone and enterodiol led to the speculation that

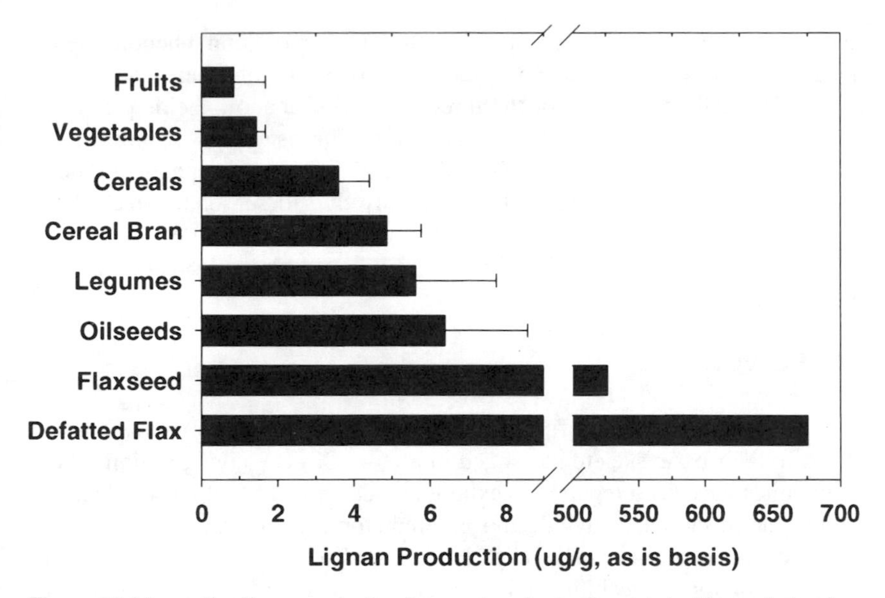

Figure 4.3 Mammalian lignan production from various foods. (Reprinted with permission from Reference [181]. Copyright, CRC Press, Boca Raton, Florida © 1994.)

these compounds when ingested may act as natural anticancer agents [105,115]. In an attempt to evaluate the potential anticancer activity of lignans, the effects of feeding flaxseed on tumour formation in the classic animal model of chemically induced colonic cancer were examined. Compared with the control group, no significant differences were found in the number, distribution or histological type of tumours in the groups of rats fed flaxseed. However, in contrast, short-term studies in rats showed a significant reduction in the total number of aberrant crypts and labelling index in animals fed flaxseed. Similar reductions in early risk markers for mammary tumours and tumour size were also demonstrated in rats fed a high-fat diet supplemented with flaxseed [116,117].

2.5. PHENOLIC ACIDS

Several bioactive functions, such as antioxidant, antimicrobial and anticancer, have been attributed to phenolic acids. In oilseed products, phenolic acids occur as hydroxylated derivatives of benzoic and cinnamic acids [118]. The levels of total and esterified phenolic acids are 81 and 73.9 mg/100 g, respectively, for dehulled, defatted flaxseed meal [119]. The major phenolic acids for dehulled, defatted flaxseed are *trans*-ferulic (46%), *trans*-sinapic (36%), *p*-coumaric (7.5%), and *trans*-caffeic (6.5%) for both total and esterified phenolic acids. Flaxseed contains 8–10 g/kg of total phenolic acids, about 5 g/kg of esterified phenolic acids and 3–5 g/kg of etherified phenolic acids. The relative amounts of the three classes of phenolic acids present in flaxseed differ significantly among cultivars. The esterified phenolic acids represents 48–66% of the total phenolic acids and are not dependent on cultivar. Variations in phenolic acids are mainly due to seasonal effect [120]. Four phenolic acids identified in defatted flaxseed powder are: ferulic acid (10.9 mg/g), chlorogenic acid (7.5 mg/g), gallic acid (2.8 mg/g), and traces of 4-hydroxybenzoic acid [121].

2.6. FLAVONOIDS

Flavonoids are a group of polyphenolic compounds that contain 15 carbon atoms in their basic skeleton arranged in a $C_6—C_3—C_6$ configuration. These compounds have been reported to exhibit a wide range of biological effects including antibacterial, antiviral, anti-inflammatory, antiallergic, and vasodilatory actions. In addition, flavonoids inhibit lipid peroxidation, platelet aggregation, capillary permeability and fragility, and the activity of enzyme systems including cyclo-oxygenase and lipoxygenase [122]. The major flavonoids in flax cotyledons are flavone C- and O-glycosides [123]. The content of flavonoids in flaxseed ranges from 35 to 71 mg/100 g and varies with cultivar and environment [124]. Genetic transformation conferring herbicide resistance to flaxseed does not appear to affect flavonoid content significantly [124].

2.7. PHYTIC ACID

Phytic acid is a natural plant inositol hexaphosphate commonly found in seeds and represents the principal form of stored phosphate. Phytic acid has hypocholesterolemic, antioxidative, anticarcinogenic, and hypolipidemic effects. It also has physiological effects similar to those of high-fiber diets and, as such, may be partly responsible for some of the health benefits attributed to high-fiber foods [125]. Phytin from defatted flaxseed flour contains 13% organic phosphorous and constitutes about 6% of the flour [126]. Defatted flaxseed contains 1.8–3.0% phytic acid, representing ≈70% of the total phosphorous [9]. Flaxseed contains 23–33 g of phytic acid per kilogram of meal, depending on cultivars and environment [127].

2.8. TOCOPHEROLS

Tocopherols are the most powerful natural fat-soluble antioxidants. A commercial flaxseed variety grown in 1994 contained 0.88, 2.42, 9.2, 0.24 of α-, β-, γ-, δ- and 12.74 mg/100 seed (wb) of total tocopherols, respectively [128]. Total tocopherol contents of flaxseed from 9 varieties grown at 13 locations

TABLE 4.6. Total Tocopherol Content (mg/100 g seed) of Flaxseed Cultivars in Different Environments.

	Location				Year		
Cultivar	Portage	Brandon	Elrose	Melfort	1991	1992	1993
AC Emerson	9.18[a]	9.22[a]	9.37[a]	8.54[b]	8.70[b]	8.76[b]	9.77[a]
AC Linora	10.86[a]	9.98[b]	9.97[b]	9.23[b]	10.25[b]	8.46[c]	11.32[a]
Flanders	8.80[b]	9.13[b]	10.02[a]	9.36[ab]	8.41[b]	8.78[b]	10.95[a]
Linola™ 947	9.49[b]	8.68[c]	10.33[a]	9.57[b]	9.39[b]	8.93[b]	10.23[a]
McGregor	10.10[a]	9.16[b]	9.00[b]	9.90[ab]	9.36[b]	9.12[b]	10.25[a]
NorLin	9.91[a]	8.47[bc]	7.86[c]	9.11[b]	9.24[a]	8.01[b]	9.16[a]
Somme	8.45[c]	8.34[c]	9.90[a]	8.90[b]	8.79[b]	8.58[b]	9.32[a]
Vimy	10.12[a]	8.03[c]	9.86[ab]	9.74[b]	9.82[a]	7.66[b]	10.83[a]
Mean of cultivars	9.61[x]	8.88[z]	9.55[x]	9.30[y]	9.25[y]	8.55[z]	10.24[x]

[a-c, x-z] Means in a row for locations or years and overall means, respectively, followed by the same letter are not significantly different by Duncan's multiple range test at the 5% level. Reprinted with permission from Reference [130].

worldwide ranged from 40 to 50 mg/100 g of oil; these differences were ascribed primarily to location [129]. Flaxseed contained an average of 9.3 mg/100 g of total tocopherol in the seed with gamma tocopherol, representing over 80% of the total. The level of tocopherol in flaxseed is cultivar-specific and regulated by environmental conditions (Table 4.6) [130]. Flaxseed hull contains approximately 26% of the total tocopherol found in the whole seed. The ratio of α, γ and δ-tocopherols of the hull [17:61:22] is different from that of the seed [1:94:5] and could be due to the preponderance of γ-tocopherol in embryo lipids and the presence of δ- and γ-tocopherol in seed coat lipids [130].

3. PROCESSING AND PRODUCTS

3.1. OIL AND MEAL

Commercial processing of flaxseed for oil and meal is similar to that of other oilseeds and includes seed cleaning, flaking, cooking, pressing, solvent extraction and solvent removal steps to yield oil and a meal. Details on modern oilseed processing have been described in recent reviews [131–133]. Generally, before flaking, the seeds are passed through shaker screens and aspirators to remove foreign material such as weed seeds, stones and soil. The clean seed, which may then be heat-conditioned, is rolled into flakes and passed to the cooker where the seed temperature is maintained at 65°C for 20 minutes.

The flakes go from the cooker to a press where oil is expelled, removing 60–70% of the oil from the flakes, which form a cake. This press cake is then extracted with hexane at 70°C to achieve rapid extraction of residual oil. After the solvent extraction, hexane is removed in a desolventizer-toaster vessel. The mechanically extracted cake usually enters the desolventizer toaster at 75°C and is discharged at 105°C, in approximately 30 minutes, then ground to produce the meal. Moisture content of the seed/meal throughout the process varies between 7 and 9%. The amount of heat used in processing of oilseeds may influence the quality of the resulting meal; excessive heating results in reduction of nitrogen digestibility and net protein utilization [134]. In most cases, undesirable factors present in the seed are removed, destroyed, or inactivated.

The protein content increases and the oil content decreases when flaxseed is processed into oil and meal (Table 4.7). The increase in protein content corresponds to the decrease in lipid content of the samples. Carbohydrate is present in the cake and meal in a much higher concentration than in the seed. Total phenolic acids decrease significantly on commercial processing of flaxseed from flakes to meal. The protein solubility decreases from 68% to 45% as the seed is processed from seed to meal, most probably due to protein aggregation as a result of heat involved during processing (Table 4.7). Protein digestibility generally increases upon processing, except at the expeller stage.

Treatment of the defatted flaxseed meal with boiling water has been used to remove undesirable constituents, especially the mucilaginous material, in order to improve the physicochemical and functional properties of the meal [79]. The resultant degummed meal showed reduced nitrogen solubility and dissociation of the high-molecular weight proteins, resulting in reduced functional properties and increased *in vitro* digestibility [77,79]. Extraction of flaxseed meal with aqueous methanol in the presence of ammonia reduces the

TABLE 4.7. Composition (%, moisture free basis) of Flaxseed at Various Processing Stages.

	Crude Protein (% N × 5.41)	Fat	Ash	Carbohydrate	Total Phenolic Acids
Seed	20.35[d]	43.79[a]	4.03[c]	9.86[c]	1.41[b]
Flake	21.34[c]	39.37[b]	3.98[c]	9.92[c]	1.59[a]
Cake	30.42[c]	17.26[c]	5.86[b]	14.97[c]	1.34[c]
Meal	34.47[a]	5.72[d]	7.25[a]	15.18[a]	0.99[d]

[a–d]Means within the same column followed by the same superscript are not significantly different ($p < 0.05$).
Data from Oomah and Mazza. 1997. Unpublished.

level of phenolic acids, tannins and soluble sugars resulting in improved nutritional and sensory qualities [135–137]. The oil extraction efficiency of this two-phase solvent system containing ammonia is high, resulting in a meal with the residual oil of about 10 g/kg [137]. Extraction of flaxseed meal with methanol, aqueous methanol and aqueous methanol-ammonia as primary extraction solvents produces significant changes in the physico-chemical characteristics of flaxseed meal. These changes are influenced by the degree of polarity of the primary extraction solvent [138]. The amount and composition of lipids extracted from flaxseed meal are also affected by these solvents [139]. Thus, the use of methanol leads to a high extraction of phospholipids which adversely affect the quality of the oil, but it can be an acceptable method for recovering phospholipids from flaxseed meal for pharmaceutical applications. Flaxseed oil for the "functional food market" is generally extracted by cold-pressing. Processing steps for the production of this type of oil involve pressing, filtration and bottling. The seed may require pretreatments such as cracking and/or flaking prior to pressing.

Since the demand for omega-3 polyunsaturated fatty acids is increasing because of the health benefits attributed to these fatty acids, novel refining techniques may be used to prepare flaxseed oil and powders with microencapsulated oils for food fortifications. The specific refining process, similar to standard techniques used for fish oils, involves neutralization and bleaching to remove free fatty acids. Special deodorizing and absorption techniques that remove peroxides, aldehydes, and ketones are keys to preventing the development of off-flavors. Finally, stabilization with an antioxidant mixture of tocopherols, ascorbyl palmitate, and lecithin protects the refined oil product from future degradation and oxidation (Figure 4.4). Packaging under an inert gas further protects the product until use [140]. The powdered forms could be used mainly in dry goods such as bakery products and milk powders. The microencapsulated powders should be dispersible in cold water and are exceptionally stable. These properties, together with neutral taste, can make them suitable for enriching foods such as reduced fat products, salad dressings, and beverages.

3.2. FLAXSEED GUM

Methods for preparing flaxseed polysaccharide gums or mucilage date back to 1932 when flax mucilage was prepared by the treatment of flaxseed with superheated steam and the extract used directly for the prevention of scale formation in boilers [141]. Reports in the late 1940s [142–143] suggested that the mucilage of flaxseed hull might affect digestibility of flaxseed meal. To test this hypothesis, flaxseed was separated into hull and cotyledon fraction in sufficient quantities to permit feeding trials [144]. In 1952, Bolley and McCormack patented a method for the preparation of gum substantially

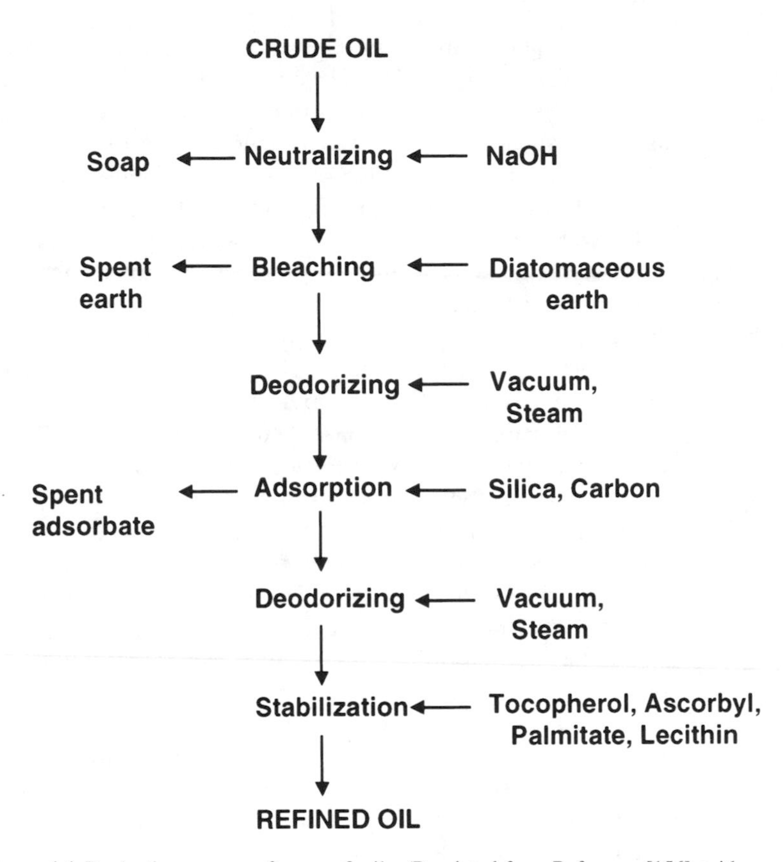

Figure 4.4 Production process of omega-3 oils. (Reprinted from Reference [156], with permission.)

free from protein and fiber contamination by extraction of an air-classified hull fraction from solvent extracted meal [145]. Solvent-extracted meal is separated by screening or air separation into a protein-rich kernel fraction and a mucilage-rich hull fraction. When the separation is carried out using an air separator, and when suitable operating steps and conditions are employed, a hull fraction can be obtained containing less than 15% protein. When screening is used as a means of separation, the hull portion needs to be further processed to obtain a concentrate containing less than 15% protein. This can be done by further screening the hull portion and retaining the oversize parts on a screen of about 35 to about 48 mesh (0.50–0.32 mm). The hull portion can also be ground in an impact-type grinding mill also known as a screen mill using screens of 3.175 mm to 0.8 mm mesh diameter. After grinding and air classification a hull fraction containing less than 7% protein can be obtained. According to this patent, the mucilage is extracted from the hull fraction by use of acidified water (pH = 4.5) in proportion of 20–50 parts water to one part hull fraction. The mixture is agitated for one hour at 60–80°C. After extraction, the fibrous residue is separated from the liquid by centrifugation and the pH of the separated liquid is adjusted to 7. The liquid is then concentrated by evaporation and spray dried to yield the dry, soluble mucilage product. Flaxseed hull has also been separated by a liquid cyclone process [9] and is purported to contain less than 10 g/kg oil, about 200 g/kg protein, and 330 g/kg total monosaccharides.

Attempts have since been made to remove mucilage by a wet process of demucilaging, followed by dehulling [75,146–148]. The wet process involves soaking of seeds in water with several changes, washing with dilute hydrochloric acid, drying and expeller pressing, followed by solvent extraction to obtain demucilaged cake/meal. The meal can be further flaked, dried and winnowed to remove hulls [147]. The procedure of Madhusudhan and Singh [75] consists of soaking the seeds in water and depulping the soaked seeds in an APV pulper to remove the mucilaginous material. The soaked seeds are directly flaked, dried, hexane-extracted, and the hulls are separated by a Satake paddy separator. The cotyledon are then ground to coarse mesh, defatted with hexane to 1% lipids and finally powdered to 60 mesh. The processed meal contains 48.9% proteins, 0.25% lipids, 10.85% fiber, 5.5% ash, 4.2% phytic acid and 34.5% carbohydrates.

Flaxseed gum or mucilage has been successfully produced by aqueous extraction using whole seed [78,88]. The method involves soaking of seeds in water, preferably at 85–90°C, separating the extracted mucilaginous material from the seed by filtration or centrifugation, concentration by ultrafiltration or vacuum evaporation, precipitation with 80% ethanol, and drying the gum. The yield and purity of extracted gum are dependent on the extraction temperature; higher temperatures extract more mucilaginous material with a high level of protein contamination [78,88]. Protein contamination can be reduced by purifying the mucilage extract with Vega clay [87] with no degradation or chemical modifications of the polysaccharides. Optimization of the aqueous extraction of the seed gum from whole seed by response surface methodology involved the following optimum conditions for gum yield and properties: temperature, 85–90°C, pH 6.5–7.0, and water to seed ratio of 13 [88]. The raw gum can be further separated into neutral (arabinoxylan) and acidic (pectin-like) fractions.

Since the mucilaginous soluble fiber has been implicated in the management of hyperglycemia and other diseases in humans [84], several new inventions have been related to the extraction of flaxseed gum as part of recent patents. Thus, the patent of Attström et al. [149] discloses the aqueous extraction of flaxseed polysaccharides with a [1 : 10] ratio of flour or whole seed to water, which may contain inorganic salts and/or flavouring agents. The extraction is typically performed for at least 3–4 hours. The process yields a polysaccharide fraction of about 4% by weight based on the solid content of the flaxseed. An aqueous solution of the polysaccharide is claimed to have the composition and characteristics that make it work extremely well as a saliva substitute. Another patent obtained by Smith-Kline Beecham [150] uses a similar extraction process where 1 part flaxseed is extracted with 10 parts water by boiling for 3 to 5 min.; then the hot extract is filtered under vacuum through a Buchner funnel with a 1 mm pore size. The resulting mucilage is oven- or freeze-dried. The mucilage obtained by this process is claimed to have mucoadherant properties and as such may be used as an artificial mucus or lubricant for topical applications in therapeutic and cosmetic utility. A third patent obtained by Kankaanpää-Anttila and Anttila [151] relates to a process for producing flaxseed proteins and mucilage. In this process, illustrated in Figure 4.5, flaxseed is cold- and/or hot-pressed and, if desired, further extracted with a suitable solvent for oil separation; the resulting pressed flaxseed is alkali extracted, the insoluble fiber is separated, and the protein and mucilage are precipitated by hydrochloric acid and ethanol, respectively. The protein and mucilage are air-dried and are used in baking. The resulting flax protein product contains 36% mucilage (with a pentosan content of 11%) and a protein content 45% of the dry matter. This patent claims that the flaxseed protein product when added at 0.6 to 5% improves bread by increasing water-binding capacity and reducing baking loss.

3.3. FLAXSEED PROTEIN

Response surface methodology has been used to optimize protein extraction from flaxseed meal [152,153]. Optimum protein extraction (97%) can be achieved using a solvent-to-meal ratio of 10 (w/v), 0.8 M NaCl, and pH 8.0. A simultaneous increase in ionic strength and decrease in solvent-to-meal ratio leads to increase in protein solubility [152]. Maximum protein extraction (78%) can also be obtained at a meal-to-solvent ratio of 1:33.6, pH 8.9, and a sodium hexametaphosphate concentration of 2.75% [153]. Isoelectric precipitation has also been used for the preparation of flaxseed protein with varying gum content [71]. The crude protein content of these preparations ranged from 56 to 86%. Generally, these flaxseed products exhibit favorable water absorption, oil absorption, emulsifying activity, and emulsion stability compared with the corresponding soybean products. The flaxseed-protein products containing varying levels of polysaccharide gums have been evaluated as additives in food systems such as canned fish sauce, meat emulsion, and ice cream [73]. Generally, flaxseed-protein products were found to have emulsion-stabilizing effects comparable with those of gelatin. The incorporation of flaxseed-protein products at a 3% level produced a smooth and creamy fish

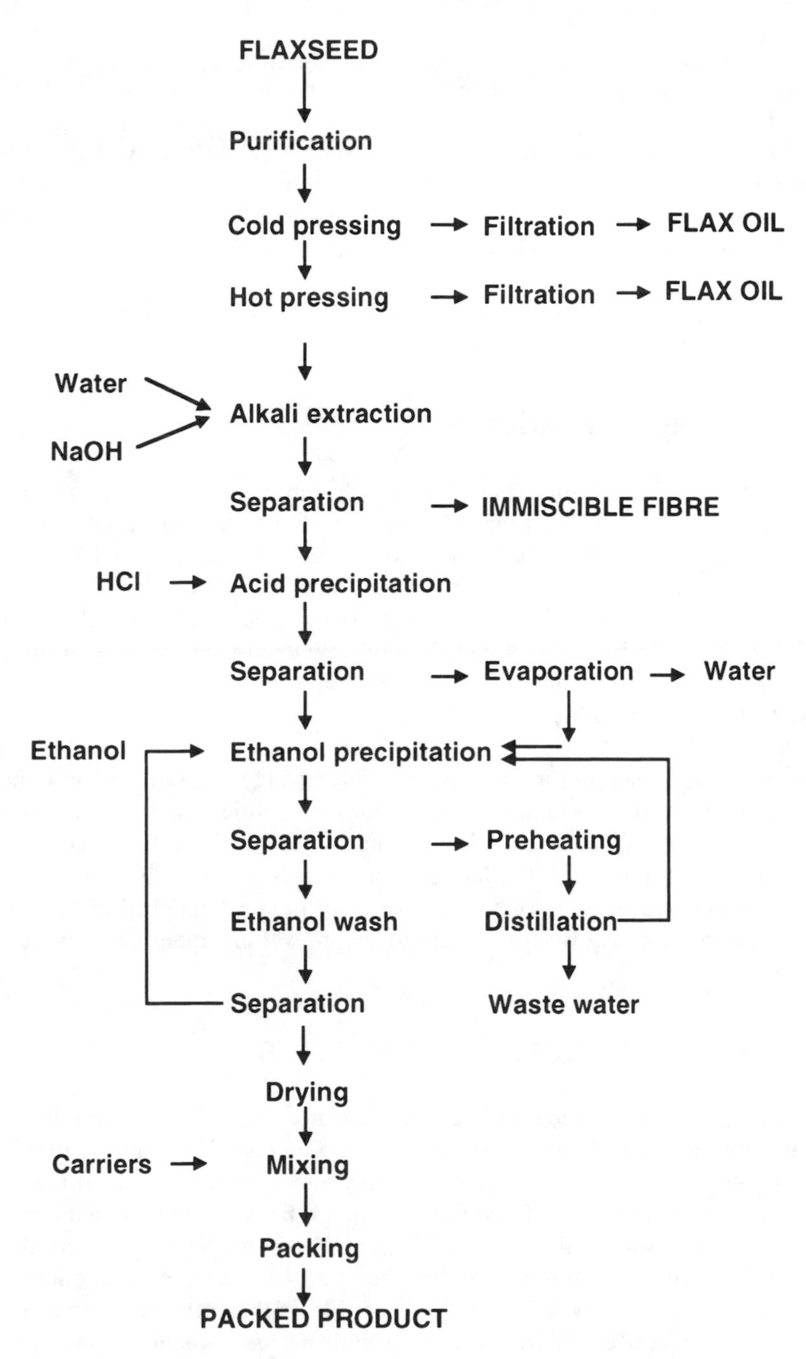

Figure 4.5 Process for separation of proteins and water-soluble carbohydrates from flaxseed. (Reprinted from Reference [151], with permission.)

sauce devoid of any undesirable flavor and a marked reduction in its red color.

Extending meat emulsions with flaxseed-protein products may lead to a reduction in fat losses during cooking and a reduction in the firmness of cooked emulsions and meaty flavour owing to their poor gelling properties. Supplementation of flaxseed-protein products in ice cream mixes increased product viscosity, specific gravity, and overrun but reduced melt-down times with an increasing level of additions from 0.5 to 1%. Thus, flaxseed-protein products have potential as emulsifiers and stabilizers in food systems.

3.4. FLAXSEED PHENOLICS

Techniques have been developed for the chromatographic separation of flaxseed phenolics [154]. Ethanolic extracts of defatted and dried flaxseed meal when applied to Sephadex LH-20 columns can be separated into four different phenolic groups. The largest number of compounds are found in a fraction (subfraction II) eluted from the RP-8 column. Fraction I is claimed to have high antioxidative activity [154], probably due to the presence of lignan in this fraction. Scale up of this process for the production of lignan-rich products may be possible.

Supercritical fluid extraction (CO_2) (Figure 4.6) has also been used for the extraction of lignan precursors present in flaxseed [155]. SDG, a plant lignan of major interest, concentrates about fourfold in dried ethanol extracts of flaxseed initially defatted by cold pressing and supercritical fluid extraction. Ethanol extraction of defatted flaxseed meal yields a SDG-rich fraction, very low in cyanogen content. This spent extract of flaxseed enriched in SDG but low in cyanogen may be appropriate for high-level incorporation into baked goods.

3.5. OTHER PRODUCTS AND PROCESSES

Attempts have been made to remove flax mucilage with dry dehulling of seeds by mechanical means. Since mucilage represents a major constraint in isolating protein from the seed in high yields, Smith et al. [156] investigated a simple process of fractionating ground flaxseed with graded sieves, and also an air-separation method. These processes consisted of grinding flaxseed, with a moisture content between 8 to 12%, between smooth rolls, mechanical separation followed by separation of the hull and embryo fraction after solvent extraction of the oil with hexane. A similar process of crushing flaxseed into a coarse meal, extracting with isopropanol at room temperature and screening the meal on a 0.25 mm sieve was used to obtain low- and high-mucilage protein products [71]. Recently, a method using a

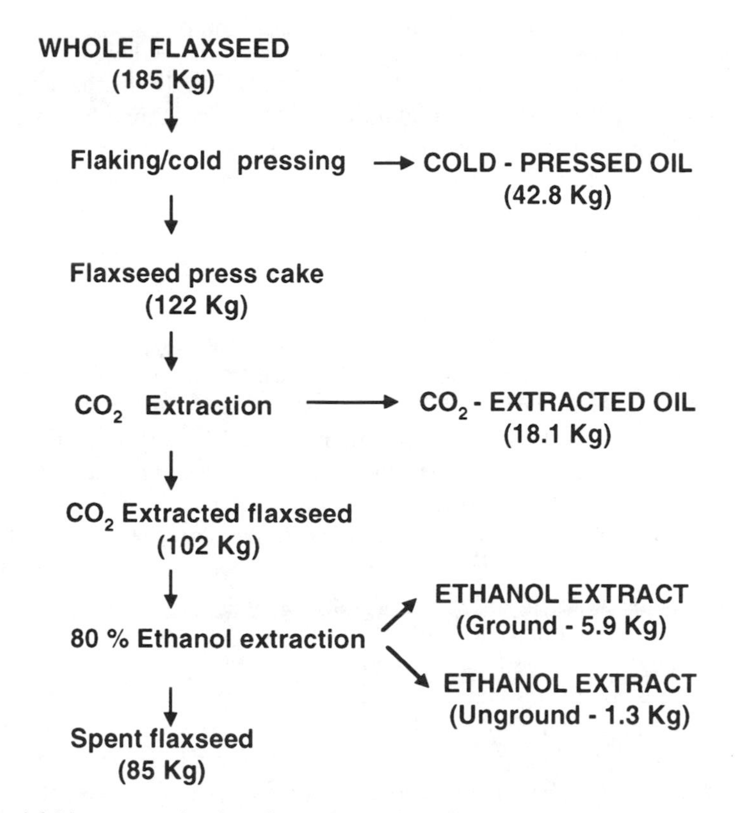

Figure 4.6 Lignan extraction from flaxseed. (Reprinted from Reference [155], with permission from AOCS Press.)

tangential abrasive dehulling device was developed to dehull flaxseed as a means of obtaining flaxseed hulls with the least amount of endosperm contamination [6].

The dehulling process proved to be very efficient, with a high percentage of actual hull removed (73%), and a relatively high endosperm recovery (76%). Subsequently, Oomah and Mazza [157] used an intermediate-sized batch dehuller to obtain four major flaxseed fractions (medium, fine, mix and hull) varying in physicochemical characteristics. In this process, flaxseed is loaded into the dehuller, equipped with 8 evenly spaced abrasive resinoid disks that are rotated at 1,725 rpm for 1–6 min. After dehulling, the sample is separated into three fractions, coarse, (i.e., material retained on an 18 mesh U.S. standard sieve, 1.00 mm), medium (material retained on a U.S. standard sieve No. 40, 0.425 mm) and fine (material passing through a U.S. standard sieve No. 40). The coarse fraction is further air-separated at constant air flow into hull, mix and unprocessed fractions.

The patent of Witt [158] discloses the use of dry flaxseed along with other ingredients in formulations of a milk-containing drink. In this patent, water, gum arabic, dry flaxseed, in an amount of 0.5 to about 0.8 part by weight per 100 parts by weight of water (5 to 8 g/L of water), and sea moss are first combined and heated to boiling, followed by filtering and blending with milk and sweetening agents. Another U.S. patent [159] discloses the use of whole flaxseed to provide a protein hydrolysate for use in beer-type beverages. The hydrolysis involves treating the whole flaxseed in water at 50–52°C with enzyme or acid to solubilize the protein. The hydrolysate is then added to converted and buffered starch and boiled for 20 to 40 minutes.

A chemically stable dry composition of flaxseed can be produced according to a process described in another U.S. patent [160]. The process involves grinding flaxseed in the presence of vitamin B-6 (75–150 parts per million parts of flaxseed) and zinc ion (in the form of zinc sulphate at 150 to 300 parts per million parts of flaxseed), at a temperature of about 70°C to just above freezing, or even at room temperature. Apparently, the addition of vitamin B-6 during the grinding step reduces the amount of cyanide produced during manufacturing, processing, packaging, and consumption. According to this invention, the ground flaxseed can be stored for over 6 months without turning rancid. The dry stable flaxseed can be used to prepare various foods such as cookies, breads, muffins, candy bars, meat analogues, processed meats, and nutritional drinks and can be sprinkled on salads and used in soups. The dry ground flaxseed can also be used to produce a stable emulsion or suspension by soaking the flaxseed about 6 to 12 parts by weight per 100 parts of an aqueous solution for about 20 min., and blending or homogenizing to form a stable emulsion or suspension. The stable emulsion or suspension is claimed to lower serum triglycerides and/or cholesterol when administered orally equivalent to 15 to 50 grams of dry flaxseed per day. This patent also describes the preparation of natural drink, flax yogurt, creamy orange drink and a carrot drink using the stable ground flaxseed.

3.6. CONSUMER PRODUCTS CONTAINING FLAXSEED

At present, the most commonly available consumer product is flaxseed bread, which generally contains about 7% ground flaxseed by weight. Replacement of six slices of regular bread with flaxseed bread containing 30% flaxseed reduced atherogenic risk factors in hyperlipemic subjects [100]. It was inferred from this study that flaxseed-soluble fibers (Table 4.8) along with lipids and other compounds may exert a more powerful hypercholesterolemic effect than wheat bran. Flaxseed has been included as whole grain in breakfast cereals [131]. Other baked products, such as muffins and cookies, are also used as vehicles for flaxseed proteins.

In a recent patent [151], flaxseed proteins and mucilaginous material are

TABLE 4.8. Composition (g/100 g) of Food Products Containing Flaxseed.

Component	Commercial Wheat Bread	Flaxseed Bread (30% flour/wt of milled flaxseed)	Flaxseed Muffin (23 g milled flaxseed per muffin)
Protein	9.2	12.3	10.0
Carbohydrate	48.0	44.8	46.3
Fat	2.6	10.7	10.4
Ash	2.0	2.7	2.1
Dietary fiber	3.9	11.6	6.1
Soluble dietary fiber	<1.4	2.9	NR
Calories (kJ)	992	1163	NR

NR = not reported.
Source: Data from Reference [100].

acid-precipitated from an alkaline extract to obtain a protein with high mucilage content. The products, which contains 40 to 50% protein and 30 to 40% mucilage, can be used in dough as an improver from 0 to 10%, preferably 0.3 to 5% of the amount of flour used. This product apparently improves dough hardness due to the proteinous part of the product, gas retention capacity, machine processability, tolerance to freezing and abuse, bread volume, and shelf life. Flaxseed finds its major application in baked items where the blending with cereals increases both the quantity and quality of the protein in the cereal products.

3.7. EFFECTS OF PROCESSING ON CHEMICAL COMPOSITION AND PROPERTIES OF FLAXSEED PRODUCTS

Different processes invariably change the chemical composition, physical properties and quality of flaxseed and its components. The composition of flaxseed lipids, for instance, is significantly affected by the extraction process and/or solvent used [139]. The use of methanol leads to a substantial extraction of phospholipids that can be easily recovered and used as lecithin for food emulsification and in human nutrition where phospholipids regulate serum lipid level and other human metabolic processes such as fat absorption, cholesterol metabolism, blood clotting, nerve, liver and lung functions, and biosynthesis of prostaglandins [161]. The effective use of solvents can also result in significant removal of cyanogenic glycosides from flaxseed meal. Extraction of cyanogenic glycosides is most effective with a multistage process involving the use of methanol-ammonia-water/hexane, especially when the extraction is repeated up to three times [136]. Products with such low cyanogenic glycoside levels have a definite potential in the functional food market. The type of extraction can also affect the composition of the resulting meal, especially the fat content, which contributes to the energy of the meal [162].

The chemical composition and physical properties of flaxseed hulls and dehulled seeds obtained by dry dehulling are different since the distribution of the major components of flaxseed (oil, protein, carbohydrate) varies within the seed [163]. The hull fraction contains low levels of oil and protein and a high concentration of carbohydrates (Table 4.9). The hulls also contain significantly higher levels of palmitic acid, and the lowest level of stearic and oleic acid compared to the whole or dehulled seed. The phenolic acids and tocopherols, known to have antioxidative activities, are present at higher concentration in dehulled seeds than in the whole seeds. The high protein content of the dehulled flaxseed makes it an attractive alternative protein source. The hull fraction, high in carbohydrate content, is recognized as having beneficial dietary effects and as such would be an important ingredient for the functional food industry. Furthermore, the hull contains over two and a half times as much lignan as the dehulled seed (23.9 and 9.0 mg SDG/g sample, respectively), thereby making flaxseed hulls a very attractive functional ingredient.

Grinding of flaxseed leads to reduced oxidative stability of the ground materials. Apparently, the oxidative susceptibility of ground seed is related to its

TABLE 4.9. Effect of Dehulling on Chemical Composition of Whole, Dehulled Seeds and Hulls of Flax (g/kg).

	Seed	Dehulled Seed	Hulls
Oil	403.8	499.7	283.9
Protein	192.0	218.0	173.1
Carbohydrate	83.4	59.4	174.9
Fatty acids			
Palmitic	52.7	53.0	78.5
Stearic	35.4	43.8	23.7
Oleic	228.6	252.9	213.3
Linoleic	152.2	148.7	150.9
Linolenic	531.3	501.0	533.5
Iodine value	185.0	178.3	184.0
Total phenolic acids	12.7	17.3	NR
Esterified phenolic acids	6.7	7.9	NR
Etherified phenolic acids	6.0	9.5	NR
Protein solubility	892.0	896.0	NR

NR = not reported.
Source: Reference [163], with permission.

particle size, with medium particle size (mesh 20–35) being more resistant to lipid oxidation. Hence, resistance to autoxidation of baked products containing ground flaxseed can be improved by choice of proper particle size [164]. The stability of flaxseed oil to oxidation is remarkably improved when it is hydrogenated with copper, although the resulting oil has low organoleptic quality [165]. The oxidative stability of flaxseed free fatty acid mixtures is improved in an aqueous solution, compared to that in air [166].

Flaxseed oil is oxidized more rapidly than other oils during heat treatment. For example, microwave heating results in a reduction of δ-tocopherol, and total biologically active tocopherol decreases due to heat degradation [167]. Reduction in moisture content of flaxseed by microwave drying is reflected in an exponential increase in the amount of hull that can be recovered [6]. Generally, microwave-treated flaxseeds produce over five times the amount of hull fraction during dehulling than untreated seeds [157]. The protein quality of flaxseed improves upon microwave heating. The proportion of acid-soluble protein decreases, while protein solubilization due to pepsin action alone increases with increasing retention time in the microwave. Microwave treatment for improving protein digestibility and easy removal of hulls makes it a potential process for innovative new product initiatives in functional and healthy foods.

4. HEALTH BENEFITS

Flaxseed is an abundant source of α-linolenic acid, viscuous fiber components and phytochemicals such as lignans and protein. These components of flaxseed are of great interest both for the food and the pharmaceutical industries. In addition, flaxseed incorporation into the diet is particularly attractive from the perspective of development of foods with specific health advantages. This topic has been covered in an excellent review [168] with the conclusion that the major determinant of the decision to purchase a flaxseed product is the perceived health benefits. An example of such flaxseed products are the omega-3 cereals and omega-3 bars introduced in 1995 [169]. These bars are cited as being the first energy bar with 1,000 mg of omega-3 in every bar. The cereal also contains 1,000 mg of omega-3 per serving.

4.1. FLAXSEED OIL

The physiological benefits of flaxseed oil is attributed primarily to the high content of ALA. However, the functional properties of ALA are not the same as those of flaxseed oil, because flaxseed oil contains other fatty acids ranging from 40 to 60%. Thus, flaxseed oil as a food ingredient has functional properties that go beyond the effects of ALA. Even low dietary levels of flaxseed oil lead to deposition of ALA and its metabolites, such as docosapentaenoic acid

(DPA; 22:5n−3), in mammary glands and tumours of carcinogen-treated rats [170]. Flaxseed oil feeding also reduces DMBA-induced mammary tumorigenesis in mice and the effect is both fat and concentration dependent [171].

Dietary ALA is converted through a series of desaturation and elongation steps to EPA and DHA (Figure 4.7). Elongation and desaturation of ALA to EPA and DHA occurs in human leukocytes and livers [172]. DHA can be synthesized from dietary ALA and can be found in membrane phospholipids of practically all cells of individuals who consume omega-3 fatty acids. DHA is one of the most abundant components of the brain structural lipids, phosphatidylethanolamine (PE), phosphatidylcholine (PC), and phosphatidyl serine (PS). Hence, an increase in the consumption of ALA is important in order to adequately provide the DHA needs of humans.

The mechanism of the inhibitory effect of ALA on tumorigenesis and metastasis is not well understood. Eicosapentaneoic acid produced *in vivo* from ALA from flaxseed [173] can compete for both the cyclooxygenase and lipoxygenase pathways, leading to decreased production of prostaglandins (PGE_2) and 4-series leukotrienes. This reduction in PGE_2 synthesis is reflected in tumour inhibition. An alternative mechanism may lie in the effects

Linoleate series	Linolenate series
C18:2ω6 Linoleic acid	C18:3ω3 Alpha-linolenic acid
⇩ Δ^6 desaturase	⇩ Δ^6 desaturase
C18:3ω6 Gamma-linolenic acid	C18:4ω3
⇩	⇩
C20:3ω6 Dihomo-gamma-linolenic acid	C20:4ω3
⇩ Δ^5 desaturase	⇩ Δ^5 desaturase
C20:4ω6 Arachidonic acid	C20:5ω3 Eicosapentaenoic acid
⇩	⇩
C22:4ω6	C22:5ω3 Docosapentaenoic acid
⇩	⇩
C22:5ω6 Docosapentaenoic acid	C22:6ω3 Docosahexaenoic acid

Figure 4.7 Essential fatty acid metabolism desaturation and elongation of ω-6 and ω-3. (Reprinted from Reference [172] with permission from Chapman & Hall, New York, NY.)

of the dietary fatty acids on cytokine production and other immunomodulatory effects of dietary ALA. It is also possible that dietary ALA may have tumour growth-retarding effects independent of its elongated, desaturated metabolites [51]. It has been suggested that the eicosanoids produced by EPA and DHA modulate the induction and proliferation of tumour cells by altering immune function and oncogene expression, exerting a direct action on growth factors [172]. Recently, secondary products of peroxidation, especially from highly unsaturated fatty acids, have been implicated in inducing profound damage when constantly in contact with cancerous cells. This inhibitory effect of fatty acids such as ALA may suppress mammary tumor growth, partly due to the formation of toxic compounds by lipid peroxidation [174].

4.2. LIGNANS

A recent review [175] attributed the protective effect of flaxseed against mammary and colon cancer to lignans and SDG, in particular (Table 4.10). The metabolic pathway for the formation of mammalian lignans involves sequential hydrolysis of the sugar moiety to release SDG, followed by dehydroxylation and demethylation by facultative bacteria to give rise to enterodiol, which is then oxidized to enterolactone (Figure 4.2). Lignans are absorbed from the intestine after synthesis by intestinal bacteria, transported to the liver, and secreted in bile [108]. Recent studies [103] suggest that the colon is the major site for metabolism and absorption of lignans. Concentrations of lignans in plasma are relatively high, especially in individuals consuming flaxseed, and elimination from the body occurring by renal clearance in urine is phenomenally high [107]. Studies in healthy men and premenopausal women have shown that both are able to produce large quantities of mammalian lignans from dietary flaxseed [103].

The mechanism by which flaxseed and its lignans influence tumorigenesis is not yet established, but several mechanisms have been suggested [175]. Lignans may stimulate plasma sex hormone-binding globulin (SHBG) synthesis in the liver and reduce the metabolic clearance rate, bioavailability and adverse effects of the steroids (Figure 4.8). The lignans have weak estrogenic/antiestrogenic effects and therefore compete with estrogens for the estrogen receptors, thereby preventing the growth of tumour cells. Lignans may have aromatase inhibitory effects; they prevent the production of oestrone from androstenedione and consequently deny the tumour a source of endogenous estrogen. Since lignans are known to suppress membrane ATPase activity [182] and to inhibit enzymes associated with cell proliferation, they may have growth inhibitory and antiproliferative effects on tumours [175]. Flaxseed extracts, as well as purified lignans, exhibit antioxidant effects *in vitro* and/or *in vivo* [183,184] and as such may protect from skin tumour and inhibit the activation of promutagens and procarcinogens [185]. Lignans may also influence

TABLE 4.10. Studies on the Anticarcinogenic and Antitumor Activities of Flaxseed Lignans.

Model	Inhibitory Action	Reference
Rats 2 g/flaxseed/d	No inhibition of chemically induced (dimethylhydrazine) colonic cancer. No differences in numbers, distribution, or histological type of tumours compared to control	176
Rats on high fat (20%) basal diet (BD) supplemented with 5 or 10% ground flaxseed (FF) or defatted flaxseed meal (FM)	Inhibit DMBA induced mammary carcinogenesis	177
Rats on high fat (20%) basal diet supplemented with 5% ground flaxseed	Inhibit DMBA induced tumour initiation and promotion	178
Rats fed 1.5 mg SDG/d equivalent to 5% ground flaxseed. Rats on high fat diet (20%) supplemented with 1.5 mg SDG/d	Inhibit DMBA induced tumour promotion	179
Basal diet supplemented with either 2.5% flaxseed, 5% flaxseed, 1.82% flaxseed oil (FO) (equivalent to ≈5% flaxseed) or 1.5 mg SDG	Inhibit DMBA induced tumour growth SDG (1.05) > 2.5% FF (3.05) > 5% FF (3.60) > BD (4.00) and FO (4.33)	179
Basal diet supplemented with 5 or 10% flaxseed or flaxseed meal	Inhibit Azoxymethane (AOM) induced colon carcinogens	180
Basal diet supplemented with either 2.5% flaxseed, 5% flaxseed meal, 5% flaxseed, 1.5 mg SDG/d	Inhibit AOM induced colon carcinogens SDG not significantly different from FM or FF diet groups	116

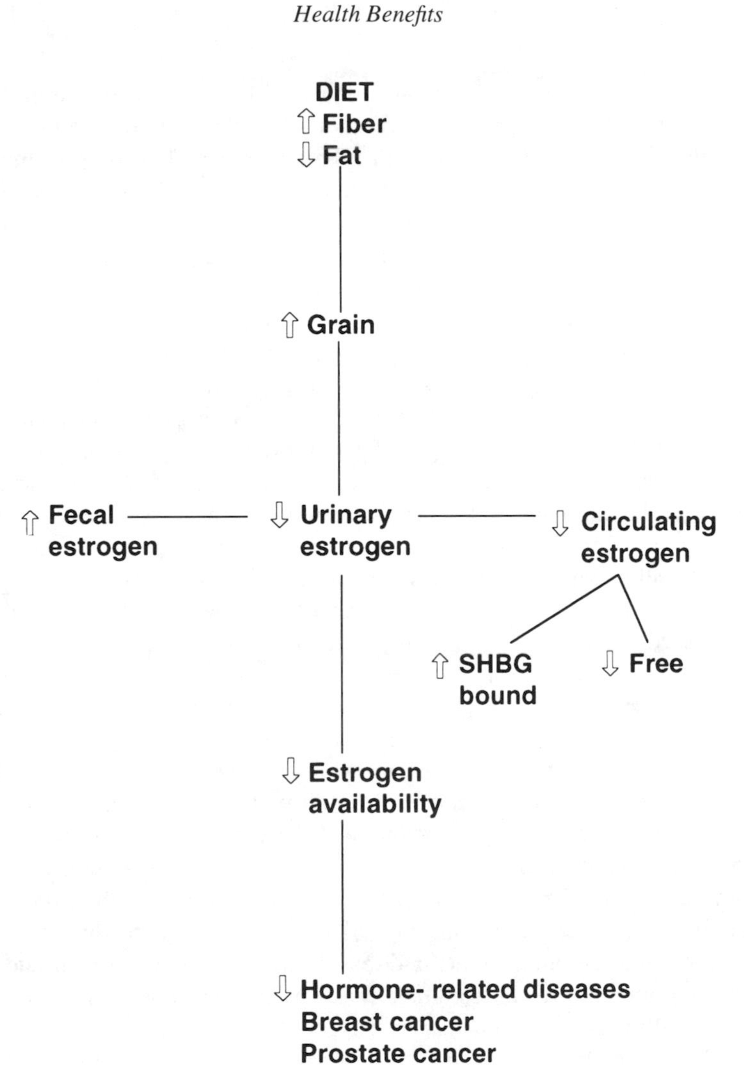

Figure 4.8 Relationship among diet, whole grain, estrogens, and hormone-related diseases. (Reprinted with permission from Reference [181]. Copyright, CRC Press, Boca Raton, Florida © 1994.)

cholesterol homeostasis [181] by inhibiting the rate-limiting enzyme in the formation of primary bile acids from cholesterol thereby reducing colon cancer risk.

The reduction in mammary and colon tumorigenesis seen in rats consuming flaxseed is thought to be partly due to the effects of lignans [178,180]. It has been proposed that lignans offer protection against breast and colon cancer due to their antiestrogenic and/or antioxidative effects [186]. Reports of lignans influencing estrogen synthesis, receptor binding, bioavailability, and action are consistent with suggestions that dietary flaxseed may exert its anticarcinogenic effects partly as a result of the antiestrogenic actions of lignans. Flaxseed is unique among grains in that the primary lignan precursor in flaxseed is secoisolariciresinol, which is metabolized by intestinal bacteria to the mammalian lignan enterodiol, which is then oxidized to enterolactone.

Evaluating the effects of flaxseed consumption on urinary lignan excretion and sex hormone metabolism in six healthy young men, Shultz et al. [187] found no significant changes in plasma testosterone, free testosterone, and SHBG concentration after 6 weeks of flaxseed consumption, despite the elevated lignan excretions, particularly of enterolactone. Alteration in the menstrual cycle of 18 young women in the Minnesota study was observed with flaxseed consumption [188]. Phipps et al. [188] concluded that the increased luteal phase length with flaxseed consumption may have been due to the increased progesterone/estradiol ratio, which appeared to be primarily due to decreased estradiol with flaxseed consumption. It is believed that increased progesterone/estradiol ratio reflects a decreased tendency toward ovarian dysfunction with flaxseed, which could lead to increased risk of breast cancer, suggesting a hormonal mechanism by which flaxseed may be cancer-preventive [188].

Flaxseed has a protective effect against both mammary and colon cancer [175]. The protective effect of flaxseed may be related to its lignans; however, the lignans may be protective only up to a point beyond which little or no beneficial effects may be expected. Short-term studies indicate that flaxseed has a cancer-protective effect, and that a high level of supplementation may not be necessary for cancer-risk reduction. The SDG from flaxseed and the mammalian lignan derived from it may exhibit a different, albeit protective effect at the tumour-promotion stage depending on the feeding regimen. Long-term studies confirm that SDG can influence tumour growth and that the reduced tumour growth from flaxseed is particularly due to the biological properties of mammalian lignans derived from SDG.

The lignans and the oil from flaxseed appear to have independent effects on carcinogenesis. For example, while both tend to reduce the growth of established tumours in the animal model, they also tend to have opposite effects on the development of new tumours. Dietary flaxseed provides a significant benefit in terms of improving renal function [189]. Reduced platelet aggregation and protection by flaxseed suggest a beneficial role for flaxseed-derived lignans [190]. Constituents of flaxseed (oil, fiber, and lignan precursors) may exert synergistic beneficial effects in this model of lupus nephritis [189]. Dietary flaxseed alternates the decline in renal function and reduces glomerular injury with favourable effects on blood pressure and plasma lipids [189]. A whole flaxseed diet confers a superior benefit compared to its oil, which in turn is superior to the defatted flaxseed diet in reducing the incidence of proteinuria, lymphadenopathy and splenic hypertrophy, and in preserving renal function.

4.3. GUMS—SOLUBLE POLYSACCHARIDES

One of the most interesting components for food processing in new product initiatives in functional foods is flaxseed gum, also referred to as *flaxseed mucilage*. Flaxseed gums can be extracted from whole flaxseed with hot water, followed by precipitation with ethanol and freeze-drying [84]. The freeze-dried material is relatively pure, free of antinutrients and stable on storage [155]. The viscosity of flaxseed gum (fiber) reduces serum cholesterol and flattens the blood glucose profile in a manner similar to guar gum, psyllium, oat gum, and other viscuous fibers intensively studied for this purpose [155]. Addition of flaxseed mucilage to a glucose-containing solution reduces the area under the blood response curve by 27% compared to oral glucose alone [101]. Soluble fiber is believed to reduce glycemic responses by increasing the viscosity of the small intestinal contents and delaying the digestion and absorption of carbohydrates [96–98].

The beneficial effects of flaxseed gum on glucose metabolism have not been completely unravelled. The hypothetical mechanism by which flaxseed reduces acute blood glucose response is by slowing carbohydrate digestion and absorption due to a combination of factors, including soluble fiber, and through the presumed effects of starch-protein interactions and antinutrients [94]. Reducing blood glucose response contributes to improving overall blood glucose control and is likely to be beneficial for individuals with glucose intolerance.

The hypolipidemic and cholesterolemic and atherogenic effects of flaxseed gum have been demonstrated in animal and human studies [100,102,191]. Although several mechanisms of action for dietary fiber have been proposed, none seems to demonstrate the simultaneous modes of action that complements the metabolic and physiological effects of fiber. The effects of flaxseed gums as a dietary fiber on serum cholesterol and lipid risk factors for coronary heart disease (CHD) may partly be due to their physicochemical properties, such as water-holding capacity, apparent solubility, binding ability, degradability, particle size and alterations by processing [192] (Table 4.11). The hypocholesterolemic effects of flaxseed gum may also be due to the high production of short-chain fatty acids from fermentation in the colon [193].

4.4. PROTEINS

Although flaxseed mucilage is known to lower blood glucose, it is unlikely that the mucilage alone has such a blood-lowering effect [95]. It has been

TABLE 4.11. Physicochemical Effects of Fiber.

Properties	Characteristics	Effect
Water-holding capacity (WHC)	Larger particle size	>WHC
Solubility	pH	↓ pH, ↑ WHC
	Ion strength	Variable effect on WHC
	Viscosity	↓ Motility
	Gelling	↓ Micelle formation
		↓ Bile acid pool size
		↓ Gastric emptying
Binding ability	Ion exchange	↑ Cation exchange, binding
	Adsorption of organic molecule	↑ Bile acid excretion
		↓ Serum and tissue cholesterol
Degradability	Fermentability	↑ Bacterial growth
		↑ Conversion to 1° to 2° bile acids
		↑ Short chain fatty acids production
Particle size	Smaller particle size	↑ Density, ↓ binding
	Larger particle size	↑ Fecal bulk, ↑ bowel effects
Processing	Temperature	Heating may alter fermentability of ↓ ion exchangeability
	Chemical texture	↑ Grinding, ↓ WHC

Source: Reprinted with permission from Reference [192]. Copyright, CRC Press, Boca Raton, Florida © 1990.

speculated that flaxseed protein may influence blood glucose in two ways. First, the protein in flaxseed may stimulate insulin secretion, which could result in reduced glycemic response [194]. Furthermore, protein may be important in determining the glycemic responses of foods due to its interaction with polysaccharides. Lignans are also known to have strong protein-binding properties [195], which may suggest some partial chemopreventive effect of flaxseed protein in conjunction with lignans.

Although the disease prevention effects of flaxseed proteins has not been studied, they may have synergistic effects with other components in flaxseed known to have protective effects. The antifungal properties of flaxseed proteins studied to date [196] may lead to its application in some food systems for weight reduction purpose (i.e., low-fat processed products) as well as for infant nutrition.

4.5. OTHER PHYTOCHEMICALS

Phytochemicals such as phytic acid and phenolic acids, present in flaxseed, have health benefits similar to those suggested for dietary fibers [185]. Phytic acid is known to lower blood glucose response by influencing the rate of starch digestion [197] and by slowing down gastric emptying [198]. In addition, phytic and phenolic acids are thought to have hypocholesterolemic effects [181]. Reduction in mammary and colon cancer risk have also been attributed to the presence of phytic acid and phenolic acids in foods. The mechanism of the inhibitory effect of these phytochemicals on carcinogenesis progress seems to be multifaceted and has been summarized elsewhere [181,185].

Flavonoids, in addition to being antioxidants, may defend cells against carcinogens via their ability to increase the pump-mediated flux of certain carcinogens from cells [199] or via induction of detoxification enzymes [122,200,201]. Flaxseed also contribute Vitamin E (tocopherols) to the diet. Tocopherols protect polyunsaturated fatty acids in cell membranes from oxidation. Furthermore, tocopherols keep selenium, which protects against oxidative tissue damage, in the reduced state, thus facilitating the antioxidant capacity of selenium. Additionally, Vitamin E has been shown to decrease the formation of nitrosamines, which may be carcinogenic, particularly in the stomach [202,203].

5. CONCLUSIONS

Functional foods are targeted to provide selective protection against some of the most common disease risks such as cardiovascular diseases, cancers, digestive disorders, and other disorders associated with lack of adequate nutrients. Some of the most important functional ingredients of flaxseeds are flaxseed oil with high α-linolenic acid content, flaxseed gum (dietary fiber), lignans, and other phytochemicals with antioxidative activities such as flavonoids, phenolic acids and tocopherols.

Although the benefits of α-linolenic acid from flaxseed oil are well known, its use in food and food products is hampered by its susceptibility to oxidation. One way of overcoming this problem is by microencapsulation of flaxseed oil to produce a dry product similar to the Dry n−3 powder [204]. This product has very high oxidative stability even after being baked or fried, and therefore has many applications in existing food systems as well as for new products with health benefits. Processes for the production of flaxseed gums have been patented especially for pharmaceutical applications [149,150]. However, availability of flaxseed gum as a product has been limited partly due to the absence of alternative efficient processing methods to-date. The application of flaxseed gums in food systems with their beneficial health effects on carbohydrate and lipid metabolism is currently underway. Further improvement in the physiological functionality of flaxseed gum can be made by enzymatically modifying its physicochemical and rheological properties to extend its application in foods and beverages with longer shelf life, improved flow, consistent viscosity, better texture and a pleasing appearance.

Many of the biological activities of flaxseed have been attributed to the high level of lignans present in the seed. However, the physiological activity of flaxseed lignan per se has not been established because of its limited availability. A prototype process for the production of a powdered concentrate and isolate containing 35% and 95% SDG, respectively, has been developed and provisional patent application and patent cooperation treaty have been filed [205,206]. Once large-scale production of flaxseed lignan is in place, studies confirming its chemopreventive effects will follow, resulting in new product initiatives in functional and healthy foods.

Although fairly abundant in flaxseed, protein has received relatively little attention. Opportunities exist in processing of flaxseed for the production of protein concentrate and protein isolate, as well as protein hydrolysates. Large-scale production of flaxseed protein is nonexistent at the present time, although several methods of protein extractions have been attempted. Different protein-extraction strategies will be required as more oilseed-extraction facilities move to mechanical, solvent-free oil extraction due to environmental pressures. These processing strategies will have to deal with the high oil content of the meal as a starting raw material. Strategies for the large-scale extraction and production of flaxseed proteins with known functionality, such as the 25 kDa antifungal protein and the oleosins, need to be developed and established. These proteins may be used to extend shelf life of food products, in addition to other physiological functions. The full potential of flaxseed and flaxseed components for production of functional foods will only be realized when processing of the individual components is in place and their physiologically activity has been tested in human studies.

6. REFERENCES

1. Caragy, A. B. 1992. "Cancer-preventive foods and ingredients," Food Technol. 46(4):65–68.
2. Cullis, C. A. and W. Cleary. 1985. "Fluidity of the flax genome," Plant Genetics, Alan R. Liss, London. pp. 303–310.
3. Judd, A. 1995. "Flax-some historical considerations," Flaxseed in Human Nutrition, S. C. Cunnane and L. U. Thompson, Champaign, IL: AOCS Press. pp. 1–10.
4. Freeman, T. P. 1995. "Structure of Flaxseed," Flaxseed in Human Nutrition, S. C. Cunnane and L. U. Thompson, Champaign, IL: AOCS Press. pp. 11–21.
5. Dorrell, D. G. 1970. "Distribution of fatty acids within the seed of flax," Can. J. Plant Sci. 50:71–75.
6. Oomah, B. D., G. Mazza and E. O. Kenaschuk. 1996. "Dehulling characteristics of flaxseed," Lebensm.-Wiss. u. -Technol. 29:245–250.
7. Growing Flax. Production, Management & Diagnostic Guide. 1996. Flax Council of Canada, Winnipeg, MB. pp. 1–56.
8. Oomah, B. D. and E. O. Kenaschuk. 1995. "Cultivars and agronomic aspects," Flaxseed in Human Nutrition, S. C. Cunnane and L. U. Thompson, Champaign, IL: AOCS Press. pp. 43–55.
9. Bhatty, R. S. and P. Cherdkiatgumchai. 1990. "Compositional analysis of laboratory-prepared and commercial samples of linseed meal and of hull isolated from flax," J. Am. Oil. Chem. Soc. 67:79–84.
10. DeClercq, D. R. 1996. 1996 Preliminary Flaxseed Quality Estimate—Report No. 2, Canadian Grain Commission, Winnipeg, MB, Canada. pp. 1–3.
11. DeClercq, D. R., J. K. Daun and K. H. Tipples. 1996. Crop Bulletin No. 231, Canadian Grain Commission, Winnipeg, MB, Canada. pp. 1–12.
12. Anonymous. 1997. Prairie Registration Recommending Committee for Grain. Oilseeds Subcommittee Report 1997. Report of Flax Co-Operative Test 1996. pp. 1–26.
13. Green, A. G. and D. R. Marshall. 1981. "Variation of oil quality and quantity in linseed (*Linum usitatissimum*)," Aust. J. Agric. Res. 32:599–607.
14. Dorrell, D. G. 1975. "Flaxseed research in Canada," Fette Seifen Anstrich. 77: 258–260.
15. Kenaschuk, E. O. 1975. "Flax breeding and genetics," Oilseed and Pulse Crops in Western Canada, J. T. Harapiak, Calgary, Alberta: Western Co-Operative Fertilizers. pp. 203–221.
16. Gill, K. S. 1987. "Linseed," Indian Council of Agricultural Research, Pusa, New Delhi. p. 386.
17. Schiefer, H. B. 1992. "In pursuit of GRAS status for flaxseed: Some practical and hypothetical considerations," In: Proceedings of the 54th Flax Institute of the U.S., Fargo, North Dakota. pp. 67–72.
18. Carter, J. F. 1993. "Potential of flaxseed and flaxseed oil in baked goods and other products in human nutrition," Cereal Foods World 38(10):753–759.
19. Green, A. G. 1986. "Effect of temperature during seed maturation on the oil composition of low-linolenic genotypes of flax," Crop Sci. 26:961.
20. Green, A. G. and D. R. Marshall. 1984. "Isolation of induced mutants in linseed

(*Linum usitatissimum*) having reduced linolenic acid content. Euphytica 33: 321–328.

21. Rowland, G. G. and R. S. Bhatty. 1990. "Ethyl methanesulphonate induced fatty acid mutations in flax," J. Am. Oil Chemists' Soc. 67(4):213–214.
22. Rowland, G. G. 1991. "An EMS-induced low-linolenic acid mutant in McGregor flax (*Linum usitatissimum* L.)," Can. J. Plant Sci. 71:393–396.
23. Miller, K. L. 1993. "High-stability oils," Cereal Foods World 38(7):478, 480–482.
24. Ntiamoah, C., G. G. Rowland and D. C. Taylor. 1995. "Inheritance of elevated palmitic acid in flax and its relationship to the low linolenic acid," Crop Sci. 35(1):148–152.
25. Rowland, G. G., A. McHughen, L. V. Gusta, R. S. Bhatty, S. L. MacKenzie and D. C. Taylor. 1995. "The application of chemical mutagenesis and biotechnology to the modification of linseed (*Linum usitatissimum* L.)," Euphytica 85:317–321.
26. Emken, E. A., R. O. Adolf, H. Rakoff, W. K. Rohwedder and R. M. Gulley. 1992. "Human metabolic studies with deuterated alpha-linolenic acid," Nutrition 8(3):213–214.
27. Ackman, R. G. and S. C. Cunnane. 1992. "Long-chain polyunsaturated fatty acids: sources, biochemistry and nutritional/clinical applications," Advances in Applied Lipid Research, F. B. Padley, London, UK: JAI Press Ltd. pp. 161–215.
28. Anding, R. H. and D. H. Hwang. 1986. "Effects of dietary linolenate on the fatty acid composition of brain lipids in rats," Lipids 21(11):697–701.
29. Machlin, L. J. 1962. "Effect of dietary linolenate on the proportion of linolenate and arachidonate in liver fat," Nature 194(4831):868–869.
30. Mohrhauer, H. and R. T. Holman. 1963. "The effect of dose level of essential fatty acids upon fatty acid composition of the rat liver," J. Lipid Res. 4:151–159.
31. Hwang, D. H., M. Boudreau and P. Chammugam. 1988. "Dietary linolenic acid and longer-chain n–3 fatty acids: comparison of effects on arachidonic acid metabolism in rats," J. Nutr. 118(4):427–437.
32. Marcel, Y. L., K. Christiansen and R. T. Holman. 1968. "The preferred metabolic pathway from linoleic acid to arachidonic acid in vitro," Biochem. Biophys. Acta 164:25–34.
33. Cunnane, S. C. 1995. "Metabolism and function of α-linolenic acid in humans," Flaxseed in Human Nutrition, S. C. Cunnane and L. U. Thompson, Champaign, IL: AOCS Press. pp. 99–127.
34. Hwang, D. H. and A. E. Carroll. 1980. "Decreased formation of prostaglandins derived from arachidonic acid by dietary linolenate in rats," Am. J. Clin. Nutr. 33:590–597.
35. Fritsche, K. L. and P. V. Johnston. 1990. "Effect of dietary alpha-linolenic acid on growth, metastasis, fatty acid profile and prostaglandin production of two murine mammary adenocarcinomas," J. Nutr. 120(12):1601–1609.
36. Henry, M. M., J. N. Moore, E. B. Feldman, J. K. Fischer and B. Russell. 1990. "Effect of dietary alpha-linolenic acid on equine monocyte procoagulant activity and eicosanoid synthesis," Circ. Shock 32(3):173–188.
37. Marshall, L. A. and P. V. Johnston. 1985. "The influence of dietary essential fatty acids on rat immunocompetent cell prostaglandin synthesis and mitogen-induced blastogenesis," J. Nutr. 115:1572–1580.
38. Morris, D. D., M. M. Henry, J. N. Moore and K. Fischer. 1989. "Effect of di-

etary linolenic acid on endotoxin-induced thromboxane and prostacyclin production by equine peritoneal macrophages," Circ. Shock 29(4):311–318.

39. Moore, J. N., J. A. Cook, M. M. Henry, H. T. Johnson, K. M. Spicer, W. C. Wise and P. V. Halushka. 1991. "Effects of linseed oil enriched diet on endotoxin-induced sequelae: differential in vitro and in vivo effects," Eicosanoids 4(1): 47–55.
40. Whelan, J., K. S. Broughton and J. E. Kinsella. 1991. "The comparative effects of dietary alpha-linolenic acid and fish oil on 4- and 5-series leukotriene formation in vivo," Lipids 26(2):119–126.
41. Calder, P. C., S. J. Bevan and E. A. Newsholme. 1992. "The inhibition of T-lymphocyte proliferation by fatty acids is via an eicosanoid independent mechanism," Immunology 75:108–115.
42. Anderson, G. T. and W. E. Connor. 1994. "Accretion of n–3 fatty acids in the brain and retina of chicks fed a low-linolenic acid diet supplemented with decosahexaenoic acid," Am. J. Clin. Nutr. 59(6):1338–1346.
43. Cook, H. W. 1991. "Brain metabolism of alpha-linolenic acid during development," Nutrition 7(6):440–442.
44. Holman, R. T., S. B. Johnson and T. F. Hatch. 1982. "A case of human linolenic acid deficiency involving neurological abnormalities," Am. J. Clin. Nutr. 35: 617–623.
45. de Lorgeril, M., S. Renaud, N. Mamelle, P. Salen, J. L. Martin, I. Monjaud, J. Guidollet, P. Touboul and J. Delaye. 1994. "Mediterranean alpha-linolenic acid-rich diet in secondary prevention of coronary heart disease," Lancet 343(8911):1454–1459.
46. Singer, P. 1992. "Alpha-linolenic acid vs. long-chain n–3 fatty acids in hypertension and hyperlipidemia," Nutrition 8(2):133–135.
47. Dyerberg, J. 1986. "Linolenate-derived polyunsaturated fatty acids and prevention of atherosclerosis," Nutr. Rev. 44(4):125–134.
48. Cunnane, S. C., Z. Y. Chen, J. Yang, A. C. Liede, M. Hamadeh and M. A. Crawford. 1991. "Alpha-linolenic acid in humans: direct functional role or dietary precursor?" Nutrition 7(6):437–439.
49. Burr, M. L., J. F. Gilber, R. M. Holliday, P. C. Elwood, A. M. Fehily, S. Rogers, P. M. Sweetnam and N. M. Deadman. 1989. "Effects of changes in fat, fish, and fiber intakes on death," Lancet 2(8666):757–761.
50. Kelly, D. S. 1995. "Immunomodulatory effects of flaxseed and other oils rich in α-linolenic acid," Flaxseed in Human Nutrition, S. C. Cunnane and L. U. Thompson, Champaign, IL: AOCS Press. pp. 145–156.
51. Johnston, P. V. 1995. "Flaxseed oil and cancer: α-linolenic acid and carcinogenesis," Flaxseed in Human Nutrition, S. C. Cunnane and L. U. Thompson, Champaign, IL: AOCS Press. pp. 207–218.
52. Levander, A. O. and A. L. Ager, Jr. 1995. "Antimalarial effects of flaxseed and flaxseed oil," Flaxseed in Human Nutrition, S. C. Cunnane and L. U. Thompson, Champaign, IL: AOCS Press. pp. 237–243.
53. Aylward, F. and B. W. Nichols. 1962. "Plant Lipids. II.—Free and combined sterols (sterol esters and glycosides) in commercial oilseed phospholipids," J. Sci. Food Agric. 13:86–91.
54. Middleditch, B. S. and B. A. Knights. 1972. "Sterols of *Linum usitatissimum* seed," Phytochemistry 11:1183–1184.

55. Oomah, B. D. and G. Mazza. 1993. "Flaxseed proteins—a review," Food Chemistry 48:109–114.

56. Oomah, B. D. and G. Mazza. 1995. "Functional properties, uses of flaxseed protein," Int. News Fats, Oils Rel. Mat. (INFORM) 6(11):1246–1252.

57. DeClercq, D. R., J. K. Daun and K. M. Tipples. 1995. "Quality of western Canadian flaxseed 1994," Crop Bulletin No. 216, Grain Research Laboratory, Winnipeg, MB. p. 10.

58. Schuster, V. W., H. Iran-Nejad and R. Marquard. 1978. "Yield performance and some quality characteristics of different linseed varieties (*Linum usitatissimum* L.) in areas with greatly varying environment," Fette, Seifen, Anstrichm. 80: 133–143.

59. Naqvi, P. A., M. Rai and A. K. Vasishtha. 1987. "Association of different components of seed and oil in linseed," J. Agric. Sci. 57(4):231–236.

60. Bajpai, M., S. Pandey and A. K. Vasishtha. 1985. "Spectrum of variability of characteristics and composition of the oils from different genetic varieties of linseed," J. Am. Oil Chem. Soc. 62:628.

61. Singh, R. A. and H. R. Singh. 1978. "Effect of nitrogen and phosphorous on yield, quality and moisture-use pattern of linseed grown on rainfed lands," Indian J. Agric. Sci. 48:583–588.

62. Sosulski, F. W. and G. Sarwar. 1973. "Amino acid composition of oilseed meals and protein isolates," Can. Inst. Food Technol. J. 6:1–5.

63. Dev, D. K., T. Sienkiewicz, E. Quensel and R. Hansen. 1986. "Isolation and partial characterization of flaxseed (*Linum usitatissimum* L.) proteins," Die Nahrung, 30:391–393.

64. Sambucetti, M. E., G. Gallegos and J. C. Sonahuja. 1973. "Isolated protein from linseed meal I. Nutritive value and toxicological tests," Arch. Latinoamericanos Nutr. 23:79–94.

65. Hossain, M. A. and K. Jauncey. 1989. "Nutritional evaluation of some Bangladeshi oilseed meals as partial substitutes for fish meal in the diet of common carp," Aquaculture and Fisheries Man. 20:255–268.

66. Bell, J. M. and M. O. Keith. 1993. "Nutritional evaluation of linseed meals from flax with yellow or brown hulls, using mice and pigs," Animal Feed Sci. Technol. 43:1–18.

67. Singh, B. and S. S. Negi. 1987. "Evaluation of peanut, mustard, linseed, and cottonseed meals for wool production in angora rabbits," J. Appl. Rabbit Res. 10: 30–34.

68. Salunkhe, D. K. and B. B. Desai. 1986. "Linseed, niger and cotton," Postharvest Biotechnology of Oilseeds, Boca Raton, FL: CRC Press, Inc. pp. 171–296.

69. Bell, J. M. 1989. "Nutritional characteristics and protein uses of oilseed meals," Oil Crops of the World, G. Röbbelon, R. K. Downey and A. Ashri, New York: McGraw-Hill Publishing Co. pp. 192–205.

70. Frank, A. W. 1987. "Food uses of cottonseed protein," Developments in Food Proteins—5, B. J. F. Hudson, London: Elsevier Applied Science Publishers. pp. 31–80.

71. Dev, D. K. and E. Quensel. 1988. "Preparation and functional properties of linseed protein products containing differing levels of mucilage," J. Food Sci. 53: 1834–1837, 1857.

72. Oomah, B. D. and G. Mazza. 1997. "Effects of processing on the physicochemical characteristics of flaxseed," (Unpublished data).
73. Dev, D. K. and E. Quensel. 1989. "Functional properties of linseed protein products containing different levels of mucilage in selected food systems," J. Food Sci. 54:183–186.
74. Panford, J. A. 1989. "Factors affecting wavelength selection for the determination of protein, oil, water and fiber in oilseeds by near-infrared reflectance (NIR) spectroscopy," Ph.D. thesis, University of Guelph, Canada.
75. Madhusudhan, K. T. and N. Singh. 1983. "Studies on linseed proteins," J. Agric. Food Chem. 31:959–963.
76. Dev, D. K. and E. Quensel. 1986. "Functional and microstructural characteristics of linseed (*Linum usitatissimum* L.) flour and a protein isolate," Lebensm.-Wiss. u. -Technol. 19:331–337.
77. Madhusudhan, K. T. and N. Singh. 1985. "Effect of detoxification treatment on the physicochemical properties of linseed proteins," J. Agric. Food Chem. 33: 1219–1222.
78. Mazza, G. and C. G. Biliaderis. 1979. "Functional properties of flaxseed mucilage," J. Food Sci. 54:1302–1305.
79. Madhusudhan, K. T. and N. Singh. 1985. "Effect of heat treatment on the functional properties of linseed meal," J. Agric. Food Chem. 33:1222–1226.
80. Bhatty, R. S. 1993. "Further compositional analyses of flax: mucilage, trypsin inhibitors and hydrocyanic acid," J. Am. Oil. Chem. Soc. 70(9):899–904.
81. Huang, A. H. C. 1992. "Oil bodies and oleosins in seeds," Ann. Rev. Plant Physiol. Plant Mol. Biol. 43:177–200.
82. Wilen, R. W., G. J. H. van Rooijen, D. W. Pierce, R. P. Pharis, L. A. Holbrook and M. M. Moloney. 1991. "Effects of jasmonic acid on embryo-specific processes in *Brassica* and *Linum* oilseeds," Plant Physiol. 95:399–405.
83. van Rooijen, G. J. H. and M. M. Moloney. 1995. "Plant seed oil-bodies as carriers for foreign proteins," Bio/Technology 13:72–77.
84. Mazza, G. and Oomah, B. D. 1995. "Flaxseed, dietary fiber, and cyanogens," Flaxseed in Human Nutrition, S. C. Cunnane and L. U. Thompson, Champaign, IL: AOCS Press. pp. 56–81.
85. Jenkins, D. J. A., T. M. S. Wolever, J. Kalmusky, S. Guidici, C. Giordani, G. S. Wong, J. N. Bird, R. Patten, M. Hail, G. Buckley and J. A. Little. 1985. "Low glycemic index carbohydrate foods in the management of hyperlipidemia," Am. J. Clin. Nutr. 42(4):604–617.
86. Cui, W., G. Mazza and C. G. Biliaderis. 1994. "Chemical structure, molecular size distribution and rheological properties of flaxseed gum," J. Agric. Food Chem. 42:1891–1895.
87. Fedeniuk, R. W. and C. G. Biliaderis. 1994. "Composition and physicochemical properties of linseed (*Linum usitatissimum* L.) mucilage," J. Agric. Food Chem. 42:240–247.
88. Cui, W., G. Mazza, B. D. Oomah and C. G. Biliaderis. 1994. "Optimization of an aqueous extraction process for flaxseed gum by response surface methodology," Lebensm.-Wiss. u. -Technol. 27:363–369.
89. Marquard, R. and W. Schuster. 1978. "Investigation of the relationship of the mucilaginous substances of linseed to genotype and source," Z. Lebensm. Unters. Forsch. 166:85–88.

90. Cui, W., E. Kenaschuk and G. Mazza. 1996. "Influence of genotype on chemical composition and rheological properties of flaxseed gums," Food Hydrocolloids 10(2):221–227.
91. Tak, G. M. and V. P. Gupta. 1993. "Studies on heterosis in linseed," Indian J. Agric. Res. 27:181–184.
92. Oomah, B. D., E. O. Kenaschuk, W. Cui and G. Mazza. 1995. "Variation in the composition of water-soluble polysaccharides in flaxseed," J. Agric. Food Chem. 43:1484–1488.
93. Wannerberg, K., T. Nylander and M. Nyman. 1991. "Rheological and chemical properties of mucilage in different varieties from linseed (*Linum usitatissimum*)," Acta Agric. Scand. 41:311–319.
94. Wolever, T. M. S. and D. J. A. Jenkins. 1993. "Effect of dietary fiber and foods on carbohydrate metabolism," CRC Handbook of Dietary Fiber in Human Nutrition, G. A. Spiller, Boca Raton, FL: CRC Press. pp. 111–152.
95. Wolever, T. M. S. 1995. "Flaxseed and glucose metabolism," Flaxseed in Human Nutrition, S. C. Cunnane and L. U. Thompson, Champaign, IL: AOCS Press. pp. 157–164.
96. Jenkins, D. J. A., T. M. S. Wolever, A. R. Leeds, M. A. Gassul, J. B. Dilawari, D. V. Goff, G. L. Metz and K. G. M. M. Alberti. 1978. "Dietary fiber, fiber analogues, and glucose tolerance: importance of viscosity," Brit. Med. J. 1:1392–1394.
97. Blackburn, N. A., J. S. Redfern, H. Jarjis, A. M. Holgate, I. Hanning, J. H. B. Scarpello, I. T. Johnson and N. W. Read. 1984. "The mechanism of action of guar gum in improving glucose tolerance in man," Clin. Sci. 66(3): 329–336.
98. Edwards, C. A., N. A. Blackburn, L. Craigen, P. Davison, J. Tomlin, K. Sugden, I. T. Johnson and N. W. Read. 1987. "Viscosity of food gums determined in vitro related to their hypoglycemic actions," Am. J. Clin. Nutr. 46(1):72–77.
99. Kritchevsky, D. 1995. "Fiber effects on hyperlipidemia," Flaxseed in Human Nutrition, S. C. Cunnane and L. U. Thompson, Champaign, IL: AOCS Press. pp. 174–186.
100. Watkins, T. R., A. C. Tomeo, M. L. Struck, L. Palumbo and M. L. Bierenbaum. 1994. "Improving atherogenic risk factors with flax seed bread," Proceedings of the 55th Flax Institute of the U.S., Fargo, ND. pp. 12–23.
101. Cunnane, S. C., S. Ganguli, C. Menard, A. C. Liede, M. J. Hamadeh, Z. Y. Chen, T. M. Wolever and D. J. Jenkins. 1993. "High alpha-linolenic acid flaxseed (*Linum usitatissimum*): some nutritional properties in humans," Br. J. Nutr. 69(2): 443–453.
102. Cunnane, S. C., M. J. Hamadeh, A. C. Liede, L. U. Thompson, T. M. S. Wolever and D. J. A. Jenkins. 1995. "Nutritional attributes of traditional flaxseed in healthy young adults," Am. J. Clin. Nutr. 61(1):62–68.
103. Setchell, K. D. R. 1995. "Discovery and potential clinical importance of mammalian lignans," Flaxseed in Human Nutrition, S. C. Cunnane and L. U. Thompson, Champaign, IL: AOCS Press. pp. 82–98.
104. Ayres, D. C. and J. D. Loike. 1990. "Lignans: chemical, biological and clinical properties," Chemistry and Pharmacology of Natural Products, J. D. Phillipson, D. C. Ayres and H. Baxter, Cambridge: Cambridge University Press. p. 402.
105. Setchell, K. D. R., A. M. Lawson, S. P. Borriello, R. Harkness, H. Gordon, D. M. L. Morgan, D. N. Kirk, L. C. Anderson, H. Aldercreutz and M. Axelson.

1987. "Lignan formation in man–microbial involvement and possible roles in relation to cancer," Lancet 1(8236):4–7.

106. Axelson, M., J. Sjövall, B. Gustafsson and K. D. R. Setchell. 1982. "Origin of lignans in mammals and identification of a precursor from plants," Nature 298: 659–670.
107. Setchell, K. D. R., A. M. Lawson, L. M. McLaughlin, S. Patel, D. N. Kirk and M. Axelson. 1983. "Measurement of enterolactone and enterodiol, the first mammalian lignans, using stable isotope dilution and gas chromatography mass spectrometry," Biomed. Mass Spectrom. 10:227–235.
108. Axelson, M. and K. D. R. Setchell. 1981. "The excretion of lignans in rats—evidence for an intestinal bacterial source for this new group of compounds," FEBS Lett. 123:337–342.
109. Bakke, J. E. and H. J. Klosterman. 1956. "A new diglucoside from flaxseed," Proc. N. Dakota Acad. Sci. 10:18–22.
110. Borriello, S. P., K. D. R. Setchell, M. Axelson and A. M. Lawson. 1985. "Production and metabolism of lignans by the human faecal flora," J. Applied Bact. 58:37–43.
111. Obermeyer, W. R., S. M. Musser, J. M. Betz, R. E. Casey, A. E. Pohland and S. W. Page. 1995. "Chemical studies of phytestrogens and related compounds in dietary supplements: flax and chaparral," Proc. Soc. Expt. Biol. Med. 208:6–12.
112. Bambagiotti-Alberti, M., S. A. Coron, C. Ghiara, V. Giannellini and A. Raffaelli. 1994. "Revealing the mammalian lignan precursor secoisolariciresinol diglucoside in flax seed by ionspray mass spectrometry," Rapid Commun. Mass Spectron. 8:595–598.
113. Bambagiotti-Alberti, M., S. A. Coron, C. Ghiara, G. Moneti and A. Raffaelli. 1994. "Investigation of mammalian lignan precursors in flax seed: First evidence of secoisolariciresinol diglucoside in two isomeric forms by liquid chromatography/mass spectrometry," Rapid Commun. Mass Spectron. 8:929–932.
114. Mazur, W., T. Fotsis, K. Wähälä, S. Ojala, A. Salakka and M. Aldercreutz. 1996. "Isotope dilution gas chromatographic-mass spectrometric method for the determination of isoflavonoids, coumesterol, and lignans in food samples," Analytical Biochem. 233:169–180.
115. Aldercreutz, H. 1995. "Phytestrogens: Epidemiology and a possible role in cancer protection," Environ. Health Persp. 103:103–112.
116. Jenab, M. and L. U. Thompson. 1996. "The influence of flaxseed and lignans on colon carcinogenesis and β-glucuronidase activity," Carcinogenesis 17:1343–1348.
117. Thompson, L. U., S. E. Rickard and M. M. Siedl. 1996. "Flaxseed and its lignan and oil components reduce mammary tumor growth at a late stage of carcinogenesis," Carcinogenesis 17(6):1373–1376.
118. Ribereau-Gayon, P. 1972. Plant Phenolics, Edinburgh: Oliver and Boyd. p. 254.
119. Dabrowski, K. J. and F. W. Sosulski. 1984. "Composition of free and hydrolizable phenolic acids in defatted flours of ten oilseeds," J. Agric. Food Chem. 32:128–130.
120. Oomah, B. D., E. O. Kenaschuk and G. Mazza. 1995. "Phenolic acids in flaxseed," J. Agric. Food Chem. 43(8):2016–2019.
121. Harris, R. K. and W. J. Haggerty. 1993. "Assays for potentially anticarcinogenic phytochemicals in flaxseed," Cereal Foods World 38:147–151.

122. Cook, N. C. and S. Samman. 1996. "Flavonoids—Chemistry, metabolism, cardioprotective effects and dietary sources," J. Nutr. Biochem. 7:66–76.

123. Ibraham, R. K. and M. Shaw. 1970. "Phenolic constituents of the oil flax (*Linum usitatissimum*)," Phytochemistry 9:1855–1858.

124. Oomah, B. D., G. Mazza and E. O. Kenaschuk. 1996. "Flavonoid content of flaxseed. Influence of cultivar and environment," Euphytica 90:163–167.

125. Thompson, L. U. 1994. "Phytic acid and other nutrients: are they partly responsible for health benefits of high fiber foods?" Dietary Fiber, D. Kritchevsky and C. Bonefield, New York: Plenum. pp. 305–317.

126. Bolley, D. S. and R. H. McCormack. 1952. "Separation of phytin from oil seed protein flours," J. Am. Oil Chem. Soc. 29:470–472.

127. Oomah, B. D., E. O. Kenaschuk and G. Mazza. 1996. "Phytic acid content of flaxseed as influenced by cultivar, growing season, and location," J. Agric. Food Chem. 44(9):2663–2666.

128. Budin, J. T., W. M. Breene and D. H. Putnam. 1995. "Some compositional properties of camelina (*Camelina sativa* L. Crantz) seeds and oils," J. Am. Oil Chem. Soc. 72:309–315.

129. Marquard, V. R., W. Schuster and H. Iran-Nejad. 1977. "Studies on tocopherol and thiamine content of linseed from worldwide cultivation and from phytotron under definite climatic conditions," Fette-Seifen-Anstrichm. 79:265–270.

130. Oomah, B. D., E. O. Kenaschuk and G. Mazza. 1997. "Tocopherols in flaxseed," J. Agric. Food Chem. 45:2076–2080.

131. Kolodziejczyk, P. P. and P. Fedic. 1995. "Processing flaxseed for human consumption," Flaxseed in Human Nutrition, S. C. Cunnane and L. U. Thompson, Champaign, IL: AOCS Press. pp. 261–280.

132. Eskin, N. A. M., B. E. McDonald, R. Przybylski, L. J. Malcolmson, R. Scartti, T. Mag, K. Ward and D. Adolph. 1996. "Canola Oil," Bailey's Industrial Oil and Fat Products, Fifth Edition, Vol. 2. Edible Oil and Fat Products: Oils and Oilseeds, Y. H. Hui, New York: John Wiley and Sons Inc. pp. 1–95.

133. Unger, E. H. 1990. "Commercial processing of canola and rapeseed: crushing and oil extraction," Canola and Rapeseed Production, Chemistry, Nutrition and Processing Technology, F. Shahidi, New York: Van Nostrand Reinhold. pp. 235–248.

134. Young, L. G. 1982. "Effects of processing on nutritive value of feeds: oilseeds and oilseed meals," Handbook of Nutritive Value of Processed Food. CRC Series in Nutrition. Vol. 2. Animal Feedstuffs, R. Miloslav, Jr., Boca Raton, FL: CRC Press. pp. 213–221.

135. Wanasundara, J. P. D. and F. Shahidi. 1994. "Functional properties and amino-acid composition of solvent extracted flaxseed meals," Food Chem. 49:45–51.

136. Wanasundara, P. K. J. P. D., R. Amarowicz, M. T. Kara and F. Shahidi. 1993. "Removal of cyanogenic glycosides of flaxseed meal," Food Chem. 48:263–266.

137. Varga, T. K. and L. L. Diosady. 1991. "Simultaneous extraction of oil and anti-nutritional compounds from flaxseed," J. Am. Oil Chem. Soc. 71:603–607.

138. Oomah, B. D. and G. Mazza. 1993. "Processing of flaxseed meal: Effect of solvent extraction on physicochemical characteristics," Lebensm.-Wiss. u. -Technol. 26:312–317.

139. Oomah, B. D., G. Mazza and R. Przybylski. 1996. "Comparison of flaxseed

meal lipids extracted with different solvents," Lebensm.-Wiss. u. -Technol. 29: 654–658.

140. Newton, J. and D. Snyder. 1977. "Nutritional aspects of long-chain omega-3 fatty acids and their use in bread enrichment," Cereal Foods World 42(3):126–131.
141. Sanftleben, J. F. 1932. "Method of making mucilaginous extract from seeds," U.S. Patent 1,841,763.
142. Mani, K. V., N. Nikolaiczuk and W. A. Maio. 1949. "Flaxseed mucilage and its effect on the feeding value of linseed oil meal in chick rations," Sci. Ag. 29: 86–90.
143. McGinnis, J. 1948. "Toxicity of linseed meal for growing chicks," Poultry Sci. 27:141–145.
144. Schlamb, K. F., C. O. Clagett and R. Bryant. 1955. "Comparison of the chick growth inhibition of unheated linseed hull and cotyledon fractions," Poultry Sci. 34:1404–1407.
145. Bolley, D. S. and R. H. McCormack. 1952. "Mucilaginous materials from flaxseed," U.S. Patent 2,593,528.
146. Singh, M. 1979. "Linseed as a protein source," Indian Food Packer 33:54–58.
147. Mandokhot, V. M. and M. Singh. 1979. "Studies on linseed (*Linum usitatissimum*) as a protein source for poultry. I. Process of demucilaging and dehulling of linseed and evaluation of processed materials by chemical analysis and with rats and chicks," Lebensm.-Wiss. u. -Technol. 16:25–31.
148. BeMiller, J. N. 1973. "Quince seed, psyllium seed, flaxseed and okra gums," Industrial Gums, 2nd ed., R. L. Whistler and J. N. BeMiller, New York: Academic Press. pp. 331–337.
149. Attström, R., P. O. Glantz, H. Hakansson and K. Larsson. 1993. "Saliva substitute," U.S. Patent No. 5,260,282. p. 14.
150. O'Mullane, J. E. and J. P. Hayter. 1993. "Linseed mucilage," International Patent No. PCT/GB93/00343.
151. Kankaanpää-Anttila, B. and M. Anttila. 1996. "Flax preparation, its use and production," International Patent No. PCT/FI96/00042.
152. Oomah, B. D., G. Mazza and W. Cui. 1994. "Optimization of protein extraction from flaxseed meal," Food Res. Int. 27:355–361.
153. Wanasundara, P. K. J. P. D. and F. Shahidi. 1996. "Optimization of hexametaphosphate-assisted extraction of flaxseed proteins using response surface methodology," J. Food Sci. 61(3):604–607.
154. Amarowicz, R. and F. Shahidi. 1994. "Application of Sephadex LH-20 chromatography for the separation of cyanogenic glycosides and hydrophylic phenolic fraction from flaxseed," J. Liq. Chromatogr. 17:1291–1299.
155. Jenkins, D. J. A. 1995. "Incorporation of flaxseed or flaxseed components into cereal foods," Flaxseed in Human Nutrition, S. C. Cunnane and L. U. Thompson, Champaign, IL: AOCS Press. pp. 281–294.
156. Smith, A. K., V. L. Johnsen and A. C. Beckel. 1946. "Linseed proteins . . . alkali dispersion and acid precipitation," Ind. Eng. Chem. 38:353–356.
157. Oomah, B. D. and G. Mazza. 1997. "Fractionation of flaxseed with an intermediate-sized batch dehuller," Lebensm.-Wiss. u. -Technol. Submitted August 29, 1997.

158. Witt, P. R. Jr. 1978. "Preparation of a beer-type beverage," U.S. Patent 4,073,947.

159. Lauredam, B. 1979. "Nutritive seamoss composition and method for preparing same," U.S. Patent 4,180,593.

160. Stitt, P. A. 1989. "Stable nutritive and therapeutic flaxseed compositions, methods of preparing the same, and therapeutic methods employing the same," U.S. Patent 4,857,326.

161. Krawczyk, T. 1996. "Lecithin: consider the possibilities," Int. News Fats, Oils Rel. Mat. (INFORM) 7(11):1158–1167.

162. Khorasani, G. R., P. H. Robinson and J. J. Kennelly. 1994. "Evaluation of solvent and expeller linseed meals as protein sources for dairy cattle," Can. J. Anim. Sci. 74:479–485.

163. Oomah, B. D. and G. Mazza. 1997. "Effect of dehulling on chemical composition and physical properties of flaxseed," Lebensm.-Wiss. u. -Technol. 30:135–140.

164. Chen, Z-Y., W. M. N. Ratnayake and S. C. Cunnane. 1994. "Oxidative stability of flaxseed during baking," J. Am. Oil Chem. Soc. 71(6):629–632.

165. Cowan, J. C., S. Koritala, K. Warner, G. R. List, K. J. Moulton and C. D. Evans. 1973. "Copper-hydrogenated soybean and linseed oils: composition, organoleptic quality and oxidative stability," J. Am. Oil Chem. Soc. 50(5):132–136.

166. Miyashita, K., N. Tateda and T. Ota. 1994. "Oxidative stability of free fatty acid mixtures from soybean, linseed, and sardine oils in an aqueous solution," Fisheries Science 60(3):315–318.

167. Yoshida, H., N. Hirooka and G. Kajimoto. 1990. "Microwave energy effects on quality of some seed oils," J. Food Sci. 55(5):1412–1416.

168. Holstun, J., D. Zetocha, L. Stearns and T. Petry. 1993. "The potential for flaxseed utilization in the U.S. baking industry," Report prepared for the North Dakota Oilseed Council and North Dakota Agricultural Products Utilization Commission, North Dakota State University.

169. McCue, N. 1995. "Showcase: fortification ingredients and functional proteins," Prepared Foods 164(11):62.

170. Serraino, M. R., L. U. Thompson and S. C. Cunnane. 1992. "Effect of low level flaxseed supplementation on the fatty acid composition of mammary glands and tumors in rats," Nutr. Res. 12(6):767–772.

171. Cameron, E., J. Bland and R. Marcuson. 1989. "Divergent effects of omega-6 and omega-3 fatty acids on mammary tumor development in C3H/Heston mice treated with DMBA," Nutr. Res. 9(4):383–393.

172. Simopoulos, A. P. 1994. "Fatty acids," Functional Foods: Designer Foods, Pharmafoods, Nutraceuticals, J. Goldberg, New York: Chapman and Hall, Inc. pp. 355–392.

173. Johnston, P. V. 1988. "Lipid modulation of immune responses," Nutrition and Immunology, R. K. Chondra, New York: Alan R. Liss, Inc. pp. 37–86.

174. Haumann, B. F. 1997. "Nutritional aspects of n–3 fatty acids," Int. News Fats, Oils Rel. Mat. (INFORM) 8(5):428–447.

175. Thompson, L. U. 1995. "Flaxseed, lignans, and cancer," Flaxseed in Human Nutrition, S. C. Cunnane, and L. U. Thompson, Champaign, IL: AOCS Press. pp. 219–236.

176. Gilbert, J. M. 1987. "Experimental colorectal cancer as a model of human disease," Ann. R. Coll. Surg. Engl. 69:48–53.
177. Serraino, M. and L. U. Thompson. 1991. "The effect of flaxseed supplementation on early risk markers for mammary carcinogenesis," Cancer Lett. 60(2): 135–142.
178. Serraino, M. and L. U. Thompson. 1992. "The effect of flaxseed supplementation on the initiation and promotional stages of mammary tumorigenesis," Nutr. Cancer, 17(2):153–159.
179. Thompson, L. U., L. Orcheson, S. Rickard and M. Seidl. 1994. "Anticarcinogenic effect of a mammalian lignan precursor from flaxseed," Proc. U.S. Flax Inst. 55:46–50.
180. Serraino, M. and L. U. Thompson. 1992. "Flaxseed supplementation and early markers of colon carcinogenesis," Cancer Lett. 63(2):159–165.
181. Thompson, L. U. 1994. "Antioxidants and hormone-mediated health benefits of whole grains," Crit. Rev. Food Sci. Nutr. 34(586):473–497.
182. Hirano, T., K. Fukuoka, K. Oka and Y. Matsumoto. 1991. "Differential sensitivity of human gastric cancer ATPase and normal gastric mucosa ATPase to the synthetic mammalian lignan analogue 2,3-dibenzyl-butane-11,4-diol (Hattalin)," Cancer Invest. 9:145.
183. Fukuda, Y., T. Osawa and M. Namiki. 1985. "Studies on antioxidative substances in sesame seed," Agric. Biol. Chem. 49:301–306.
184. Osawa, T., M. Nagata, M. Namiki and Y. Fukuda. 1985. "Sesamolinol, a novel antioxidant isolated from sesame seeds," Agric. Biol. Chem. 49:3351–3352.
185. Thompson, L. U. 1993. "Potential health benefits and problems associated with antinutrients in foods," Food Res. Int. 26:131–149.
186. Adlercreutz, H. 1984. "Does fiber-rich food containing animal lignan precursors protect against color and breast cancer? An extension of the 'fiber hypothesis,'" Gastroenterology 86:761.
187. Shultz, T. D., W. R. Bonorden and W. R. Seaman. 1991. "Effect of short-term flaxseed consumption on lignan and sex hormone metabolism in men," Nutr. Res. 11(10):1089–1100.
188. Phipps, W. R., M. C. Martini, J. W. Lampe, J. L. Slavin and M. S. Kurzer. 1993. "Effect of flax seed ingestion on the menstrual cycle," J. Clin. Endocrinol. Metab. 77(5):1215–1218.
189. Parbtani, A. and W. F. Clark. 1995. "Flaxseed and its components in renal disease," Flaxseed in Human Nutrition, S. C. Cunnane and L. U. Thompson, Champaign, IL: AOCS Press. pp. 244–260.
190. Hall, A. V., A. Parbtani, W. F. Clark, E. Spanner, M. Keeney, I. Chin-Yee, D. J. Philbrick and B. J. Holub. 1993. "Abrogation of MRL/lpr lupus nephritis by dietary flaxseed," Am. J. Kidney Dis. 22(2):326–332.
191. Ranhotra, G. S., J. A. Gelroth, B. K. Glaser and P. S. Potnis. 1993. "Lipidemic responses in rats fed flaxseed oil and meal," Cereal Chem. 70(3):364–368.
192. Anderson, J. W., D. A. Deakins, T. L. Floore, B. M. Smith and S. E. Whitis. 1990. "Dietary fiber and coronary heart disease," Crit. Rev. Food Sci. Nutr. 29(2):95–147.
193. Berggren, A. M., I. M. E. Björck, E. M. G. L. Nyman and B. O. Eggum. 1993. "Short-chain fatty acid content and pH in caecum of rats given various sources of carbohydrates," J. Sci. Food Agric. 63:397–406.

194. Nuttall, F. Q., A. D. Mooradian, M. C. Gannon, C. Billington and P. Krezowski. 1984. "Effect of protein ingestion on the glucose and insulin response to a standardized oral glucose load," Diab. Care 7:465–470.

195. Adlercreutz, H., T. Fotsis, J. Lampe, K. Wahala, T. Makela, G. Brunnow and T. Hase. 1993. "Quantitative determination of lignans and isoflavonoids in plasma of omnivorous and vegetarian women by isotope dilution gas chromatography-mass spectrometry," Scan. J. Clin. Lab. Invest. 53:5–18.

196. Borgmeyer, J. R., C. E. Smith and O. K. Huynh. 1992. "Isolation and characterization of a 25 kDa antifungal protein from flaxseeds," Biochem. Biophys. Res. Com. 187:480–487.

197. Yoon, J. H., L. U. Thompson and D. J. A. Jenkins. 1983. "The effect of phytic acid on in-vitro rate of starch digestibility and blood glucose response," Am. J. Clin. Nutr. 38:835–842.

198. Sognen, E. 1965. "Apparent depression in the absorption of strychnine, alcohol, sulphanilamide after oral administration of sodium fluoride, sodium oxalate, tetracemin and sodium phytate," Acta Pharmacol. Toxicol. 22:8–18.

199. Phang, J. M., C. M. Poore, J. Lopaczynska and G. C. Yeh. 1993. "Flavonol-stimulated efflux of 7,12-dimethylbenz(a) anthracene in multidrug-resistant breast cancer cells," Cancer Res. 53:5977–5981.

200. Dragsted, L. O., M. Strube and J. C. Larsen. 1993. "Cancer-protective factors in fruits and vegetables: biochemical and biological background," Pharmacol. Toxicol. 72 (Suppl. 1):116–135.

201. Steinmetz, K. A. and J. D. Potter. 1996. "Vegetables, fruit, and cancer prevention: A review," J. Am. Diet. Assoc. 96(10):1027–1039.

202. Bertram, J. S., L. N. Kolonel and F. L. Meyskens. 1987. "Rationale and strategies for chemoprevention of cancer in humans," Cancer Res. 47:3012–3031.

203. Fiala, E. S., B. S. Reddy and J. H. Weisburger. 1985. "Naturally occurring anticarcinogenic substances in foodstuffs," Ann. Rev. Nutr. 5:295–321.

204. Laurintzen, D. 1994. "Food enrichment with marine omega-3 fatty acids," Int. Food Ing. 1/2:41–44.

205. Wescott, N. D. and A. D. Muir. 1995. "Improved process for extracting lignans from flaxseed," U.S. Patent 08/415050.

206. Wescott, N. D. and A. D. Muir. 1996. "Process for extraction and purifying lignans and cinnamic acid derivatives from flaxseed," International Patent PCT/CA 96/00192.

CHAPTER 5

Functional Grape and Citrus Products

B. GIRARD[1]
G. MAZZA[1]

1. GRAPES

1.1. INTRODUCTION

GRAPES are the world's largest temperate fruit crop with approximately 65 million metric tons produced annually [1]. About 80% of the total crop is used in wine making, 13% is sold as table grapes and the balance is grown largely for raisins, juice and other products. Most grapes are grown in Europe, with Italy, France and Spain accounting for approximately 40% of the world's 9,000,000 hectares of grapevines [1,3]. California produces about a fifth of the world's raisins and 10% of the world's table grapes [2].

There are two major types of grapes: European and North American. European grapes belong to the species *Vitis vinifera* L., and over 95% of all the grapes produced are of this species. These grapes are characterized by a relatively thick skin that adheres to a firm pulp that is sweet throughout. Most *viniferas* grow best in a Mediterranean-type of climate with long, relatively dry summers and mild winters [2,3]. Certain varieties are used principally for wine; others for raisins or for table use. Leading wine varieties include 'Cabernet Sauvignon,' 'Chardonnay,' 'Pinot Noir,' 'Zinfandel' and 'Carignane.' Table grapes are large and tasty and have an attractive color. The chief varieties include 'Emperor' and 'Tokay,' which grow in large clusters of red berries. Other table grapes include the greenish-white, seedless 'Perlete' and

[1]Agriculture and Agri-Food Canada, Pacific Agri-Food Research Centre, Summerland, BC, Canada.

the black 'Ribier.' Most raisin grapes are seedless, and have a soft texture when dried. Leading raisin varieties include 'Thompson Seedless,' 'Black Corinth' and 'Muscat of Alexandria' [2,3].

North American grapes belong to two main species: *Vitis labrusca* and *V. rotundifolia*. Both species can be consumed fresh or processed into juice, wine, or jelly. The *labrusca* grapes are grown principally in the lower Great Lakes region of the United States and Canada. The most important variety is the 'Concord,' which has large purple berries. The *rotundifolia* or 'Muscadine' grapes grow throughout the southeastern United States, from North Carolina to eastern Texas. They are exemplified by the 'Scuppernong' variety, which is long-lived, disease-resistant and vigorous [3].

The components of grapes and grape products believed to play a significant role in preventing or delaying the onset of diseases including cancer and cardiovascular diseases are the phenolic compounds [4–7]. These compounds are secondary plant metabolites that contribute in an important manner to the flavor and color characteristics of grapes, grape juices and wines. The phenolic compounds of grapes include phenolic acids, anthocyanins, flavonols, flavan-3-ols, and tannins (Table 5.1). The flavonoids (C_6—C_3—C_6), which include the anthocyanins, flavanols and flavan-3-ols, are powerful antioxidants [5–10], and are found in high concentration in grapes and grape products [11]. These compounds exhibit a wide range of biochemical and pharmacological effects, including antiinflammatory and antiallergic effects [11]. Grape flavonoids such as quercetin, kaempferol, and myricetin also inhibit carcinogen-induced tumors in rats and mice [12–15]. Quercetin and other polyphe-

TABLE 5.1. Phenolic Components of Red and White Grapes.

	Content (mg/100 g F.W.)		
Compound	Red	White	Reference
Anthocyanins	8–388	—	33, 34, 35, 36
Flavonols	1.85–9.75	0.81–8.19	37
Flavan-3-ols[a]	22–37 ppm (juice); 2.5–16.7 (skin)	1.4–52.7 (skin)	38, 39, 40
Tannins[b]	32.1–78.1 (skin)	17.2 (skin)	38
Hydroxybenzoic acid derivatives	24.73 mg/100 g DW (skin)	0.4 mg/100 g DW (skin)	42
Hydroxycinnamic acid derivatives	10–109 (skin)	1.33–86.55 (skin)	43
Total phenolics	900–950	350 (skin); 100 (pulp)	33, 41

[a](+)-Cathechin (5) and (−)-epicatechin (13).
[b]Proanthocyanidins (85:15 procyanidin: prodelphinidin units).
Source: Adapted from Reference [11].

nolic flavonoids in wine have been shown to inhibit the oxidation and cytotoxicity of low-density lipoprotein (LDL) [6], and Frankel et al. [7] showed that red wine protects LDL from oxidation.

Anthocyanins have known pharmacological properties and are used by humans for therapeutic purposes. Applied orally or by intravenal or intramuscular injection, pharmaceutical preparations of *Vaccinium myrtillus* anthocyanins (VMA) reduce capillary permeability and fragility [16,17]. This anti-inflammatory activity of VMA accounts for their significant anti-edema properties and their action on diabetic microangiopathy [17–20]. It has also been reported that anthocyanins possess anti-ulcer activity [21] and provide protection against UV radiation [22].

Recently, the antioxidative activity of several anthocyanins including malvidin 3-*p*-coumaroylglucoside-5-glucoside, cyanidin 3-glucoside and cyanidin as well as crude extracts of grapes, currants, raspberries, and blueberries has been reported [23–27]. Malvidin 3-*p*-coumaroylglucoside-5-glucoside has been found to be twice as effective as commercially available antioxidants such as (+)-catechin and α-tocopherol. Cyanidin 3-*O*-β-D-glucoside and cyanidin have antioxidative activity in linoleic acid autoxidation, liposome, rabbit erythrocyte membrane, and rat liver microsomal systems. Cyanidin has a stronger activity than cyanidin 3-*O*-β-D-glucoside and the same activity as α-tocopherol in the liposome and rabbit erythrocyte membrane systems.

Two other components alleged to reduce the risk of cancer and coronary heart diseases are ellagic acid and resveratrol [28,29]. Ellagic acid ($C_{14}H_6O_8$) is an acid hydrolytic product of ellagitannin found in grape juice and wine [30]; and resveratrol (3,5,4′-trihydroxystilbene) is a stilbene phytoalexin produced in the leaves and fruit of grape in response to UV irradiation and to infections by the fungus *Botrytis cinerea* and by the powdery and downy mildew fungi [31]. The concentration of resveratrol in grape products ranges from about 0.5 to 15 mg/kg in fresh grape skins, and from 1.5 to 3 mg/L in wines. Grape juices contain less than 0.01 μg/L of resveratrol [31,32]. Ellagic acid content in 'Muscadine' grape juice varies from 1.6 to 23.1 μg/ml [30]. Factors that influence the amount and composition of biologically active compounds present in grapes and grape products vary greatly with the species, variety, maturity, seasonal conditions, production area, and yield of the fruit. Also, conditions of processing and storage affect the concentration of phenolic compounds in grapes and grape products such as wine and juice [11, 30–43].

1.2. PROCESSING OF GRAPE PRODUCTS

Grapes are currently processed primarily into wine, juice, raisins, and brandy. Other products include grapeseed oil, grape pomace, hydrocolloids, and anthocyanins [44–46].

1.2.1. Wine

Wine is a moderately alcoholic drink made by fermentation of juice extracted from fresh, ripe grapes. Wines may be classified by varietal names such as 'Cabernet Sauvignon,' 'Chardonnay,' 'Pinot Noir,' and 'Merlot,' or by generic names, which refer to regions in Europe where wines of that general type were first produced. Generic names include 'Burgundy,' 'Chianti,' and 'Chablis.'

The six main classes of wine are: red table wines, white table wines, rosé table wines, dessert wines, sparkling wines, and appetizer wines. The difference between these classes of wines is not only in their color or when they should be served; they differ significantly in production methods, composition, sensory quality, and physiological characteristics. For instance, red wines, which are produced by fermentation on the skins, contain 2–3 times more phenolics than white wines [47] (Table 5.2). White wines are usually

TABLE 5.2. Gross Phenolic Composition (in Gallic Acid Equivalent per Liter) for Typical Red and White Wines from *Vitis vinifera* Grapes.

		White Wine		Red Wine	
Phenolic Compound	Source[a]	Young	Aged	Young	Aged
Nonflavonoids, total		175	160–260	235	240–500
Cinnamates, derivatives	G, D	154	130	165	150
Low volatility benzene derivatives	D, M, G, E	10	15	50	60
Tyrosol	M	10	10	15	15
Volatile phenols	M, D, E	1	5	5	15
Hydrolyzable tannins, etc.	E	0	0–100	0	0–260
Macromolecular complexes					
Protein-tannin	G, D, E	10	5	5	10
Flavonoids, total		30	25	1060	705
Catechins	G	25	15	200	150
Flavanols	G, D	tr	tr	50	10
Anthocyanins	G	0	0	200	20
Soluble tannins, derivatives	G, D	5	10	550	450
Other flavonoids, derivatives	G, D, E, M			60	75
Total phenols		215	190–290	1,300	955–1,216

[a]D = degradation product; E = environment; cooperage, G =grapes; M = microbes, yeast.
Source: Adapted from Reference [11].

more delicate in flavor than red, and because of the lack of anthocyanins and very low levels of tannins [47], defects in taste and appearance are more apparent in them [40,44].

Figure 5.1 shows a flow diagram for the production of red and white wine from grapes. The major difference in the making of the two wine types is in the pre-fermentation operations, with white wine being produced by the fermentation of the pressed grape juice, and red wine being produced by the fermentation of the juice on the skins in order to extract the red color. The process of white wine production seeks to avoid direct or enzymatic breakdown of the components of the skin, seed, or stalk; therefore, pressing and filtration precede the fer-

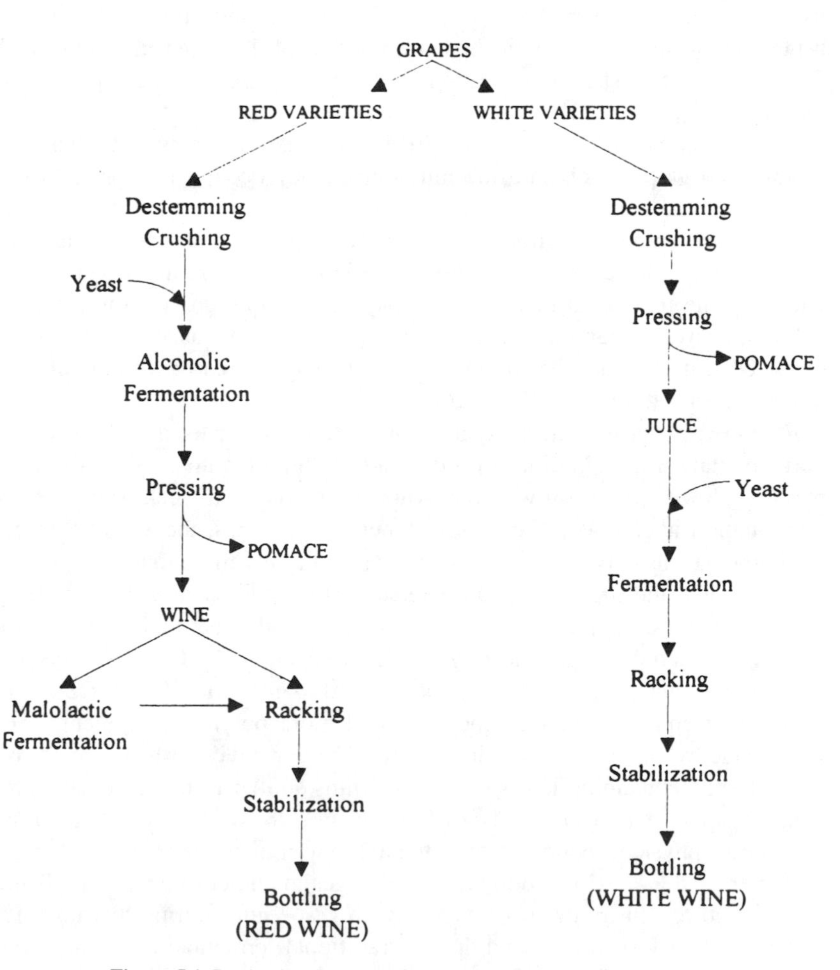

Figure 5.1 Production flowchart for red and white wine from grapes.

mentation processes. In the production of red wine, the extraction of anthocyanins and related phenolics from the grape solids begins with the crushing of grapes and continues through the fermentation and pressing operations. Raising the temperature to 50–60°C prior to fermentation of the mash, or to 30–40°C after the alcoholic fermentation, may be carried out to increase extraction of red pigments, as well as other phenolics and flavor components that contribute to the character of red wines.

Vigorous crushing enhances the extraction and diffusion of the anthocyanins and other phenolic compounds [48]; however, the resultant wines are frequently too astringent and bitter. Furthermore, enzymatic oxidation of phenolic compounds is enhanced, which may lead to browning of the must or juice and development of undesirable sensory characteristics of the wine. The use of sulfur dioxide (SO_2) as an antioxidant and antiseptic is widely accepted as an indispensable aid in wine making [49]. However, if too much SO_2 is added to musts, fermentation may be incomplete, and the color will be bleached [50].

Maceration, characterized by the diffusion of anthocyanins and other phenolics from grape solids into the must-wine, may occur either prior to fermentation as in thermovinification or during the alcoholic fermentation, either with crushed grapes (traditional vinification) or with whole grapes (carbonic maceration). In all cases, maceration time is most important. In wines produced by the traditional method, 5–6 days of maceration is sufficient for a colored, fruity, low-tannin wine for early drinking. If the maceration period is extended, anthocyanin content and color intensity decrease, while total phenolics continue to increase [36,51,52].

Extended pomace contact or maceration time is practised in France and northern Italy, where in order to secure a very high tannin content, the wine may be allowed to remain with the skins and seeds for a week or more after fermentation is completed. In North American wineries, the crushed grapes are in the vats usually only about 3–4 days and rarely more than 5 days [44].

Timberlake and Bridle [53] compared wines from Cascade grapes made by carbonic maceration, thermovinification, and the traditional vinification methods. They found that wine made by thermovinification (60°C for 30 min) was much more colored than that fermented on its skin (10 to 15°C for 2 days); however, it contained less anthocyanin and more polymeric pigments. The wine made by carbonic maceration (30 to 35°C for 7 days) was the least colored, despite containing levels of anthocyanins similar to those of wine produced by thermovinification. The differences in color were attributed to variations in the physicochemical state of the anthocyanins.

Somers and Evans [54] followed the changes in anthocyanins, total phenolics, and color density of heat-treated Syrah grape juice during thermovinification at pH 3.40 and 3.83 and during traditional fermentation on the skins. Their results reveal that by the end of fermentation at pH 3.83, color density

(E_{420} + E_{520}) had decreased fivefold, whereas the anthocyanin content and total phenolics had declined only by approximately 30%. At pH 3.4, the color density decreased threefold and the total anthocyanins and total phenolics declined by 20%. The authors attributed the majority of the loss in color density to the destructive effect of ethanol on structures of deeply colored pigment aggregates present in the juice prior to fermentation [54].

The changes in 15 anthocyanins in musts and wines from three cultivars of grapes from southern Italy were reported by Leone et al. [55]. Table 5.3 gives the evolution of the anthocyanins in Troia must and wine produced by the conventional fermentation method. As in other *Viniferas*, malvidin 3-glucoside and its acetate and coumarate derivatives were the major anthocyanins of Troia grapes. Within 24 hours from crushing of the grapes, the percentage of malvidin 3-glucoside had changed from 28.6 to 44.4%, malvidin 3-acetylglucoside remained near 20%, and malvidin 3-*p*-coumaroylglucoside decreased from 26.6 to 12.3% of total anthocyanin content. Seven days after the beginning of wine making, at the time of drawing off the must and pressing of the pomace, the total anthocyanin content of the must had increased from 445 mg/L at the beginning of maceration to 1079 mg/L, and the percent distribution of the pigments had undergone only limited variations. In wine at the third racking, 7 months after vinification, the malvidin-derived anthocyanins accounted for 85% of the total anthocyanins in the wine. At this stage, the delphinidin, cyanidin, petunidin, and peonidin derivatives were only minor components or had completely disappeared from the wine. The amount of the major anthocyanins transferred from the grapes to the 7-month-old wine were 41% malvidin 3-glucoside, 39% malvidin 3-acetylglucoside, and only 9% malvidin 3-*p*-coumaroylglucoside. The corresponding values for a 20-day old 'Syrah' wine are 31%, 32% and 8.5%, respectively [56].

The polyphenol composition of wines produced by carbonic maceration is closely linked to the combination of temperature and duration of the fermentation. It has been reported that it requires 10 days at 30–32°C to obtain wines rich in tannins and 6 days at 32°C or 13 days at 25°C to obtain a wine more colored than tannic [57].

Changes in anthocyanins and other phenolics as a result of their adsorption/desorption by grape solids and yeast have been reported [58]; however, such effects are minimal. Nonetheless, seed and stalk phenols are qualitatively and quantitatively different from those of the berry, and under conditions of vigorous crushing and extended pomace contact they will contribute to the quality of the finished product [58–61].

Champagne and other sparkling wines are produced by carbonation under pressure or by being allowed to continue fermentation (to produce CO_2) in the bottle. Dessert wines are generally produced by fortification with alcohol so that they retain some of the sugars present in the grapes. They develop their special quality by being allowed to undergo a prolonged, slow oxidation [44].

TABLE 5.3. Changes in Anthocyanin Composition During Making of Red Wine.[a,b]

	Fermentation								Racking					
	Grapes		24 h		72 h		Pressing		1		2		3	
Anthocyanin	ppm	%	mg/L	%	mg/L	%	mg/L	%	mg/L	%	mg/L	%	mg/L	%
Dp	85	4.9	26	5.8	40	3.2	32	3.0	22	2.0	21	2.7	12	2.7
Cn	8	0.5												
Pt	83	4.8	24	5.4	68	5.4	60	5.6	53	4.9	41	5.2	24	5.4
Pn	55	3.1	16	3.6	13	1.0	21	1.9	15	1.4	6	0.8	6	1.3
Mv	500	28.6	198	44.4	551	43.7	464	43.0	523	48.1	362	45.8	206	46.3
Dp acetate	18	1.0			14	1.1	29	2.7			6	0.8	6	1.3
Cy acetate	tr.						13	1.2	23	2.1	5	0.6	6	1.3
Pt acetate	19	1.1	8	1.8	33	2.6	20	1.9	23	2.1	17	2.1	6	1.3
Pn acetate	13	0.7	6	1.3	32	2.5	12	1.1	14	1.3	6	0.8	6	1.3
Mv acetate	335	19.2	93	20.9	300	23.8	256	23.7	261	24.0	204	25.8	129	29.0
Dp cumarate	67	3.8			11	0.9	6	0.5	13	1.2	6	0.8		
Mv caffeoate	15	0.9												
Pt cumerate	42	2.4	13	2.9	30	2.4	20	1.9	19	1.8	14	1.8		
Pn cumerate	25	1.4	7	1.6	16	1.3	16	1.5	9	0.8	9	1.1		
Mv cumarate	482	27.6	55	12.3	153	12.1	130	12.0	112	10.3	94	11.9	44	9.9
Total	1,747		446		1261		1079		1087		791		445	

[a]Crushing of grapes: 19-10-82; Pressing: 23-10-82; Racking: 27-10-82; Second racking: 30-11-82; Third racking: 5-5-83.
[b]Dp = delphinidin 3-glucoside; Cy = cyanidin 3-glucoside; Pt = petunidin 3-glucoside; Mv = malvidin 3-glucoside.
Source: Adapted from Reference [55].

1.2.2. Juice

Grape juice, the liquid expressed from suitably ripened grapes, differs little in composition from the grapes except for the content of crude fibre and the oils, which are present primarily in the seed. In North America, the majority of red grape juice is prepared from Concord grapes (*V. labrusca*) [62,63]. *Vinifera* grapes are much higher in sugar, lower in acidity and not as flavorful as *labrusca* grapes. This lack of tartness and flavor is believed to be the reason for the limited quantity of *vinifera* grapes processed into juice [62,63].

A typical purple-red color is associated with high quality in grape juice, and changes in color during processing and storage from purple-red to brown result in a drastic decline in quality [64]. The color of 'Concord' juice is largely due to over 30 anthocyanin pigments located in and adjacent to the skin. Maturity influences the color of the grapes and, consequently, the juice made from them. Mature grapes yield juice with superior sensory quality and more desirable color than unripe grapes.

Concord juice is acceptable only when hot-pressed. In this process, the stemmed/crushed grapes are heated to 60°C by passing through a heat exchanger. The heating step is followed by addition of 50–100 ppm of pectinase enzyme and a press aid to reduce the slipperiness of the pulp, thus permitting the effective use of a screw press. The mash is generally hot-pressed to maximize yield and color extraction. Potassium metabisulphite may be used to prevent browning. The juice is flash pasteurized at 85°C and stored in bulk at approximately 0°C for a few weeks to precipitate the excess potassium bitartrate. The tartrate precipitates are known as argols and constitute approximately 4 kg/tonne of original grape juice. Unlike the tartrates from wine, which tend to appear in the form of large pure crystals (wine stones), tartrates from grape juice are much smaller and contain substantial amounts of occluded pigments [63]. The detartrated juice that is to be preserved by pasteurization must be treated with bentonite in order to remove proteins which form an undesirable haze upon heating. The juice may be further depectinized, filtered, and concentrated or bottled utilizing a pasteurization procedure to prevent microbial spoilage. Grape juice is most often concentrated by evaporation or freezing of water; however, concentration is also possible using a combination of reverse osmosis and evaporation [63].

Few studies on the content of flavonoids and other phenolics of grape juice have been published. However, recent results reported by Hertog et al. [65] show that the contents of the potentially anticarcinogenic flavonoids, quercetin and myricetin, in red wines and red grapes vary from 4 to 16 mg/L and from 7 to 9 mg/L, respectively (Table 5.4).

TABLE 5.4. Quercetin and Myricetin Contents of Wines and Fruit Juices.

Beverage	Concentration (mg/L)[a]	
	Quercetin	Myricetin
Wine		
Red Rioja Otonal 1990	4.1	9.3
Red Chianti 1990	16	8.0
Red California Dry Pinot Noir 1990	8.8	6.9
White Bordeaux St. Loubes Rineaux 1990	<0.5	<0.5
Fruit juice		
Apple juice (Albert Heijn, Zaandam)	2.5	<0.5
Grape juice (Riedel, Ede)	4.4	6.2
Tomato juice	13	<0.5
Grapefruit juice (fresh)	4.9	<0.5
Lemon juice (fresh)	7.4	<0.5
Orange juice (fresh)	3.4	<0.5
Orange juice	5.7	<0.5
Other beverages		
Beer (Heineken)	<0.5	<0.5
Chocolate milk (semi-skimmed milk)	1.3	<0.5
Coffee	<0.5	<0.5

[a]Mean of duplicate determination; <0.5 below the limit of detection.
Source: Adapted from Reference [65].

1.2.3. Grape Pomace

Grape pomace or marc consists of pressed skins, seeds and stems, and represents as much as 20% of the weight of grapes processed into wine and juice [44,45]. Table 5.5 gives the composition of Concord and De Chaunac pomace samples from commercial wineries and juice processing operations in the Niagara Peninsula of Canada [46].

In the past, grape pomace was disposed of in a number of ways. Some wineries have dehydrated the pomace to low moisture content and ground it for use in feeding livestock, particularly dairy cows [44]. Growers have also spread it on vineyards as a soil conditioner, but this practice is declining although growers may be paid to truck the pomace away from wineries. Consequently, considerable quantities of pomace are taken to disposal sites, and these sites are becoming more difficult to locate and expensive to operate. A variety of products including ethanol, tartrates, citric acid, grape seed oil, grape seed tannins, hydrocolloids, and anthocyanins can be produced from grape pomace [44–46]. Figure 5.2 shows a scheme for the production of anthocyanin pigments, and grapeseed tannins and oil. The first step is the separation of the seeds from grape pomace for oil recovery by mechanical press-

TABLE 5.5. Composition of Concord and De Chaunac Pomace Samples Obtained from Commercial Pressing Operations.

	Concord			De Chaunac		
Component	Cold Pressed	Hot Pressed	Fermented Skins	Cold Pressed	Hot Pressed	Fermented Skins
Seed (%)	15	22	18	30	36	37
Total soluble solids (%)	13	12	5	10	9	4
Total acidity (g/L)	13	9	11	7	7	8
Tannin (mg/100 g)[a]	391	254	178	444	120	120
Alcohol (%)	tr	tr	6	tr	tr	2.4
Methyl anthranilate (ppm)	8	5	5	—	—	—
Total volatile esters (ppm)	57	52	75	3	3	38
Volative acidity (g/L)	0.2	0.1	0.3	1	1	1
Total anthocyanin (mg/100 g)	460	200	360	425	79	211

[a]Does not include tannin from the seed; tr, trace.
Source: Adapted from Reference [46].

ing or by solvent extraction of the ground seeds. Fermentation of pomace can yield ethanol, which may be used for fortification of dessert wines, for fuel alcohol and other uses. Tartrates can be extracted by a continuous method or batch process [44].

Anthocyanins are probably the most valuable components of grape pomace and a large number of methods for their extraction have been reported. Enocyanin or "enocianina," a deeply colored extract of red grape pomace, has been produced commercially in Italy since 1879 [66–69]. The general method for the commercial production of enocyanin involves three major steps: (1) maceration of the pomace in a mild solution of sulfur dioxide for 48–72 hours, (2) separation of the water phase from the spent pomace, and (3) vacuum concentration of the water extract, with or without recovery of ethanol. The maceration or steeping process is normally carried out by mixing one part of pomace with one part of 0.1–0.2% aqueous sulfur dioxide solution or its equivalent in bisulfite or metabisulfite. To maximize the extraction of anthocyanins, the pomace-SO_2 solution is thoroughly mixed several times over the 48–72 hour maceration period. Aqueous sulfur dioxide is used to improve the extraction of the anthocyanins, and to protect the pigments

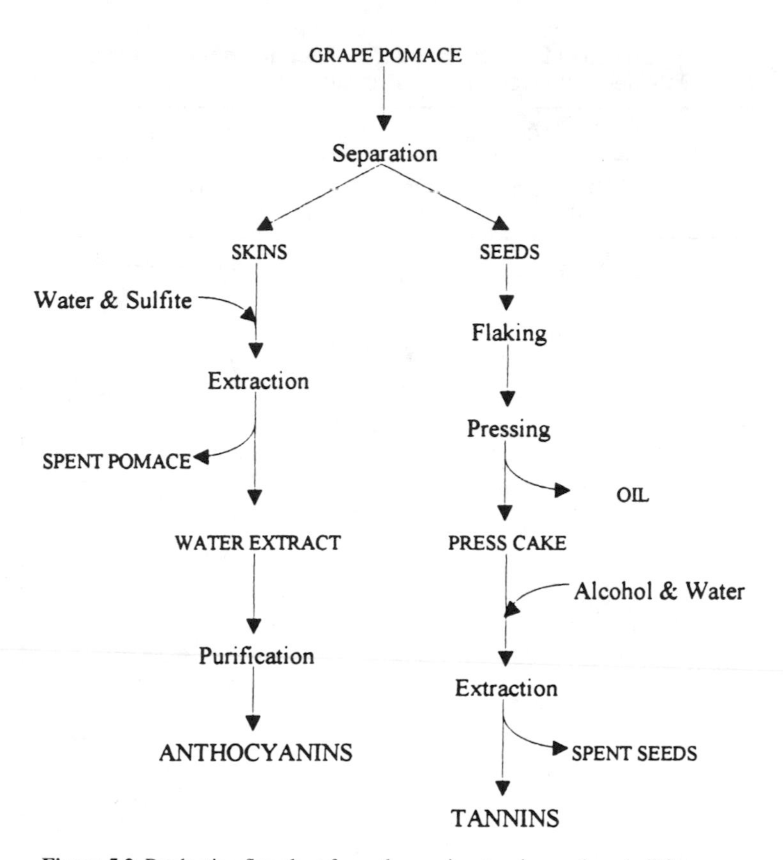

Figure 5.2 Production flowchart for anthocyanins, tannins, and seed oil from grape pomace.

from oxidation and microbial spoilage. The separation of the aqueous pigment extract from the pomace is normally achieved by allowing the free-run extract to flow into a tub and pumping it to a storage tank. The pomace is then pressed using a vertical or a horizontal basket or a Willmes press, and both the press and free-run extracts are combined to give a practically colorless liquid which remains as long as sufficient SO_2 is present. This diluted, aqueous, pigment extract is then filtered, desulfurized and concentrated by vacuum evaporation at 40–45°C to produce an intensely colored concentrate, or spray-dried to produce a dark-red water-soluble powder.

Langston [70] has patented a process for production of a pigment extract free of sugars, organic acids, polymerized anthocyanins, and other water-soluble material. This product is obtained using an aqueous extraction solvent containing bisulfite, followed by chromatographic separation on a nonionic adsorbent. Fuleki and Babjak [46] developed a process for the production of a liquid or dry food colorant from grape pomace. The product, which is completely soluble in water and alcohol, has an anthocyanin concentration of 40 g/kg in the powder and 10 g/kg in the liquid form. The colors produced depend on the pH and the concentration of the colorant, with color intensification from light red to deep red occurring with decreasing pH. Canada, the United States, Japan and countries in the European Economic Community permit the use of this colorant in food. The manufacturer recommends it for use in beverages, jams, jellies, syrups, drink-mix crystals, ice creams, pastries, confectioneries, and also some cosmetics and pharmaceuticals [46].

Grape seed tannins are primarily condensed or non-hydrolysable tannins, and can be considered as dimers or higher oligomers of variously substituted flavan-3-ols. The monomeric units are usually linked by carbon-carbon bonds, normally between carbon-4 on one flavan-3-ol molecule and carbon-8 on the adjacent molecule. On heating with strong acids, the condensed tannins polymerize further to produce red amorphous compounds known as phlobaphenes and also yield small quantities of anthocyanins. This has resulted in a third generic name for the condensed tannins, namely, proanthocyanidins [71–73]. The content and composition of condensed tannins and flavan-3-ols can vary with the variety, the degree of maturity and the part of the berry studied [38,74–76]. Table 5.6 lists the proanthocyanidins and monomeric flavan-3-ols isolated from grape seeds and skins by HPLC. As can be noted, the composition of the seeds is much more diverse than that of the skins, with the former containing 27 different compounds. The content of the monomeric and oligomeric flavan-3-ols are also much higher in seeds, whereas there are only traces of flavan-3-ol derivatives in pulp.

Oil is a major component of grape seeds. On a dry-weight basis, whole seeds contain 11 to 15% oil of which 62 to 71% is linoleic acid (18:2), 14 to 28% is oleic acid (18:1), and 10 to 14% saturated fatty acids [44]. The oil also contains 0.03 to 0.07% tocopherols, which markedly protect the oil quality during storage.

1.3. PHYSIOLOGICAL PROPERTIES

In traditional medicine, grapes and other fruits are used in the preparation of extracts including infusions, tinctures, juices, and syrups. In 1939, Rusznyàk and Szent-Györgyi observed that a mixture of two flavanones decreased capillary permeability and fragility in humans and proposed the name vitamin P [77]. The term vitamin P had to be abandoned because ultimately the flavonoids did not meet the definition of vitamins. However, in recent years numerous studies have shown that flavonoids and other phenolics, present in grapes and grape products, possess anticarcinogenic, anti-inflammatory, antihepatotoxic, antibacterial, antiviral, antiallergic, antithrombotic, and antioxidant effects [11,12,16,17].

TABLE 5.6. Proanthocyanidins in Grape Seeds and Skins.

Compounds isolated from seeds:

- Catechin-(4$\alpha \rightarrow$8)-catechin-(4$\alpha \rightarrow$8)-catechin (C2)
- Catechin-(4$\alpha \rightarrow$8)-catechin (B3)
- Epicatechin-(4$\beta \rightarrow$8)-epicatechin (B1)
- (+)-Catechin
- Epicatechin-(4$\beta \rightarrow$8)-epicatechin-(4$\beta \rightarrow$8)-catechin
- Catechin-(4$\alpha \rightarrow$8)-epicatechin (B4)
- Catechin-(4$\alpha \rightarrow$8)-catechin-(4$\alpha \rightarrow$8)-epicatechin
- Epicatechin-(4$\beta \rightarrow$6)-epicatechin-(4$\beta \rightarrow$6)-catechin
- Catechin-(4$\alpha \rightarrow$6)-catechin (B6)
- Epicatechin-(4$\beta \rightarrow$6)-epicatechin-(4$\beta \rightarrow$8)-epicatechin
- Epicatechin-(4$\beta \rightarrow$8)-epicatechin (B2)
- Epicatechin-(4$\beta \rightarrow$8)-epicatechin-3-*O*-gallate-(4$\beta \rightarrow$8)-catechin
- Epicatechin-3-*O*-gallate-(4$\beta \rightarrow$8)-epicatechin(B2-3-*O*-gallate)
- (−)-Epicatechin
- Catechin-(4$\alpha \rightarrow$8)-epicatechin-3-*O*-gallate (B4-3′-*O*-gallate)
- Epicatechin-(4$\beta \rightarrow$8)-epicatechin-(4$\beta \rightarrow$6)-catechin
- Epicatechin-3-*O*-gallate-(4$\beta \rightarrow$8)-catechin (B1-3-*O*-gallate)
- Epicatechin-(4$\beta \rightarrow$6)-catechin (B7)
- Epicatechin-(4$\beta \rightarrow$8)-epicatechin-(4$\beta \rightarrow$8)-epicatechin (C1)
- Epicatechin-(4$\beta \rightarrow$8)-epicatechin-(4$\beta \rightarrow$8)-epicatechin-(4$\beta \rightarrow$8)-epicatechin
- (−)-Epicatechin-3-*O*-gallate
- Epicatechin-3-*O*-gallate-(4$\beta \rightarrow$6)-catechin (B7-3-*O*-gallate)
- Epicatechin-3-*O*-gallate-(4$\beta \rightarrow$8)-epicatechin-3-*O*-gallate (B2-3,3′-*O*-digallate)
- Epicatechin-(4$\beta \rightarrow$8)-epicatechin-(4$\beta \rightarrow$8)-epicatechin-3-*O*-gallate
- Epicatechin-(4$\beta \rightarrow$8)-epicatechin-3-*O*-gallate-(4$\beta \rightarrow$8)-epicatechin-3-*O*-gallate
- Epicatechin-(4$\beta \rightarrow$6)-epicatechin (B5)

Compounds isolated from skin:

- Catechin-(4$\alpha \rightarrow$8)-catechin (Dimer B3)
- Epicatechin-(4$\beta \rightarrow$8)-catechin (Dimer B1)
- (+)-Catechin
- Epicatechin-(4$\beta \rightarrow$8)-epicatechin-(4$\beta \rightarrow$8)-catechin
- Catechin-(4$\alpha \rightarrow$8)-epicatechin (Dimer B4)
- Epicatechin-(4$\beta \rightarrow$8)-epicatechin-3-*O*-gallate (B2-3′*O*-gallate)
- Epicatechin-(4$\beta \rightarrow$8)-epicatechin-(4$\beta \rightarrow$8)-epicatechin (Trimer C1)
- (−)-Epicatechin-3-*O*-gallate

Source: Adapted from References [74, 75].

1.3.1. Anticarcinogenic Effects

The anticarcinogenic activity of phenolics has been correlated with the inhibition of colon, esophagus, lung, liver, mammary, and skin cancers [78]. Examples of grape phenolics that inhibit carcinogenesis include resveratrol [29], quercetin [13,15,79], caffeic acid [80,81], ellagic acid [28,82,83], and flavan-3-ols [84,85]. Resveratrol has been shown to have cancer chemopreventive activity in assays representing three major stages of carcinogenesis [29]. It has been found to act as an antioxidant and antimutagen and to induce phase II drug-metabolizing enzymes (anti-initiation activity); it mediated anti-inflammatory effects and inhibited cyclooxygenase and hydroperoxidase functions (antiprogression activity); and it induced human promyelocytic leukemia cell differentiation (antiprogression activity). In addition, resveratrol inhibited the development of preneoplastic lesions in carcinogen-treated mouse mammary glands in culture and inhibited tumorigenesis in a mouse skin cancer model [29].

Flavonoids and polyphenols have been shown to impact on the initiation step of cancer development by protecting the cells against direct-acting carcinogens such as nitrosamines [13] or altering their metabolic activation [83]. Particularly active polyphenols are the monomeric flavan-3-ols [84,85] and ellagic acid [28,82]; for the latter compound, a mechanism based on the structural similarity to polycyclic aromatic compounds has been proposed [86]. Antitumor-promoting activity of flavonoids has been connected to the inhibition of various cellular DNA and RNA polymerases [87] and/or the inactivation of ornithine decarboxylase [88]. In addition, some flavonoids such as quercetin appear to be effective in assisting cell cycle progression.

1.3.2. Anti-Atherogenic Effects

The association between grape phenolics and coronary heart disease (CHD) has been ascribed in part to the presence of flavonoids and resveratrol in red wine [7–9,89–92]. In addition, several epidemiological studies have shown that coronary heart disease mortality can be decreased by moderate consumption of alcohol, especially red wine [93–95]. The primary mechanisms believed to be responsible for this reduced risk factor include reduced platelet coagulability [96,97] and higher circulatory high-density lipoprotein cholesterol (HDL), which is increased by ethanol in a dose-response manner [94,95]. Other mechanisms such as inhibition of lipoprotein oxidation, free-radical scavenging and modulation of eicosanoid metabolism [98–101] are also thought to play a role in the reduction of atherosclerosis and its sequelae, including CHD, in moderate drinkers. Consumption of wine and beer has been associated with greater decreases in cardiovascular disease than consumption of spirits [102], possibly because wine and beer are rich in phenolic compounds that inhibit oxidative reactions.

1.3.3. Anti-Inflammatory Activity

This was the first known pharmacological effect of the flavonoids [77]. Several prescription and non-prescription pharmaceutical products containing anthocyanins from bilberry (*Vaccinium myrtillus*) as the active principle are used to control capillary permeability and fragility [16,19,20]. The anti-inflammatory activity of these anthocyanin extracts accounts for their significant anti-edema properties and their action on diabetic microangiopathy [20]. Flavan-3-ols, (+)-catechin, and (−)-epicatechin, found at concentrations as high as 52.7 mg/100 g of the dry weight of grape skins (Table 5.1), have been isolated from several traditional drugs that inhibit various biological events that are linked to inflammation. Two such drugs are *Asoka Aristha,* used in Sri Lanka to treat menorrhagia (excessive menstrual discharge), and *Cinnamoni Cortex,* used in Chinese medicine for analgesia or absence of the sense of pain without loss of consciousness [103].

1.3.4. Antibacterial and Antiviral Activity

Grape phenolics, especially caffeic acid, (−)-epicatechin and chlorogenic acid, possess antibacterial or antiviral activities [103]. Hydroxybenzoic, salicylic, gallic, and protocatechuic acids have also been reported to possess an antibacterial effect [104,105]. The antiviral potential of epicatechin observed *in vitro* has been suggested to be due to inhibition of the reverse transcriptase derived from Moloney murine leukaemia virus [103]. Reverse transcription inhibitors can be very specific for retroviruses because the action of reverse transcriptase is different from cellular enzymes, including DNA polymerase [103]. Chlorogenic acid has been found to be active against the Epstein-Barr and the HIV viruses [103]. Most of the phenolic compounds tested for antimicrobial properties, however, have been shown to display considerably lower activity than products such as antibiotics [17].

1.3.5. Antioxidant Activity

Antioxidation is one of the most important mechanisms for preventing or delaying the onset of major degenerative diseases of aging, including cancer, heart disease, cataracts, and cognitive disfunction. The antioxidants are believed to exert their effects by blocking oxidative processes and free radicals that contribute to the causation of these chronic diseases [106–107]. Several grape phenolics, especially catechins, flavonols, anthocyanins, and tannins, have been shown to perform these functions [78,89,106–110].

1.4. CONCLUSIONS

From the foregoing, it is evident that grapes and grape products are rich in phenolic compounds, particularly flavonoids, which have demonstrated a wide range of biochemical and pharmacological effects, including anticarcinogenic, antiatherogenic, anti-inflammatory, antimicrobial, and antioxidant activities. The available information suggests that regular consumption of currently available grape products should have a long-term health benefit. However, for increased concentration of grape phenolics, such as resveratrol, ellagic acid and flavonoids, new food products rich in these phytochemicals need to be developed. The by-products of wine making, grape skins, seeds and cluster stems are rich in catechins, proanthocyanidins and/or anthocyanins and provide opportunities for producing concentrates rich in these powerful natural antioxidants, which can then be incorporated in a variety of foods such as breakfast cereals, bakery products, and confectionaries. Novel methods for processing grape pomace into anthocyanins, seed tannins and seed oils are presented. Also, the influence of type of grapes and winemaking techniques on the content of physiologically active catechins and proanthocyanidins and other phenolics in wine is discussed. There is, however, a need for a better understanding of the chemistry and *in vivo* functions of grape phenolics. Research is needed not only to define mechanisms of these compounds as they can be used effectively in food systems, but also to establish their safety, and fully understand their potential health benefits when added to food systems.

2. CITRUS FRUITS

2.1. INTRODUCTION

Citrus are the world's largest subtropical and tropical fruit crop with approximately 74 million metric tons produced annually [1]. Oranges account for 70% of this total production. The major producing countries of oranges are Brazil (17.5 million tons), the United States (7.5 million tons) and China (4.7 million tons) [1]. In recent years, Brazil has accounted for about half of the oranges processed in the world, with the United States contributing for about 30%. Florida is the dominant orange processor in the United States while California is the largest U.S. supplier of fresh oranges [111].

Anatomically, citrus fruits such as orange (*Citrus sinensis*), tangerine (*Citrus reticulata*), lemon (*Citrus limon*), and grapefruit (*Citrus paradisi*) consist of an outer peel or rind, which includes epidermis, flavedo, and albedo (Figure 5.3). The flavedo in the subepidermal region contains chromoplasts imparting green, yellow, or orange color to the fruit, and numerous oil glands filled with aromatic essential oils. The albedo (mesocarp) is made up of spongy layers of parenchymatous cells rich in pectin. The inner flesh or endocarp consists of segments (carpels) distributed around a soft pithy core forming the central axis of the fruit. Surrounded by a thin wall (carpellary membrane called *septum*), each segment is filled with closely compacted juice vesicles from which citrus juice is primarily derived. Seeds may be found within the segments adjacent to the core.

The recognition of physiologically active components in citrus fruits and

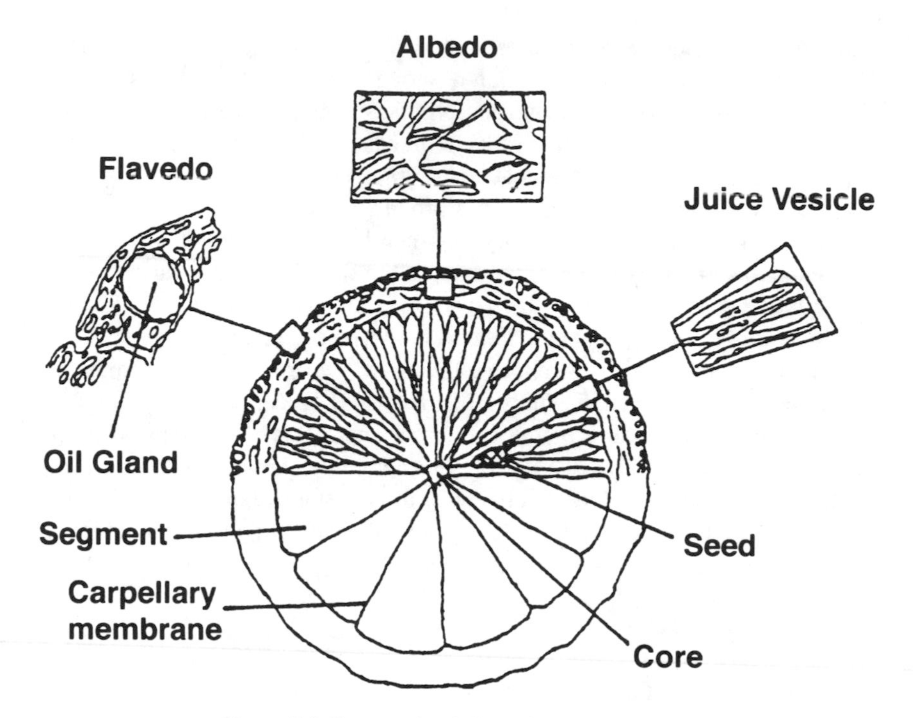

Figure 5.3 Cross-sectional illustration of a citrus fruit.

their contribution to human health has proved to be a growing area of research. A large number of constituents in citrus products have been shown to be capable of preventing or alleviating diseases and promoting health [112–114]. Vitamin C, E, and carotenoids, for instance, are thought to play a role in preventing or delaying the onset of major degenerative diseases of aging such as cancer, cardiovascular disease, and cataracts by counteracting oxidative processes. Similarly, several "non nutrient" components of citrus, including limonoids and flavonoids, appear to inhibit carcinogenesis by acting as blocking and/or suppressing agents.

2.2. COMPONENTS AND THEIR EFFECTS ON HEALTH

2.2.1. Flavonoids

Citrus flavonoids and limonoids are two main classes of compounds that have been extensively investigated not only because of their flavor impact on citrus juices but also because of their pharmacological activity, their potential for use as taxonomic markers, and their high value as by-products of the citrus industry. Four types of flavonoids occur in citrus: flavanones, flavones, flavonols and anthocyanins (Table 5.7). The flavanones predominate among the citrus flavonoids; the flavones and the flavonols are present in considerably smaller amounts. Naringin is the major flavanone glycoside in grapefruit, narirutin and hesperidin in sweet orange, and eriocitrin and hesperidin in lemon [115,116]. Anthocyanins are only found in certain red varieties (e.g., 'Moro') from which the name "blood oranges" is derived [117].

Purified flavanoid extracts of citrus peel have been manufactured by citrus processors and utilized as food supplements for both human and animal use for several decades. Once claimed to possess vitamin-like activity for their effects on capillary permeability and fragility, some bioflavonoids have sufficient antibacterial, antifungal, and antiviral activity to be considered for use in combatting infection [118]. The benefits of flavonoids in the human diet have been increasingly studied for numerous aspects associated with health and diseases.

Recently, it has been determined that grapefruit juice increased the systemic bioavailability of certain drugs such as felodipine and other related dihydropyridine calcium antagonists [119]. Similarly, daily consumption of grapefruit juice increased plasma cyclosporin concentrations in patients who had received an allographic kidney transplant [120]. Since drug interactions did not occur with orange juice, these pharmacokinetic effects may be attributed to a substance(s) specific to grapefruit juice (i.e., naringin and/or other bioflavonoids) [121].

It is now well established that cells involved in immunity and inflammation can be affected by several flavonoids such as quercetin, tangeritin, fisetin, and others. Quercetin has been widely studied and found to affect the secretory, motile, and mitogenic responses of various cells, including the inhibition of phytomitogenic stimulants on lymphocytes [122], the inhibition of LDL uptake into macrophages [123], the inhibition of the respiratory burst in stimulated neutrophils [124], the inhibition of mast cell and basophils mediator release [125], and the inhibition of aggregation and release reaction of platelets stimulated by secretogogues [114].

There is further concrete evidence to indicate that selected citrus and other naturally occurring flavonoids possess anticancer activities. It has been established that inhibition of *in vivo* carcinogenesis can be achieved by treating animals with certain flavonoids [126]. Quercetin or one of its metabolites appears to cross the gastrointestinal mucosal barrier and affect the induction and progression of the carcinogen-induced mammary tumors. Quercetin has also been shown to inhibit the activity of tumor promoters [127] and inhibit a multidrug-resistance gene that cancer cells activate to pump chemotherapeutic agents out of the tissue [128]. Polyhydroxylated flavonoids such as luteolin, fisetin, and quercetin as well as the polymethoxylated flavonoids nobiletin and tangeretin possess antiproliferative activity against a number of different cancer cell lines

TABLE 5.7. Structures of Selected Citrus Flavonoid Compounds.

Flavanone — Flavone and Flavonol — Anthocyanin

	Position of Radicals[a]							
Flavonones[a]	3	5	6	7	8	3′	4′	5′
Flavonones								
Naringin		OH		O-neo			OH	
Naringenin		OH		OH			OH	
Hesperidin		OH		O-rut		OH	OCH_3	
Hesperetin		OH		OH		OH	OCH_3	
Eriocitrin		OH		O-rut		OH	OH	
Nariutin		OH		O-rut			OH	
Flavones								
Tangeritin		OCH_3	OCH_3	OCH_3	OCH_3		OCH_3	
Nobiletin		OCH_3	OCH_3	OCH_3	OCH_3	OCH_3	OCH_3	
Luteolin		OH		OH		OH	OH	
Flavonols								
Quercetin	OH	OH		OH		OH	OH	
Rutin	O-rut	OH		OH		OH	OH	
Quercetrin	O-rut	OH		OH		OH	OH	
Kaempferol	OH	OH		OH			OH	
Anthocyanins								
Cyanidin 3-glu	O-glu	OH		OH		OH	OH	
Cyanidin 3,5-glu	O-glu	O-glu		OH		OH	OH	
Delphinidin 3-glu	O-glu	OH		OH		OH	OH	OH
Delphinidin 3,5-glu	O-glu	O-glu		OH		OH	OH	OH
Cyanidin 3-(4″-HAc)-glu	O-(4″-HAc)-glu	OH		OH		OH	OH	

[a]Neo, neohesperidose; rut, rutinose; rha, rhamnose; glu, glucose; Hac, acetyl.
Source: Adapted from Reference [116].

(e.g., leukemia, gastric, colon, mammary, ovarian) as determined by *in vitro* studies [129–131]. In the presence of ascorbic acid, the antiproliferative activity of fisetin and quercetin against squamous cell carcinoma was augmented by 100% [132]. It is interesting to note that ascorbic acid may have flavonoid-sparing activity by inhibiting the oxidative degradation of quercetin *in vitro,* indicating a potentiating interaction. Certain isoflavones (genistein and orobol) and flavones (fisetin and quercetin) can induce mammalian DNA cleavage *in vitro* [133]. Genistein has also been demonstrated to have the capacity to convert undifferentiated malignant cells to a differentiated mature phenotype [133]. Tangeritin is one flavonoid found to have antimetastatic activity that relates to an effect on adhesion between tumor cells and organs [134,135]. Clearly, flavonoids are common dietary constituents which, through various modes of action, may participate in cancer prevention/inhibition.

2.2.2. Limonoids

Limonoids are a group of chemically related triterpene derivatives present in orange, grapefruit, lemon, and lime. Limonin followed by nomilin are the predominant members of this group (Figure 5.4). These citrus limonoids have certain biological activities that may be used as chemopreventive agents. For

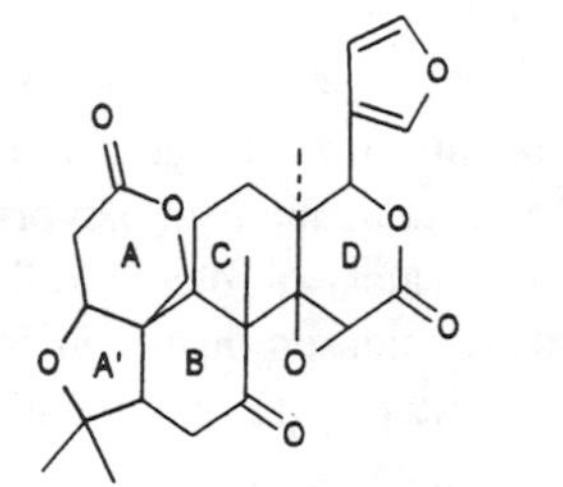

Limonin

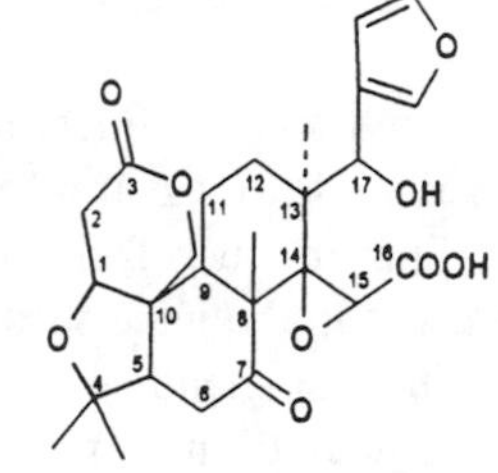

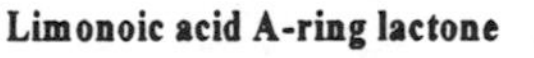

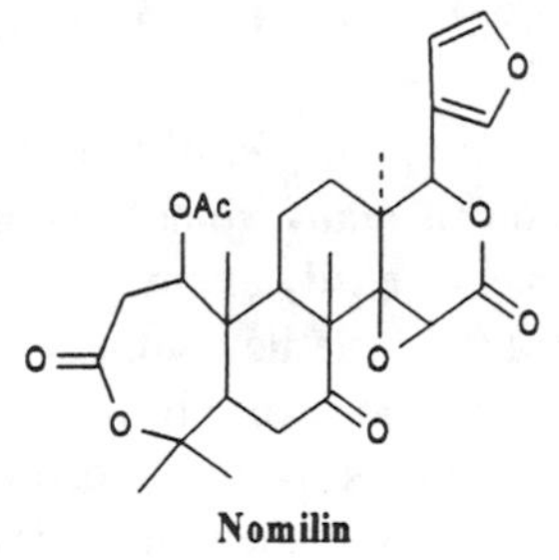

Nomilin

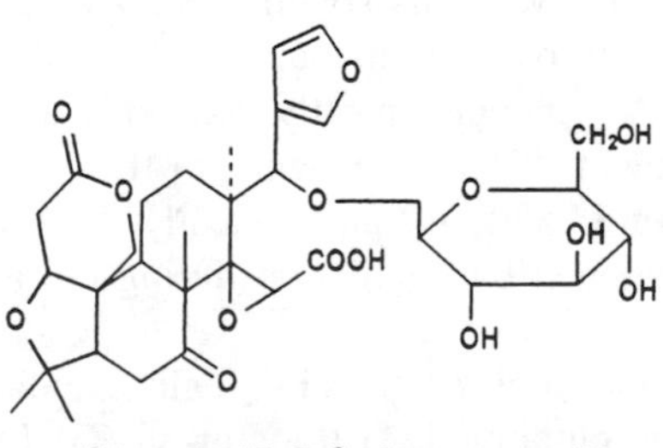

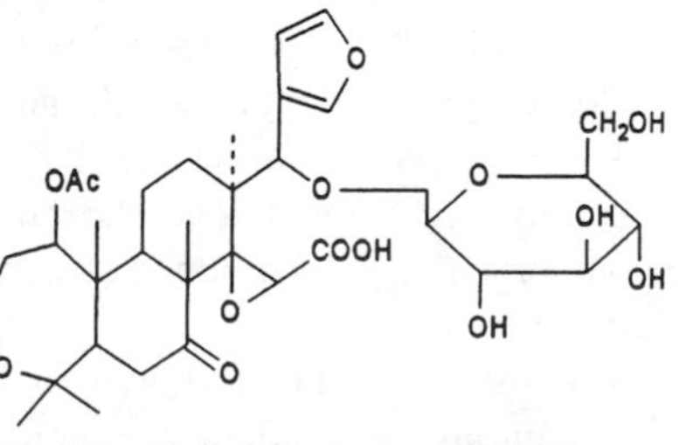

Limonin 17-O-β-glucopyranoside **Nomilin 17-O-β-D-glucopyranoside**

Figure 5.4 Structure of several citrus limonoids.

example, limonin and nomilin possess a characteristic furan moiety substituted at the C-3 position [136]. As with many other furan-containing natural products, nomilin and limonin have been found to induce the enzyme activity glutathione S-transferase (GST) when administered to animals [137]. GST is a major detoxifying enzyme system that catalyses the conjugation of glutathione with electrophiles that include activated carcinogens [138], and generally become less reactive and more water soluble, thus facilitating excretion. This protection mechanism against the effects of xenobiotics by nomilin and limonin was correlated with the inhibition of forestomach, lung, and skin tumor formation. Although these bitter aglycones and many other structure-related limonoids such as ichangin, isobacunoic, and obacunone were also found to be good GST inducers [137], their content in citrus juice is low. However, citrus juices contain higher concentration of mostly tasteless, water-soluble limonoid glycosides (Figure 5.4). For example, the average concentration of limonin 17-β-D-glucopyranoside (LG) in orange juice is 176–180 ppm as compared to a combined concentration of limonin and nomilin of 1–2 ppm [139,140]. A number of species of bacteria are known to be capable of hydrolysing limonoid glycosides; therefore, limonin aglycones may be liberated in the human intestinal tract [141]. LG was also found to be an effective antineoplastic agent in an oral tumour model. Since limonoid glycosides exist at high concentrations in juices, the total exposure to these compounds may be expected to be substantial.

2.2.3. Limonene and Selected Essential Oils

The perceived flavor of fruits and fruit products results from the contribution of many volatile components. However, mild and delicate fruit flavors may be easily altered by processing. In citrus fruits, the water-soluble and oil-soluble volatile components present in the juice sacs are released during juice extraction. Peel oil, located in ductless glands on the outer portion (flavedo) of the fruit, is introduced into the juice during extraction, and contributes significantly to the unique flavor of citrus juice. The balance of both juice and oil components is necessary for good flavor quality. Citrus volatiles contain approximately 95–96% terpene hydrocarbon (mostly *d*-limonene), 1.6% aldehydes (largely octanal and decanal), 0.8% alcohols (mostly linalool), and 0.3% esters (largely octyl and neryl acetates) [142]. *d*-Limonene or (4R)-(+)-4-isopropenyl-1-methylcyclohexene (Figure 5.5) is an optically active monoterpene hydrocarbon that can be obtained by distillation during citrus juice processing.

Limonene has been shown to block and suppress carcinogenic events. Endogenous antioxidant systems such as glutathione S-transferase (GST) are involved in the detoxification pathways of carcinogens. As blocking agents, the addition of limonene and limonene-rich citrus oils (orange,

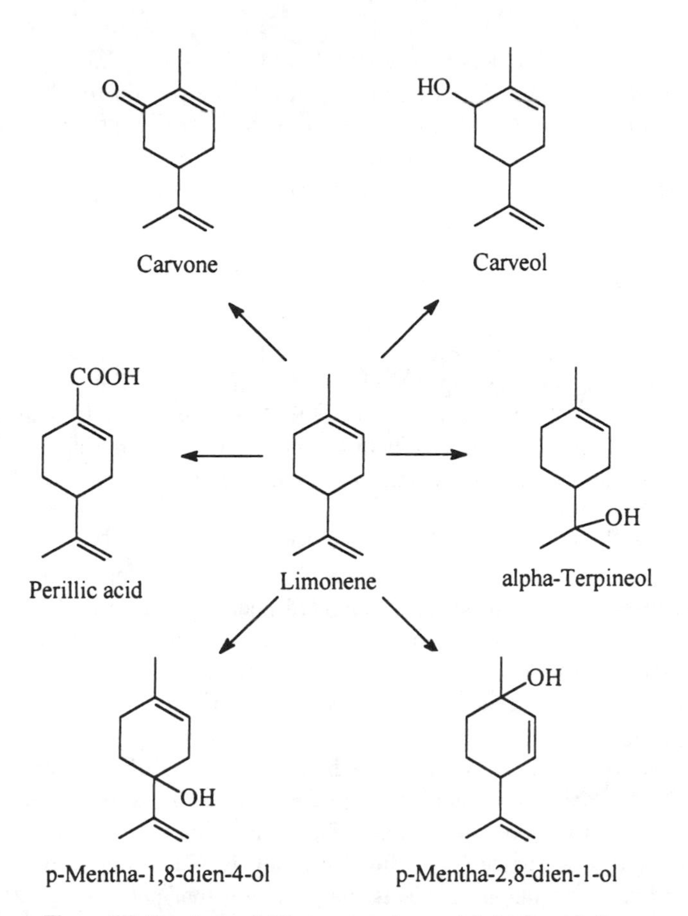

Figure 5.5 Structures of *d*-limonene and several derived metabolites.

lemon, grapefruit or tangerine) to a semi-purified diet resulted in induction of GST activity in the liver and small bowel mucosa. Feeding of these oils further resulted in inhibition of forestomach, lung, and mammary tumors [143,144].

Limonene has been studied as a possible suppressing agent by directly counteracting the mechanistic consequences of genotoxic events. As a common early event in the carcinogenic process, the *ras* family of mutated proto-oncogenes codes for proteins such as p21. To exert its transforming properties on the regulation of cellular growth and differentiation, $p21^{ras}$ must undergo farnesylation in order to be translocated to the plasma membrane. Limonene and orange oil can reduce the amount of the active mutated gene product by inhibiting isoprenylation of the $p21^{ras}$ protein in mammalian cells cultured *in vitro* and also *in vivo* mammary tissue [145–147]. Other terpenes such as

(±)-menthol and 1,8-cineole were also found to act in a similar manner by inhibiting HMG-CoA reductase activity, an enzyme pivotal for the synthesis of farnesol [148]. Nerolidol, a naturally occurring compound structurally related to and a putative analogue of farnesol, has been reported to inhibit azomethane-induced large bowel neoplasia and, therefore, impact on the consequences of oncogene activation [149].

2.2.4. Pectin and Dietary Fibre

Consumer interest in dietary fibre has continued to increase as more information about its potential impact on health has become available. Citrus fruits constitute one of the richest sources of high-quality pectin. Although soluble in water, pectin is classified as a dietary fibre because it is resistant to hydrolysis by enzymes of the human small intestine. Pectin, cellulose, and hemicellulose, with only trace amounts of lignin, are the predominant components of dietary fibre from most fruits, including oranges and apples. Pectic substances are constituents of plant cell walls where they function as bonding and lining substances in intracellular spaces. Extracted pectins are a group of heterogeneous polysaccharides with high molecular weight consisting of linear chains of $(1 \rightarrow 4)$ linked α-D-anhydrogalacturonic acid units with portions rich in L-rhamnose and with variable side chains containing arabinose, galactose, and xylose [150].

The function of dietary fibre has been an active area of research since the mid-1970s. Dietary incorporation of pectin appears to affect several metabolic and digestive processes; those of principal interest are the effects on lowering glucose absorption and cholesterol levels. Numerous studies, both in animal models and human subjects, have shown that pectin (20–30 g/day) added to a test meal significantly reduces the rate of glucose uptake, with concomitant reduction of serum insulin production [151–156]. Evidence suggests that pectin exerts its effect on postprandial serum glucose and insulin responses by delaying gastric emptying and decreasing absorption rates. For individuals with noninsulin-dependent diabetes mellitus, this could facilitate dietary management.

Epidemiological data suggest that an elevated level of low-density lipoprotein (LDL) cholesterol is a primary risk factor for coronary heart disease (CHD). The mechanism by which dietary fibre intake protects against CHD appears to be by lowering cholesterol. Both human and animal model studies have shown that pectin is a major component of fibre responsible for this activity, and that pectin supplementation of the diet (15–20 g/day) is effective in reducing LDL serum cholesterol levels rather than the HDL fraction [157–161]. Pectin fortification significantly increases fat [162], bile acid, and cholesterol [163] excretion in patients.

Beside pectin, other soluble (e.g., psyllium) and insoluble fibre (e.g., cellulose, hemicellulose, noncellulosic polysaccharides, and lignin) have been studied for their physiological effects. Many soluble fibres tend to delay gastric emptying, slow passage of food through the small intestine, lower serum cholesterol, and decrease the glycemic response to food [164]. In contrast, insoluble fibres have an effect on bowel regularity by hastening passage of food through the intestine and increase fecal bulk. Mixtures of both soluble and insoluble fibres may have the greatest therapeutic effects in diabetes and hypertriglyceridemia [165].

2.2.5. Carotenoids and Vitamin A

Carotenoids are a large group of fat soluble, C-40 plant pigments that are synthesized by plants [166]. Fruits and vegetables of green, orange, and red color are the most important sources of carotenoids in human diet. Over 600 carotenoids have been identified and are classified into (a) hydrocarbon carotenoids, with β-carotene and lycopene being the most prominent members, and (b) oxycarotenoids (xanthophylls) to which belong β-cryptoxanthin, lutein, zeaxanthin, canthaxanthin, and astaxanthin [167] (Figure 5.6). Among the 50–60 carotenoids considered to be vitamin A precursors, β-carotene is the most prevalent followed by β-cryptoxanthin, and the α-, and γ-carotenes. In all cases, it is a requirement for vitamin A activity that the plant carotenoid is cleaved enzymatically in the body and transformed into retinol. Red grapefruit, cantaloupe and apricot are considered good supplemental fruit sources of vitamin A activity (Table 5.8).

Vitamin A plays a central role in many essential biological processes. Its function as a chromophore in the visual process has been recognized for decades. It is also involved in fetal development and in the regulation of proliferation and differentiation of many types of cells throughout life. However, it has become increasingly clear that carotenoids mediate cellular functions in addition to serving as vitamin A precursors. Much interest has been generated in attempting to relate the known carotenoid functions to the possible mechanism whereby β-carotene or other carotenoids might serve as dietary chemopreventive agents. The beneficial effects of β-carotene are thought to occur through one of several modes: singlet oxygen quenching (photoprotection), antioxidant protection, and enhancement of the immune response. β-Carotene is approved for the general treatment of erythropoietic protoporphyria, a genetically inherited, light-sensitive skin disease [169]. It has been shown to be effective in protecting lipid membranes from free radical damage [170] particularly under low oxygen partial pressure [171]. Thus, β-carotene might complement other protective antioxidants such as vitamin C and vitamin E, which are most effective at normal oxygen pressures. The antioxidative properties of carotenoids are not restricted to β-carotene. Of a range of lipophilic agents, the most efficient singlet oxygen quencher is lycopene [172]. Zeaxan-

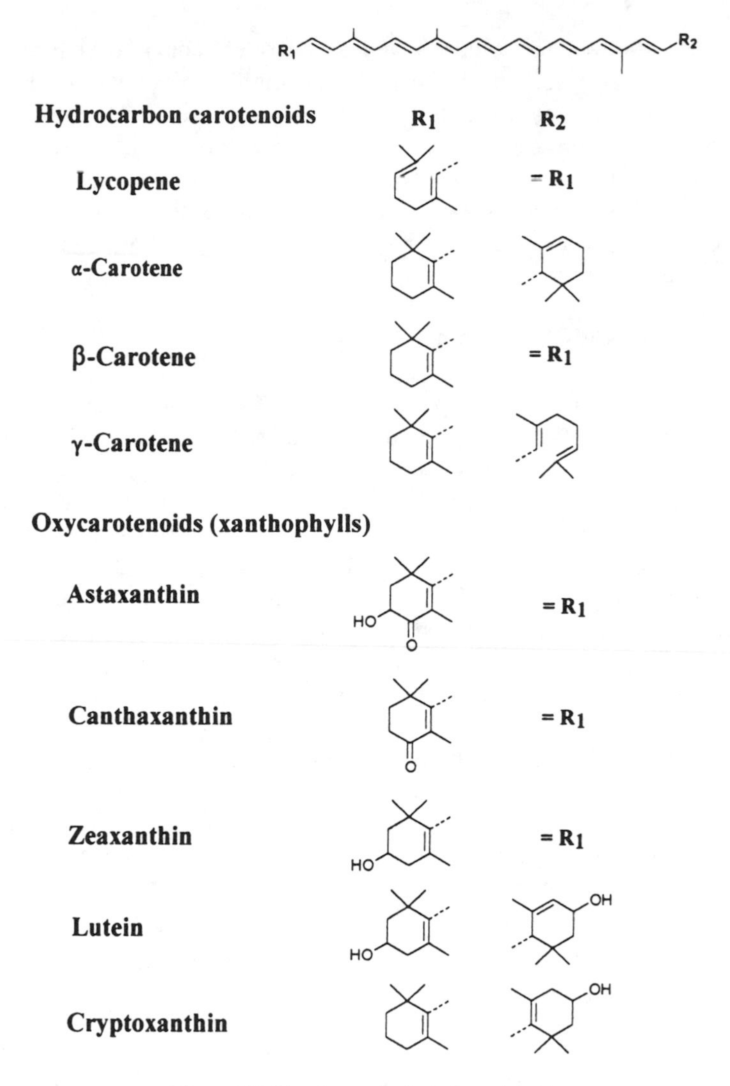

Figure 5.6 Structures of selected carotenoids.

thin and lutein are also more generally effective than *β*-carotene as scavengers of oxidative species [173].

Carotenoids have been shown to enhance both specific and nonspecific immune functions [172]. A number of modulating immunological reactions can increase the tumoricidal activity of cytotoxic T-cells, macrophages, and/or natural killer cells and enhance traditional antimicrobial, immunological functions [174]. Retinoic acid has antiproliferative and differentiative effects

TABLE 5.8. Concentration of Provitamin A Carotenoids in Selected Fruits.

Fruit	Concentration (μg/100 g)			Vitamin A Activity (IU/100 g)
	Alpha-Carotene	Beta-Carotene	Beta-Cryptoxanthin	
Grapefruit	1.03	248.23	6.72	422
Orange	19.56	40.04	7.23	88
Cantaloupe	8.99	1642.79	5.85	2750
Apricot	0.00	615.16	22.46	1046
Peach	2.88	76.68	3.39	133
Nectarine	0.00	49.22	34.38	111

Source: Adapted from Reference [168].

and may act on oncogene expression [175]. Carotenoids without provitamin A activity, such as canthaxanthin, have also been shown to possess antimutagenic and anticarcinogenic properties [176–178]. β-Carotene has also been found to reduce the incidence of cardiovascular events [179].

2.2.6. F olic Acid

Folic acid and its derivatives are water soluble compounds collectively referred to as folate or folacin. Oranges, tangerines, and their juices contain only moderate amounts of folic acid, but are major contributors to the diet because of their high level of consumption (Table 5.9). The principal form of folate in citrus is the reduced 5-methyl tetrahydrofolate (monoglutamate form), which can readily be absorbed in the upper part of the small intestine (jejunum). Polyglutamate derivatives are also present but must first be converted to the monoglutamate form by conjugase enzymes associated with the

TABLE 5.9. Vitamin C and Folic Acid Content in Single-Strength Orange and Grapefruit Juices.

Vitamin	RDI (mg)	RDI (%): 8-fl oz Serving	
		Orange	Grapefruit
Vitamin C	60.0	120–190	85–180
Folic acid	0.4	7–10	13–24

Source: Adapted from Reference [113].

intestinal mucosa [180,181]. Folic acid is light- and oxygen-sensitive and quite heat labile, since up to 50% of this vitamin can be destroyed following blanching for an extended period of time. The destruction of folic acid parallels that of ascorbic acid; however, significant amounts of ascorbic acid present in foods such as in citrus can stabilize and protect folic acid [182].

Total folate content in the average diet has been found to be below the recommended daily allowances, and mild to moderate folic acid deficiency is thought to be relatively prevalent in the general population [183]. Folates play an important metabolic role as co-enzymes that transport single carbon fragments during amino acid metabolism and nucleic acid synthesis. Severe deficiency causes megaloblastic anemia, and deficiency during pregnancy may lead to neural tube defects [184]. Folic acid has been linked to other pathological disorders such as cardiovascular disease and cancer. Since an inverse relationship has been observed between serum homocysteine and folate levels [185], patients with cardiovascular disease who have elevated blood homocysteine levels may benefit from a nutritional intervention with folic acid. In addition, *in vitro* and animal studies have shown that folic acid deficiency causes increased micronuclei formation and chromosomal damage [112]. The expression of certain chromosomal fragile sites, which are associated with oncogenes and breakpoints thought to be relevant to specific cancers, has also been shown to be increased in folic acid deficiency. Furthermore, cellular dysplasia exhibited by cervical and lung cells may be reversed by administration of folic acid [186]. The potential role of folate continue to be examined in terms of the chemopreventive mechanisms and dietary/serum levels to provide protection [183].

2.2.7. Vitamin C

Vitamin C is present in greatest amounts in fruits and vegetables, especially citrus fruits and juices (Table 5.9). The most active antiscurvy forms of vitamin C are L-ascorbic acid (the reduced form) and its interconvertible derivative, dehydroascorbic acid (the oxidized form). The water solubility and strong reducing properties of L-ascorbic acid are attributable to its enediol structure, which is conjugated with the carbonyl group in a lactone ring. The greatest proportion (over 60%) of vitamin C content in citrus is located in the flavedo and albedo [187]. It is interesting to note that the concentration of vitamin C in the pulp is approximately twice that found in the peel and 10 times the level found in the juice. Vitamin C can be adversely affected by oxygen, light, and heat. In foods that are particularly rich in ascorbic acid, such as fruit products, loss is usually associated with nonenzymatic browning [188].

Some of the principal biochemical functions of vitamin C in humans are to maintain a reducing environment for enzyme systems involved in the hydroxylation of lysine and proline in the synthesis of connective tissue. However, evidence has emerged from recent nutritional studies that dietary vitamin C may exert a protective action in the diet beyond prevention of scurvy. Within the last few decades, epidemiological and experimental evidence have indicated that other important health-promoting and disease-preventative properties might be due to vitamin C [189]. Vitamin C has been categorized as a potential cancer-inhibiting agent by preventing the formation of carcinogens from precursor compounds. Biochemical studies suggested that vitamin C impedes the reaction of nitrites with amines and amides to form potent carcinogenic nitrosamines within the digestive tract [190], and prevents oxidation of specific chemicals to their active carcinogenic forms [191]. Protective associations have been found between vitamin C-rich foods and cancers of the esophagus [192], stomach [193], and cervix [194]. Ascorbic acid has been shown *in vitro* to reduce mutagenicity of gastric juices, as determined by the Ames test [195]. In other *in vitro* studies, vitamin C has been shown to cause regression of tobacco-induced malignant changes in hamster lung cells and to increase survival of ovarian tumor cells exposed to radiation [196]. While many studies support the role of vitamin C in reducing cancer risk, the possibility remains that other protective factors in vitamin C-containing foods may function synergistically with vitamin C and/or be specifically responsible for some anticancer effects.

2.3. PROCESSING OF CITRUS PRODUCTS

Citrus fruits are widely marketed as fresh commodities. Large volumes of citrus fruits are also produced primarily for processing either as single-strength juice or concentrate. Other products include essence and oil, pigments, pectin, and flavonoids and limonoids such as naringin and limonin. An overview of the processing operations and products for citrus fruits is shown in Figure 5.7.

2.3.1. Juice

Since its development in the 1940s, frozen concentrated orange and grapefruit juices have become prominent frozen food items. Large quantities of fruits are converted into juice concentrates for economic ways of storage, packaging and distribution to consumers throughout the year. Orange juice is defined as an unfermented juice obtained from mature oranges of the species *Citrus sinensis*. Maturity standards for oranges in terms of soluble solids ($\geq$8%) and Brix/acid ratio ($\geq$8.1 to 10) have been established for manufacturing concentrated orange products [197]. Many process operations and equipment are equally applicable to oranges, tangerines, lemons, and grapefruit. Weighing, grading and washing are the front-end operations, which also include material selection, preparation, handling, and testing.

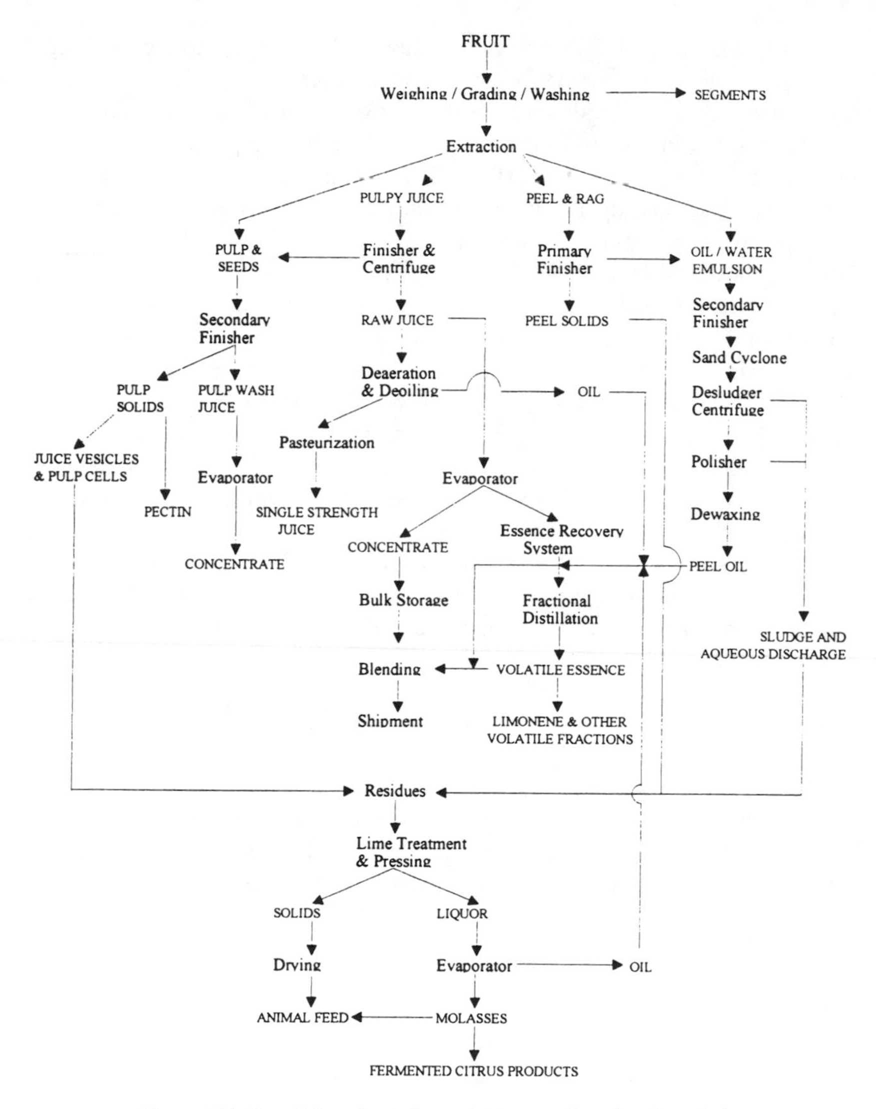

Figure 5.7 Overall flowchart of processing operations for citrus fruit.

2.3.1.1. Juice Extraction

The two types of extractors commercially encountered around the world are the FMC Citrus Juice Extractor and the Brown Extractor [197]. The unique aspect of the FMC machine is the extraction of juice from the whole fruit without first cutting it in half. A tube with an internal perforated strainer is inserted into the fruit held between two cups. Upon pressure applied by the interlocking cups, juice is channelled through the strainer and into a manifold. The pulp, membrane section and seed residues larger than the prefinisher tube holes are discharged through the center of the plunger. At the end of the stroke, the shredding action of the cups' intermeshing fingers causes the peel to flex and tear, and the oil-bearing glands of the flavedo are ruptured. The released peel oil is captured in a spray of water and collected separately as oil emulsion. The disintegrated peel from the extracted fruit is discharged into the waste conveyor. At the end of the operation, four streams are generated: the juice, the peel, the center part containing rag, pulp and seeds, and the oil emulsion. By comparison, with the Brown extractor, the fruit enters the machine and is sliced in half. The halves are oriented and picked up by synthetic rubber cups. Serrated plastic reamers penetrate the fruit with a rotary movement. Juice collects in a bottom pan and each peel half is ejected.

2.3.1.2. Adjustment of Solids Content

Finishers may differ in design but the main function is to remove excess pulp, peel particles, seed fragments, and segment membrane residues from the extracted juice. The process is usually accomplished by forcing the juice through a screen with perforations of about 0.5 mm in diameter by the action of a screw or other means. A standard juice finisher is generally capable of lowering pulp content of juice to about 12%. If a lower level is desired (3% to 5%), centrifugation becomes necessary.

The excess pulp and tissue by-products of extracted juice leaving the primary finishers are processed through a series of secondary finishers. About 5–7% of additional soluble solids can be recovered using a countercurrent pulp wash system (1 to 8 stages) and represents 60 to 90% of the pulp's soluble solids content [197]. The quality of the pulp wash juice is considered inferior to the regular juice, and may be added back to the main juice stream if governing regulations allow it. Alternately, pulp wash solids can be treated with pectolytic enzymes to reduce their viscosity and concentrated. Pasteurized frozen pulp may be used to adjust the pulp content of juices, juice concentrates, juice-containing drinks, and beverages that contain no juices.

2.3.1.3. Pasteurization

As part of the steps leading to pasteurization, deaeration is often carried out in the same operation as deoiling. Gases such as oxygen that may oxidize vitamin C and cause flavor deterioration are easily removed by subjecting the juice to vacuum. For optimum flavor and storage life, excessive citrus oil content is reduced by means such as vacuum flash evaporation. Deaeration and deoiling evaporation are generally carried out continuously in a vacuum of

660 mm Hg or higher. The vaporized oils and water are condensed, the oil is separated and the water recombined with the original juice [142]. For optimum flavor and storage life, citrus juice should contain between 0.008 and 0.020% recoverable oil.

Pasteurization of fresh extracted raw citrus juice is carried out to denature the pectinesterase enzyme, which causes sedimentation or gelation of concentrate, and to inactivate spoilage microorganisms. Typical commercial heat treatments to achieve stability vary from 90 to 95°C for 15 to 60 sec [197]. Flash pasteurization is generally accomplished in tubular or plate-type heat exchangers using either steam or hot water as the heating medium. Single-strength juices may be packaged by filling containers with hot pasteurized juice (minimum 77°C) and chilling quickly or filling with cold pasteurized juice and packaging aseptically.

2.3.1.4. Concentration

Juice from extractors and finishers may also be conveyed to an evaporator where the juice is concentrated to a desired solids level, generally 65–70°Brix. In this operation, the juice is simultaneously deaerated, deoiled, pasteurized and concentrated. Evaporators are designed to incorporate a high-temperature short-time (HTST) pasteurization with either tubular or plate-heat exchangers. The highest juice temperature regime in the evaporator system is in the range of 95°C to 105°C, with typical residence time of 6 to 10 minutes varying with the type of system. One of the dominant evaporators used commercially is the multistage, multieffect thermal-accelerated-short-time-evaporator (TASTE). An "effect" defines the heat flow through the evaporator. The first effect receives energy for driving the evaporator. Vapor from the first effect is used to supply evaporation heat for the second effect and so on for the next 2–5 effects [198]. The number of effects determines the energy efficiency of the unit. The stages of an evaporator define the product flow. In a forward-flow evaporator, the single-strength juice enters the first stage and parallels the heat flow through the effects. The juice in each stage flows down the internal surface as a film. The heat supplied from the exterior surface causes evaporation of the juice held under vacuum conditions. The useful energy contained in the separated water vapor is directed to the next stage to be used further as a heat source. The concentrate emerging from the last stage is flash-cooled to 12°C and pumped to blending tanks for standardization. Concentrate may be shipped in bulk form at 65°Brix to reconstitution plants or packaged at a minimum of 38°Brix and frozen at about −18°C before transportation.

2.3.2. Volatile Oil and Essence

In the first stage of an evaporator, the essence-bearing vapors are boiled off under vacuum, pass through the next effect, and can be directed to an essence recovery system (ERS). ERS consists of a series of fractionators, condensers, scrubbers, and chillers. The condensed volatiles are drained into a decanter where the concentrated flavor components are separated into an aqueous phase (aroma) and oil phase (essence oil). These essence oils possess the aroma and flavor characteristics of fresh juice and are quite different from the peel oils. Since concentrates from evaporators are devoid of most juice volatiles, blending is an important operation that affects end product quality. Techniques to restore natural flavour and quality include the use of condensed volatile fractions (aqueous and oil), orange pulp, and pressed citrus peel oil.

Peel oil is obtained either prior to or during juice extraction depending on the type of manufacturing system used. The crude oil emulsion is produced from the rupture by pressure or abrasion of oil glands in the peel and washed away in a slurry. The peel particles and the oil-water emulsion are then separated through a finisher. The finished emulsion passes through a sand cyclone and is fed to a desludger centrifuge to produce an oil-rich emulsion, which is sent to a polisher that recovers the clear oil. The oil is referred to as *cold-pressed oil* or *essential oil* and contains high concentrations of d-limonene. In addition to the cold-pressed peel oil recovery process and the essential oil generated from the deaeration/deoiling or concentration operations of the juice by vacuum flash evaporation, limonene-rich oil is also decanted from evaporator condensate streams during the concentration of press liquor to molasses (Figure 5.7). Dilute concentrations of oil containing *d*-limonene can be recovered from citrus plant waste streams using membrane technology. High ultrafiltration membrane rejection (78–97%) has been reported for mixtures with low initial limonene concentrations (0.04–0.6% v/v) [199]. Citrus oils are generally winterized to remove waxy materials that could produce a hazy or cloudy appearance in the final product. The dewaxing process is a function of temperature and time. If the oil is held at −29°C, the precipitated wax is centrifuged after 3 to 5 days. When held for 4 to 5 weeks at −12°C to −4°C, the clear oil is normally decanted off tall and narrow tanks with conical bottoms to facilitate separation. Dewaxed oils are then stored at 15–22°C under an inert gas atmosphere.

Fractional distillation under vacuum can be used to separate selected components such as *d*-limonene. Concentrated or "folded" citrus oils enhance the contribution of the aromatic aldehydes and other components with lighter peel notes and reduce the harsher taste associated to terpenes. Terpeneless (C-10) and sesquiterpeneless (C-15) orange oils may also be produced by aqueous alcohol extraction [200] and by adsorption chromatography [201].

The reduction in *d*-limonene content improves the water solubility of essences and the oxidative stability of citrus products. *d*-Limonene and other terpenes oxidize readily in the presence of air, leading to undesirable flavors resembling a terebinthic taste [202]. The microflora of oil emulsions can also hydrolyze *d*-limonene to α-terpineol contributing to the development of off-odor [203–205]. A number of microorganisms (e.g., *Pseudomonas* and *Penicilium* strains) can metabolize *d*-limonene to several products, including p-menthadienol, carveol, carvone, and perillic acid (Figure 5.5) [206].

2.3.3. Pigments

Using differential centrifugation, orange/red carotenoid pigment granules can be recovered from orange and tangerine juices. These granules can be added to poorly colored commercial, reconstituted frozen concentrated orange juices and can be used to intensify the color of products other than citrus [207]. During standard fruit-processing operations, neither pasteurization, concentration nor drying has an appreciable effect on carotenoid content [208–210]. However, they can be adversely affected by oxygen, light, and heat. Carotenoids are found primarily in the more stable *trans*-form even though *cis*-isomers do occur naturally. Varying amounts of *cis*-isomers can be found in processed products and their formation as a consequence of heat treatment has been reported by several authors [211–214]. Hydrocarbon carotenoids are generally more heat resistant than other classes of carotenoids such as xanthophylls [215,216]. If oxygen is present during processing or storage, extensive losses of carotenoids may occur, stimulated by light, enzymes, and co-oxidation with lipid hydroperoxides [188].

2.3.4. Pectin and Dietary Fibre

Being a structural component, pectin is concentrated in those fruit fractions highest in cell wall content, such as peel, membranes, juice sacs and cores [217,218]. Pectin content in orange juice (44.5 to 103 mg/100 ml) is distributed between the pulp (156 to 426 mg/100 ml) and serum (12.5 to 51 mg/100 ml). Levels of pectin in oranges consumed as peeled fruit or in juice are normally too low to provide significant pharmacological benefit. In combination with other pectin-containing fruits and vegetables, citrus fruit supplements to the diet could help achieve total pectin levels equalling those effective in controlled tests. Although peel and membranes are unsuited for consumption due to excessive levels of naringin, limonin, and other bitter compounds, juice sacs are a palatable by-product that can be used to formulate specialty juices or synthetic beverages with significant levels of pectin and dietary fibre. Only 125 g of juice sacs would be required to supply 6 g of pectin and 13 g of total dietary fibre [219]. Thus, such pulpy citrus juice with a natural appearance may offer an alternative to the consumption of pectin as a powder, slurry or gel.

Citrus fruit peel, particularly the albedo portion, serves as a major raw material for pectin manufacture destined to the production of jams, jellies and preserves. Pectin content in the peels of citrus fruits ranges from 30 to 33% on dry-weight basis. Pectin manufacturers aim at producing water-soluble pectin preparations with specified degree of methylation (DM) and degree of acetylation (DA), which are able to form gels under specific conditions. Figure 5.8 shows an overall process for production of pectins. Raw materials primarily employed in industrial practice are citrus and apple pomaces. Among the citrus fruits, lemon is the major source, but lime, orange and grapefruit are also used. The peel of these fruits is available subsequent to the extraction of juice and essential oils. After a size-reduction operation, the peel pomace may be washed in a two-step countercurrent fluming process that removes at least 20% of the total dry peel solids [220]. The residual reducing sugar should be low because of potential browning of the product in the dryer. Browning defects can be carried over to affect pectin recovery and quality at the refinery. It may also have a detrimental impact on the cholesterol-lowering effect of the fibre [221]. Excess water is separated by passing the peel pomace over a stationary screen and through a screw press. The moisture content of the press cake is reduced to 8–10% in a dryer to arrest pectinesterase activity and minimize the shipping expense to the pectin production plants.

Extraction conditions (pH, temperature, time) must be optimized with respect to mass yield, gelling capacity, and desired DM. After rehydration at a typical ratio of 1:35 citrus pomace-to-water, the pH of the raw material is adjusted with a mineral acid (e.g., sulfurous, sulfuric, hydrochloric, nitric) [222]. Fast-gelling ("rapid-set") pectins (DM $>$ 70%) are typically extracted at pH 2.5 and 100°C for 45 min. Medium-fast and "slow-set" pectins (DM 60–70%) are extracted at lower temperatures for longer periods of time (e.g., 60°C, 4 h) because deesterification at lower temperature proceeds faster than depolymerization [223].

The separation of the viscous extract from the strongly swollen and partly disintegrated pomace can be carried out by vibrating screens, decanter centrifuges, vacuum drum filters and various types of presses, often in combination with pressing aids such as diatomaceous earth, wood meal, or cellulose fibres. The depectinated pomace is mostly used as cattle feed. To prevent degradation and demethylation of the extracted pectin by acid hydrolysis of glycosidic and ester bonds, the pH is raised to values between 3 and 4 using weak alkali such as sodium carbonate or ammonia.

For the recovery of pectin from the clarified extracts, the metal ion precipitation method (aluminium, copper) has largely been replaced by alcohol precipitation (methanol, ethanol, and isopropanol) for environmental reasons [223]. Pectins precipitate at alcohol concentrations higher than 45% (w/v). To minimize the volume of alcohol, the clarified extract is first concentrated in multistage evaporators from 0.3–0.5% to 3–4% pectin content. By acid treatment

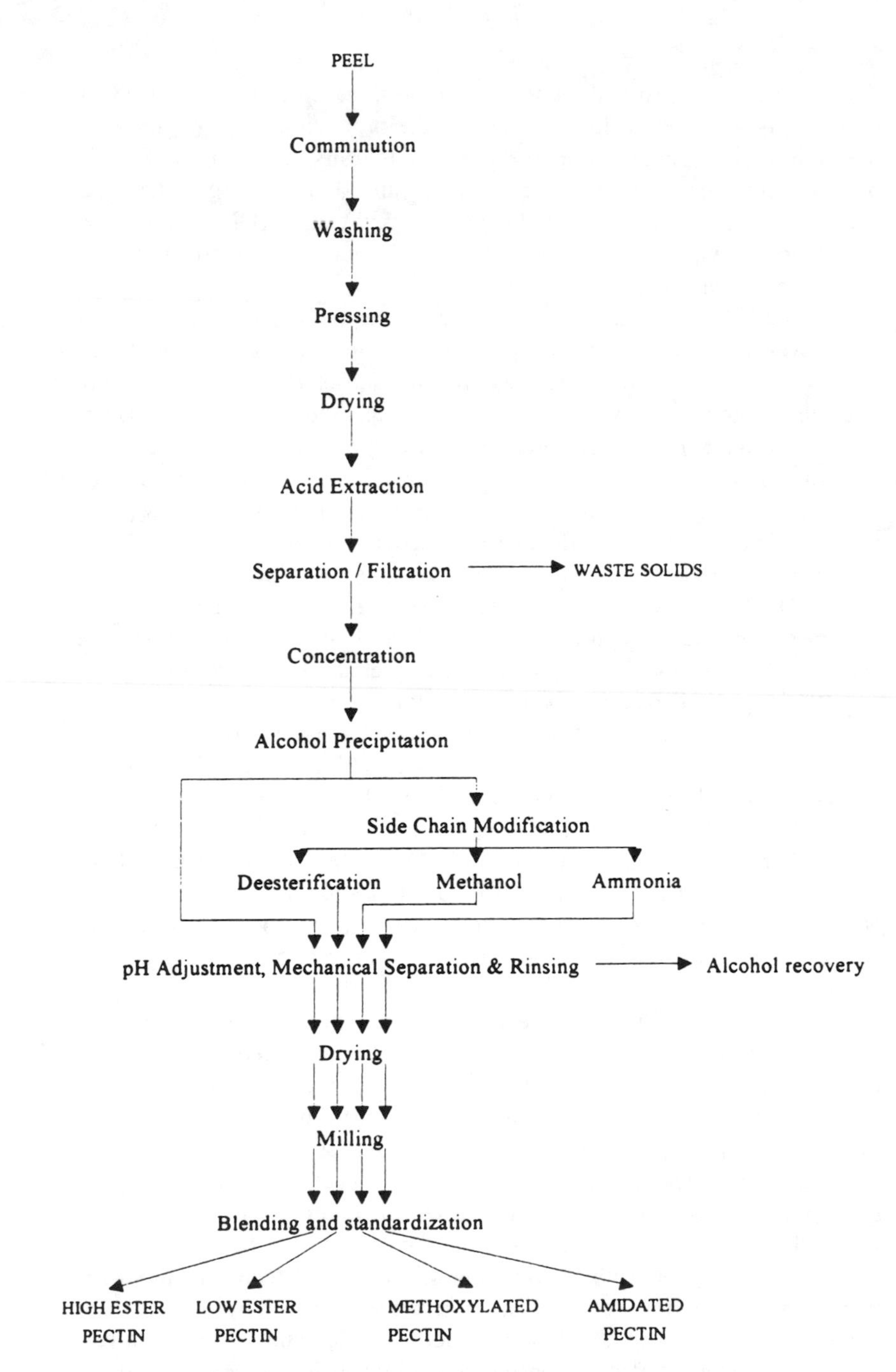

Figure 5.8 Overall flowchart of a pectin production process.

concurrently with ethanol or isopropanol, the pectin suspension can be hydrolyzed to a desired DM under conditions of low pH and temperatures not exceeding 50°C. Neutral sugar side chains are removed, thus raising the content of galacturonic acid and producing HM pectins with various setting temperatures as well as LM pectins. Alternatively, an often-desired methoxylation can be achieved with methanol. By contrast, on adding ammonia to alcoholic suspensions, methyl ester groups are replaced by amide, giving amidated pectins. Temperatures must be kept below 10°C to prevent β-eliminative pectin degradation. Termination of acid deesterification or ammonical amidation is achieved by pH adjustment to 3–4 or by rapid mechanical separation of the suspended pectin. The precipitate is further rinsed with alcohol, dried and milled. Due to variations in the raw materials, there are large differences in the gelling power of pectin preparations. Batches are therefore blended and standardized with sugar such as sucrose, glucose or lactose.

2.3.5. Naringin and Limonin

A moderate amount of bitterness is desirable in citrus juices, but some processed products have excessive bitterness that adversely affects the flavor and therefore the marketability of products made from these juices. Naringin and limonin are primarily responsible for the objectionable bitterness in early-season navel oranges and grapefruits. Grade A grapefruit juice must contain less than 600 ppm naringin or less than 7 ppm limonin [226].

Naringin is an intensely bitter, white, crystalline solid that is only slightly soluble in cold water, but quite soluble in warm water. This compound is present in all parts of the fruit, with the highest concentrations found in the peel albedo, core and rag (segment membranes) (Table 5.10). It is the 7β-neohesperidoside

TABLE 5.10. Distribution of Bitter Compounds in White Grapefruit.

Fruit Part	Naringin[a] (ppm)	Limonin[b] (ppm)
Juice vesicle	471	7
Flavedo	4,882	25
Albedo	11,647	74
Section membrane	7,412	107
Core	9,647	296
Seed	411	9,270

[a] *Source:* Reference [224].
[b] *Source:* Reference [225].

of the aglycone, naringenin, and the linkage of the two sugars (rhamnose and glucose) that determine its bitter quality. As for all citrus flavonoids, naringin has a bitterness threshold in water of approximately 20 ppm, ranging from 300 to 1900 ppm in juice [227]. Naringin also acts synergistically with limonin present in processed juice to cause bitterness even at subthreshold levels for both compounds individually [228].

Limonin is a white, crystalline solid sparingly soluble in water [229]. This 22-carbon tetranortriterpenoid dilactone is 20 times more bitter than naringin, with an average taste threshold of 1 ppm in water and 6–10 ppm in orange juice. Intact fruits contain limonoic acid A-ring lactone, a more water-soluble and relatively tasteless glucoside precursor of limonin. Limonin does not have time to develop if the fruit is consumed fresh and thus does not affect the fresh-market quality. When the fruit is macerated, the acidic medium and subsequent heat treatments cause the conversion of the monolactone to the intensely bitter dilactone form. Limonin is found primarily in the seeds, with smaller amounts in the central core and segment membranes (Table 5.10). It is important to avoid high extraction pressures which might rupture the seeds during juice extraction.

Various research efforts have attempted to find suitable and efficient processes for reducing bitterness in citrus juices. Techniques for removal of limonoids and naringin from juices were reviewed by Dekker [230], who reported uses of resins, enzymes, and supercritical extraction. The naringin level can be reduced through treatment with commercial naringinase enzymes, which hydrolyze naringin to the less bitter prunin plus rhamnose and, because of the flavanoid glucosidase present, further hydrolyze prunin to the nonbitter naringenin plus glucose. Combining immobilization of naringinase with use of cellulose triacetate resulted in a useful process to remove both naringin and limonin from grapefruit juice [231]. So far, enzymatic methods have experienced limited industrial impact.

Recent application of solid-phase extraction technology to orange and grapefruit juices allowed the possibility of extending the use of debittered juices and by-products without significantly altering most chemical components or juice properties and has become the preferred method for commercial processors (Figure 5.9). To avoid oil saturation and fouling of the adsorbent, freshly extracted juice requires the common practice of vacuum deoiling; this operation also occurs during evaporation when processing juice into concentrates. Excess pulp that can clog the adsorbent may be removed by centrifugation or membrane filtration. Two columns containing the resin (neutral adsorbent such as styrene divinylbenzene or ion exchange) are used alternatively for treatment and regeneration in a continuous process. The pulp is reblended with the debittered juice prior to concentration, adding about 15% of the original bitterness back to the finished juice.

Several other fractions recovered during fruit extraction and processing can

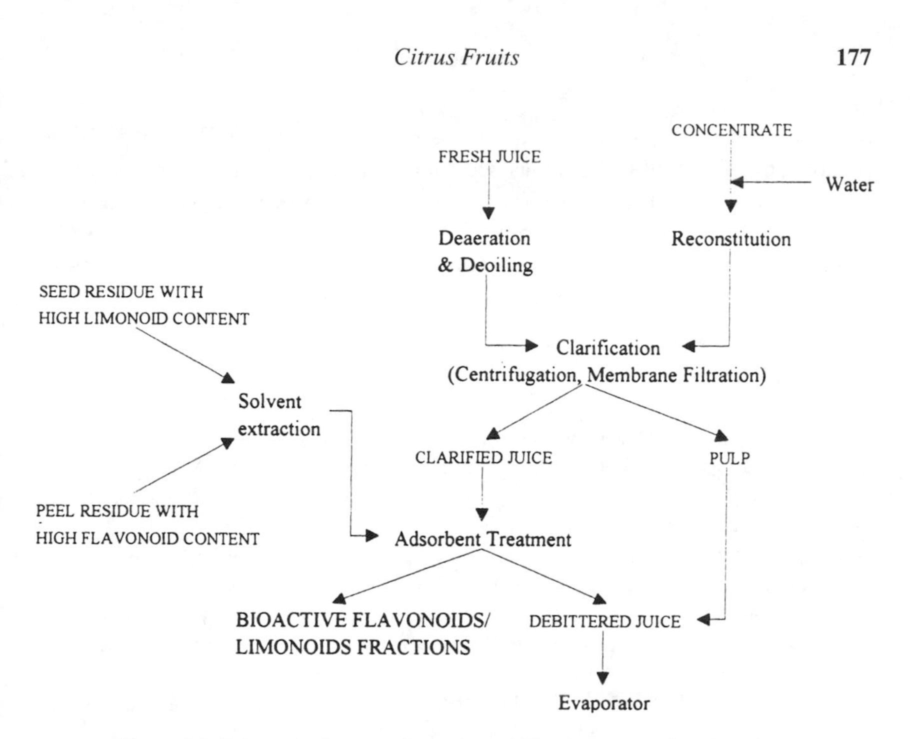

Figure 5.9 Schematic diagram of adsorbent debittering process for citrus juice.

benefit greatly from debittering. Besides utilization of debittered juices, there is considerable interest in flavonoid by-products recovered during regeneration of adsorbents used for debittering. Pulp wash can contain up to twice the limonin content in juice, and core wash can contain 3–5 times the limonin level in juice [232]. Further, peel, seed, and other residues are rich sources of flavonoids, which could be extracted and purified for alternate functional use.

2.4. CONCLUSIONS

A variety of biologically active constituents may contribute to the protective health effects of diets rich in fruits and vegetables. As with most other plant products, citrus fruits make up a complex food system containing a broad mixture of secondary metabolites that include nutrient and non-nutrient phytoprotectants. These common dietary constituents participate in disease prevention and health promotion through several different mechanisms. The precise role that these phytochemicals play under the various conditions of current dietary selection, or that they could play under optimal conditions, remains to be established. Since these agents could mediate biological responses in a dose-dependent manner, consumption as part of the normal diet may not yield a sufficient dose to be effective. Knowledge about individual phytochemicals is increasing but the potential synergistic effects of different phytochemicals should be emphasized. In addition, changes that are known to occur in the chemical composition of foods during processing or through enzymatic action must be taken into consideration. Ultimately, some of these compounds may be useful as chemopreventive agents to be taken as dietary supplements and/or incorporated in processed foods.

3. REFERENCES

1. FAO Production Yearbook. 1990. FAO Statistics Series No. 44. Food and Agriculture Organization of the United Nations, Rome. pp. 286.
2. Nelson, K. E. 1991. "The grape," Quality and Preservation of Fruits. N. A. M. Eskin, Boca Raton, FL: CRC Press Inc. pp. 125–167.
3. Childers, N. F. 1976. Modern Fruit Science. New Brunswick, NJ: Horticultural Publications, Rutgers University. pp. 666–713.
4. Hertog, M. G. L., P. C. H. Hollman, M. B. Katan and D. Kromhout. 1993a. "Intake of potentially anticarcinogenic flavonoids and their determinants in adults in the Netherlands," Nutr. Cancer, 20:21–29.
5. Hertog, M. G. L., E. J. M. Feskens, P. C. H. Hollman, M. B. Katan and D. Kromhout. 1993b. "Dietary antioxidant flavonoids and risk of coronary heart disease: the Zutphen elderly study," Lancet, 342:1007–1011.
6. DeWhalley, C. V., S. M. Rankin, R. S. Hoult, W. Jessup and D. S. Leake. 1990. "Flavonoids inhibit the oxidative modification of low density lipoproteins by macrophages," Biochem. Parmacol., 39:1743–1748.
7. Frankel, E. N., J. Kanner and J. E. Kinsella. 1993. "Inhibition *in vitro* of oxidation of human low density lipoproteins by phenolic substances in wine," Lancet, 341:454–457.
8. Kanner, J., E. Frankel, R. Granit, B. German and J. E. Kinsella. 1994. "Natural antioxidants in grapes and wines," J. Agric. Food Chem., 42:64–69.
9. Kinsella, J. E., E. Frankel, B. German and J. Kanner. 1993. "Possible mechanisms for the protective role of antioxidants in wine and plant foods," Food Technol., 47(4):85–89.
10. Maxwell, M., A. Cruickshank and G. Thorpe. 1994. "Red wine and the antioxidant activity of serum," Lancet, 334:193–196.
11. Macheix, J. J., A. Fleuriet and J. Billot. 1991. Fruit Phenolics. Boca Raton, FL: CRC Press Inc. pp. 1–103.
12. Middleton, E. and C. Kandaswami. 1992. "Effects of flavonoids on immune and inflammatory cell functions," Biochem. Pharmacol., 43:1167–1179.
13. Verma, A. K., J. A. Johnson, M. N. Gould and M. A. Tanner. 1988. "Inhibition of 7, 12-dimethylbenz(a)anthracene and N-nitrosomethylurea induced rat mammary cancer by dietary flavonol quercetin," Cancer Res., 48:5754–5788.
14. Wei, H., L. Tye, E. Bresnick and D. F. Birt. 1990. "Inhibitory effect of apigenin, a plant flavonoid, on epidermal ornithine decarboxylase and skin tumor promotion in mice," Cancer Res., 50:499–502.
15. Deschner, E. E., J. Ruperto, G. Wong and H. L. Newmark. 1991. "Quercetin and rutin as inhibitors of azoxymethanol-induced colonic neoplasia," Carcinogenesis, 7:1193–1196.

16. Wagner, H. 1979. "Phenolic compounds in plants of pharmaceutical interest," Biochemistry of Plant Phenolics. T. Swain, J. B. Harborne and C. F. Van Sumere, New York, NY: Plenum Press. pp. 581.
17. Wagner, H. 1985. "New plant phenolics of pharmaceutical interest," Ann. Proc. Phytochem. Soc. Eur., Vol. 15. C. F. Van Sumere and P. J. Lea, Oxford UK: Clarendon Press. pp. 409–425.
18. Mabry, T. J. and A. Ulubelen. 1980. "Chemistry and utilization of phenylpropanoids including flavonoids, coumarins and lignans," J. Agric. Food Chem. 28:188–196.
19. Beretz, A. and J.-P. Cazahave. 1988. "The effect of flavonoids on blood vessel wall interactions," Plant Flavonoids in Biology and Medicine II. V. Cody, E. Middleton, J. B. Harborne and A. Beretz, New York, NY: Alan R. Liss, Inc. pp. 187–200.
20. Boniface, R., M. Miskulin, L. Robert and A. M. Robert. 1986. "Pharmacological properties of *Myrtillus* anthocyanosides: correlation with results of treatment of diabetic microangiopathy," Flavonoids and Bioflavonoids. L. Farkas, M. Gabor and F. Kallay. Amsterdam: Elsevier. pp. 193–201.
21. Cristoni, A. and M. J. Magistretti. 1987. "Antiulcer and healing activities of *Vaccinium myrtillus* anthocyanosides," Farmaco Prat., 42:29–40.
22. Kano, E. and J. Miyakoshi. 1976. "UV protection effect of keracyanin an anthocyanin derivative on cultured mouse fibroblast L cells," J. Radiat. Res., 17:55–65.
23. Igarashi, K., K. Takanashi, M. Makino and T. Yasui. 1989. "Antioxidative activity of major anthocyanin isolated from wild grapes (*Vitis coignetiae*)," Nippon Shokuhin Kogyo Gakkaishi, 36:852–856.
24. Costanino, L., A. Albasini, G. Rastelli and S. Benvenuti. 1992. "Activity of polyphenolic crude extracts as scavengers of superoxide radicals and inhibitors of xanthine oxidase," Plant Med., 58:342–344.
25. Tsuda, T., K. Ohshima, S. Kawakishi and T. Osawa. 1994. "Antioxidative pigments isolated from the seeds of *Phaseolus vulgaris* L.," J. Agric. Food Chem., 42:248–251.
26. Tsuda, T., M. Watanabe, K. Ohshima, S. Norinobu, S.-W. Choi, S. Kawakishi and T. Osawa. 1994. "Antioxidative activity of the anthocyanin pigments cyanidin 3-*O*-β-D-glucoside and cyanidin," J. Agric. Food Chem., 42:2407–2410.
27. Tamura, H. and A. Yamagami. 1994. "Antioxidant activity of monoacylated anthocyanins isolated from Muscat Baily A grape," J. Agric. Food Chem., 42: 1612–1615.
28. Maas, J. L., G. I. Galletta and G. D. Stoner. 1991. "Ellagic acid, an anticarcinogen in fruits, especially strawberries: A review," HortScience, 26:10–14.
29. Jang, M., L. Cai, G. O. Udeani, K. V. Slowing, C. F. Thomas, C. W. W. Beecher, H. S. Fong, N. R. Farnsworth, A. D. Kinghorn, R. G. Mehta, R. C. Moon and J. M. Pezzuto. 1997. "Cancer chemopreventive activity of resveratrol, a natural product derived from grapes," Science, 275:218–220.
30. Boyle, J. A. and L. Hsu. 1990. "Identification and quantification of ellagic acid in muscadine grape juice," Amer. J. Enol. Vitic., 41:43–47.
31. Okeda, T. and K. Yokotsuka. 1996. "Trans-resveratrol concentrations in berry skins and wines from grapes grown in Japan," Am. J. Enol. Vitic., 47:93–99.
32. Jeandet, P., R. Bessis, B. F. Maume, P. Meunier, D. Peyron and P. Trollat. 1995. "Effect of enological practices on the resveratrol isomer content of wine," J. Agric. Food Chem., 43:316–319.

33. Crippen, D. D., Jr., and J. C. Morrisson. 1986. "The effects of sun exposure on the phenolic content of Cabernet Sauvignon berries during development," Am. J. Enol. Vitic., 37:243–247.
34. Lamikanra, O. 1988. "Development of anthocyanin pigments in muscadine grapes," HortScience, 23:597–599.
35. Peynaud, E. and P. Ribereau-Gayon. 1971. "The grape," The Biochemistry of Fruits and Their Products, Vol. 2. A. C. Hulme, London: Academic Press. pp. 172–205.
36. Mazza, G. 1995. "Anthoycanins in grapes and grape products," CRC Crit. Rev. Food Sci. Nutri., 35:341–371.
37. Cheynier, V. and J. Rigaud. 1986. "Identification et dosage de flavonols du Raisin," Bull. Liaison Groupe Polyphénols, 13:442–447.
38. Bourzeix, M., D. Weyland and N. Heredia. 1986. "Etude des catechines et des procyanidols de la grappe de raisin, du vin et d'autres dérivés de la vigne," Bull. O.I.V., 669–670, 1171.
39. Nagel, C. W. and L. W. Wulf. 1979. "Changes in the anthocyanins, flavonoids and hydroxycinnamic acid esters during fermentation and aging of Merlot and Cabernet Sauvignon," Am. J. Enol. Vitic., 30:111–116.
40. Singleton, V. L. and E. Trousdale. 1983. "White wine phenolics: varietal and processing differences as shown by HPLC," Am. J. Enol. Vitic., 34:27–34.
41. Van Buren, J. 1970. "Fruit phenolics," The Biochemistry of Fruits and Their Products, Vol. 1. A. C. Hulme, London: Academic Press. pp. 269–304.
42. Ribereau-Gayon, P. 1964. "Les composés phénoliques du raisin et du vin. I. Les acides phénols," Ann. Physiol. Vég., 6:119–139.
43. Boursiquot, J. M. 1987. "Contribution à l'étude des esters hydroxycinnamoyltartriques chez le genre *Vitis*. Recherche d'application taxonomique." Thèse Doct. Ing., ENSA, Montpellier, France.
44. Amerine, M. A., H. W. Berg and W. V. Cruess. 1967. The technology of wine making, 2nd ed. Westport, CT: AVI. pp. 367, 288, 658, 659.
45. Hang, Y. D. 1988. "Recovery of food ingredients from grape pomace," Process Biochem., 23:2–4.
46. Fuleki, T. and L. J. Babjak. 1986. "Natural food colorants from Ontario grapes," Highlights Agric. Res. Ont., 9(3):6–9.
47. Singleton, V. L. 1980. "Grape and wine phenolics, background and prospects," C. R. Coll. Centenaire Paris. pp. 215.
48. Riva, M., C. Cantarelli and L. Cassani. 1980. "Estrazione dei polifenoli dalla bacca dell'uva e riduzione delle dimensioni," Industrie Bevande, 10:33–36.
49. Somers, T. C. and M.E . Evans. 1975. "Color composition and red wine quality—the importance of low pH and low SO_2," Aust. Grape Grower Wine Maker, 136:1–10.
50. Markakis, P. 1982. "Stability of anthocyanins in foods," Anthocyanins as Food Colors. P. Markakis, New York, NY: Academic Press. pp. 245–253.
51. Macheix, J. J., A. Fleuriet and J. Billot. 1991. "Phenolic compounds in fruit processing," Fruit Phenolics. Boca Raton, FL: CRC Press. pp. 295–360.
52. Ribéreau-Gayon, P. 1982. "The anthocyanins of grapes and wines," Anthocyanins as Food Colors. P. Markakis. New York, NY: Academic Press Inc. pp. 209–244.

53. Timberlake, C. F. and P. Bridle. 1976. "The effect of processing and other factors on the color characteristics of some red wines," Vitis, 15:37–49.
54. Somers, T. S. and M. E. Evans. 1979. "Grape pigment phenomena: interpretation of major color losses during vinification," J. Sci. Food Agric., 30:623–633.
55. Leone, A. M., E. La Notte and G. Gambacorta. 1984. "Gli antociani nelle fasi de macerazione e di elaborazione del vino. L'influenza della tecnica diffusiva sulla loro estrazione," Vignevini, 11(4):17–31.
56. Roggero, J. P., B. Rogonnet and S. Coen. 1984. "Analyse fine des anthocyanines des vins et des pellicules de raisin par la technique HPLC," Vignes et Vins, 327: 38–42.
57. Flanzy, C., M. Flanzy and P. Benard. 1987. La vinification par macération carbonique. INRA, Paris.
58. Ribéreau-Gayon, P. 1974. "The chemistry of red wine color," The Chemistry of Wine Making. A. E. Webb, Washington, DC: American Chemical Society. pp. 50–65.
59. Haslam, E. 1980. "In vino veritas: oligomeric procyanidins and the aging of red wines," Phytochemistry, 19:2577–2582.
60. Kovac, V., E. Alonso, M. Mourziex and E. Revilla. 1992. "Effect of several enological practices on the content of catechins and procyanidins in red wines," J. Agric. Food Chem., 40:1953–1957.
61. Ricardo-da-Silva, J. M., V. Cheynier, A. Samson and M. Bourzeix. 1993. "Effect of pomace contact, carbonic maceration, and hyperoxidation on the procyanidin composition of Grenache blanc wines," Am. J. Enol. Vitic., 44: 168–172.
62. Pederson, C. S. 1971. "Grape juice," Fruit and Vegetable Juice Processing Technology. D. K. Tessler and M. A. Joslyn, New York, NY: Van Nostrand Reinhold/AVI. pp. 234–271.
63. McLelland, M. R. and E. J. Rau. 1990. "Grape juice processing," Production and Packaging of Non-Carbonated Fruit Juices and Beverages. D. Hicks, Glasgow, UK: Blackie and Sons. pp. 226–242.
64. Morris, J. R., W. A. Sistrunk, J. Junek and C. A. Sims. 1986. "Effects of fruit maturity, juice storage, and juice extraction temperature on quality of Concord grape juice," J. Am. Soc. Hort. Sci., 111:742–746.
65. Hertog, M. G. L., P. C. H. Hollman and B. van de Patte. 1993. "Content of potentially anticarcinogenic flavonoids in tea infusions, wines and fruit juices," J. Agric. Food Chem., 41:1242–1246.
66. Dieci, E. 1967. "Sull'enocianina tecnica," Riv. Vitic. Enol., 12:567–572.
67. Garoglio, P. G. 1953. Nuovo trattato di enologia. Vol. III. Sansoni, Florence, Italy. pp. 64.
68. Garoglio, P. G. 1965. "La nuova enologia," Instituto di Industrie Agrarie, Florence, Italy. pp. 502–570.
69. Garoglio, P. G. 1980. "L'enocianina," Enciclopedia Vitivinicola Mondiale, AEB, Brescia, 130:427–431.
70. Langston, M. S. K. 1985. Anthocyanin colorant from grape pomace. U.S. Patent No. 4,500,556.
71. Foo, L. Y. and L. J. Porter. 1980. "The phytochemistry of proanthocyanidin polymers," Phytochemistry, 19:1747–1754.

72. Foo, L. Y. and L. J. Porter. 1981. "The structure of tannins of some edible fruits," J. Sci. Food Agric., 32:711–716.
73. Haslam, E. 1981. "Vegetable tannins," The Biochemistry of Plants, Vol. 7. E. E. Conn, New York, NY: Academic Press. pp. 527–537.
74. Santos-Buelga, C., E. M. Francia-Aricha and M. T. Escribano-Bailón. 1995. "Comparative flavan-3-ol composition of seeds from different grape varieties," Food Chemistry, 53:197–200.
75. Escribano-Bailón, M. T., M. T. Guerra, J. C. Rivas-Ganzalo and C. Santos-Buelga. 1995. "Proanthocyanidins in skins from different grape varieties," Z. Lebensm. Unters Forsch., 200:221–224.
76. Czochanska, Z., L. Y. Foo and L. J. Porter. 1979. "Compositional changes in lower molecular weight flavans during grape maturation," Phytochemistry, 18: 1819–1822.
77. Rusznyàk, S. and A. Szent-Györgyi. 1936. "Vitamin P: flavonols as vitamins," Nature, 138:27.
78. Decker, E. A. 1995. "The role of phenolics, conjugate linoleic acid, carinosine, and pyrrologlunolinc quinone as nonessential antioxidants," Nutrition Reviews, 53(3):49–58.
79. Verma, A. K. 1992. "Modulation of mouse skin carcinogenesis and epidermal phospholipid biosynthesis by the flavonol quercetin," Phenolic Compounds in Food and Their Effects on Health, Vol. II. Antioxidants and Cancer Prevention. C.-T. Ho, C. Y. Lee, and M-T Huang, Washington, DC: American Chemical Society. pp. 250–264.
80. Hirose, M., T. Hoshiya, K. Akagi, S. Takahashi, Y. Hara and N. Ito. 1993. "Effects of green tea catechins in a rat multiorgan carcinogenesis model," Carcinogenesis, 14:1549–1553.
81. Kuenzig, W., J. Chan and E. Norkus. 1984. "Caffeic acid and ferulic acid as blockers of nitrosoamine formation," Carcinogenesis, 5:309–314.
82. Mandel, S. and G. D. Stoner. 1990. "Inhibition of *N*-nitrosobenzyl-methylamine-induced esophageal tumorigenesis by ellagic acid," Carcinogenesis, 11:55–61.
83. Chang, R. L., T. Huang and A. W. Wood. 1985. "Effect of ellagic acid and hydroxylated flavonoids on the tumorigenicity of benzo(a) pyrene and (±)-7β,8-dihydroxy-9,10-epoxy, 7,8,9,10-tetrahydrobenzo(a)pyrene on mouse skin in the newborn mouse," Carcinogenesis, 6:1127–1133.
84. Yoshizawa, S., T. Horiuchi and I. Suganuma. 1992. "Penta-*o*-galloyl-β-D-glucose and (−)-epigallocatechin gallate: cancer preventive agents," Phenolic Compounds in Food and Their Effects on Health, Vol. II. Antioxidants and Cancer Prevention. C.-T., Ho, C. Y. Lee, M-T Huang, Washington, DC: American Chemical Society. pp. 316–325.
85. Liu, L. and A. Castonguay. 1991. "Inhibition of the metabolism and genotoxicity of 4-(methylnitrosamino)-1-(3-pyridyl)-1-butanone (NNK) in rat hepatocytes by (+)- catechin," Carcinogenesis, 12:1203–1208.
86. Sayer, J. M, H. Yagi, A. W. Wood, A. H. Connery and D. M. Jerina. 1982. "Extremely facile reaction between the ultimate carcinogen benzo[a]pyrene-7,8-diol 9,10-epoxide and ellagic acid," J. Am. Chem. Soc., 104:5562–5564.
87. Ohno, K. and H. Nakane. 1990. "Mechanism of inhibition of various cellular DNA and RNA polymerases by several flavonoids," J. Biochem., 108:609–613.
88. Agarual, R., S. K. Katiyar, S. I. A. Zaidi and H. Mukthar. 1992. "Inhibition of

skin tumor promoter-caused induction of epidermal ornithine decarboxylase in SENCAR mice by polyphenolic fraction isolated from green tea and its individual epicatechin derivatives," Cancer Res., 52:3582–3588.

89. St. Léger, A. S., A. L. Cochrane and F. Moore. 1979. "Factors associated with cardiac mortality in developed countries with particular reference to the consumption of wine," Lancet, 1017–1020.
90. Renaud, S. and M. de Lorgeril. 1992. "Wine, alcohol, platelets and the French paradox for coronary heart disease," Lancet, 339:1523–1526.
91. Frankel, E. N., J. Kanner, J. B. German, E. Parks and J. E. Kinsella. 1993a. "Inhibition of human low-density lipoprotein by phenolic substances in red wine," Lancet, 341:454–457.
92. Frankel, E. N., A. L. Waterhouse and J. E. Kinsella. 1993b. "Inhibition of human LDL oxidation by resveratrol," Lancet, 341:1103–1104.
93. Rimon, E. B., E. L. Giovanucci and W. C. Willett. 1991. "Prospective study of alcohol consumption and risk of coronary disease in men," Lancet, 338:464–468.
94. Klatsky, A.L. 1994. "Epidemiology of coronary heart disease—influence of alcohol," Alcohol Clin. Exp. Res., 18:88–96.
95. Graziano, J. M., J. E. Buring and J. L. Breslow. 1993. "Moderate alcohol intake: increased levels of high-density lipoprotein and its subfractions and decreased risk of myocardial infarction," N. Engl. J. Med., 329:1829–1834.
96. Elwood, P. C., S. Renaud, D. S. Sharp, A. D. Beswick, J. R. O'Brien and J. W. G. Yarnell. 1991. "Ischemic heart disease and platelet aggregation," Circulation, 83: 38–44.
97. Renaud, S. C., A. D. Beswick, A. M. Fehily, D. S. Sharp and P. C. Elwood. 1992. "Alcohol and platelet aggregation: the Caerphilly prospective heart disease study," Am. J. Clin. Nutr., 55:1012–1017.
98. Steinberg, D., S. Parsatharathy, T. E. Carew, J. C. Khoo and J. L. Witztum. 1989. "Beyond cholesterol. Modifications of low-density lipoprotein that increase its atherogenicity," N. Engl. J. Med., 320:915–924.
99. Esterbauer, H., J. Gebicki, H. Puhl and G. Jurgens. 1992. "The role of lipid peroxidation and antioxidants in oxidative modification of LDL," Free Radic. Biol. Med., 13:341–390.
100. Bors, W. and M. Saran. 1987. "Radical scavenging by flavonoid antioxidants," Free Rad. Res. Commun., 2:289–294.
101. Afanas'ev, I. B., A. I. Dorozhko, A. V. Brodskii, V. A. Kostyuk and A. I. Potapovitch. 1989. "Chelating and free radical scavenging mechanisms of inhibitory actions of rutin and quercetin in lipid peroxidation," Biochem. Pharmacol., 38:1763–1769.
102. Friedman, L. A. and A. W. Kimball. 1986. "Coronary heart disease mortality and alcohol consumption in Framingham," Am. J. Epidemiology, 24:481–489.
103. Pisha, E. and J. M. Pezzuto. 1994. "Fruits and vegetables containing compounds that demonstrate pharmacological activity in humans," Economic Med. Plant Res., 6:189–233.
104. Dumenil, G., M. Vasquez, A. Cremieux and G. Balansard. 1980. "Action antibactérienne des acides phénols de la série benzoique," Bull. Biaison Groupe Polyphénols, 10:302–308.
105. Balansard, G., D. Zamble, G. Dumenil and A. Cremieux. 1980. "Mise en évidence des propriétés antimicrobiennes du latex obtenu par incision du tronc de

Alafia multiflora Stapf. Identification de l'acide vanillique," Plant. Med. Phytother., 2:99–104.

106. Ames, B. N. 1983. "Dietary carcinogens and anticarcinogens. Oxygen radicals and degenerative diseases," Science 221:1256–1264.
107. Block, G. 1992. "The data support role for antioxidants in reducing cancer risk," Nutrition Reviews 50(7):207–213.
108. Mackerras, D. 1995. "Antioxidants and health," Food Australia (Supplement) 47(11):1–23.
109. Bors, W., W. Heller, C. Michel and K. Stettmaier. 1996. "Flavonoids and polyphenols," Chemistry and Biology Handbook of Antioxidants. New York, NY: Marcel Dekker, Inc. pp. 409–465.
110. Mazza, G. 1997. "Anthocyanins in edible plant parts: A qualitative and quantitative assessment,"Antioxidant Methodology *In vivo* and *In vitro* Concepts, Champaign, IL: AOCS Press. pp. 119–140.
111. Brown, M. G., R. L. Kilmer and K. Bedigian. 1993. "Overview and trends in the fruit juice processing industry," Fruit Juice Processing Technology. Auburndale, FL: AgScience. pp. 1–22.
112. Tillotson, J. E., S. M. Gershoff, A. M. Humber and M. C. Crim. 1993. "Review of the medical and nutritional literature pertaining to the health and benefits of citrus fruits and juices." Food Policy Institute, Tufts Univ., Medford, MA.
113. Rouseff, R. L. and S. Nagy. 1994. "Health and nutritional benefits of citrus fruit components," Food Technol., 11:125–132.
114. Middleton, E. and C. Kandaswami. 1994. "Potential health-promoting properties of citrus flavonoids," Food Technol., 11:115–119.
115. Rouseff, R. L. 1988. "Liquid chromatographic determination of naringin and hesperidin as a detector of grapefruit juice in orange juice," J. Assoc. Anal. Chem., 71:798–802.
116. Park, G. L., S. M. Avery, J. L. Byers and D. B. Nelson. 1983. "Identification of bioflavonoid from citrus," Food Technol., 37:98–105.
117. Mazza, G. and E. Miniati. 1993. Anthocyanins in Fruits, Vegetable and Grains. Boca Raton, FL: CRC Press. pp. 211–212.
118. Huet, R. 1982. "Constituants des agrumes à effet pharmacodynamique: les citroflavonoides," Fruits, 37:267–271.
119. Bailey, D. G., J. Malcolm, O. Arnold, A. Strong, C. Munoz and J. D. Spence. 1993. "Effect of grapefruit juice and naringin on nisoldipine pharmacokinetics," Clin. Pharmacol. Therap., 54(6):589–594.
120. Ducharme, M. P., R. Provenzo, M. Dehoorne-Smith and D. J. Edwards. 1993. "Trough concentrations of cyclosporine following administration with grapefruit juice," Brit. J. Clin. Pharmacol., 36:457–459.
121. Bailey, D. G., J. Malcolm, O. Arnold and J. D. Spence. 1994. "Grapefruit juice and drugs—how significant is the interaction?" Clin. Pharmacokinet., 26(2):91–98.
122. Mookerjee, B. K., T.-P. Lee, H. A. Lippes and E. Middleton. 1986. "Some effects of flavonoids on lymphocyte proliferative responses," J. Immunolopharmacol., 8:371–392.
123. De Whalley, C. V., S. M. Rankin, R. S. Hoult, W. Jessup and D. S. Leake. 1990. "Flavonoids inhibit the oxidative modification of low density lipoproteins by macrophages," Biochem. Pharmacol., 39:1743–1750.

124. Busse, W. W., D. E. Kopp and E. Middleton. 1984. "Flavonoid modulation of human neutrophil function," J. Allergy Clin. Immunol., 73:801–809.
125. Middleton, E. and G. Drzewiecki. 1984. "Flavonoid inhibition of human basophil histamine release stimulated by various agents," Biochem. Pharmacol., 33:3333–3338.
126. Verma, A. K., J. A. Johnson, M. N. Gould and M. A. Tanner. 1988. "Inhibition of 7,12-dimethylbenz[a]anthracene and N-nitrosolmethylurea-induced rat mammary cancer by dietary flavonol quercetin," Cancer Res., 48:5754–5758.
127. Fujiki, H., T. Horiuchi, K. Yamashita, H. Hakii, Y. Hirata and T. Şugimura. 1986. "Inhibition of tumor promotion by flavonoids," Plant Flavonoids in Biology and Medicine: Biochemical, Pharmacological and Structure-Activity Relationships. V. Cody, E. Middleton and J. B. Harborne, New York, NY: Alan R. Liss Inc. pp. 429–440.
128. Kioka, N., N. Hosokawa, T. Komano, K. Hirayoshi, K. Nagata and K. Ueda. 1992. "Quercetin, a bioflavonoid, inhibit the increase of human multidrug resistance gene (MDRI) expression caused by arsenite," FEBS Lett., 301:307–309.
129. Ranelletti, F. O., R. Ricci, L. M. Larocca, N. Maggiano, A. Capelli, G. Scambia, P. Benedetti-Panini, S. Mancuso, C. Rumi and M. Piantelli. 1992. "Growth-inhibitory effect of quercetin and presence of type-II estrogen-binding sites in human colon-cancer cell lines and primary colorectal tumors," Int. J. Cancer, 50: 486–492.
130. Markaveritch, B. M., R. R. Roberts, M. D. Alejandro, G. A. Johnson and J. H. Clark. 1988. "Bioflavonoid interaction with rat uterine type II binding sites and cell growth inhibition," J. Steroid Biochem., 30:71–78.
131. Kandaswami, C., E. Perkins, D. S. Soloniuk, G. Drzewiecki and E. Middleton, Jr. 1991. "Antiproliferative effects of citrus flavonoids on a human squamous cell carcinoma *in vitro,*" Cancer Letters, 56:147–152.
132. Kandaswami, C., E. Perkins, D. S. Soloniuk, G. Drzewiecki and E. Middleton, Jr. 1993. "Ascorbic acid-enhanced antiproliferative effect of flavonoids on squamous cell carcinoma *in vitro,*" Anti-Cancer Drugs, 4:91–96.
133. Yamashita, Y., S. Kawada and H. Nakano. 1990. "Induction of mammalian topoisomerase II dependent DNA cleavage by nonintercalative flavonoids, genistein, and orobol," Biochem. Pharmacol., 39:737–744.
134. Bracke, M. E., G. DePestel, V. Castronovo, B. Vyncke, J.-M. Foidart, L. C. A. Vakaet and M. M. Mareel. 1988. "Flavonoids inhibit malignant tumors invasion in vitro," Plant Flavonoids in Biology and Medicine II: Biochemical, Cellular and Medicinal Properties. V. Cody, E. Middleton, J. B. Harborne, and A. Beretz, New York, NY: Alan R. Liss Inc. pp. 219–233.
135. Bracke, M. E., B. M. Vyncke, N. A. Van Larebeke, E. A. Bruyneel, G. K. DeBruyn, G.H. De Pestel, W. J. De Coster, M. Espeel and M. M. Mareel. 1989. "The flavonoid tangeretin inhibits invasion of MO4 mouse cells into embryonic chick heart in vitro," Clin. Exptl. Metastasis, 7:283–300.
136. Dreyer, D. L. 1968. "Limonoid bitter principles," Fortsch. Chem. Org. Nat., 26: 190–244.
137. Lam, L. K. T., Y. Li and S. Hasegawa. 1989. "Effects of citrus limonoids on glutathione *S*-transferase activity in mice," J. Agric. Food Chem., 37:878–880.
138. Chasseaud, L. F. 1979. "The role of glutathione-S-transferases in the metabolism

of chemical carcinogens and other electrophilic agents," Adv. Cancer Res., 29: 175–227.

139. Fong, C. H., S. Hasegawa, Z. Herman and P. Ou. 1990. "Limonoid glucosides in commercial citrus juices," J. Food Sci., 54:1505–1506.
140. Herman, Z., C. H. Fong, P. Ou and S. Hasegawa. 1990. "Limonoid glucosides in orange juices by HPLC," J. Agric. Food Chem., 38:1860–1861.
141. Hasegawa, S. 1987. "Limonoid debittering of citrus juices using immobilized bacterial cell systems," Food Biotech., 1:249–261.
142. Redd, J. B. and C. M. Hendrix, Jr. 1993. "Processing of natural citrus oils and flavors," Fruit Juice Processing Technology. S. Nagy, C. S. Chen and P. E. Shaw, Auburndale, FL: AgScience, pp. 83–109.
143. Hocman, G. 1989. "Prevention of cancer: vegetables and plants," Comp. Biochem. Physiol., 93:201–12.
144. Wattenberg, I. W., A. B. Hanley, G. Barany, V. L. Sparnins, L. K. T. Lam and G. R. Fenwick. 1986. "Inhibition of carcinogenesis by some minor dietary constituents," Diet, Nutrition, and Cancer. Y. Hayashi, Tokyo, Japan: Sci. Soc. Press. pp. 193–203.
145. Crowell, P. L., R. R. Chang, Z. Ren, C. E. Elson and M. N. Gould. 1991. "Selective inhibition of isoprenylation of 21–26 kDa proteins by the anticarcinogen d-limonene and its metabolites," J. Biol. Chem., 266:17679–17685.
146. Wattenberg, L. W. 1983. "Inhibition of neoplasia by minor dietary constituents," Cancer Res., 43:2448s–2453s.
147. Maltzman, T. H., L. H. Hort, C. E. Elson, M. A. Tanner and M. N. Gould. 1989. "The prevention of nitrosomethylurea induced mammary tumors by *d*-limonene and orange oil," Carcinogenesis, 10(4):781–783.
148. Clegg, R. J., B. Middleton, C. D. Bell and D. A. White. 1982. "The mechanism of cyclic monoterpene inhibition of hepatic 3-hydroxy-3-methylglutaryl coenzyme A reductase *in vivo* in the rat," J. Biol. Chem., 257:2294–2299.
149. Nagahara, A., H. Benjamin, J. Stockson, J. Krewson, K. Sheng, W. Liu and M. W. Pariza. 1992. "Inhibition of benzo[α]pyrene-induced mouse forestomach neoplasia by a principal flavour component of Japanese-style fermented soysauce," Cancer Res., 52(7):1754–1756.
150. Aspinal, G.O. 1980. "Chemistry of cell wall polysaccharides," The Biochemistry of Plants. J. Preiss, New York, NY: Academic Press. p. 473.
151. Jenkins, D. J. A., D. V. Goff, A. R. Leeds, K. G. M. M. Alberti, T .M. S. Wolever, M. A. Gassull and T. D. R. Hockaday. 1976. "Unabsorbable carbohydrates and diabetes: decreased postprandial hyperglycaemia," Lancet, 2:172–1174.
152. Kanter, Y., N. Eitan, G. Brook and D. Barzilai. 1980. "Improved glucose tolerance and insulin response in obese and diabetic patients on a fibre-enriched diet," Israel J. Med. Sci., 16:1–6.
153. Levitt, N. S., A. I. Vink, A. A. Sive, P. T. Child and W. P. V. Jackson. 1980. "The effect of dietary fibre on glucose and hormone responses to a mixed meal in normal subjects and in diabetic subjects with and without autonomic neuropathy," Diabetes Care, 3:515–519.
154. Poynard, T., G. Slama, A. Delage and G. Tchobroutsky. 1980. "Pectin efficacy in insulin-treated diabetics assessed by the artificial pancreas," Lancet, 1:58.
155. Schwartz, S. E., R. A. Levine, R. S. Weinstock, S. Petokas, C. A. Mills and F. D. Thomas. 1988. "Sustained pectin ingestion: effect on gastric emptying and glu-

cose tolerance in non-insulin-dependent diabetic patients," Am. J. Clin. Nutr., 48:1413–1417.

156. Vaaler, S., K. F. Hanssen and Ø. Aagenaes. 1980. "Effects of different kinds of fibre on postprandial blood glucose in insulin-dependent diabetes," Acta Med. Scand., 208:389–391.
157. Bell, L. P., K. J. Hectorn, H. Reynolds and D. B. Hunninghake. 1990. "Cholesterol-lowering effects of soluble-fibre cereals as part of a prudent diet for patients with mild to moderate hypocholesterolemia," Am. J. Clin. Nutr., 52(6): 1020–1026.
158. Cerda, J. J., F. L. Robbins, C. W. Burgin, T. G. Baumgartner and R. W. Rice. 1988. "The effects of grapefruit pectin on patients at risk for coronary heart disease without altering diet or lifestyle," Clin. Cardiol., 11:589–594.
159. Jenkins, D. J. A., D. Reynolds, A. R. Leeds, A. L. Waller and J. H. Cummings. 1979. "Hypocholesterolemic action of dietary fibre unrelated to fecal bulking effect," Am. J. Clin. Nutr., 32:2430–2435.
160. Nakamura, H., T. Ishikawa, N. Tada, A. Kagami, K. Kondo, E. Miyazima and S. Takeyama. 1982. "Effect of several kinds of dietary fibres on serum and lipoprotein lipids," Nutr. Repts. Intl., 26(2):215–221.
161. Stasse-Wolthius, M., H. F. F. Albers, J. G. C. van Jeveren, J. W. deJong, J. G. A. J. Hautvast, R. J. J. Hermus, M. B. Katan, W. G. Brydon and M. A. Eastwood. 1980. "Influence of dietary fibre from vegetables and fruits, bran or citrus pectin on serum lipids, and colonic function," Am. J. Clin. Nutr., 33:1745–1756.
162. Sandberg, A.-S., R. Ahderinne, H. Andersson, B. Hallgren and L. Hultén. 1983. "The effect of citrus pectin on the absorption of nutrients in the small intestine," Human Nutr. Clin. Nutr., 37C:171–183.
163. Bosaeus, I., N. G. Carlsson, A. S. Sandberg and H. Andersson. 1986. "Effect of wheat bran and pectin on bile acid and cholesterol excretion in ileostomy patients," Hum. Nutr. Clin. Nutr., 40C:429–440.
164. Anderson, J. W. 1990. "Dietary fibre and human health," HortScience 25(12): 1488–1495.
165. Anderson, J. W. 1985. "Physiological and metabolic effects of dietary fibre," Fed. Proc., Fed. Amer. Soc. Expt. Biol., 44:2902–2906.
166. Briton, G. and T. W. Goodwin. 1982. Carotenoid chemistry and biochemistry. Elmsford, NY: Pergamon Press. p. 398.
167. Straub, O. 1987. Key to Carotenoids. H. Pfander, 2nd ed. Birkhauser Verlag, Basel.
168. Bureau, J. L. and R. J. Bushway. 1986. HPLC determination of carotenoids in fruits and vegetables in the United States. J. Food Sci., 51:128–130.
169. Mathews-Roth, M. M., M. A. Pathak, T. B. Fitzpatrick, L. C. Harber and E. H. Kass. 1970. "Beta-carotene as a photoprotective agent in erythropoietic protoporphyria," New Engl. J. Med., 282:1231–1234.
170. Krinsky, N. I. and S. M. Deneke. 1982. "Interaction of oxygen and oxy-radicals with carotenoids," J. Nat. Cancer Inst., 69:205–210.
171. Burton, G. W. and G. W. Ingold. 1984. "Beta-carotene: an unusual type of lipid antioxidant," Science, 224:569–573.
172. Bendich, A. 1990. Carotenoids: Chemistry and Biology. N. I. Krinsji, M. M. Mathews-Roth, and R. F. Taylor. New York, NY: Plenum Press. pp. 323–336.

173. Micozzi, M. S., G. R. Beecher, P. R. Taylor and F. Khachik. 1990. "Carotenoid analyses of selected raw and cooked foods associated with a lower risk for cancer," J. Natl. Cancer Inst., 82: 282-285.
174. Mathews-Roth, M. M. 1991. "Recent progress in the medical application of carotenoids," Pure and Appl. Chem., 63:147–156.
175. Prasad, K. N. and J. Edwards-Prasad. 1990. "Expressions of some molecular cancer risk factors and their modification by vitamins," J. Am. Coll. Nutr., 9:28–34.
176. Pung, A., J. E. Rundhaug, C. N. Yoshizawa and J. S. Bertram. 1988. "β-Carotene and canthaxanthin inhibit chemically- and physically-induced neoplastic transformation in 10T1/2 cells," Carcinogenesis, 9:1533.
177. Bertram, J. S., A. Pung, M. Churley, J. Kappock, L. R. Wilkens and R. V. Cooney. 1991. "Diverse carotenoids protect against chemically induced neoplastic transformation," Carcinogenesis, 12:671.
178. Zhang, L. X., R. V. Cooney and J. S. Bertram. 1991. "Carotenoids enhance gap junctional communication and inhibit lipid peroxidation in C3H/10T1/2 cells: relationship to their cancer chemopreventive action," Carcinogenesis, 12:2109.
179. Gaziano, J. M., J. E. Manson, P. M. Ridker, J. E. Buring and C. H. Hennekens. 1990. "Beta-carotene therapy for chronic stable angina," Circulation, 82(4)(Suppl. III):201.
180. Abad, A. R. and J. F. Gregory. 1987. "Determination of folate bioavailability with a rat bioassay," J. Nutr., 117:866–873.
181. Halsted, C. H., C. M. Baugh and C. E. Butterworth. 1974. "Jejunal uptake of conjugated folate in man," Gastroenterology, 66:706.
182. White, D. R., H. S. Lee and R. E. Kruger. 1991. "Reversed-phase HPLC/EC determination of folate in citrus juice by direct injection with column switching," J. Agric. Food Chem., 39:714–717.
183. Steinmetz, K. A. and J. D. Potter. 1991. "Vegetables, fruits, and cancer. II. Mechanisms," Cancer Causes and Control, 2:427–442.
184. Hawkes, J. G. and R. Villota. 1989. "Folates in foods: reactivity, stability during processing, and nutritional implications," Crit. Rev. Food Sci. Nutr. 26(6):439–538.
185. Kang, S. S., P. K. W. Wong and M. Norusia. 1987. "Homocysteinemia due to folate deficiency," Metabolism, 36:458–462.
186. Potischman, N. 1983. "Nutritional epidemiology of cervical neoplasia," J. Nutr., 123:424–429.
187. Eaks, I. L. 1964. "Ascorbic acid content of citrus during growth and development," Bot. Gaz., 125:186–191.
188. Tannenbaum, S. R., V. R. Young and M. C. Archer. 1985. "Vitamins and minerals," Food Chemistry, O. R. Fennema. New York, NY: Marcel Dekker Inc. pp. 477–544.
189. DHHS, 1988. The Surgeon General's Report on Nutrition and Health, U.S. Dept. Of Health and Human Services, Superintendent of Documents, U.S. Govt. Print. Off., Washington, DC.
190. Mirvish, S. S., A. Cardesa, L. Wallcave and P. Shibik. 1975. "Induction of mouse lung adenomas by amines or ureas plus nitrite and N-nitroso compounds. Effect of ascorbate, gallic acid, thiocyanate and caffeine," J. Natl. Cancer Inst., 55:633–636.
191. Pipkin, G. E., J. U. Schlegel, R. Nishimura and G. N. Shultz. 1969. "Inhibitory effect of L-ascorbate on tumor formation in urinary bladders implanted with 3-hydroxyanthranilic acid," Proc. Soc. Exp. Biol. Med., 131:522–524.

192. Ackerman, L. V., I. B. Weinstein and H. S. Kaplan. 1978. "Cancer of the esophagus," Cancer in China, H. S. Kaplan and P. J. Tsuchitaui, New York, NY: Alan R. Liss Inc., pp. 111–136.
193. Kolonel, L. N., A. M. Y. Noura, T. Hirohata, J. H. Hankin and M. W. Hinds. 1981. "Association of diet and birth of place with stomach cancer incidence in Hawaii, Japanese and Caucasians," Am. J. Clin. Nutr., 34:2478–2485.
194. Wassertheil-Smoller, S., S. L. Romney, J. Wylie-Rosett, S. Slagle, G. Miller, D. Lucido, C. Duttagupta and P. R. Palan. 1981. "Dietary vitamin C and uterine cervical dysplasia," Am. J. Epidem., 114:714–724.
195. O'Connor, H. J., N. Habibzedah, C. J. Schorah, A. T. Axon, S. E. Riley and R. C. Gamer. 1985. "Effect of increased intake of vitamin C on the mutagenic activity of gastric juice and intragastric concentrations of ascorbic acid," Carcinogenesis, 6:1175–6.
196. Willett, W. C. and B. MacMahon. 1984. "Diet and cancer—an overview," N. Engl. J. Med., 310:633–8.
197. Chen, C. S., P. E. Shaw and M. E. Parish. 1993. "Orange and tangerine juices," Fruit Juice Processing Technology, S. Nagy, C. S. Chen and P. E. Shaw. Auburndale, FL: AgScience, pp. 111–165.
198. Rebeck, H. M. 1990. "Processing of citrus juices," Production and Packaging of Non-carbonated Fruit Juices and Fruit Beverages, D. Hicks. London: Blackie and Son Ltd., pp. 1–32.
199. Braddock, R. J. 1982. "Ultrafiltration and reverse osmosis recovery of limonene from citrus processing waste streams," J. Food Sci., 47:946–948.
200. Owusu-Yaw, J., R. F. Matthews and P. F. West. 1986. "Alcohol deterpenation of orange oil," J. Food Sci., 51(5):1180–1182.
201. Ferrer, O. J. 1984. "Frontal analysis displacement chromatography of terpene-reduced orange oil," M.Sc. Thesis, University of Florida, Gainsville, FL.
202. Blair, J. S., E. M. Godar, J. E. Masters and D. W. Riester. 1952. "Flavor deterioration of stored canned orange juice," Food Res., 17:235–260.
203. Murdock, D. I. and G. L. K. Hunter. 1970. "Bacteriological contamination of some citrus oils during processing," J. Food Sci., 35:652–655.
204. Askar, V. A., H. J. Bielig and H. Treptow. 1973. "Aroma changes in orange juice," Dtsch. Lebensm.-Rundsch., 69:360–367.
205. Tatum, J. H., S. Nagy and R. E. Berry. 1975. "Degradation products formed in canned single-strength orange juice during storage," J. Food Sci., 40:707–709.
206. Gabrielyan, K. A., I. Menyailova and L. A. Nalhapetyan. 1992. "Biocatalytic transformation of limonene," (review), Appl. Biochem., 28(3):241.
207. Fellers, P. J. and R. W. Barron. 1987. "A commercial method for recovery of natural pigment granules from citrus juices for color enhancement purposes," J. Food Chem., 52:994–995, 1005.
208. Higby, W. K. 1963. "A simplified method of determination of some aspects of the carotenoid distribution in natural and carotene fortified orange juice," J. Food Sci., 27:42–49.
209. Ting, S. V. 1961. "The total carotenoid and carotene content of Florida orange concentrate," Proc. Fla. State Hort. Soc., 74:262–267.
210. Khachik, F., G. R. Beecher and W. R. Lusby. 1989. "Separation, identification, and quantification of the major carotenoids in extracts of apricots, peaches, can-

taloupe, and pink grapefruit by liquid chromatography," J. Agric. Food Chem., 37:1465–1473.

211. Gortner, W. A. and V. L. Singleton. 1961. "Carotenoid pigments of pineapple fruit. II. Influence of fruit ripeness, handling and processing on isomerization," J. Food Sci., 26:53–55.
212. Panalaks, T. and T. K. Murray. 1970. "The effect of processing on the content of carotene isomers in vegetables and peaches," Can. Inst. Food Sci. Technol. J., 3: 145–151.
213. Ogunlesi, A. T. and C. Y. Lee. 1979. "Effect of processing on the stereoisomerization of major carotenoids and vitamin A value of carrots," Food Chem., 4: 311–318.
214. Chandler, L. A. and S. J. Schwartz. 1987. "HPLC separation of cis-trans carotene isomers in fresh and processed fruits and vegetables," J. Food Sci., 52: 669–672.
215. Khachik, F., G. R. Beecher and N. E. Whittaker. 1986. "Separation, identification, and quantification of the major carotenoids and chlorophyll constituents in extracts of several green vegetables by liquid chromatography," J. Agric. Food Chem., 34:603–616.
216. Khachik, F., G. R. Beecher and W. R. Lusby. 1988. "Separation and identification of carotenoids and carotenol fatty acid esters in some squash products by liquid chromatography. II. Isolation and characterization of carotenoids and related esters," J. Agric. Food Chem., 36:938–946.
217. Braddock, R. J. and P. G. Crandall. 1981. "Carbohydrate fibre from orange albedo," J. Food Sci., 46:650–651, 654.
218. Braddock, R. J. and T. R. Graumlich. 1981. "Composition of fibre from citrus peel membranes, juice vessels and seeds," Lebensm.-Wiss. u.- Technol., 14:229–231.
219. Baker, R. A. 1984. "Potential dietary benefits of citrus pectin and fibre," Food Technol., 11:133–139.
220. Braddock, R. J. and P. G. Crandall. 1978. "Properties and recovery of waste liquids from citrus pectin pomace manufacture," J. Food Sci., 387–388.
221. Horigome, T., E. Sakaguchi and C. Kishimoto. 1992. "Hypocholesterolaemic effect of banana (*Musa sapientum* L. Var. Cavendishii) pulp in the rat fed on a cholesterol-containing diet," Brit. J. Nutr., 68:231–244.
222. Rouse, A. H. and P. G. Crandall. 1978. "Pectin content of lime and lemon peel as extracted by nitric acid," J. Food Sci., 43:72–73.
223. Voragen, A. G. J., W. Pilnik, J. F. Thibault, M. A. V. Axelos and C. M. G. C. Renaud. 1995. "Pectins," Food Polysaccharides and Their Applications, A. M. Stephen. New York, NY: Marcel Dekker, Inc. pp. 287–340.
224. Barthe, G. A., P. S. Jourdan, C. A. McIntosh and R. L. Mansell. 1988. "Radioimmunoassay for the quantitative determination of hesperidin and analysis of its distribution in *Citrus sinensis*," Phytochemistry, 27:249–254.
225. Mansell, R. L. and E. W. Weiler. 1980. "Radioimmunoassay for the determination of limonin in citrus," Phytochemistry, 19:1403–1407.
226. Johnson, R. L. and B. V. Chandler. 1982. "Reduction of bitterness and acidity in grapefruit juice by adsorptive processes." J. Sci. Food Agric., 56:287–293.
227. Rouseff, R. C. 1980. "Flavonoids and citrus quality," Citrus Nutrition and Quality, S. Nagy and J. A. Attaway. Washington, DC: American Chemical Society, pp. 83–108.

228. Guadagni, D. G., V. F. Maier and J. G. Turnbaugh. 1974. "Effect of subthreshold concentrations of limonin, naringin and sweeteners on bitterness perception," J. Sci. Food Agric., 25:1349–1354.
229. Guadagni, D. G., V. F. Maier and J. G. Turnbaugh. 1973. "Effect of some citrus juice constituents on taste thresholds for limonin and naringin bitterness," J. Sci. Food Agric., 24:1199–1205.
230. Dekker, R. F. H. 1988. "De-bittering of citrus fruit juices: specific removal of limonin and other bitter principles," Austr. J. Biotechnol., 2(1):65–67.
231. Tsen, H. Y. and G. K. Yu. 1991. "Limonin and naringin removal from grapefruit juice with naringinase entrapped in cellulose triacetate fibres," J. Food Sci., 56: 31–34.
232. Kimball, D. A. 1991. Citrus Processing: Quality Control and Technology, New York, NY: Van Nostrand Reinhold. pp. 473–474.

CHAPTER 6

Functional Vegetable Products

P. DELAQUIS[1]
G. MAZZA[1]

THE term *vegetable* embraces a large and diverse category of plants and parts thereof. Table 6.1 shows a classification of vegetables based upon the gross morphology of plant organs. Since this is a book on functional foods and nutraceuticals, we have restricted our attention to those vegetables known to contain components that have been shown to serve functional and nutraceutical roles, such as anticancer and heart-protective affects.

1. THE CRUCIFERAE

1.1. INTRODUCTION

The Cruciferae is a large, homogeneous plant family consisting of well over 2000 species, including several important food crops (Table 6.2). Some Cruciferae are used in the preparation of condiments or garnishes, such as mustard and horseradish sauces, and do not contribute significant nutrients to the diet. In contrast, crucifers that are eaten as vegetables provide concentrated sources of nutrients such as vitamins, minerals and fibre, and nonnutrient phytochemicals such as sulfur-containing compounds. Cruciferous vegetables are often referred to as cole crops and include broccoli, brussel sprouts, cabbage, cauliflower, collards, kale, and kohlrabi. The leaves, buds and flowers of cole crops may be consumed raw or cooked, fermented and

[1]Agriculture and Agri-Food Canada, Pacific Agri-Food Research Centre, Summerland, BC, Canada.

TABLE 6.1. Classification of Vegetables Based on Morphology of Plant Organs.

Type	Examples
Roots	Sweet potatoes, carrots
Modified stems	
Corms	Toro
Tubers	Potatoes
Modified buds	
Bulbs	Onions, garlic
Leaves	Cabbage, spinach, lettuce
Petals (less stalk)	Celery, rhubarb
Flower buds	Cauliflower, artichoke
Sprouts, shoots (young stems)	Asparagus, bamboo shoots
Legumes	Peas, green beans
Cereals	Sweet corn
Vine fruits	Squash, cucumbers
Berry fruits	Tomato, eggplant

TABLE 6.2. Crop Species from the Cruciferae Family.

Species	Common name
Brassica oleracea L. var. *capita* L.	White cabbage
Brassica oleracea L. var. *botrytis* L. subvar. *cymosa*	Broccoli
Brassica oleracea L. var. *botrytis* L. subvar. *cauliflora*	Cauliflower
Brassica oleracea L. var. *gemmifera* DC	Brussel sprouts
Brassica oleracea L. *gongylodes* L.	Kohlrabi
Brassica oleracea L. var. *acephala* DC	Kale
Brassica campestris L. ssp. *rapifera* (Metzg.) Sinsk.	Turnip
Brassica napus L. var. *napobrassica* (L.) Reichenb.	Rutabaga, swede
Brassica nigra (L.L.) Koch	Black mustard
Brassica juncea (L.) Czern et Cross	Brown mustard
Sinapis alba L.	Yellow mustard
Raphanus sativus L.	Radish
Armoracia lapathifolia Gilib	Horseradish
Wasabi japonica Matsum.	Wasabi, Japanese horseradish
Crambe maritima L.	Sea kale
Nasturtium officinalis R. Br.	Water cress
Lepidium sativum L.	Golden cress

occasionally dried. Rutabaga and turnip are also considered coles but, unlike other members of this group, the root is harvested and consumed.

Remedies containing plant materials from the Cruciferae have long been used by practitioners of folk medicine. Their effectiveness in the treatment of infectious disease has been substantiated by the discovery and characterization of antimicrobial phytochemicals from these plants [1]. Convincing experimental evidence also exists for their role in the prevention of degenerative diseases. An early report by Spector et al. [2] revealed that mortality rates for laboratory animals exposed to X-rays could be reduced significantly by feeding of broccoli and cabbage. Epidemiological investigations later revealed that some cancers, particularly cancers of the colon, occur less frequently in individuals who regularly consume vegetables such as brussel sprouts, cabbage and broccoli [3,4]. Pioneering work by Wattenberg [5] eventually led to the identification of sulfur-containing compounds in cole crops that provide protection against cancer. Several groups of compounds in Cruciferae, including the glucosinolates, isothiocyanates, dithiolthiones, indoles, sulfonates, and vitamins, have been reported to be capable of preventing or alleviating diseases and promoting health.

1.2. BIOLOGICALLY ACTIVE COMPONENTS OF CRUCIFERS

1.2.1. Glucosinolates and Their Metabolites

All species of Cruciferae contain glucosinolates—vacuole-bound glycosides consisting of a β-thioglucose group, R side chain and oxime moiety. More than 100 of these compounds have been identified to date. They are grouped as aryl, alkyl, aromatic, or indole glucosinolates according to the structure of the side chain. Examples of each type of glucosinolate and the chemical nature of their side chain are given in Table 6.3.

TABLE 6.3. Major Glucosinolates in Cole Crops.

R-Side Chain	Trivial Name	Major Source
3-Butenyl	Gluconapin	Cabbage, broccoli
Allyl	Sinigrin	Cabbage, broccoli, brussel sprouts
2-Phenylethyl	Gluconasturtiin	Turnips, watercress
3-Indolylmethyl	Glucobrassicin	Cabbage, broccoli, brussel sprouts
1-Methoxy-3-indolylmethyl	Neoglucobrassicin	Cabbage, broccoli, brussel sprouts, rutabaga
Benzyl	Glucotropaeolin	Garden cress
(R)-2-hydroxy-3-butenyl	Progoitrin	Rutabaga

Upon release from the vacuole, as a result of injury or mechanical disruption, glucosinolates are readily hydrolyzed by a group of enzymes referred to as myrosinases (thioglucoside glucohydrolase EC 3:2:3:1). The structure of reactants and products of this reaction are shown in Figure 6.1. Some of these products, particularly the isothiocyanates and indoles, contribute significantly to the flavour of processed cole crops. The tissues of freshly harvested plants do contain low levels of these compounds. Some release may occur as a result of senescence during storage, as a consequence of food processing operations that disrupt the cell, or through thermal degradation during cooking. Differences in myrosinase activity between cultivars and within plant tissues may also lead to variable isothiocyanate concentrations [6].

Glucosinolate content and the relative proportion of individual glucosinolates are species specific. The most concentrated source of glucosinolates in the human diet appears to be brussel sprouts, which may contain between 600–3900 μg glucosinolate/g wet tissue [7]. From a practical point of view, differences due to cultivar and agronomic practice are probably more important, since glucosinolate content has a considerable impact on the quality of stored and processed cole crops. Breeding and selection of cultivars for more desirable organoleptic properties has led to considerable variation in the glucosinolate profiles of vegetables such as cabbage [8] and brussel sprouts [7]. Climate and horticultural practice also influence the accumulation of these compounds in the plant, and the effects of plant spacing, irrigation and fertilizer have been described in cabbage [8]. In addition, glucosinolate content may increase during storage [9,10].

Digestion of glucosinolates and absorption of hydrolytic products have been demonstrated in humans, but the fate of these compounds is not well known. Dose-dependent excretion of metabolites following ingestion of glucosinolate rich meals was reported by Chung et al. [11]. Purified aromatic isothiocyanates administered by the oral route are also quickly absorbed [12]. Unfortunately, there are little data on the fate of other isothiocyanates in the digestive tract. Enzymatic hydrolysis and release of the glucosinolate reaction products may occur during chewing, but myrosinase activity is expected to decline rapidly under the adverse conditions encountered in the stomach. A more likely mechanism for the absorption of hydrolytic products of dietary glucosinolates involves release through the action of myrosinase-producing enteric microorganisms and rapid uptake in the colon [13–16].

1.2.2. Non-glucosinolate Sulfur Compounds

At least one substituted sulfoxide, *S*-methyl cysteine sulfoxide (SMCSO), occurs in Cruciferae [17,18]. Marks et al. [19] measured SMCSO concentrations in several cole crops including broccoli (19.1 mg/100 g

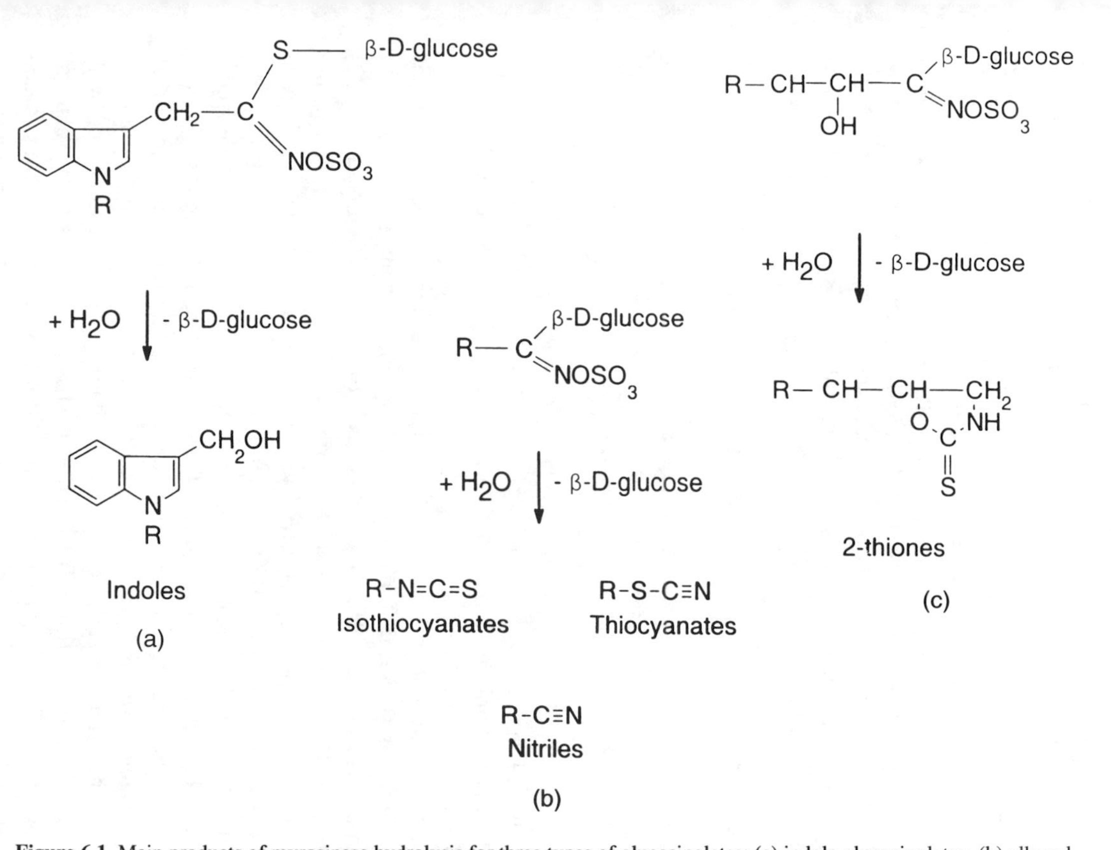

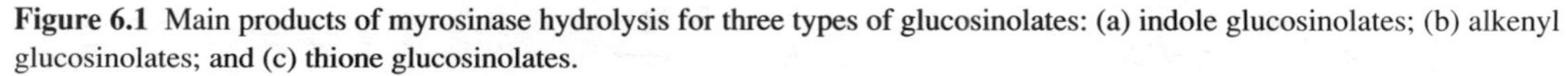

Figure 6.1 Main products of myrosinase hydrolysis for three types of glucosinolates: (a) indole glucosinolates; (b) alkenyl glucosinolates; and (c) thione glucosinolates.

fresh weight), cabbage (18.5 mg/100 g), cauliflower (14.3 mg/100 g) and brussel sprouts (68.0 mg/100 g). In a more recent study, Nakamura et al. [20] found higher concentrations in broccoli (198 mg/100 g), cabbage (101 mg/100 g) and cauliflower (122 mg/100 g). SMCSO content in *Allium* sp. is known to be cultivar dependant and subject to differences in soil fertility [21]. Levels in Cruciferae are probably influenced by similar factors.

Substituted cysteine sulfoxides are rapidly degraded by cysteine lyases in macerated tissues to yield a variety of rearrangement products including thiosulfinates and sulfides. These compounds contribute to the characteristic odor and flavor of raw onions, garlic, and, to a lesser extent, cole crops. Cysteine lyase activity is optimal at pH 6.5 and declines rapidly under acidic conditions. One of the main products of the reaction in Cruciferae is *S*-methyl methane thiosulfinate (MMTSO).

1.2.3. Vitamins

Cole crops have long been recognized as important sources of vitamin C and other water-soluble vitamins in the diet including riboflavin, niacin and thiamine (Figure 6.2). Crucifers are also a good source of the fat-soluble vitamins generally grouped together as vitamin A, which refers to a class of compounds with similar structure and activity that includes beta-carotene, retinol and retinal (vitamin A aldehyde). The fat-soluble vitamin K_1 (phytonadione) is also found in cole crops.

Dietary contributions of individual vitamins differ between species of Cruciferae, as shown in Table 6.4 [22]. The relative concentration of each vitamin also varies within the plant. For example, Branion et al. [23] showed that the highest levels of vitamin C in cabbage are found in the outer green leaves and the core, while the area between the core and green leaves contains significantly lower amounts. In addition, vitamin contents differ between cultivars of the same species. Burrell et al. [24] measured a range of concentrations between 48.0 and 180.9 mg/100 g among 31 cabbage cultivars grown under the same conditions, and found that concentrations changed over the growing season. The latter report also served to illustrate the effect of soil fertility, since vitamin C content increased with high nitrogen applications. Toivonen et al. [25] showed a similar relationship in broccoli, although climactic conditions during the growing season had far more impact on vitamin C. Cabbage and kale have been reported to contain appreciable amounts of the fat-soluble vitamin K_1 [26]. Climate, soil fertility, growing conditions, maturity, and location within the plant also influenced the level of vitamin K_1.

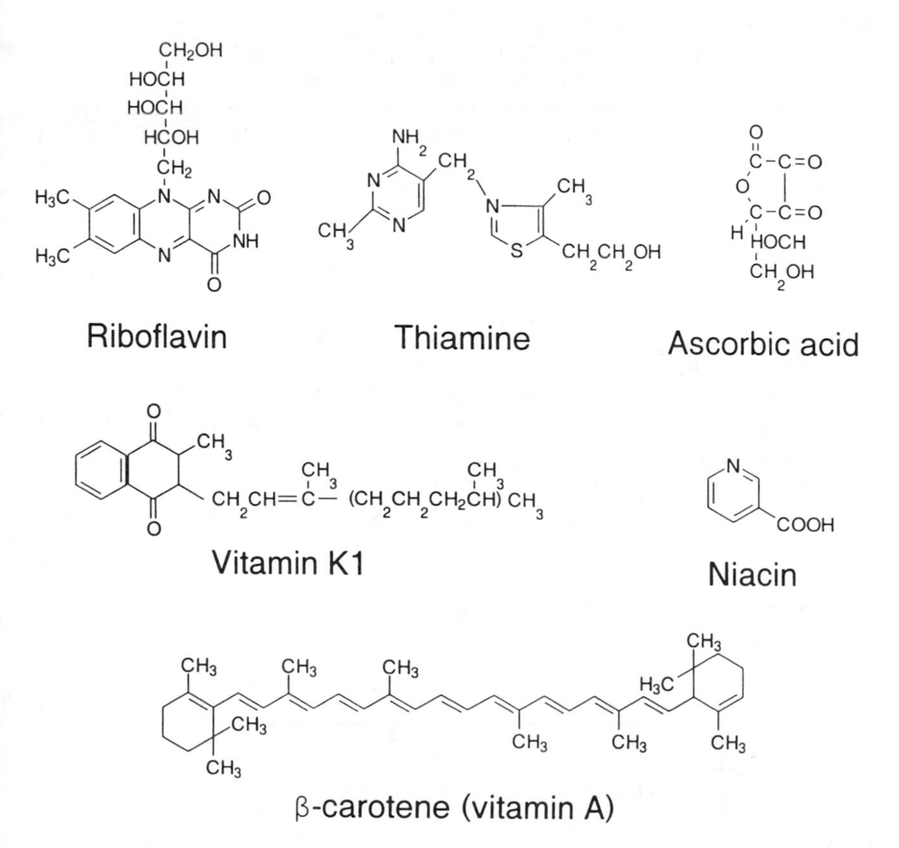

Figure 6.2 Chemical structures of vitamins found in Cruciferous crops.

1.3. HEALTH BENEFITS

1.3.1. Isothiocyanates

Several isothiocyanates have been shown to inhibit or block tumours induced by chemical carcinogens. Tumours of the mammary gland [27], digestive tract [28], and nitrosamine-induced lung tumours [29] occur at lower frequencies in laboratory animals fed aromatic isothiocyanates (phenethyl, benzyl and the synthetic phenyl derivative) prior to exposure to the carcinogen. A potent isothiocyanate inhibitor of mammary tumours, 1-isothiocyanate-4-(methylsulfinyl)butane (sulforaphane), was isolated from broccoli and characterized by Zhang et al. [30,31]. Synthetic analogues of sulphoraphane were

TABLE 6.4. Water-Soluble Vitamins in Various Raw and Processed Cole Crops.

Source	Vitamin A (RE[a])	Vitamin C (mg)	Thiamine (mg)	Niacin (NE[b])	Riboflavin (mg)
Cabbage, fresh	13.51	56.8	.06	.54	.03
Cabbage, boiled, drained	8.86	24.0	.06	.38	.06
Sauerkraut, canned	2.01	14.9	.02	.32	.02
Cauliflower, fresh	1.9	71.6	.08	1.06	.06
Cauliflower, boiled, drained	.8	51.1	.06	.99	.05
Rutabaga, fresh	0	25.0	.09	.95	.04
Rutabaga, boiled, drained	0	21.7	.07	.83	.04
Radish, fresh	trace	22.2	.29	.44	.04
Turnip, fresh	0	21.2	.04	.58	.03
Turnip, boiled, drained	0	9.1	.03	.41	.02
Broccoli, fresh	154.3	93.4	.07	1.13	.12
Broccoli, boiled, drained	140.8	62.8	.08	1.28	.21

[a]Retinol equivalents.
[b]Niacin equivalents.
Source: Data from Reference [22].

also chemoprotective [32]. Additional evidence suggests that some isothiocyanates may play a direct role in the suppression of tumour growth. Phenethyl isothiocyanate was shown to inhibit the growth of human leukemia cells [33]. Allyl isothiocyanate is believed to play a role in both chemoprevention and suppression of tumour growth [34,35].

Although experimental evidence for the protective role of isothiocyanates is extensive, the mechanisms responsible for these effects have not been fully elucidated. Chemoprotective isothiocyanates or their metabolites can reduce the toxic effects of carcinogens in two ways. They may interfere with a group of enzymes generally referred to as phase 1 enzymes (cytochrome P-450 dependant monooxygenases). These enzymes activate carcinogens by forming reactive electrophiles that may bind to DNA. Such a mechanism is believed to be responsible for the inhibition of nitrosamine-induced lung tumorigenesis by aromatic isothiocyanates [31,36]. A second type of mechanism effected by sulforaphane and structurally related isothiocyanates, is the induction of phase 2 detoxifying enzymes (glutathione transferases, NAD(P)H:quinone oxidoreductase, UDP-glucoronosyl transferases), which convert carcinogens to easily excreted products [37].

Whether these chemoprotective effects are due to the undenatured isothiocyanates or to secondary metabolites formed within the cell is unclear. The isothiocyanates likely do not survive long in the cell since reactions with oxygen, sulfur or nitrogen-centered nucleophiles readily occur due to the strongly electrophilic central carbon of the isothiocyanate group. Products of these reactions may include carbamates, thiocarbamates or thiourea derivatives. Some of these compounds, particularly the carbamates, have been shown to offer protection against cancer in animal trials [5]. Proteins can react directly through free amino groups or sulfhydryl side chains [38]. Such reactions may lead to modification of enzyme activity and could be implicated in chemoprevention. Evidence exists to support a role for secondary metabolites in this type of reaction. Recent studies by Adesida et al. [33] have shown that thiocarbamyl metabolites of phenylethyl isothiocyanate are more efficient inhibitors of human leukemia cell growth than the parent molecule.

1.3.2. Indoles

Epidemiological evidence suggests that indolyl glucosinolates or their metabolites play a significant role in cancer prevention. Rats fed glucobrassicin prior to exposure to potent carcinogens demonstrate substantially reduced incidences and multiplicities of chemically induced tumours [31]. The chemoprotective effect of indolyl glucosinolates is due to the hydrolytic products of myrosinase activity, more specifically, the rearrangement products of the indolyl moiety: indole-3-carbinol, 3,3′-diindolyl methane and indole-3-acetonitrile. Chemoprotective effects have been demonstrated for each of these compounds, and indole-3-carbinol is usually reported to exert the greatest activity [39]. Indole-3-carbinol is known to be a potent inducer of phase 2 enzymes [40] and a variety of other hepatic enzymes [41]. It has also been shown to inhibit DNA binding of benzopyrene and *N*-nitrosodimethylamine, two potent cancer inducers and mutagens. Recent investigations have suggested that indole-3-carbinol may be a useful chemoprotective agent against hormone-induced cancers, particularly estrogen-related uterine and breast cancers [17]. In addition, animal studies indicate that this compound may inhibit the initiation of aflatoxin B1-induced carcinogenesis [42], although it may act as a tumour promoter after initiation [43].

1.3.3. Dithiolthiones

Cabbage is reported to contain another group of potent inhibitors of carcinogenesis that are believed to derive from glucosinolates: the dithiolthiones. The structure of an unsubstituted 1,2-dithiole-3-thione is provided in Figure 6.3. Al-

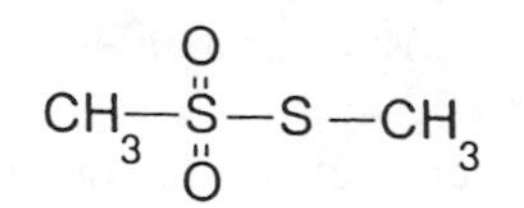

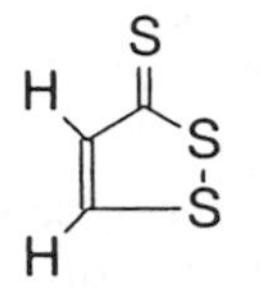

Figure 6.3 Chemical structures of *S*-methyl methanesulfonate and 1,2-dithiole-3-thione.

though the presence of these compounds was reported in cabbage over 30 years ago, analytical difficulties have hindered investigations on the occurrence or distribution of these compounds in cabbage or other cruciferous vegetables. Using available methods, Marks et al. [19] were unable to detect 1,2-dithiole-3-thiones in cabbage purchased from a local supermarket. Nonetheless, there is continued interest in the biological activity of dithiolthiones due to their ability to protect against known cancer-inducing chemicals, including aflatoxins [44]. One of the synthetic dithiolthiones, 5-(2-pyrazinyl)-4-methyl-1,2-dithiole-3-thione or Oltipraz, has been widely investigated and has been shown to inhibit tumorigenesis of the breast, skin, lung, colon, trachea, forestomach, liver, and urinary bladder in rodents [45]. This compound has also been reported to inhibit the replication of the human immunodeficiency virus, which is believed to induce acquired immune deficiency syndrome [46].

1.3.4. Other Sulfur-Containing Compounds

Both SMCSO and MMTSO have been reported to inhibit chemically and uv-induced mutagenesis [17,19]. Oral administration has also been reported to inhibit chemically induced colon carcinogenesis in the rat [20].

1.3.5. Vitamins

Both vitamins C and A have been reported to protect against cancer in laboratory studies, but their mode of action remains unclear [47]. In addition, vitamin C is essential for the formation of collagen and is required for the development of cartilage, bone and teeth, proper wound healing, formation of hemoglobin and erythrocytes, and immunological reactions. Vitamin A plays a significant role in vision and in the synthesis of glycoproteins. Vitamin K_1 is essential for synthesis of blood-clotting factors in the liver.

1.4. PRODUCTS FROM CRUCIFERS

1.4.1. Food Products

Fresh cruciferous vegetables develop characteristic pungent, sulfuraceous odors and flavors during preparation by cutting or slicing. Flavor and odor development is the consequence of complex enzymic and non-enzymic reactions that usually involve the physiologically active sulfur-containing compounds. The hydrolytic products of myrosinase activity shown in Figure 6.1, notably isothiocyanates and nitriles, have a significant impact on the sensory characteristics of cruciferous vegetables. An important volatile component in cooked cabbage, dimethyl disulfide, is released upon enzymic hydrolysis of SMCSO [48]. Isothiocyanates and indoles induce hot, bitter flavors and odors ranging from pungent to sulfurous. Accumulation of isothiocyanates (chiefly allyl isothiocyanate) in coleslaw is responsible for occasional development of undesirable "hot" and bitter flavors during storage [49]. Alterations in the glucosinolate profile of cabbage can therefore have a significant impact on the sensory quality of products derived from this vegetable. Increases in glucosinolate content have been demonstrated in other stored raw or processed products and may also lead to quality defects. The appearance of hot flavors in broccoli florets stored aerobically have been linked to increased glucosinolate content. Conversely, the appearance of off-flavors is delayed under atmospheres containing elevated (20%) CO_2 [50]. It is unclear whether such differences result from reduced glucosinolate content alone or from changes in myrosinase activity over time.

Most cruciferous plant foods are consumed raw in salads, or immediately after cooking in the home. Some, such as broccoli and brussel sprouts, may be preserved for this purpose by freezing, which is an effective means for the preservation of typical brassica flavors. On the other hand, few cole crops are dehydrated or canned. Heat treatment leads to formation of glucosinolate breakdown products and development of undesirable cooked flavors. Destruction of myrosinase and other enzyme activities are responsible for the lack of desirable flavor development, while non-enzymic thermal reactions may lead to the synthesis of undesirable flavors and odors [6,7]. Attempts have been made to restore the flavor profile of heat-processed cabbage by addition of myrosinase, but this does not appear to have been widely adopted by the industry [51]. More recently, Shim and Lindsay [52] showed that treatment with sulfhydryl oxidase prevents the development of undesirable odors in cooked cabbage and broccoli.

Extended storage in cold and controlled atmospheres (CA) tends to lower the vitamin content of cole crops. For example, Vitamin C in cabbage has been reported to decrease by 10% within a few days after harvest due to autolytic reactions, and a further 25% upon long-term storage under CA at 0°C [53]. Tadokoro et al. [54] observed thiamin, riboflavin and vitamin C losses in cabbage after 60 days of storage. In contrast, vitamin C content in whole broccoli and broccoli spears remained stable under aerobic storage at 4°C in a study by Paradis et al. [55], but significant losses were observed at 20°C. The effect of long-term storage on the vitamins of other cole crops does not appear to have been studied in detail.

Most vitamins are susceptible to heat. Thus, application of heat for blanching or cooking of cole crops may lower vitamin content either though thermal degradation or leaching. Vitamin C, vitamin A, niacin and thiamine are thermolabile and destruction by heat may be extensive, while riboflavin is stable under most cooking conditions. Vitamin levels in raw and cooked cabbage given in Table 6.4 illustrate the extent of loss incurred through boiling, a common method of preparation in the home. According to this source, vitamin C losses in boiled cabbage are greater than 50%. Similar losses have been reported in broccoli, but vitamin C retention was improved by cooking in steam or in a sous vide (boil-in-bag) package, possibly due to a reduced leaching [56].

Considerable tonnage of cabbage is devoted to production of a fermented product, sauerkraut, which is occasionally pasteurized for long-term preservation. Fermentation of salted cabbage is initiated by several species of homofermentative and heterofermentative lactic acid bacteria. The final acid content of sauerkraut reaches 1.5–2.0%, expressed as lactic acid. Vitamin concentrations tend to be significantly lower in pasteurized sauerkraut than in fresh cabbage (Table 6.4), although some vitamins are likely consumed by bacteria during fermentation. This, however, is probably not the main cause of overall losses. Indeed, microbial growth may contribute a variety of vitamins to the product. The overall reduction in vitamin content is more likely a consequence of thermal processing. Similar reductions are expected in pickled cabbage and cauliflower, which are heat-processed after being mixed with vinegar brines. Cabbage is also used extensively in the commercial production of coleslaw, a prepared salad made by mixing raw cabbage with a vinegar-based dressing, either mayonnaise or vinaigrette. There is no evidence that this process leads to reductions in vitamin content in excess of those expected for stored fresh cabbage.

2. ONIONS AND GARLIC

2.1. INTRODUCTION

There are more than 250 members of the genus *Allium*, the onion family. Two of these, onions (*A. cepa*), and garlic (*A. sativum*), have been used in traditional and folk medicine for over 4,000 years [57–61]. Disorders for which both garlic and onions have been used include asthma, arthritis, arteriosclerosis, chicken pox, the common cold, diabetes, malaria, tumors, and heart problems [60] (Table 6.5). Modern science has shown that alliums and their constituents have several therapeutic effects, including antiplatelet aggregation activity, fibrinolytic activity, anticarcinogenic effects, antimicrobial activity, and anti-inflammatory and antiasthmatic effects [57,60–62]. Some important garlic and onion-derived compounds and their biological activities are given in Table 6.6.

2.2 BIOLOGICALLY ACTIVE COMPONENTS OF ALLIUMS

2.2.1. Sulfur Compounds

Volatile sulfur compounds are not present as such in intact cells. The reaction between the enzyme allinase and the volatile precursors [*S*-alk(en)yl cysteine sulfoxide and sulfonic acid] takes place when cells are ruptured, resulting in the formation of different thiosulfinates and related sulfonic acid derived compounds [20,57–59,63] (Figure 6.4). Decomposition of thiosulfinates such as allicin (diallyl thiosulfinate) proceeds by several pathways. One interesting pathway involves three molecules of allicin that combine, producing two molecules of ajoene, which is apparently at least as potent as aspirin in preventing the aggregation of blood platelets and thus in keeping blood

TABLE 6.5. Some of the Diseases and Ailments Against Which Onion and Garlic Have Been Claimed to Be Effective.

Arteriosclerosis	Epilepsy	Measles
Arthritis	Epistaxis	Meningitis
Asthma	Eye burns	Phthisis
Bronchitis	Fits	Piles
Catarrh	Gangrene	Rheumatism
Chicken Pox	Hypertension	Scurvy
Cholera	Influenza	Septic poisoning
Common cold	Jaundice	Smallpox
Diabetes	Laryngitis	Splenic enlargement
Dropsy	Lead poisoning	Tobacco poisoning
Dysentery	Lip, mouth disorders	Tuberculosis
Dyspepsia	Malaria	Typhoid

Source: Reprinted with permission from Reference [60]. Copyright CRC Press, Boca Raton, Florida © 1985.

TABLE 6.6. Some Bioactive Compounds of Onion and Garlic Products.

Compound	Biological Activity	Reference
Allicin	Antimicrobial	Block [57]
Alliin	Hypolipidaemic	Sumiyoshi and Wargovich [77]
	Antimicrobial	Sumiyoshi and Wargovich [77]
	Hypoglycaemic	Sumiyoshi and Wargovich [77]
Ajoene	Antithrombotic	Sumiyoshi and Wargovich [77]
Diallyl sulfide	Chemopreventive	Sumiyoshi and Wargovich [77]
	Insecticidal	Sumiyoshi and Wargovich [77]
Thiosulfinates	Antiinflammatory	Breu and Dorsch [62]
	Antiasthmatic	Breu and Dorsch [62]
Cepaenes	Antiphlogistic	Breu and Dorsch [62]
	Antiasthmatic	Breu and Dorsch [62]
Saponin	Antihyperlipaemic	Breu and Dorsch [62]
Ascorbic acid	Antioxidant	Pisha and Pezzuto [64]
Caffeic acid	Antitumor	Pisha and Pezzuto [64]
	Antimutogenic	Pisha and Pezzuto [64]
	Antioxidant	Pisha and Pezzuto [64]
	Antiviral	Pisha and Pezzuto [64]
Linoleic acid	Immunomodulation	Pisha and Pezzuto [64]
S-methyl methanethiosulfonate	Antimutogenic	Kanamure et. al. [20]

from clotting [57]. Through other non-enzymatic degradation pathways, thiosulfonates are converted into sulfur-containing compounds such as thiosulfinates, cepaenes, mono-, di- tri- and tetrasulfides, thiols, thiophenes, and sulfur dioxide.

The types and concentrations of sulfur compounds extracted from onions and garlic are affected by plant maturity, production practices, cultivar, location in the plant, and processing conditions. Freeman [65] used both gas-liquid chromatography and chemical analysis of thiosulfinate, pyruvate and sulfur to investigate the distribution of flavor components in onion, garlic, and leek. His results for onion show that dried outer scales were virtually free of volatile sulfur-containing compounds, the concentrations of which (on a fresh-weight basis) increased progressively from a minimum value in the outer leaf to the innermost tissue and the stem. The latter often contained more than twice the concentration present in the outer leaf. Sulfate addition to the soil was found to affect the levels of sulfur-containing compounds in the mature plant, with low levels of sulfate nutrition being associated with low

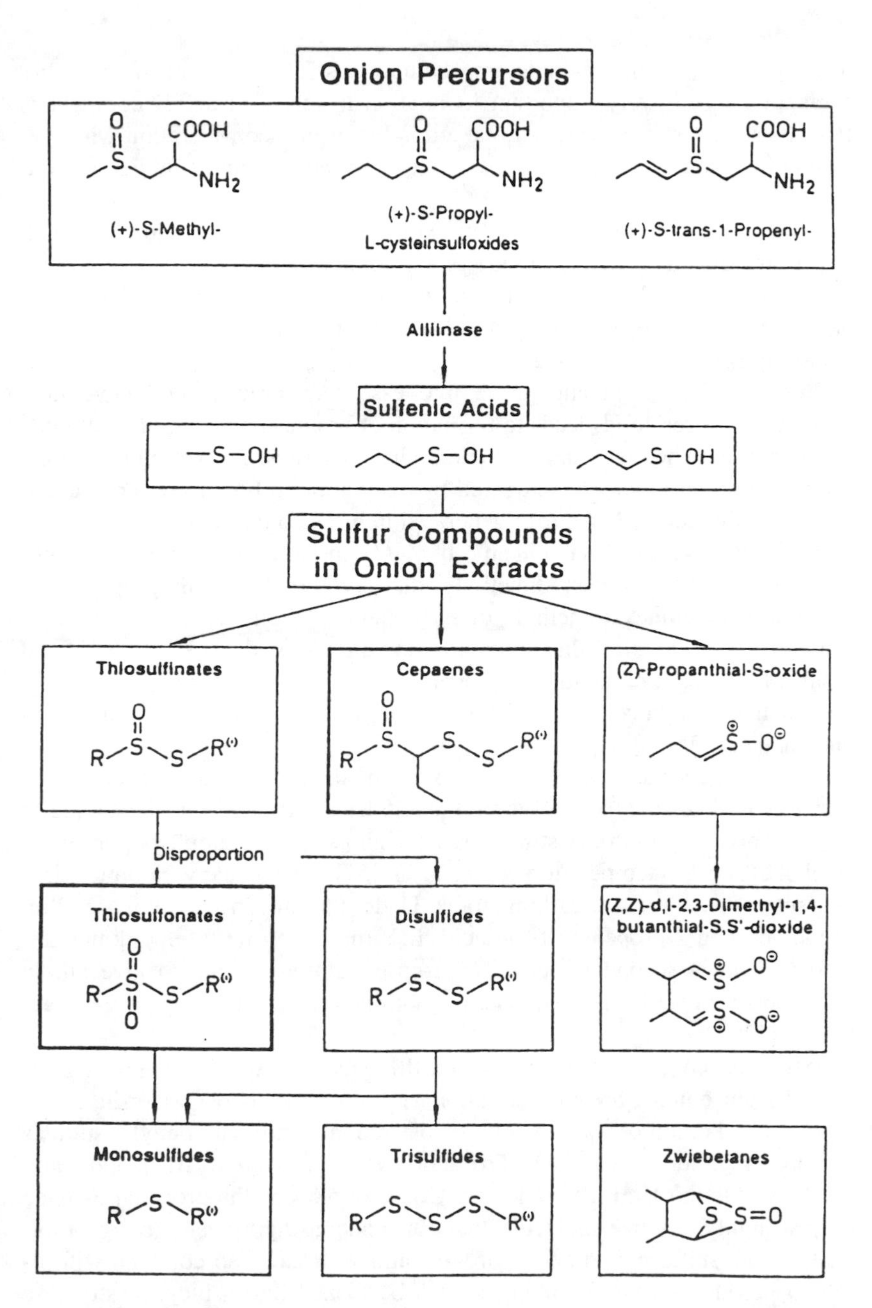

Figure 6.4 Sulphur compounds in extracts of *Allium cepa* L. (Reprinted from Reference [62], by permission of the publisher Academic Press Limited, London.)

levels of volatile sulphur-containing compounds [66,67]. Plant maturity has been found to be very important in relation to levels of sulfur compounds [68], therefore, it is necessary to take this factor into consideration when selecting for pungency, flavor or bioactive compounds in onion and garlic products.

Storage and processing have been extensively studied in conjunction with flavor strength. In general, storage of onion and garlic seems to lead to increased levels of sulfur-containing compounds, probably because of the gradual formation of the *S*-alk(en)yl-L-cysteine sulfoxides from γ-glutamyl precursors during storage [69–72].

Processing of onion and garlic into essence, extracts, and dehydrated, canned and frozen foods leads to formation of products with significantly different physico-chemical and biological characteristics. For example, the essential oil of garlic may be extracted by distillation in boiling water in a still or by introduction of live steam generated in a separate steam boiler. The extracted volatiles are collected in an oily mass consisting of dimethyl-, diallyl-, and methyl allyl sulfides; dimethyl-, dipropyl-, diallyl-, allylpropyl-, and methylallyl disulfides; dimethyl-, diallyl-, and methylallyl trisulfides; methylpropyl trisulfide; diallyl thiosulfinate; and sulfur dioxide [73,74]. Garlic oil obtained by steam distillation has been shown to possess biological properties, such as antioxidant effects. However, it lacks bactericidal and antithrombotic activity [75,76].

When garlic is subjected to extraction with ethanol and water at room temperature, it yields the oxide of diallyl disulfide, allicin, which is the source of garlic odor (Figure 6.5). A still gentler technique, which employs pure ethyl alcohol at subzero temperature, yields alliin [57], a molecule with optical isomerism at the sulfur and carbon atoms. Under the influence of allinase alliin decomposes to 2-propenesulfenic acid. In turn, 2-propenesulfenic dimerizes, or pairs with a second molecule of 2-propenesulfenic acid, to give allicin [57], which possesses hypolipidaemic, antimicrobial and hypoglycaemic activities [77].

Extraction conditions also influence the nature of sulfur compounds extracted from onions. Steam distillation yields a dark-yellow water-insoluble liquid, called onion oil, which consists of predominantly alkyl-enyl disulfides and higher sulfides [73,78–81]. Extraction with a mixture of freon and water at 0°C yields the lacrimatory factor, $C_2H_5CH{=}SO$ or thiopropanal *S*-oxide [57], a highly reactive molecule that can undergo hydrolysis giving propionaldehyde, sulfuric acid and hydrogen sulfide. It can also combine with itself to produce a four-atom ring or can be locked into a bicyclic structure [57, 62,82]. Extraction of onion with ethyl alcohol at subzero temperatures yields the lacrimatory precursor, trans-(+)-*S*-(1-propenyl)-L-cystein sulfoxide, which is a positional isomer of alliin that is converted by the enzyme allinase

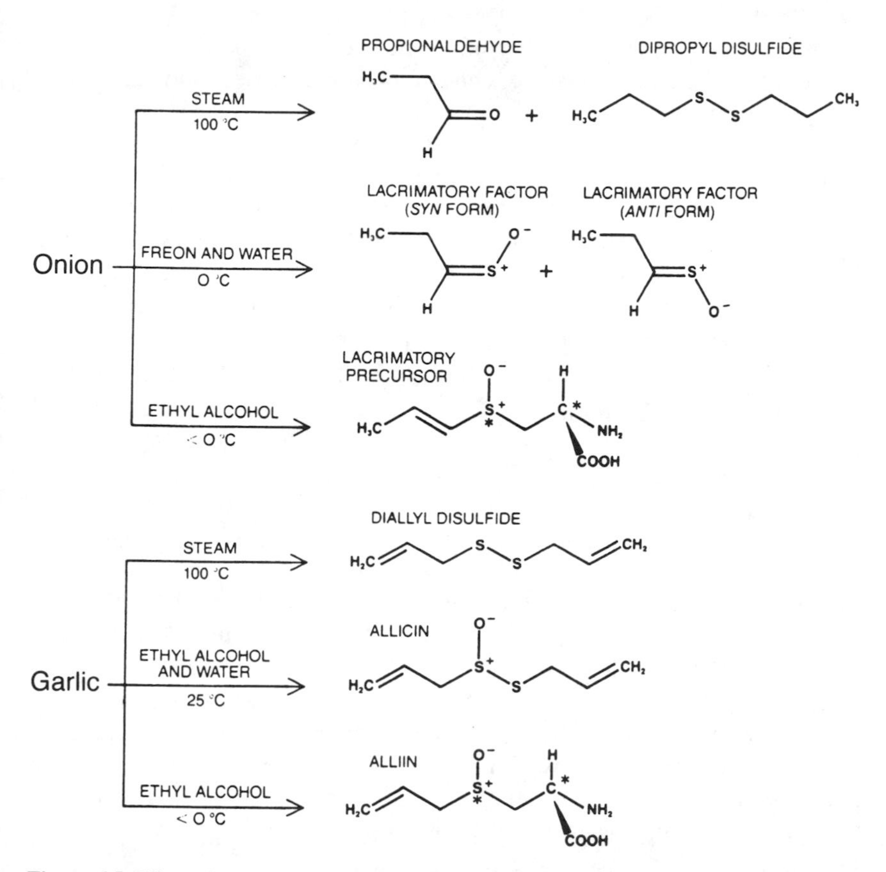

Figure 6.5 Effect of processing method on the type of physiologically active compounds extracted from onion and garlic. (Reprinted from Reference [57], with permission. ©Jerome Kuhl, 1998.)

into the lacrimatory factor [57,82]. Supercritical carbon dioxide extraction of flavor components present in onion juice that had been held at 20–22°C for 15 h has yielded 28 sulfur-containing compounds, including diallyl thiosulfinate, propyl methanethiosulfonate, dithiin derivatives, diallyl sulfide, and diallyl trisulfide [83].

Onion juice can contain an undesirable bitter component(s) that is eliminated if the juice is initially acidified to pH 3.9, then adjusted to normal pH 5.5–6.0 [84]. The component(s) responsible for the bitter flavor is unknown, although the action of allinase on the lacrimatory precursor *trans*-(+)-*S*-(1-propenyl)-L-cystein sulfoxide has been reported to lead to bitterness in homogenated onion [85].

Determination of pyruvate, thiosulphinate and headspace volatiles in fresh, dehydrated, freeze-dried, pickled, canned, boiled, and fried onion has shown that processed products contain only a fraction of the sulfur-containing compounds present in the fresh vegetables [68,86,87]. Taste threshold determinations indicated a 95% reduction in flavor intensity, while analysis by gas chromatography revealed component losses ranging from 25% for enzymatically produced pyruvate, 26% for the lachrymator, and an overall 57% reduction in total peak areas [68,70]. Freeze-drying yields a product that retains more of the characteristic flavor components of fresh onion, as judged by sensory tests, than the other processes.

2.2.2. Non-sulfur Compounds

2.2.2.1. Flavonoids

Flavonoids are present in the bulbs as well as the leaves of alliums. The flavonoids found in onion include eight quercetin glucosides, the 4′-glucoside, the 7,4′-diglucoside, the 3-4′-diglucoside, the 3-glucoside, the 7-glucoside, the 3,7-diglucoside, the 3-rutinoside (rutin), the 3-rhamnoside (quercitrin), the 7,4′-, and 3-glucosides of kaempferol, isorhamnetin 4′-glucoside, and eight anthocyanins [88,89]. Most of these flavonoids are potent antioxidants with a wide array of biochemical functions. They are involved in immune function, gene expression, capillary and cerebral blood flow, liver function, enzyme activity, platelet aggregation, and collagen, phospholipid, cholesterol and histamine metabolism [89,90].

2.2.2.2. Prostaglandins

Onion has been suggested as a potential source of prostaglandins [91,92]. To date, nine prostaglandins have been isolated and characterized. They are prostaglandin A_1, A_2, B_1, E_1, $F_{1\alpha}$, $F_{2\alpha}$, D_2, E_2, and 6-keto-prostaglandin $F_{1\alpha}$ [93, 94].

2.2.2.3. Sterols and Steroid Saponins

Sterols and steroidal glycosides have been found in various alliums, and saponin levels of 0.1% in leek, 0.021% in garlic and 0.095% in onion have been reported [95]. The content of sterols and their glycosides has been determined in leaves and bulbs of onion, with levels of 2.7% free sterols and sterol esters, 1.7% sterol glycosides and 0.8% acetyl sterol glycosides in leaves reported. In bulbs, the amount of these sterol derivatives is lower than in leaves [61].

2.2.2.4. *Oligofructans*

Onion bulbs contain a high concentration (35–40% dry wt) of fructans, which constitute a major portion of the water-soluble carbohydrates and have been associated with the storage life of bulbs [96–98]. Fructans are fructosyl polymers, which consist of linear chains of D-fructose molecules joined by β(2→1) linkages. This chain is terminated by a D-glucose molecule linked to fructose by an α (1→2) bond as in sucrose. A number of health benefits result from ingestion of oligofructans or oligosaccharides. These include proliferation of bifidobacteria and reduction of detrimental bacteria in the colon, reduction of toxic metabolites and detrimental enzymes, prevention of pathogenic and otogenous diarrhea, prevention of constipation, protection of liver function, reduction of serum cholesterol, reduction of blood pressure, and anticancer effects [99,100].

2.3. HEALTH BENEFITS

Alliums are used in traditional and folk medicine for many major and minor disorders. Modern science can recognize many of the symptoms alleviated by garlic and onion as indicative of certain diseases and disorders. However, hard experimental data are available to support only a few of the claims of their healing properties. This section will deal briefly with the major medicinal aspects of alliums, emphasizing chemical evidence concerning the active principle(s).

2.3.1. Anticarcinogenic Effects

A number of alliums have been found to possess significant anticarcinogenic activity with garlic being the most effective [101–105]. The effect has been attributed primarily to the interaction of the sulfur components of garlic with tumor cell metabolism [106–108]. Glutathione-*S*-transferases and glutathione increased following feeding of processed garlic to rats [108–110]. Glutathione-*S*-transferases are important detoxifying enzymes that remove various deleterious chemical species, produced from carcinogenic substances, by binding them to reduced glutathione [106,110]. Any agent that promotes the activity of glutathione-*S*-transferases would conceivably have a chemopreventive effect. Oral administration of allyl methyl trisulfide promoted glutathione-*S*-transferase activity in the forestomach, small bowel mucosa, liver, and lung of mice. Similarly, three other garlic-derived sulfur compounds, allyl methyl disulfide, diallyl trisulfide and diallyl disulfide, stimulated the glutathione-*S*-transferase activity in these organs, whereas the saturated propyl analogues failed to do so [108]. *S*-allyl cysteine has also been found to increase glutathione and glutathione-*S*-transferase activity in liver and mammary tissue [109,110]. The induction of these enzymes and the increase in glutathione concentration indicate increased detoxification of carcinogenic compounds and may account for the ability of garlic and its constituents to reduce experimentally induced cancer of the breast and liver [109,111].

Topical application of garlic oil substantially reduced skin cancers induced by the carcinogen 7,12-dimethylbenze(a)anthracene (DMBA) in mice [105], and dietary garlic and its constituents inhibited the development of skin cancer produced by DMBA and 12-*O*-tetradecanoylphorbol-13-acetate (TPA) [112,113]. In mice, injection of a garlic extract suppressed cancer development of transplanted cancer cells [114]. With Murphy-Sturm lymphosarcoma in rats, it was found that pre-incubation of tumor cell suspension with thiosulphinate prior to subcutaneous transplantation resulted in complete inhibition of tumor growth [101,102].

That alliums provide protection against cancer has also been shown by at least two epidemiological studies [115–117]. In one of these studies conducted by researchers at the National Cancer Institute in Bethesda, Maryland, in collaboration with Chinese investigators, 564 patients with stomach cancer were compared with 1,113 controls from an area of China where stomach cancer rates are high. They found that consumption of garlic, onions, and scallions is inversely proportional to the occurrence of stomach cancer [116, 117].

2.3.2. Cardiovascular Protective Effects

2.3.2.1. Antiplatelet Aggregation Activity

Platelet aggregation induced by collagen, arachidonic acid, ADP, adrenaline, and the thrombin has been shown to be suppressed/inhibited by garlic and onions and their components, and the effect is dose dependent [118–120]. Several mechanisms appear to be involved in this process. They include modification of the platelet membrane properties, inhibition of calcium mobilization and inhibition of several steps of the arachidonic acid cascade in blood platelets [121].

In a placebo-controlled double-blind study, the effects of administering 800 mg of garlic powder to humans over a period of 4 weeks was studied. It was found that spontaneous platelet aggregation disappeared, the microcirculation of the skin increased by 47.6%, the plasma viscosity decreased by 3.2%, the diastolic blood pressure decreased by 9.5%, and blood glucose concentration decreased by 11.6% [122].

2.3.2.2. Thromboxane Biosynthesis

Part of the antiaggregation activity of onion and garlic preparations seems to be mediated by the inhibition of thromboxane biosynthesis in blood platelets.

Thromboxane A_2 is produced in the platelets and causes the release of ADP, which acts on the platelets in concert with the thromboxane. In a 1986 study by Ali and Mohammad [123], aqueous extract of garlic inhibited thromboxane A_2 formation in clotting blood and in blood vessel preparations of rabbits. In another study, garlic provided protection against thrombo-cytopenia and hypotension after intravenous injection of collagen or arachidonic acid in rabbits [124]. In this latter study, all animals that were pretreated with garlic survived the lethal dose of collagen and arachidonic acid, while those in the untreated group died [124].

2.3.2.3. Fibrinolytic Activity

The effects of onion and garlic products on fibrinolytic activity, plasma fibrinogen levels and blood-clotting time have been studied in rabbits and healthy and diseased humans. Studies on animals have shown that alliums enhance the blood's fibrinolytic activity, suppress blood fibrinogen concentration, and increase blood coagulation time [125–127]. In humans with myocardial infarction treated with garlic oil (equivalent to 1 g raw garlic per kilogram body weight), the fibrinolytic activity has been found to increase by 63 to 96% above the postinfarction value [128]. It has been suggested that much of the activity derives from the sulfur-containing components. Cycloalliin has been found to increase the fibrinolytic activity of venous blood without having any effect on platelet aggregation [129].

2.3.2.4. Effects on Blood and Tissue Lipids

A large number of studies have been conducted to assess the importance of garlic and onion in lowering serum cholesterol levels in both animals [130–133] and humans [134–138]. The results generally show that alliums lower cholesterol and triglycerides levels in the blood. The range of reduction is significant but relatively small.

2.3.3. Other Effects

Consumption of both garlic and onion bulbs can reduce the level of blood sugar, and exert beneficial effects on diabetes [139,140]. (Prop-2-enyl) propyl disulfide has been proposed as the active agent in onion [139], and di(prop-2-enyl) disulfide and di(prop-2-enyl) thiosulfinate are believed to be responsible for the activity displayed by garlic [141,142].

Alliums also reduce hypertension [143], and apparently stimulate the body's immune system [59]. Many of the other pharmacological effects of onion and garlic (Table 6.5) can be ascribed to their antimicrobial activity, as a range of bacteria and fungi are inhibited by treatment with garlic and onion extracts [144–146].

2.4. ALLIUM-BASED PRODUCTS

Allium-based products are currently marketed in a variety of forms. They include for onion: dehydrated onion pieces, onion powder, onion flavoring, encapsulated flavors, oleoresins and essential oils, onion salt, pickled onions, canned, frozen and packaged onion; for garlic: dehydrated garlic powder, garlic salt, garlic juice, and garlic flavoring, encapsulated flavors, oleoresins and essential oils. The processed products have considerable advantages to the food industry. The reduction in bulk means lower transport and distribution costs, the products are not subject to seasonal fluctuation in availability and prices, are more reproducible in organoleptic quality, and are more readily dispersed in food products than is the case with the chopped, sliced or blended fresh or stored vegetable [60].

The primary function of existing allium products is to provide consumers with the characteristic pungent flavor imparted by volatile sulfur compounds. The value of both garlic and onion in disease prevention and health promotion has been of little consideration in the development of consumer products from alliums. In recent years, the therapeutic properties of alliums have been recognized in the processing of onion and garlic capsules, tablets, and even the development of odorless products. These products, however, are more like drugs than true functional foods. Significant progress has been made in designing lower salt-, lower calorie-, lower cholesterol-, and higher fiber- and calcium-containing foods, using new food ingredients, such as artificial sweeteners and carbohydrate or protein-based fat substitutes and new processing methods [147,148]. Thus, one possible approach in development of novel value-added allium-based functional foods involves incorporation of garlic and/or onion into food products such as bakery products, imitation meats and sausages, and meat pies. The key to the more widespread and increased consumption of alliums, and consequently to the increased exploitation of their medicinal and physiological properties, is improvement or elimination of the flavor of these vegetables. A solution for flavor improvement would be inactivation of the enzyme allinase and production of onion and garlic products rich in alliin and non-sulfur compounds. Freezing is a suitable method for the destruction of the allinase in onion or garlic [149]. Products manufactured from frozen alliums would lack the volatile sulfur-containing compounds normally found in these products. However, the high concentration of alliin (0.24% of the weight of typical garlic bulb), flavonoids, saponins, oligofructans and prostaglandins present in frozen or freeze-dried products would still provide considerable health benefits. The frozen or freeze-dried alliums could serve as raw material for the production of numerous new products including purified fructo-oligosaccharides and S-alk(en)yl-cysteine sulfoxides.

3. VEGETABLES RICH IN NONDIGESTIBLE OLIGOSACCHARIDES

3.1. INTRODUCTION

Oligosaccharides are one of the most popular functional food components in Japan, used primarily as sucrose substitutes in many consumer products including soft drinks, cookies, breakfast cereals, cakes, chocolates, and candies [150]. Physiologically functional oligosaccharides are short-chain polysaccharides that have unique chemical structures (Figure 6.6) and that are not di-

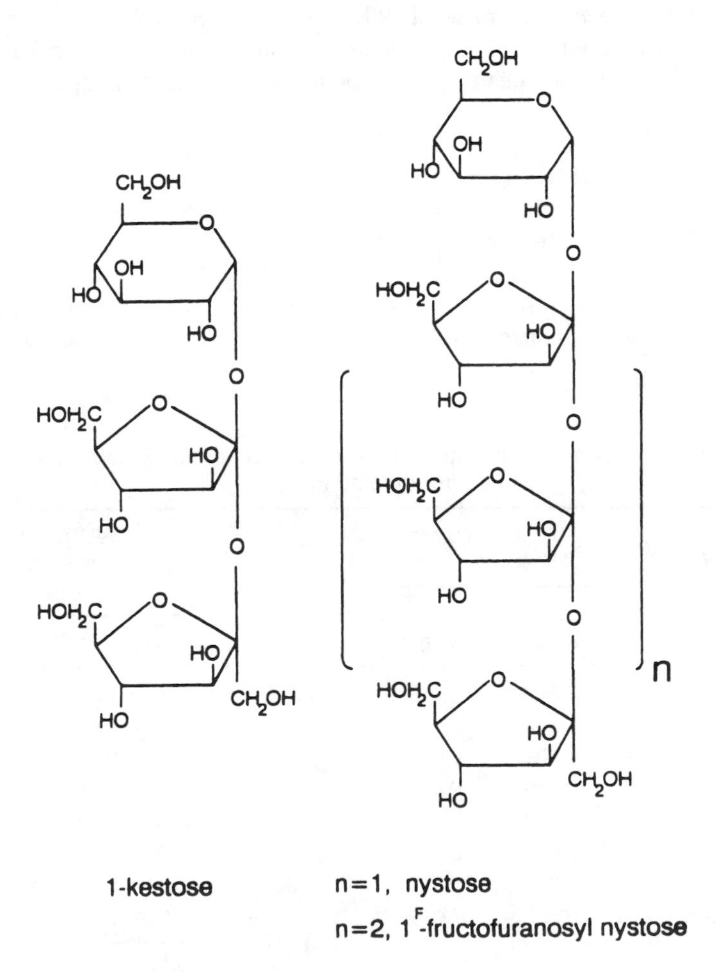

Figure 6.6 Chemical structure of fructo-oligosaccharides.

gested by humans. Rather, they are selectively utilized by the bifidobacteria, a group of microorganisms that are antagonistic toward undesirable bacteria in the digestive tract [99,100,150–153]. The health benefits of oligosaccharide consumption arise primarily from increased numbers of bifidobacteria in the colon.

Several vegetables are known to contain oligosaccharides. Chicory roots, Jerusalem artichoke tubers, asparagus, banana, tomatoes, alliums, and burdock are rich in fructo-oligosaccharides (FOS) [96,98,151,154,155]. However, the estimated average daily ingestion of these oligosaccharides from natural sources has been estimated at only 13.7 mg/kg/day or 806 mg/day (Table 6.7) [151]. Thus, consumption of supplemental fructo-oligosaccharides has been recommended [99, 151]. The health benefits associated with the consumption of these sugars include reduction of constipation, blood lipids, blood cholesterol, blood pressure, and intestinal toxins [99,100,150–152].

3.2. HEALTH BENEFITS

3.2.1. Improved Intestinal Microflora

Human and animal studies have shown that addition of fructo-oligosaccharides to the diet stimulates proliferation of *Bifidobacterium* species and other

TABLE 6.7. Concentration and Consumption of Fructo-oligosaccharides in Selected Foods.

Food	Daily Consumption of Food (g/kg/day)		Wet Weight FOS (%)	Wet Weight Average Daily Consumption of FOS	
	Dry Weight	Wet Weight		g/kg/day	mg/day
Banana	0.224	0.933	0.30	2.80×10^{-3}	164.95
Barley	0.057	0.064	0.15	9.66×10^{-5}	5.69
Garlic	0.001	0.002	0.60	1.17×10^{-5}	0.69
Honey	0.015	0.018	0.75	1.38×10^{-4}	8.11
Onion	0.002	0.018	0.23	4.00×10^{-5}	2.36
Rye	0.004	0.005	0.50	2.26×10^{-5}	1.33
Brown sugar	0.011	0.011	0.30	3.22×10^{-5}	1.90
Tomato	0.492	7.029	0.15	1.05×10^{-2}	620.99
			Total	1.37×10^{-2}	806.02

Source: Reprinted from Reference [151], with permission from *Food Technology*.

useful bacteria while suppressing the growth of harmful bacteria, such as *Clostridium* species [99,100]. Enhanced bifidobacterial growth results in the production of acetic and lactic acids, lower intestinal pH and inhibition of bacteria that produce toxic, malodorous substances, such as amines, ammonia, and hydrogen sulfide. Amines contribute to high blood pressure and can react with nitrites to form carcinogenic nitrosamines. Bifidobacteria are known to degrade nitrosamines. Protection against infection may be also due to direct antagonism through secretion of antimicrobial compounds. A high-molecular weight substance effective against *Shigella flexneri* 5503-DI, *S. faecalis*, *E. coli*, and other bacteria has been described [156,157]. Bifidin, an antibiotic produced by *Bifidobacterium bifidum*, is effective against *Shigella dysenteriae*, *Salmonella typhosa*, *Staphylococcus aureus*, and *E. coli* [99, 100].

3.2.2. Noncariogenic

Fructo-oligosaccharides and other oligosaccharides, such as erythritol, sorbitol, maltitol, and lactitol, are noncariogenic sucrose substitutes. These sweeteners are not utilized by dental cariogenic bacteria, such as *Streptococcus mutans,* that normally form the acids and insoluble β-glucans that lead to formation of dental caries [158].

3.2.3. Reduction of Serum Cholesterol

Consumption of 6–12 g of oligosaccharides/day for 2–3 months can reduce total serum cholesterol by 20–50 dl [159]. The reduction has been attributed to increased populations of the intestinal bacterium *Lactobacillus acidophilus*, which has been shown to assimilate cholesterol *in vitro* [160]. At least one strain (*L. acidophilus* 2056) has been reported to inhibit absorption of cholesterol micelles through the intestinal wall [161].

3.2.4. Anticonstipation Effect

Daily consumption of 3–10 g of oligosaccharides produces an anticonstipation effect within a week. This effect has been attributed to increased levels of short-chain fatty acids and increased intestinal peristalsis produced by increased population of bifidobacteria in the intestines [99,100,162]. On the other hand, consumption of large amounts of nondigestible oligosaccharides causes diarrhea, abdominal distention and flatulence. The reported maximum dose of small-size fructo-oligosaccharides (GF, GF_2, GF_3, GF_4, G_1 glucose and F_1 fructose) that does not cause diarrhea in humans is 0.3 and 0.4 g/kg body weight/day for men and women, respectively [100]. The corresponding nondiarrhea-causing doses for soybean oligosaccharides are 0.64 g/kg for men and 0.96 g/kg for women [163]. The effective daily doses of pure oligosaccharides are 3.0 g for fructo-oligosaccharides, 2.0–2.5 g for galacto-oligosaccharides, 2.0 g for soybean oligosaccharides, and 0.7 g for xylo-oligosaccharides [100,150].

3.3. OLIGOSACCHARIDES-RICH PRODUCTS

At least one Japanese company, Meiji Seika Ltd. of Kanagana, has commercialized production of fructo-oligossacharides, mainly consisting of GF_1, GF_2, GF_3, and GF_4, by enzymatic transformation of sucrose [100]. Mixtures of these small fructo-oligosaccharides, marketed under the name of Neosugar, are widely used as food ingredient, and as feed ingredient to reduce diarrhea and increase food efficiency in piglets, and as pet food ingredient to reduce faecal odour [164,165]. Neosugar is produced from sucrose by the action of the enzyme β-fructofuranosidase produced from *Aspergillus niger*. More recently, Yun et. al. [166] developed a continuous process that uses immobilized cells of *Aureobasidium pollulans* entrapped in calcium alginate gel to produce fructo-oligosaccharides from sucrose solutions. Table 6.8 illustrates some of the recent processes for the enzymatic production of fructo-oligosaccharide-rich syrups. The composition of Neosugar and Neosugar G is shown in Table 6.9. These products have been found to be nondigestible by human and animal enzymes but selectively utilized by bifidobacteria [99,100].

TABLE 6.8. Recent Processes for the Enzymatic Production of Fructo-oligosaccharides.

Enzyme Source	Substrate	Process[a]	Stability[b]	Reference
A. pullulans	770 g L^{-1} sucrose	Semibatch (IC)	60 days	[167]
A. pullulans	770 g L^{-1} sucrose	Continuous (IC)	100 days	[166]
A. pullulans	770 g L^{-1} sucrose	Semibatch (IE)	20 days	[168]
Aureobasidium sp.	400 g L^{-1} sucrose	Continuous (IE)	30 days	[169]
A. phoenicis	750 g L^{-1} sucrose	Batch (M)	—	[170]
A. pullulans	Sugar beet molasses	Continuous (IC)	25 days	[171]

[a]IC, IE, and M indicate immobilized cells, immobilized enzyme, and intact mycelium, respectively.
[b]Stability was evaluated by the maximum operation period without loss of the initial enzyme activity.
Source: Reprinted from Reference [172], with permission from Elsevier Science, Inc., 655 Avenue of the Americas, New York, NY 10010-5107.

TABLE 6.9. Composition (%) of Two Fructo-oligosaccharide-rich Products, Neosugar and Neosugar G.

Component	Neosugar	Neosugar G
Monosaccharides[a]	0	35
Sucrose	0	10
GF_2[b]	30	25
GF_3[c]	57	25
GF_4[d]	13	5
Total of fructo-oligosaccharides[e]	100	55

[a]Glucose and fructose.
[b]1-Kestose.
[c]Nystose.
[d]1^F-Fructosylnystose.
[e]GF_2, GF_3, GF_4.
Source: Reprinted from Reference [100] with permission from the Japan Bifidus Foundation.

The enzymatic processes used to prepare fructo-oligosaccharides from sucrose yield a large amount of glucose in addition to fructo-oligosaccharides. Removal of the glucose is required to prepare dry powder or glucose-free products, and this requires relatively expensive chromatographic processes [172]. On the other hand, it is possible to prepare fructo-oligosaccharide-rich flour [173,174] and/or syrup [175,176] by partially hydrolizing the Jerusalem artichoke or chicory fructans either with acid or with endo inulase (Figure 6.7). Jerusalem artichoke tubers contain about 200 g solids/kg fresh weight, which consists of 680–830 g fructans, 150–160 g protein, 130 g insoluble fibres, and 50 g ash/kg dry matter [177]. Once diced or sliced, the tubers develop brown coloration and off-flavor because they are rich in polyphenols and polyphenol oxidases. Therefore, for the production of dietary fructo-oligosaccharides-rich flour and/or syrup the oxidases are inactivated by heating at a temperature ranging from 90°C (water blanching) to 150°C (steam heating) (Figure 6.7). Table 6.10 illustrates examples of syrup preparations produced by hydrolysis at 100°C and pH 2.5. As expected, longer heating times led to greater hydrolysis, which resulted in sweeter syrup of lower fructo-oligosaccharide content.

Whether produced enzymatically or from plant sources, fructo-oligosaccharides have found use in a wide range of food applications. One effective use of FOSs can be achieved by blending them with other sweeteners such as high-fructose syrup and tabletop sugars, and using the mixture to formulate food products with enhanced health benefits. Addition of fructo-oligosaccharides to some food products may also enhance consumer preference for the products. Recent results of sensory testing with yogurt-containing FOSs, for

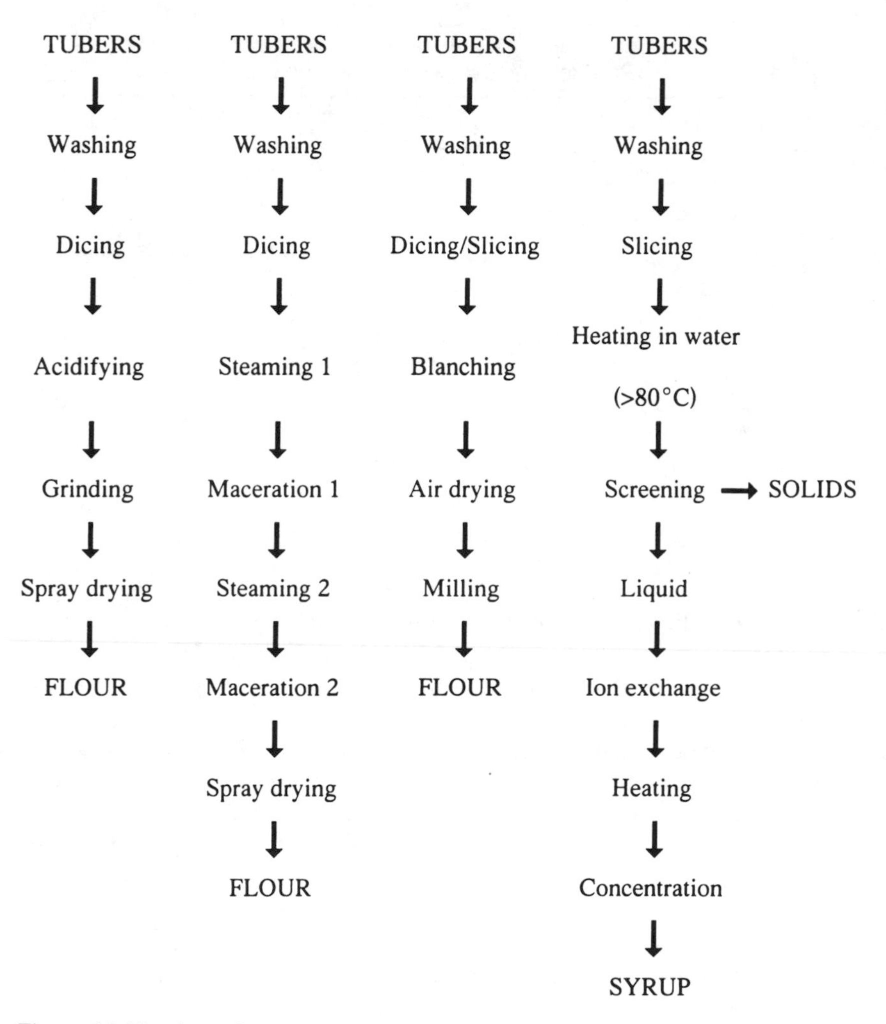

Figure 6.7 Flowsheets for production of fructo-oligosaccharides-rich flour and syrup from Jerusalem artichoke tubers.

instance, have indicated a slight flavour and texture preference for the FOS-enhanced yogurt. The FOS-containing product was identified as being creamier and less chalky in texture, and sweeter, with less sour/fermented taste and aftertaste [151].

4. OTHER VEGETABLES

It is now well established that consumption of the so-called yellow-green vegetables offers protection against cancer [178] and heart disease [179]. Epi-

TABLE 6.10. Composition of Carbohydrates in Fructo-oligosaccharide-rich Syrup from Jerusalem Artichoke Tubers.

Heating Time (min)	Composition (%)						
	G[a]	F	DP 2	DP 3	DP 4	DP 5	DP > 5
2.5	4.6	16.4	44.9	11.9	8.6	6.0	7.6
5	7.2	26.2	38.1	8.1	6.6	4.6	9.3
10	13.5	45.1	36.7	3.3	1.6	0.6	tr
15	22.1	63.8	12.1	tr	tr	tr	tr

[a]G = glucose; F = fructose; DP = degree of polymerization (DP = *n* contains F_n or GF_{n-1}); tr = trace.

Source: Reprinted from Reference [165] with kind permission of Elsevier Science—NL, Sara Burgerhartstraat 25, 1055 KV Amsterdam, The Netherlands.

demiological investigations have revealed significant risk reduction in populations favouring diets rich in vegetables such as carrots, spinach, lettuce, peppers and tomato. These plants are good and varied sources of carotenoids, a diversified group of yellow-to-red plant pigments that includes α- and β-carotene, lutein, lycopene and various xanthophylls.

The role of β-carotene in protection against cardiovascular disease has been substantiated by clinical studies [180]. Protection against skin and lung cancer, particularly in smokers, is enhanced in populations that consume foods rich in β-carotene [178,179]. Some investigators have suggested that beneficial effects are due to complex interactions between plant carotenoids rather than to single site reactions involving individual compounds [181]. Several mechanisms have been proposed to account for the physiological activity of the carotenoids. The most plausible involves the potent antioxidant properties exhibited by these compounds and their ability to deactivate harmful chemical species such as singlet oxygen, free radicals, lipid peroxy radicals. Evidence also exists for direct stimulation of the immune system and immune response by various carotenoids. Readers are referred to the review of Thurnham [179] for a description of these effects.

Although the beneficial effects of several vegetables on human health have long been recognized, the identity and properties of the physiologically active compound(s) are often unclear. For example, sporadic reports in the literature suggest that celery is a cancer-preventive food, although it does not contain significant amounts of the better-known cancer-protective phytochemicals. Investigations by Zheng et al. [182] have shown that celery seed oil contains a phthalide that induces the detoxifying glutathione transferase enzyme. Shinohara et al. [183] extracted a heat-stable glycoprotein from spinach that modulates the growth of human cancer cells.

5. CONCLUSIONS AND FUTURE PROSPECTS

Crucifers, alliums, and many other vegetables contain a variety of biologically active phytochemicals. Scientific evidence for their role in the prevention of disease, such as cancer, is growing rapidly. Despite recent advances, however, much remains to be learned about the role of these compounds in human health.

The impact of food handling and processing on nutrients such as vitamins and minerals are well known. Unfortunately, the stability and fate of phytochemicals such as sulfur-containing compounds in processed foods have not been investigated to the same extent. Despite this paucity of data, there is widespread but unsubstantiated belief that beneficial phytochemicals or the bioactive compounds derived from them are depleted by processing, particularly where thermal treatments are employed. Further research in this area is necessary for the development of processes or techniques that will lead to optimal retention of desirable compounds during food preparation, both in the home and in large-scale food processing operations.

Classical plant breeding methods and biotechnological techniques are routinely used to enhance desirable traits in crop plants. It is tempting to think that new cultivars of Cruciferae, Alliums and other vegetables with new or elevated levels of beneficial phytochemicals could be created. Such an approach is fraught with difficulties, however, since many of these compounds are highly odoriferous and may impart undesirable sensory characteristics to the plant. In fact, it has been suggested that current cabbage cultivars are largely the result of early attempts to reduce sulfurous odors in cooked cabbage. In addition, several of the sulfur-containing compounds discussed above have been shown to exert toxic effects at higher concentrations.

Further research on the physiological properties, stability and safety of seemingly beneficial phytochemicals occurring in vegetables is clearly required. Past research efforts have focussed largely on the occurrence and physico-chemical properties of these molecules. In future, more effort should be devoted to the physiological properties and stability of biologically active phytochemicals in fresh and processed foods.

6. REFERENCES

1. Delaquis, P. J. and G. Mazza. 1995. "Antimicrobial properties of the isothiocyanates and their role in food preservation." Food Technology 49:73–84.
2. Spector, H. 1959. "Reduction of X-radiation mortality by cabbage and broccoli." Exp. Biol. Med. 100:405–407.
3. Graham, S., H. Dayal, M. Swanson, A. Mittelman and G. Wilkinson. 1978. "Diet in the epidemiology of cancer of the colon and rectum." J. Natl. Cancer Inst. 61:709–714.

4. Manousos, O., N. E. Day, D. Trichopoulos, F. Gerovassilis, A. Tnozou and A. Polychronopoulos. 1983. "Diet and colorectal cancer: a case control study in Greece." Int. J. Cancer. 32:1–5.
5. Wattenberg, L. W. 1978. "Inhibitors of chemical carcinogenesis." Adv. Cancer Res. 26:197–226.
6. Pocock, K., R. K. Heaney, A. P. Wilkinson, J. E. Beaumont, J. G. Vaughan and G. R. Fenwick. 1987. "Changes in myrosinase activity and isoenzyme pattern, glucosinolate content and the cytology of myrosin cells in leaves of heads of three cultivars of English white cabbage." J. Sci. Food Agric. 41:245–257.
7. Heaney, R. K. and G. R. Fenwick. 1980. "Glucosinolates in *Brassica* vegetables: analysis of 22 varieties of brussel sprouts." J. Sci. Food Agric. 31:785–793.
8. Pritchard, M. K and R. F. Becker. 1989. "Cabbage," Quality and Preservation of Vegetables, Eskin, N. A. M., Boca Raton, FL: CRC Press, Inc. pp. 265–284.
9. Guffy, S. K. and J. R. Hicks. "Effect of cultivar, maturity and storage on respiration, dry weight and glucosinolate content of cabbage." Acta Hortic. 157:211–218.
10. Bérard, L. S. and Chong, C. 1984. "Influence of storage on glucosinolate fluctuations in cabbage." Acta Hortic. 157:203–210.
11. Chung, F.-L., M. A. Morse, K. I. Ecklind and J. Lewis. 1992. "Quantitation of human uptake of the anticarcinogen phenethyl isothiocyanate after a watercress meal." Cancer Epidemiol. Biomarkers & Prev. 1:383–388.
12. Mennicke, W. H., K. Görler, G. Krumbiegel, D. Lorenz and N. Rittman. 1988. "Studies on the metabolism and excretion of benzyl isothiocyanate in man." Xenobiotica 18:441–447.
13. Oginsky, E. L., A. E. Stein and M. A. Greer. 1965. "Myrosinase activity in bacteria as demonstrated by the conversion of progoitrin to goitrin." Proc. Soc. Exp. Med. 119:360–364.
14. Tani, N., M. Ohtsuru and T. Hata. 1974. "Isolation of myrosinase producing microorganism." Agric. Biol. Chem. 38:1617–1622.
15. Nugon-Baudon, L., O. Szylit and P. Raibaud. 1988. "Production of toxic glucosinolate derivatives from rapeseed meal by intestinal microflora of rat and chicken." J. Sci. Food Agric. 43:299–308.
16. Nugon-Baudon, L., S. Rabot, J.-M. Wal and O. Szylit. 1990. "Interactions of the intestinal microflora with glucosinolates in rapeseed meal toxicity: first evidence of an intestinal Lactobacillus posessing a myrosinase-like activity." J. Sci. Food Agric. 52:547–559.
17. Stoewsand, G. S. 1995. "Bioactive organosulfur phytochemicals in *Brassica oleracea* vegetables—a review." Food Chem. Toxicol. 33:537–543.
18. VanEtten, C. H. and I. A. Wolff. 1973. "Natural sulfur compounds," Toxicants Occurring Naturally in Foods, Washington, DC: National Research Council, Food Protection Committee, National Academy of Sciences. pp. 210–234.
19. Marks, H. S., H. C. Leichtweiss and G. S. Stoewsand. 1991. "Analysis of a reported organosulfur, carcinogenesis inhibitor: the 1,2-dithiole-3-thione in cabbage." J. Agric. Food Chem. 39:893–895.
20. Nakamura, Y. K., T. Matsuo, K. Shimoi, Y. Nakamura and I. Tomita. 1996. "*S*-methyl methanethiosulfonate, bio-antimutagen in homogenates of Cruciferae and Liliaceae vegetables." Biosci. Biotech. Biochem. 60:1439–1443.
21. Randle, W. M., J. E. Lancaster, M. L. Shaw, K. H. Sutton, R. L. Hay and M. L. Bussard. 1995. "Quantifying onion flavor compounds responding to sulfur

fertility—sulfur increases levels of alk(en)yl cysteine sulfoxides and biosynthetic intermediates." J. Am. Soc. Hort. Sci. 120:1075–1081.

22. Health and Welfare Canada. 1988. Nutrient Value of Some Common Foods, Ottawa, ON: Canadian Government Publishing Services.
23. Branion, L. D., S. J. Roberts, C. R. Cameron and A. M. McCready. 1948. "The ascorbic acid content of cabbage." J. Am. Diet. Assoc. 24:101–106.
24. Burrell, R. C., H. D. Brown and V. R. Elbright. 1940. "Ascorbic acid content of cabbage as influenced by variety, season and soil fertility." Food Res. 5:247–252.
25. Toivonen, P. M. A., B. J. Zebarth and P. A. Bowen. 1994. "Effect of nitrogen fertilization on head size, vitamin C content and storage life of broccoli (*Brassica oleracea* var. *Italica*)." Can. J. Plant Sci. 74:607–610.
26. Ferland, G. and J. A. Sadowski. 1992. "Vitamin K1 (phylloquinone) content of green vegetables: effect of plant maturation and geographical growth location." J. Agric. Food Chem. 40:1874–1877.
27. Wattenberg, L. W. 1977. "Inhibition of the carcinogenic effects of polycyclic hydrocarbons by benzyl isothiocyanate and related compounds." J. Natl. Cancer Inst. 58:395–398.
28. Stoner, G. D., D. T. Morrissey, Y.-H. Heur, E. M. Daniel, A. J. Galati and S. A. Wagner. 1991. "Inhibitory effects of phenethyl isothiocyanate on *N*-nitrosobenzylmethylamine carcinogenesis of the rat esophagus." Cancer Res. 51:2063–2068.
29. Morse, M. A., S. G. Amin, S. S. Hecht and F.-L. Chung. 1989. "Effects of aromatic isothiocyanates on tumorigenicity, *O*-methylguanine formation, and metabolism of the tobacco-specific nitrosamine 4-(methylnitrosamino)-1-(3-pyridyl)-1-butanone in A/J mouse lung." Cancer Res. 49:2894–2897.
30. Zhang, Y., P. Talalay, C.-G. Cho and G. H. Posner. 1992. "A major inducer of anticarcinogenic protective enzymes from broccoli: isolation and elucidation of structure." Proc. Natl. Acad. Sci. 89:2399-2403.
31. Zhang, Y., T. W. Kensler, C.-G. Cho, G. H. Posner and P. Talalay. 1994. "Anticarcinogenic activities of sulforaphane and structurally related synthetic norbornyl isothiocyanates." Proc. Natl. Acad. Sci. 91:3147–3150.
32. Zhang, Y. and P. Talalay. 1994. "Anticarcinogenic activities of organic isothiocyanates: chemistry and mechanisms." Cancer Res. (Suppl.) 54:1976s–1981s.
33. Adesida, A., L. G. Edwards and P. J. Thornalley. 1996. "Inhibition of human leukemia 60 cell growth by mercapturic acid metabolites of phenylethyl isothiocyanate." Food Chem. Toxicol. 34:385–392.
34. Bogaards, J. J. P., B. Van Ommen, H. E. Falke, M. I. Willems and P. J. Van Bladeren. 1993. "Glutathione *S*-transferase subunit induction patterns of brussel sprouts, allyl isothiocyanate and goitrin and rat liver and small intestine mucosa: a new approach for the identification of inducing xenobiotics." Food Chem. Toxicol. 28:81–88.
35. Nastruzzi, C., R. Cortesi, E. Esposito, E. Menegatti, O. Leoni, R. Iori and S. Palmieri. 1996. "*In vitro* cytotoxic activity of some glucosinolate-derived products generated by myrosinase hydrolysis." J. Agri. Food Chem. 44:1014–1021.
36. Jiao, D., K. I. Ecklund, C.-I. Choi, D. H. Desai, S. G. Amin and F.-L. Chung. 1994. "Structure-activity relationships of isothiocyanates as mechanism-based

inhibitors of 4-(methylnitrosamino)-1-(3-pyridyl)-1-butanone-induced lung tumorigenesis in A/J mice." Cancer Res. 54:4327–4333.

37. Posner, G. H., C.-G. Cho, J. V. Green, Y. Zhang and P. Talalay. 1994. "Design and synthesis of bifunctional analogs of sulforaphane: correlation between structure and potency as inducers of anticarcinogenic detoxication enzymes." J. Med. Chem. 37:170–176.
38. Kroll, J. and H. Rawel. 1996. "Chemical reactions of benzyl isothiocyanate with myoglobin." J. Sci. Food Agric. 72:376–384.
39. Wattenberg, L. W. and W. D. Loub. 1978. "Inhibition of polycyclic aromatic hydrocarbon induced neoplasia by naturally occurring indoles." Cancer Res. 38:1410–1416.
40. Babisch, J. L. and G. S. Stoewsand. 1978. "Effect of dietary indole-3-carbinol on the induction of mixed function oxidases of rat tissue." Food Cosm. Toxicol. 16:151–155.
41. Shertzer, H. G. and M. Sainsbury. 1991. "Chemoprotective and hepatic enzyme induction properties of indole and indenoindole antioxidants in rats." Food Chem. Toxicol. 29:391–400.
42. Stoewsand, G. S., J. B. Babisch and H. C. Wimberly. 1978. "Inhibition of hepatic toxicities from polybrominated biphenyls and aflatoxin B1 in rats fed cauliflower." J. Environ. Pathol. Toxicol. 2:399–405.
43. Dashwood, R. H., A. T. Fong, D. E. Williams, J. D. Hendricks and G. S. Bailey. 1991. "Promotion of aflatoxin B1 carcinogenesis by the natural tumour modulator indole-3-carbinol: influence of dose, duration and intermittent exposure on indole-3-carbinol promotional potency." Cancer. Res. 51:2362–2368.
44. Kensler, T. W., N. E. Davidson, P. A. Egner, K. Z. Guyton, J. D. Groopman, T. J. Curphey, Y. L. Liu and B. D. Roebuck. 1993. "Chemoprotection against aflatoxin induced hepatocarcinogenesis by dithiolthiones." Rev. Med. Vet. Mycol. 1:238–252.
45. Maxuitenko, Y. Y., D. L. MacMillan, T. W. Kensler and B. D. Roebuck. 1993. "Evaluation of the post-initiation effects of oltipraz on aflatoxin B1-induced preneoplastic foci in a rat model of hepatic tumorigenesis." Carcinogenesis 14: 2423–2425.
46. Prochaska, H. J., Y. Yeh, P. Baron and B. Polsky. 1993. "Oltipraz, an inhibitor of human immunodeficiency virus type 1 replication." Proc. Natl. Acad. Sci. 90: 3953–3957.
47. Greenwald, P. 1996. "Chemoprevention of cancer." Sci. Am. 275:96–99.
48. Dateo, G. P., R. C. Clapp, D. A. M. Mackey, E. J. Hewitt and T. Hasselstrom. 1957. "Identification of the volatile sulfur components of cooked cabbage and the nature of the precursors in the fresh vegetable." Food Res. 22:440–446.
49. West, L. G., A. F. Badehop and J. L. McLaughlin. 1977. "Allyl isothiocyanate and allyl cyanide production in cell-free cabbage leaf extracts, shredded cabbage and coleslaw." J. Agric. Food Chem. 25:1234–1237.
50. Hansen, M., P. Moller, H. Sorensen and M. Cantwell de Trejo. 1995. "Glucosinolates in broccoli stored under controlled atmosphere." J. Am. Soc. Hort. Sci. 120:1069–1074.
51. Srisangnam, C., D. K. Salunke, N. R. Reddy and G. G. Dull. 1980. "Quality of cabbage. II. Physical, chemical and biochemical modification in processing

treatment to improve flavor of branched cabbage (*Brassica oleracea* L.)." J. Food Qual. 3:233–239.

52. Shim, K. H. and R. C. Lindsay. 1990. "Suppression of undesirable sulfurous aromas of cruciferous vegetables with caraway sulfhydryl oxidase." Kor. J. Food Sci. Technol. 22:555–561.
53. Henze, J. 1977. "Influence of CA storage on fermentation of white cabbage (*Brassica oleracea* L.)." Acta Hortic. 62:77–80.
54. Tadokoro, T., M. Wada, K. Yamaka, T. Iijima, O. Baba, A. Karimata, A. Yoneyasu and A. Maekawa. 1993. "Loss of vitamins from cabbage." J. Jap. Soc. Nutr. Food Sci. 46:175 –178.
55. Paradis, C., F. Castaigne, T. Desrosiers and C. Willemot. 1995. "Evolution of vitamin C, beta-carotene and chlorophyll content in broccoli heads and florets during storage in air." Sci. Alim. 15:113–123.
56. Petersen, M. A. 1993. "Influence of sous vide processing, steaming and boiling on vitamin retention and sensory quality in broccoli florets." Zeitsch. Lebensm. Unter. Forsch. 197:375–380.
57. Block, E. 1985. "The chemistry of garlic and onions." Sci. Am. 252:114–119.
58. Block, E. 1986. "Antithrombotic agent of garlic: A lesson from 5000 years of folk medicine," Folk Medicine: The Art and the Science, Steiner, R. P., Washington, DC: American Chemical Society. pp. 125–137.
59. Srivastava, K. C., A. Bordiov and S. K. Verma. 1995. "Garlic (*Allium sativum*) for disease prevention." South African J. Sci. 91:68–77.
60. Fenwick, G. R. and A. B. Hanley. 1985. "The genus *Allium* Part 1." CRC Crit. Rev. Fd. Sci. Nutr. 22:199–271.
61. Hanley, A. B. and G. R. Fenwick. 1985. "Cultivated alliums." J. Plant Foods 6:211–238.
62. Breu, W. and W. Dorsch. 1994. "*Allium cepa* L. (onion): Chemistry analysis and pharmacology." Econ. Med. Plant Res. 6:116–147.
63. Block, E., S. Naganathan, D. Putman, and S.-H. Zhao. 1992. "*Alium* chemistry: HPLC quantitation of thiosulfinates from onion, garlic, wild garlic, scallions, shallots, elephant (great-headed) garlic, chives and chinese chives. Uniquely high allyl to methyl ratios in some garlic samples." J. Agric. Food Chem. 40:2418–2430.
64. Pisha, E. and J. M. Pezzuto. 1994. "Fruits and vegetables containing compounds that demonstrate pharmacological activity in humans." Econ. Med. Plant Res. 6:189–233.
65. Freeman, G. G. 1975. "Distribution of flavour components in onion (*Allium cepa* L.), leek (*Allium porrum*) and garlic (*Allium sativum*)." J. Sci. Food Agric. 26: 471–481.
66. Freeman, G. G. and N. Mossadeghi. 1970. "Effect of sulphate nutrition on flavour components of onion (*Allium cepa*)." J. Sci. Food Agric. 21:610–615.
67. Freeman, G. G. and N. Mossadeghi. 1971. "Influence of sulphate nutrition on the flavour components of garlic (*Allium sativum*) and wild onion (*Allium vineale*)." J. Sci. Fd. Agric. 22:330–335.
68. Lancaster, J. E., B. J. McCallion and M. L. Shaw. 1984. "The levels of precursors, the *S*-alk(en)yl-L-cysteine sulphoxides during the growth of the onion (*Allium cepa* L.)." J. Sci. Fd. Agr. 35: 415–421.
69. Freeman, G. G. and R. J. Whenham. 1974. "Changes in onion (*Allium cepa* L.)

flavour components resulting from some postharvest processes." J. Sci. Fd. Agric. 25:499–515.

70. Freeman, G. G. and R. J. Whenham. 1974. "Flavour changes in dry bulb onions during over-winter storage at ambient temperature." J. Sci. Fd. Agric. 25:517–522.
71. Freeman, G. G. and R. J. Whenham. 1976. "Nature and origin of volatile flavour components of onion and related species." Flavours 910:222–229.
72. Schwimmer, S. and S. J. Austin. 1971. "γ-Glutamyl transpeptidase of sprouted onion." J. Food Sci. 36:807–808.
73. Abraham, K. O., M. L. Shankaranarayana, B. Raghaven and C. P. Natarajan. 1976. "Alliums—varieties, chemistry and analysis." Lebensm.-Wiss. u. -Technol. 9:193–200.
74. Pino, J., A. Rosado and A. Gonzalez. 1991. "Volatile flavour components of garlic essential oil." Acta Alimentaria 20:163–171.
75. Ariga, T., H. Suzuki, S. Oshiba, S. Imai, H. Sawai, T. Seiki and K. Saito. 1989. Platelet aggregation inhibition by essential oil components of garlic (Abstract 942). XIIth Congress of the International Society on Thrombosis and Haemostasis, Tokyo.
76. Makheja, A. N. and J. M. Bailey. 1990. "Antiplatelet constituents of garlic and onion." Agents Actions 29:360–363.
77. Sumiyoshi, H. and M. J. Wargovich. 1989. "Garlic (*Allium sativum*): A review of its relationship to cancer." Asia Pacific J. Pharmac. 4:133–140.
78. Brodnitz, M. H., C. L. Pollock and P. P. Vallon. 1969. "Flavor components of onion oil." J. Agric. Food Chem. 17:760–763.
79. Brodnitz, M. H. and D. L. Pollock. 1970. "Gas chromatographic analysis of distilled onion oil." Food Technol. 24:78–81.
80. Boelens, M., P. J. deValois, H. J. Wobben and A. van der Gen. 1971. "Volatile flavor compounds from onion." J. Agric. Food Chem. 19:984–991.
81. Farkas, P., P. Hradsky and M. Kovac. 1992. "Novel flavour components identified in steam distillate of onion (*Allium cepa* L.)." Z. Lebensm. Unters Forsch. 195:459–462.
82. Block, E. 1994. "Flavorants from garlic, onion and other alliums and their cancer preventive properties," Food Phytochemicals for Cancer Prevention, Huang, M. T., T. Osawa, C.-T. Ho and R. T. Rosen, Washington, DC: American Chemical Society, ACS Symposium Series 546. pp. 84–96.
83. Sinha, N. K., D. E. Guyer, D. A. Gage and C. T. Liva. 1992. "Supercritical carbon dioxide extraction of onion flavours and their analysis by gas chromatography-mass spectrometry." J. Agric. Food Chem. 40:842–845.
84. Schwimmer, S. and D. G. Guadagui. 1967. "Cysteine-induced odour intensification in onions and other foods." J. Food Sci. 32:405–408.
85. Schwimmer, S. 1968. "Enzymatic conversion of *trans*-(+)-*S*-(1-propenyl)-L-cysteine-*S*-oxide to the bitter and odour-bearing components of onion." Phytochm. 7:401–404.
86. Bernhard, R. A. 1968. "Comparative distribution of volatile aliphatic disulphides derived from fresh and dehydrated onions." J. Fd. Sci. 33:298–304.
87. Mazza, G., M. LeMaguer and D. Hadziyev. 1980. "Headspace sampling procedures for onion (*Allium cepa* L.) aroma assessment." Can. Inst. Fd. Sci. Tech. J. 13:87–96.

88. Hermann, K. 1976. "On the contents and localization of phenolics in vegetables." Qual. Plant. Plant Foods Human Nutr. 25:231–240.
89. Mazza, G. and E. Miniati. 1993. Anthocyanins in Fruits, Vegetables and Grains. Boca Raton, FL: CRC Press, Inc. pp. 269–270.
90. Stavric, B. and T. I. Matula. 1992. "Flavonoids in foods: Their significance for nutrition and health." Lipid-Soluble Antioxidants, Augustine et al., Basel, Switzerland: Birkhäuser Verlag. pp. 274–294.
91. Pobozsny, K., P. Tetenyi, I. Hethelyi, L. Kocsar and V. Mann. 1979. "Investigations into the prostaglandin content of *Allium* species." Herba Hungarica 18:71–75.
92. Attrep, K. A., W. P. Bellman Sr., M. Attrep Jr., J. P. Lee and W. E. Braselton Jr. 1980. "Separation and identification of prostaglandin A_1 in onion." Lipids 15: 292–296.
93. Ustünes, L., M. Claeys, G. Laekeman, G. Herman, A. J. Vlietinck, and A. Ozer. 1985. "Isolation and identification of two isomeric trihydroxyoctadecenoic acids with prostaglandin E—like activity from onion bulbs (*Allium cepa*)." Prostaglandins 29:847–851.
94. Ali, M., M. Afzal, R. A. H. Hassan, A. Farid and J. F. Burka. 1990. Gen. Pharmacol. 21(3):273.
95. Smoczkiewicz, M. A., D. Nitschke and H. Wieladek. 1982. "Microdetermination of steroid and triterpene saponin glycosides in various plant materials. I. *Allium* species." Mikrochim. Acta 11:42–50.
96. Darbyshire, B. and R. J. Henry. 1978. "The distribution of fructans in onions." New Phytol. 81:29–34.
97. Rutherford, P. P. and E. W. Weston. 1968. "Carbohydrate changes during cold storage of some inulin containing roots and tubers." Phytochem. 7:175–178.
98. Suzuki, M. and J. A. Cutcliffe. 1989. "Fructans in onion bulbs in relation to storage life." Can. J. Plant Sci. 69:1327–1333.
99. Tomomatsu, H. 1994. "Health effects of oligosaccharides." Food Technol. 48: 61–65.
100. Hideka, H., T. Eida and T. Takizawa. 1986. "Effects of fructooligosaccharides on intestinal flora and human health." Bifidobacteria Microflora 5:37–50.
101. Weisberger, A. S. and J. Pensky. 1957. "Tumour inhibiting effects derived from an active principle of garlic (*Allium sativum*)." Science 126:1112–1115.
102. Weisberger, A. S. and J. Pensky. 1958. "Tumour inhibition by a sulphydryl-blocking agent related to an active principle of garlic (*Allium sativum*)." Cancer Res. 18:1301–1307.
103. Kroning, F. 1964. "Garlic as an inhibitor for spontaneous tumours in mice." Acta Unio Contra Camcrum 20:855–859.
104. Kimura, Y. and K. Yamamoto. 1964. "Influence of crude extracts from garlic and some related species on MTK-sarcoma III." Gann 55:325–329.
105. Belman, S. 1983. "Onion and garlic oils inhibit tumour promotion." Carcinogenesis 4:1063–1066.
106. Jakoby, W. B. 1978. "The glutathione *S*-transferase: A group of multifunctional detoxification protein." Adv. Enzymol. 46:383–414.
107. Sparnins, V. L., A. W. Mott and L. W. Wattenberg. 1986. "Effects of allyl methyl trisulfide on glutathione *S*-transferase activity and PB-induced neoplasia in the mouse." Nutr. Cancer 8:211–215.

108. Sparnins, V. L., G. Barany and L. W. Wattenberg. 1988. "Effects of organosulfur compounds from garlic and onion on benzo(a)pyrene-induced neoplasia and glutathione *S*-transferase activity in the mouse." Carcinogenesis 9:131–134.
109. Liu, J. Z., R. I. Lin and J. A. Milner. 1992a. "Inhibition of 7,12-dimethylbenz(a)-anthracene induced mammary tumors and DNA adducts by garlic powder." Carcinogenesis 13:1847–1851.
110. Liu, J. Z., X. Y. Lin and J. A. Milner. 1992b. "Dietary garlic powder increases glutathione content and glutathione *S*-transferase activity in rat liver and mammary tissues." FASEB J. 6:a1493.
111. Amagase, H. and J. A. Milner. 1993. "Impact of various sources of garlic and their constituents on 7,12-dimethylbenz(a)anthracene binding to mammary cell DNA." Carcinogenesis 14:1625–1631.
112. Nishino, H., A. Iwashima, Y. Itakura, H. Matsuura and T. Fuwa. 1989. "Antitumor-promoting activity of garlic extracts." Oncology 46:277–280.
113. Nishino, H., A. Nishino, J. Takayasu, A. Iwashima, Y. Itakura, Y. Kodera, H. Matsuura and T. Fuwa. 1990. "Antitumor-promoting activity of allixin, a stress compound produced by garlic." Cancer J. 3:20–21.
114. Lamm, D. L., D. R. Riggs and J. I. DeHaven. 1990. "Intralesional immunotherapy of murine transitional cell carcinoma using garlic extract," Garlic in Biology and Medicine, Irvine, CA: Nutrition International Co.
115. Mei, X., M. C. Wang, H. X. Xu, X. P. Pan, C. Y. Gao, N. Han and M. Y. Fu. 1982. "Garlic and gastric cancer—the effect of garlic on nitrite and nitrate in gastric juice." Acta Nutr. Sinica 4:53–58.
116. You, W. C., W. J. Blot, Y. S. Chang, A. Ershow, Z. T. Yang, Q. An, B. E. Hendersen, J. F. Fraumeni and T. G. Wang. 1989. "*Allium* vegetables and reduced risk of stomach cancer." J. Natl. Cancer Inst. 81:162–164.
117. Horwitz, N. 1981. "Garlic as a plat du jour. Chinese study finds it could prevent G.I. cancer." Med. Trib. (August) 12.
118. Ariga, T., S. Oshiba and T. Tamada. 1981. "Platelet aggregation inhibitor in garlic." Lancet 2:150–154.
119. Apitz-Castro, R., S. Cabrera, M. R. Cruz, E. Ledezma and M. K. Jain. 1983. "The effects of garlic extract and of three pure components isolated from it on human platelet aggregation, arachidonate metabolism, release activity and platelet ultrastructure." Thromb. Res. 32:155–162.
120. Apitz-Castro, R., J. Escalante, R. Vargas and M. K. Jain. 1986. "Ajoene, the antiplatelet principle of garlic, synergistically potentiates the antiaggregatory action of prostacyclin, forskolin, indomethacin and dipyridamole on human platelets." Thromb. Res. 42:303–311.
121. Mustafa, T. and K. C. Srivastava. 1990. "Possible leads for arachidonic acid metabolism altering drugs from natural products." J. Drug Dev. 3:47–60.
122. Kiesewetter, H., F. Jung, G. Pindur, E. M. Jung, C. Mrowietz and E. Wenzel. 1991. "Effect of garlic on thrombocyte aggregation, microcirculation, and other risk factors." Int. J. Clin. Pharmac. Toxic. 29:151–155.
123. Ali, M. and S. Y. Mohammad. 1986. "Selective suppression of platelet thromboxane formation with sparing prostacyclin synthesis by aqueous extract of garlic in rabbits." Prostagl. Leukotr. Med. 25:139–146.
124. Ali, M., M. Thomson, M. A. Alnaqeeb, J. M. Al-Hassan, S. H. Khater and S. A. Gomes. 1990. "Antithrombotic activity of garlic: its inhibition of the synthesis of

thromboxane B_2 during infusion of arachidonic acid and collagen in rabbits." Prost. Leuk. Essen. Fatty Acids 41:95–99.

125. Bordia, A., S. K. Arora, L. K. Kothari, R. C. Jain, B. S. Rathore, A. S. Rathore, M. K. Dube and N. Bhu. 1975. "The protective action of essential oils of onion and garlic in cholesterol-fed rabbits." Atherosclerosis 22:103–109.
126. Bordia, A. K. and S. K. Verma. 1978. "Garlic on the reversibility of experimental atherosclerosis." Indian Heart J. 30:47–50.
127. Bordia, A. and S. K. Verma. 1980. "Effect of garlic feeding on regression of experimental atherosclerosis in rabbits." Artery 7:428–437.
128. Bordia, A. K., H. K. Joshi, Y. K. Sandhya and N. Bhu. 1977. "Effect of essential oil of garlic on serum fibrinolytic activity in patients with coronary artery disease." Atherosclerosis 28:155–159.
129. Agarwal, R. K., H. A. Dewar, D. J. Newell and B. Das. 1977. "Controlled trial of the effect of cycloalliin on the fibrinolytic activity of venous blood." Atherosclerosis 27:347–351.
130. Jain, R. C. 1975. "Onion and garlic in experimental cholesterol atherosclerosis I. Effect on serum lipids and development of atherosclerosis." Artery 1:155–160.
131. Jain, R. C. 1978. "Effect of alcoholic extract of garlic in atherosclerosis." Am. J. Clin. Nutr. 31:1982–1987.
132. Qureshi, A. A., N. Abuirmeileh, Z. Z. Din, C. E. Elson and W. C. Burger. 1983. "Inhibition of cholesterol and fatty acid biosynthesis in liver enzymes and chicken hepatocytes by polar fractions of garlic." Lipids 18:343–345.
133. Qureshi, A. A., N. Abuirmeileh, W. C. Burger, T. Ahmad and C. E. Elson. 1983. "Suppression of avian hepatic lipid metabolism by solvent extracts of garlic. Impact on serum lipids." J. Nutr. 113:1746–1751.
134. Wilcox, B. F., P. K. Joseph and K. T. Augusti. 1984. "Effects of allylpropyldisulphide isolated from *Allium cepa* Linn. on high-fat fed rats." Ind. J. Biochem. Biophys. 21:214–219.
135. Sainani, G. S., D. B. Desai, S. M. Natu, D. V. Pise and P. G. Sainani. 1979a. "Dietary garlic, onion and some coagulation parameters in Jain community." J. Assoc. Phys. Ind. 27:707–712.
136. Sainani, G. S., D. B. Desai, N. H. Gorhe, S. M. Satu, D. V. Pise and P. G. Sainani. 1979b. "Effect of dietary garlic and onion on serum lipid profile in Jain community." Ind. J. Med. Res. 69:776–782.
137. Sucur, M. 1980. "Effect of garlic on serum lipids and lipoproteins in patients suffering from hyperlipoproteinemia." Diabetal. Croatica 9:323–329.
138. Qureshi, N., R. I. S. Lin, N. Abuirmeileh and A. A. Qureshi. 1990. "Dietary kyolic (aged garlic extract) and *S*-allyl cysteine reduces the levels of plasma triglycerides, thromboxane B_2 and platelet aggregation in hypercholesterolemic model," Garlic in Biology and Medicine, Irvine, CA: Nutrition International Co.
139. Augusti, K. T. 1974. "Effect on alloxan diabetes of allyl propyl disulphide obtained from onion." Die Naturwissenschaften 61:172–173.
140. Jain, R. C. and C. R. Vyas. 1975. "Garlic in alloxan-induced diabetic rabbits." Am. J. Clin. Nutr. 28:684–685.
141. Pushpendran, C. K., T. P. A. Devasagayam and J. Eapen. 1982. "Age-related hyperglycaemic effect of diallyl disulphide in rats." Ind. J. Exp. Biol. 20:428–429.
142. Mathew, P. T. and K. T. Augusti. 1973. "Studies on the effect of allicin (diallyl disulphide oxide) on alloxan diabetes, I. Hyperglycaemic action and enhance-

ment of serum insulin effect and glycogen synthesis." J. Ind. Biochem. Biophys. 10:209–212.

143. Foushee, D. B., J. Ruffin and U. Banerjee. 1982. "Garlic as a natural agent for the treatment of hypertension: a preliminary report." Cytobios 34:145–152.
144. De Wit, J. C., S. H. W. Notermans and N. Gorin. 1979. "The antimicrobial effect of onion and garlic extracts." Antonie van Leeuwenhoek 45:156–160.
145. Agrawal, P. and B. Rai. 1984. "Effect of bulb extracts of onion and garlic on soil bacteria." Acta Bot. Ind. 12:45–49.
146. Awasthi, P. B. and C. R. Leathers. 1984. "Effect of aqueous garlic extract on growth of *Coccidioides immitis* and two arthroconidia-producing fungi." Acta. Bot. Ind. 12:22–25.
147. Schmidl, M. K. and T. P. Lobuza. 1985. "Low calorie formulations: cutting calories and keeping quality." Proc. Prep. Foods 154(11):118–120.
148. Schmidl, M. K. and T. P. Labuza. 1994. "Medical foods," Functional Foods, Goldberg, I., New York, NY: Chapman and Hall. pp. 151–179.
149. Schwimmer, S. and D. G. Guadagni. 1968. "Kinetics of the enzymatic development of pyruvic acid and odor in frozen onions treated with cysteine C-S-lyase." J. Food Sci. 33:193–196.
150. Oku, T. 1994. "Special physiological functions of newly developed mono- and oligosaccharides," Functional Foods, Goldberg, I., New York, NY: Chapman and Hall. pp. 202–218.
151. Spiegel, J. E., R. Rose, P. Karabell, V. H. Frankos and D. F. Schmitt. 1994. "Safety and benefits of fructooligosaccharides as food ingredients." Food Technol. 48(1): 85–89.
152. Hosoya, N., B. Dhorranintra and H. Hidaka. 1988. "Utilization of [U—^{14}C] fructooligosacharides in man as energy resources." J. Clin. Biochem. Nutr. 5:67–74.
153. Fuchs, A. 1986. Processing and Utilization of Insulin-Containing Plants. European Federation of Biotechnology. Report on the 2nd Workshop on Agricultural Surpluses, Part 3. pp. 171–205.
154. Chubey, B. B. and D. G. Dorrell. 1977. "Chicory, another potential-fructose crop." Can. Inst. Food Sci. Technol. J. 10:331–332.
155. Shiomi, J. I., J. Yamada and M. Izawa. 1976. "Isolation and identification of fructooligosaccharides in roots of asparagus (*Asparagus officinalis* L.)." Agric. Biol. Chem. 40:567–575.
156. Nakaya, R. 1984. "Role of *Bifidobacterium* in enteric infection." Bifidobacteria Microflora 3:3–9.
157. Okamura, N., R. Nakaya, H. Yokota, N. Yamai and T. Kariashima. 1986. "Interaction of *Shigella* and *Bifidobacteria*." Bifidobacteria Microflora 5:51–55.
158. Ikeda, T., T. Shiota, I. R. McChee, J. Otaka, S. M. Michalek, K. Ochiai, M. Hirasawa and K. Sugiruoto. 1978. "Virulence of *Streptococcus mutants:* comparison of the effects of coupling sugar and sucrose on certain metabolic activities and canogenicity." Infect. Immun. 19:477–480.
159. Yamashito, K., K. Kawai and M. Itakura. 1984. "Effects of fructo-oligosaccharides on blood glucose and serum lipids in diabetic subjects." Nutr. Res. 4: 961–966.
160. Gilliland, S. E. and D. K. Walker. 1990. "Factors to consider when selecting a culture of *Lactobacillus acidophilus* as a dietary adjunct to produce a hypocholesterolemic effect in humans." J. Dairy Sci. 73:905–911.

161. Suzuki, Y., H. Kaizu and Y. Yamaguchi. 1991. "Effect of cultured milk on serum cholesterol concentrations in rats fed high-cholesterol diets." Animal Sci. Technol. (Japan). 62(6):565–571. In Japanese.

162. Hosono, A. 1990. "Functionality of milk by fermentation." New Food Industry 32(10):51–52. In Japanese.

163. Hata, Y., K. Nakajima, Y. Hosono and M. Yamamoto. 1989. "Effects of soybean *o*-oligosaccharides on human digestive organs." J. Japan Soc. Clin. Nutr. 11(1):42–46.

164. Farnworth, E. R., N. Oilawri, H. Yamazaki, H. W. Modler and J. D. Jones. 1991. "Studies on the effect of adding Jerusalem artichoke flour to pig milk." Can. J. Animal Sci. 71:531–536.

165. Yamazaki, H. and K. Matsumoto. 1994. "Purification of Jerusalem artichoke fructans and their utilization by bificobacteria." J. Sci. Food Agric. 64:461–465.

166. Yun, J. W., Jung, K. H., Jeon, Y. J. and Lee, J. H. 1992. "Continuous production of fructo-oligosaccharides from sucrose by immobilized cells of *Aureobasidium pullulans*." J. Microbiol. Biotechnol. 2:98–101.

167. Yun, J. W., K. H. Jung, J. W. Oh and J. H. Lee. 1990. "Semibatch production of fructo-oligosaccharides from sucrose by immobilized cells of *Aureobasidium pullulans*." Appl. Biochem. Biotechnol. 24/25:299–308.

168. Yun, J. W. and Song, S. K. 1993. "Production of high-content fructo-oligosaccharides by the mixed-enzyme system of fructosyltransferase and glucose oxidase." Biotechnol. Lett. 15:573–576.

169. Hayashi, S., Kinoshita, J., Nonoguchi, M., Takasaki, Y. and Imada, K. 1991. "Continuous production of 1-kestose by β-fructofuranosidase immobilized on *Shirasu* porous glass." Biotechnol. Lett. 13:395–398.

170. van Balken, J. A. M., T. J. G. M. van Dooren, W. J. J. van den Tweel, J. Kamphuis and E. M. Meijer. 1991. "Production of 1-kestose with intact mycelium of *Aspergillus phoenicic* containing sucrose-1^F-fructosyltransferase." Appl. Microbiol. Biotechnol. 35:216–221.

171. Fujisaki, H., T. Muratsubaki, T. Kamada and K. Sayama. 1989. "Production of sweetener containing fructo-oligosaccharides from sugar beet molasses." Proc. Res. Soc. Jpn. Sugar Refineries Technol. 37:27–32.

172. Yun, J. W. 1996. "Fructooligosaccharides—Occurrence, preparation, and application." Enzyme Microb. Technol. 19:107–117.

173. Yamazaki, H., H. W. Modler, J. D. Jones and J. I. Elliot. 1989. "Process for preparing flour from Jerusalem artichoke tubers." US Patent No. 4,871,574.

174. Mazza, G. 1984. "Sorption isotherms and drying rates of Jerusalem artichokes (*Helianthus tuberosus* L.)." J. Food Sci. 49:384–388.

175. Yamazaki, H. and K. Matsumoto. 1993. "Production of fructo-oligosaccharide-rich fructose syrup," Inulin and Inulin-Containing Crops, Fuchs, A., Amsterdam, The Netherlands: Elsevier Science Publishers. pp. 355–358.

176. Tamatami, H., K. Takahashi, K. Sato, K. Mizushima and F. Yoshimi. 1989. "Additive for stock feeds, stock feed containing additive, and process for preparation of additive." U.S. Patent No. 4,865,852.

177. Fleming, S. E. and J. W. D. GrootWassik. 1979. "Preparation of high fructose syrup from tubers of Jerusalem artichoke." CRC Crit. Rev. Food Sci. Nutr. 12:1–45.

178. Muscat, J. E. and M. Huncharck. 1996. "Dietary intake and the risk of malignant mesothelioma." Br. J. Cancer 73:1122–1125.
179. Thurham, D. I. 1994. "Carotenoids: functions and facclacies." Proc. Nutr. Soc. 53:77–87.
180. Gaziano, J. M., J. E. Manson, P. M. Ridker, J. E. Buring and C. H. Hennekens. 1990. "Beta carotene therapy for chronic stable angina." Circulation 82:201–204.
181. Wahlqvist, M. L., N. Wattanapenpaiboon, F. A. Macrae, J. R. Lambert, R. MacLennan and B. H.-H. Hsu-Hage. 1994. "Changes in serum carotenoids in subjects with colorectal adenomas after 24 mo of beta carotene supplementation." Am. J. Clin. Nutr. 60:936–943.
182. Zheng, G., P. M. Kenney, J. Zhang and L. K. T. Lam. 1993. "Chemoprevention of benzo[a]pyrene-induced forestomach cancer in mice by natural phthalides from celery seed oil." Nutr. Cancer 19:77–86.
183. Shinohara, K., M. Kobori and Z. L. Kong. 1993. "Desmutagenic effect of vegetables on mutagens and carcinogens and growth-inhibiting effect of spinach components on cultured human cancer cells." Camb. Roy. Soc. Chem. 123:238–242.

CHAPTER 7

Processing and Properties of Mustard Products and Components

W. CUI[1]
N. A. M. ESKIN[2]

1. INTRODUCTION

MUSTARD seeds have been used as condiments for thousands of years. The earliest recorded use is found in Sandscrit and Sumerian texts dating back almost 3000 years. The English word mustard is derived from the Latin "mustum ardens," which means "burning must." Mustard was originally used to mask the taste of degraded perishables. The development of improved culinary and storage techniques, however, eliminated the need for using it as a masking agent for spoiled foods. Today, mustard is the largest volume spice in international trade, accounting for 160,000 tons per year [1]. Because the crop requires long days, its production is concentrated in the northern hemisphere, with Canada as one of the major producers and exporters of mustard seeds for the spice market.

The two principal botanical species of mustard are *Sinapis alba* and *Brassica juncea*. *Sinapis alba*, commonly referred to as "white" or "yellow" mustard; it contains less oil but is higher in mucilage. *Brassica juncea,* commonly referred to as "brown" or "oriental" mustard, is much richer in oil and considered an important oilseed crop on the Indian subcontinent. Other constituents present in mustard seeds include isothiocyanates, erucic acid, phenolics, phytin, and dithiolthiones. This chapter will review the processing of

[1]Food Processing and Quality Improvement Program; Agriculture and Agri-Food Canada; Guelph, ON, Canada.
[2]Department of Foods and Nutrition, University of Manitoba, Winnipeg, MB, Canada.

mustard products as well as the properties of selected mustard seed components.

2. MUSTARD PROCESSING AND PRODUCTS

2.1. PROCESSING OF MUSTARD

Mustard seeds for processing must be dried soon after harvest to prevent the growth of moulds. Drying is carried out initially on the farm and then completed at the factory. The maximum temperature recommended for drying is 32°C [2]. Higher temperatures may destroy myrosinase, the enzyme responsible for releasing isothiocyanates from glucosinolates. The milling of mustard seeds is designed to separate the bran (testa and aleurone layer) from the flour (embryo and cotyledons), followed by size reduction using different shaped rollers. The flour is then carefully sifted to separate the fine and coarse fractions The sifted flour or powdered mustard may still contain some testa fragments. In England, oil is not removed from mustard seeds prior to milling. In North America and the rest of Europe, however, seeds are often partially deoleated before crushing to aid the milling process. In Canada, a process for deheating yellow mustard seeds was developed by UFL Foods to provide an ingredient with thickening, stabilising and emulsifying properties. In this process, myrosinase is deactivated by a controlled heat treatment, cooled and then finely ground.

Commercial processing of mustard seed into various products is outlined in Figure 7.1. Only small portions of mustard seeds are cold pressed for extracting the oil with remaining product referred to as "press cake." The essential oil of *Brassica juncea* is obtained by steam distillation of the press cake after myroinase has been allowed to release allyl isothiocyanate from sinigrin glucoside. In contrast, the essential oil of yellow mustard (*Sinapis alba*) is obtained by solvent extraction of the cake because 4-hydroxybenzyl isothiocyanate enzymically formed from sinalbin glucoside is nonvolatile. Enzymic hydrolysis, in both cases, is brought about by maceration of the cake with warm water [3].

2.2. MUSTARD OIL

Brassica juncea provides one of the major edible oils in India. The oil is brownish yellow in colour and accounts for 29–46% of the total seed weight [2]. Extraction of the oil is carried out by village "ghapis" rotary mills, expeller and hydraulic processes. In the north-eastern region of India, the oil is used in its crude state as a frying medium for several food preparations. It is also used for body massaging, as a hair oil, illuminant and lubricant.

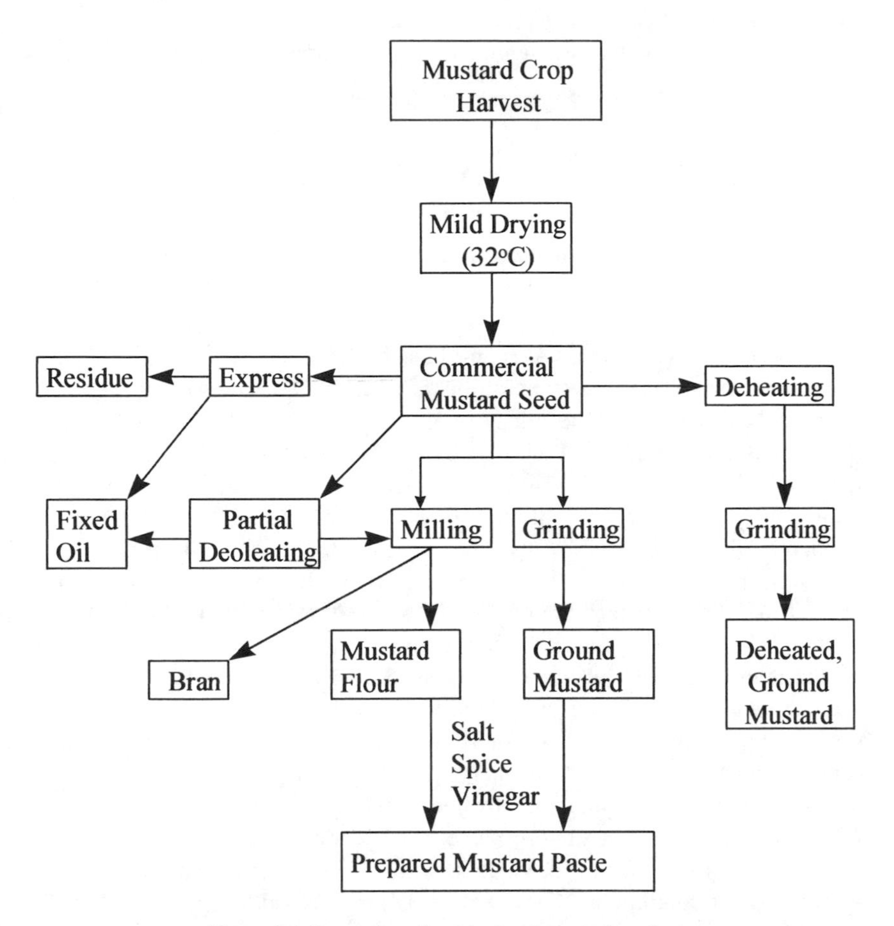

Figure 7.1 Processing of mustard and mustard products.

Sinapis alba oil has a golden yellow colour characterized by a mild taste. The content of the seed oil ranges from 20 to 35% and is also used as a lubricant and illuminant. The oil is a by-product of the condiment industry in countries where the seeds are partially deoleated before milling (Figure 7.1). In Sweden, the oil is also used in the production of mayonnaise.

An important commercial aspect of the crushing of any oilseed is the disposal of the seed residue. Mustard meals are comparatively rich in protein, but their pungency makes them unsuitable for feedstock purposes. All the residues described here can be used as fertilisers, although the commercial value of a meal used as fertiliser is far less than its use as a feed. Further research is needed to better utilise mustard meal in order to stimulate the crushing industry.

2.3. MUSTARD FLOUR, GROUND MUSTARD AND PREPARED MUSTARD

Mustard flour is a fine powder derived from the endosperm or interior portion of the seed. The flour can be made from either straight yellow or oriental mustard seeds or a blend of the two. Mustard flour is generally retailed directly or sold to industry as an ingredient for products such as salad dressings, mayonnaise, barbecue sauces, pickles, and processed meats.

Ground mustard, a powder made by grinding whole yellow mustard seeds, is used primarily in the meat industry as an emulsifier, water binder, and inexpensive bulking agent. It is also used in seasonings for frankfurters, bologna, salami, and lunch loaf. In addition, ground mustard is used in salad dressings, pickled products and condiments. The water-binding and emulsifying properties of ground mustard is largely attributed to the mucilaginous material present in yellow mustard bran (see Section 3.3 for details). Ground mustard is an excellent bulking agent for the meat industry as it is a cheaper protein source than meat with excellent water absorbing and fat binding properties. The amount of ground mustard added to processed meat was limited, at one time, by its hot flavour. This problem, however, has been resolved by the recent introduction of deheated mustard, produced by a process that deactivates the enzyme myrosinase under controlled temperature conditions.

Prepared mustard is a smooth paste usually composed of ground mustard and/or mustard flour with salt, vinegar, with or without sugar and/or dextrose, spices or other condiments. For example, Dijon mustard is a paste made from sifted or sieved products of which the total dry matter (including salt and sugar) must not be less than 28%. Other popular prepared mustard products, such as French and German mustards, can be found in practically every grocery store in North America and Europe.

2.4. YELLOW MUSTARD BRAN

Yellow mustard bran used to be a by-product in the preparation of mustard flour. Recently, however, the demand for bran has increased, and mustard seed bran is often more requested than mustard flour. Research conducted in our laboratories has shown that yellow mustard bran contained about 20–25% water-soluble polysaccharides, which exhibit unique rheological and interfacial properties (see Section 3.3 for details). These properties were responsible for the stabilising, emulsifying, water-binding and fat-absorbing properties of yellow mustard bran and bran-containing products.

3. MUSTARD COMPONENTS: NATURE, CHEMISTRY AND PROPERTIES

Mustard seeds are composed of protein (23–30%), fixed oil (29–36%), and carbohydrate (12–18%) together with minor constituents including minerals (4%), essential oil (isothiocyanates, 0.8–2.3%), phytin (2–3%), as well as phenolic compounds (Table 7.1). Processed mustard flour is usually enriched with fixed oil (30–42%) and protein (30–35%). In contrast, bran products contain much less oil and protein (7 and 13–16%, respectively), but are rich in fibre (15%).

3.1. ISOTHIOCYANATES

Both mustard and canola contain significant amounts of glucosinolates. The high content of glucosinolates is desirable in mustard as they are the precursors of flavour components, also called "essential oil." When mustard seeds are crushed and exposed to liquids such as water, vinegar or grape juice, an enzyme called myrosinase (thioglucoside glucohydrolase, EC 3.2.3.1) hydrolyses glucosinolates to isothiocyanates as shown in Figure 7.2. Isothiocyanates are responsible for the hot spiciness of prepared mustard

TABLE 7.1. Chemical Composition of Mustard Seed and Its Products.

Mustard Product	Isothiocyanates: Allyl- (%)	Isothiocyanates: 4-Hydroxybenzyl (%)	Fixed Oil (%)	Protein[a] (%)	Crude Fiber (%)	H_2O (%)	Ash (%)
Whole yellow seed		2.3	29	30	9	6	4
Whole brown seed	0.80		32	26	7	6	4
Whole oriental seed	0.78		36	23	6	6	4
Yellow flour		0.0	30	35	3.5	6	4
Brown flour	0.95		40	35	3.5	6	4
Oriental flour	0.90		42	30	3.5	6	4
Yellow bran			7	16	15	10	4
Brown bran	0.20		7	13	15	10	4
Oriental bran	0.35		7	15	15	10	4

[a]Protein = $N \times 6.25$.

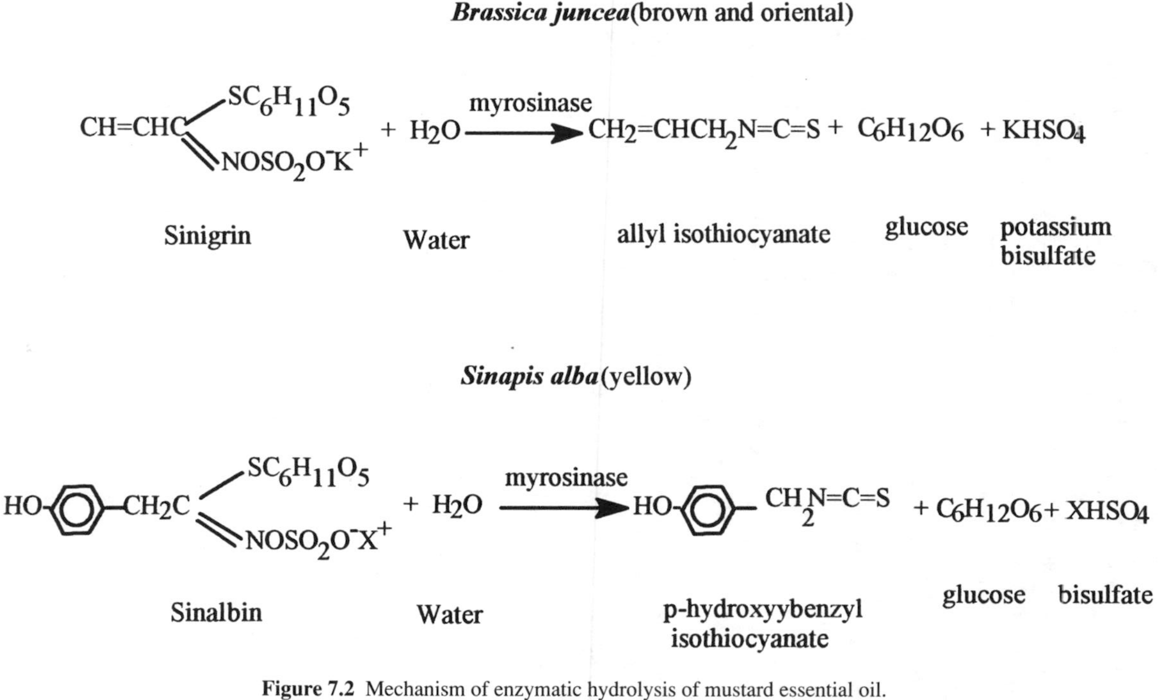

Figure 7.2 Mechanism of enzymatic hydrolysis of mustard essential oil.

products but differ in flavor depending on their structure. Oriental and brown mustard release a volatile compound, ally isothiocyanate (AIT), which produces a sharp taste sensation and pungent aroma similar to horseradish. Yellow mustard releases a nonvolatile compound, 4-hydroxybenzyl isothiocyanate (PHBIT), which elicits a hot mouthfeel in condiments.

3.2. MUSTARD OIL AND FATTY ACIDS

Mustard oil is second only to soybean oil as an edible oil in India. The content of fixed oil in *Brassica juncea* seeds (32–36%) is significantly higher than that of *Sinapis alba* seeds (29%) (Table 7.1). The major fatty acids of mustard seed oils are erucic, oleic, linoleic, linolenic, eicosenoic and palmitic (Table 2). Erucic acid accounts for 18–51% of the total fatty acids of mustard oil. *Sinapis alba* seeds tend to be higher in monounsaturated fatty acids (oleic and erucic acids) and lower in polyunsaturated fatty acids (linoleic and linolenic acids). It is worth noting that mustard oil contains 9–15% omega-3 fatty acids, which is much higher than most of the commonly used vegetables oils (canola, 10.5%; soybean, 7.8% and corn, 1.5%)[4].

Erucic acid (C22:1), a long-chain monounsaturated fatty acid, exhibits high fire and smoke points (217°C). These properties permit erucic acid to withstand high frying temperatures and remain liquid at room temperature [5]. Oils containing high levels of erucic acid, such as crambe and industrial rapeseed, have found extensive uses as lubricants or in lubricant formulations [6]. High erucic acid oils have found clinical applications in the treatment of a rare children's disease known as adrenoleukodystrophy.

Nonedible uses of high erucic acid oils are based on the industrial applications of erucic acid and its cleavage products. These include the hydrogenated derivative behenic acid, erucyl and behenyl alcohols and their esters, amides and amine derivatives.

TABLE 7.2. Variation in Fatty Acids (%) in Mustard Seed Oils.

Fatty Acid	*Sinapis alba*	*Brassica juncea*
Palmitic	2–3	2–4
Oleic	16–18	7–22
Linoleic	7–10	12–24
Linolenic	9–12	10–15
Eicosenoic	6–11	6–14
Erucic	33–51	18–49

Source: Adapted from Reference [1].

These compounds are used in industry as emulsifiers, processing aids, antistatic agents, stabilisers, and corrosion inhibitors [6]. Behenic acid and esters are also used to enhance the performance of pharmaceuticals, cosmetics, fabric softeners and hair conditioners.

Erucamide ($CH_3(CH_2)_7CH{=}CH(CH_2)_{11}CONH_2$), the amide derivative of erucic acid, acts as a processing aid and antiblock agent in plastic films by lubricating and forming a thin layer on the surface of the plastic.

In addition to these applications, oxidative products of erucic acid are used in the production of plastics, resins and nylons. These include brassylic acid, $HOOC(CH_2)_{11}COOH$, a 13-carbon dicarboxylic acid, and pelagonic acid, $CH_3(CH_2)_7COOH$. Brassylic acid is used in the preparation of long-chain nylons and in automotive parts and products [7,8].

Based on the extensive applications of erucic acid, mustard species with high levels of this acid could be grown to meet industrial demands for this component.

3.3. YELLOW MUSTARD MUCILAGE

3.3.1. Nature and Extraction

When yellow mustard seeds are exposed to water, the surface of the seeds become sticky. If the seeds are dried immediately after wetting, some of them will glue together. This phenomenon is due to the presence of mucilaginous material in yellow mustard seeds. The mucilage is deposited in the epidermal layer of the seed coat which is readily exuded in a high moisture environment [9,10]. The release of mucilage from the seeds when immersed in water can be observed with the naked eye. If the dampened seeds are allowed to dry, the exuded mucilage forms a whitish layer on the surface.

Extraction and characterization of yellow mustard mucilage (YMM) have received considerable attention over the years. Back in 1932, Bailey and Norris [11] used a seed-to-water ratio of 1 : 10 and stirring and shaking for 24 hr to extract the mucilaginous material from yellow mustard seeds. The viscous extract was filtered through a thin cotton cloth and the seed returned for two additional extractions. The three extracts were combined and filtered through a bed of glass wool and cotton cloth to remove foreign particles, while the filtrate was poured into alcohol to precipitate the mucilage, as a fibrous gelatinous product. Filtration, redissolving and reprecipitation of the mucilage were repeated several times with the product dried in successive increasing concentrations of alcohol and finally under vacuum over phosphorus pentoxide [11]. The prepared mucilage was a white fibrous product corresponding in yield of about 2% of the dry seed. More recently, Woods and Downey [12] found that addition of a small amount of chloroform to the water (2.5 ml/L) prevented undesirable fermentation during extraction of yellow mustard mucilage. The extraction was carried out by shaking the whole seed (5 g) slowly in 90 ml of chloroform water overnight. The whole seeds were removed by straining through cheesecloth and the mucilage precipitated in acidified acetone (2.5 ml conc. HCl/L). The mucilage was collected using preweighed filters and dried under vacuum at room temperature. The content of mucilage extracted by this procedure varied from 0.3 to 2.1%, with an average of 1.3%. The relative low yields reported by Woods and Downey [12] could be attributed to a single extraction compared to Bailey and Norris's three sequential extractions [11]. Woods and Downey [12] also found that mucilage content in yellow mustard seeds was significantly affected by maturity, cultivar, location, and year. An improved extraction procedure developed in our laboratory increased the yield of mucilage from yellow mustard to 5% of seed weight [13]. The final mucilage product, obtained by alcohol precipitation of filtrate from three successive extractions, was snow-white and cotton-like in appearance and represented 93% of the total extractable mucilage (Table 7. 3).

Using whole yellow mustard seeds as a source of mucilage is not economically feasible as there are no practical applications for the seeds following extraction of mucilage. In North America, a number of food companies currently process mustard meats as food ingredients with the bran as a by-product. Since mucilage is deposited mainly in the epidermal layer of the seed coat, extraction of mucilage from yellow mustard bran appears to be a better way of producing the gum. The reported yield of mucilage obtained from the bran varies from 15–25% depending on the extraction conditions [14–16]. The extraction process generally involves defatting the bran with a mixture of hexane, ethanol and water. The defatted, dried bran is then water extracted (1:20 ratio) and separated by centrifugation with the mucilage precipitated with two volumes of 95% ethanol and then dried (freeze-dried or vacuum-dried). Siddiqui and co-workers [10] modified the above method by extracting yellow mustard hulls with boiling water (1:16 w/v) for 35 min. The extract was separated by centrifugation and precipitated by adding isopropanol to a final concentration of 70% w/v. The precipitate was then separated by filtration through a thin cotton cloth, washed with 70% isopropanol,

TABLE 7.3. Yield of Mucilage from Yellow Mustard Seeds upon Sequential Aqueous Extraction (100 g seeds/600 g H_2O).

Extraction	1	2	3	4	5	6
Weight (g)	3.45	0.93	0.54	0.25	0.12	5.29
Percent (%)	65.2	17.6	10.2	4.7	2.3	100

Source: Adapted from Reference [13].

air-dried and pulverised. Recently, Cui and Eskin [17] used response surface methodology to optimize this extraction process. The improved extraction yielded 20–25% mucilage.

3.3.2. Composition

Yellow mustard mucilage was first reported to be composed of cellulose (50%) together with acidic polysaccharides, which yielded arabinose, galactose, rhamnose, galacturonic, and glucuronic acids on hydrolysis, as well as methoxyl groups [11]. Another study suggested that galactose, arabinose and galacturonic acid were major constituents with xylose, glucose, mannose, and rhamnose as minor components [16]. Theander et al. [18] found that mustard mucilage contains 39.3% glucose, 25.4% arabinose, 17.9% galactose, 7.5% xylose, 5.4% mannose, 4% xylose and 1% fructose. Cui et al. [13] showed that crude mucilage contains 80.4% carbohydrates, 4.4% protein and 15% ash. Dialysis reduces the ash content to 4.8% with a corresponding increase in carbohydrates from 80.4 to 91.1% (Table 7.4). Of the monosaccharides,

TABLE 7.4. Chemical Compositions of Yellow Mustard Seed Mucilage and Its Fractions.

Component	(dwb)	CM[c]	CM[d]	WS	WI
Water	(%)	6.9	8.7	10.2	8.1
Ash	(%)	15.0	4.8	4.3	1.7
Protein[a]	(%)	4.4	4.1	2.2	4.2
Fat	(%)	0.2	n.d.[e]	n.d.	n.d.[e]
Carbohydrate[b]	(%)	80.4	91.1	93.5	94.1
Potassium	(%)	2.1	0.04	0.01	0.02
Calcium	(%)	2.2	1.2	1.6	0.48
Magnesium	(%)	1.3	0.6	0.4	0.16
Phosphorus	(%)	2.1	0.6	0.4	0.09
Sulphur	(%)	1.4	0.29	0.16	0.02
Iron	(ppm)	212.5	260.0	223.0	358.0
Zinc	(ppm)	53.5	70.0	123.0	208.0
Manganese	(ppm)	73.0	70.0	72.0	27.0
Copper	(ppm)	13.5	12.0	34.0	18.0

[a] $N \times 6.25$.
[b] By difference.
[c] Crude mucilage before dialysis.
[d] Crude mucilage after dialysis.
[e] Not determined.
CM = crude mucilage; WS = water-soluble fraction; WI = water-insoluble fraction.
Source: Adapted from Reference [13].

glucose (23.5%) is the predominant neutral sugar followed by galactose (13.8%), rhamnose (3.2%), arabinose (3.0%), and xylose (1.8%) together with 14.7% uronic acids.

3.3.3. Heterogeneity and Structures

Yellow mustard mucilage is a complex mixture of polysaccharides containing six neutral sugars and two uronic acids. The crude mucilage is easily separated into water-soluble (WS) and water-insoluble (WI) fractions by centrifugation. WS, the major fraction responsible for the rheological properties of yellow mustard mucilage [13], can be further fractionated into CTAB-precipitated (WSCP) and CTAB-soluble (WSCS) fractions [19]. CTAB (hexadecyltrimethyl-ammonium bromide) is a quaternary ammonium cation that can complex with acidic polysaccharides to form a precipitate. Using anion chromatography, WSCP and WSCS were fractionated into five relatively pure subfractions as represented in Figure 7.3. Of the 10 fractions obtained, only 3 polysaccharide fractions (i.e., WSCP-I, WSCP-III and WSCS-I) were found to exhibit the unique shear thinning flow behaviour of yellow mustard mucilage [20]. The WSCP-I and WSCS-I fractions were characterized as neutral polysaccharides typical of cellulose-like structures. Some of the hydroxyl groups at C2, 3 and 6 can be substituted by ether groups (ethyl and propyl). The ethyl group may be randomly distributed in the C2, 3 and 6 positions while the propyl ether is predominant at the 6 position. These ether groups along the cellulose-like backbone chain may act as "kinks" that can alter the conformational regularity of the 1,4-linked β-D-glucose backbone chain and favour the solubilization of the polymer in an aqueous medium. Alternatively, for steric reasons, these groups hinder interchain associations among the cellulose chains, thus enhancing the solubility of the polysaccharide. The WSCP-II fraction is a pectic polysaccharide composed of 2,4-linked and 2-linked L-rhamnose, 6-linked D-galactose, a terminal nonreducing D-glucuronic acid and 4-linked D-galacturonic acid [23]. A possible average repeating unit, 2D NMR, has been proposed for WSCP-III (Figure 7.4).

3.3.4. Functional Properties

3.3.4.1. Rheological Properties

The consistency of prepared mustard products, such as salad dressings and food pastes, is attributed to the presence of mucilage [15]. Research conducted in our laboratory during the past decade has led to a better understanding of the structure-property relationship of yellow mustard mucilage [13,19–25]. Generally, our results show that mustard mucilage has rheologi-

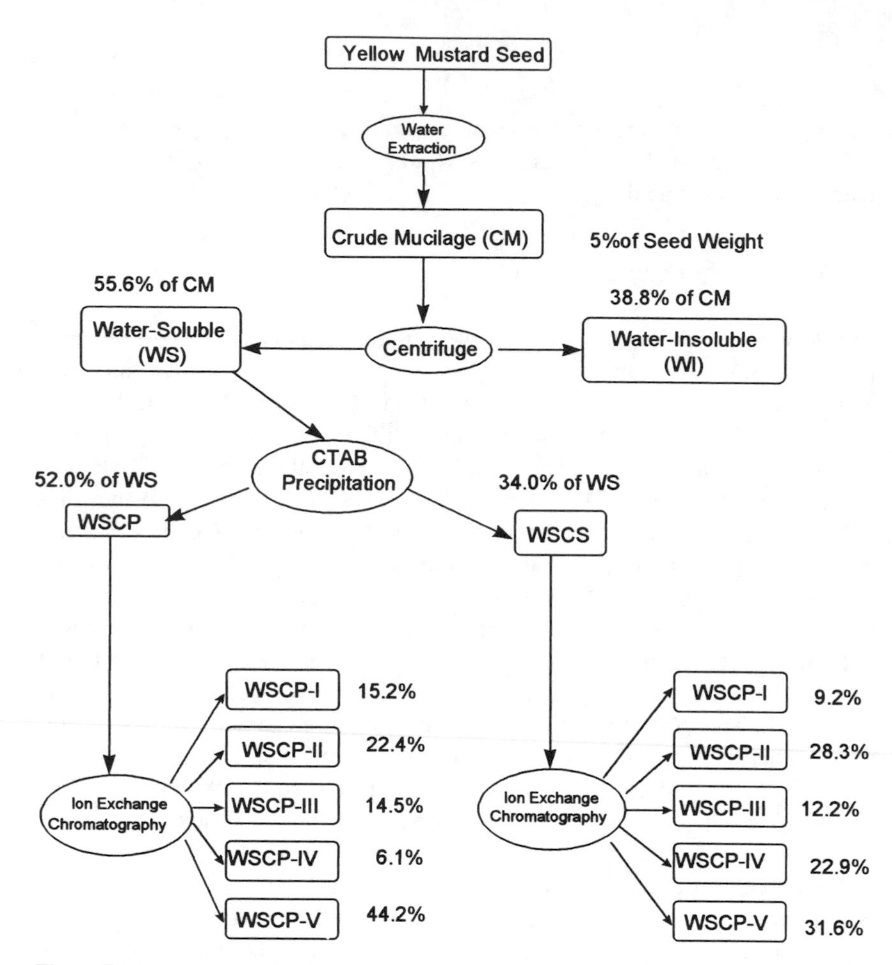

Figure 7.3 Extraction and fractionation of yellow mustard mucilage. (Reprinted with permission from Reference [20]. Copyright 1994 American Chemical Society.)

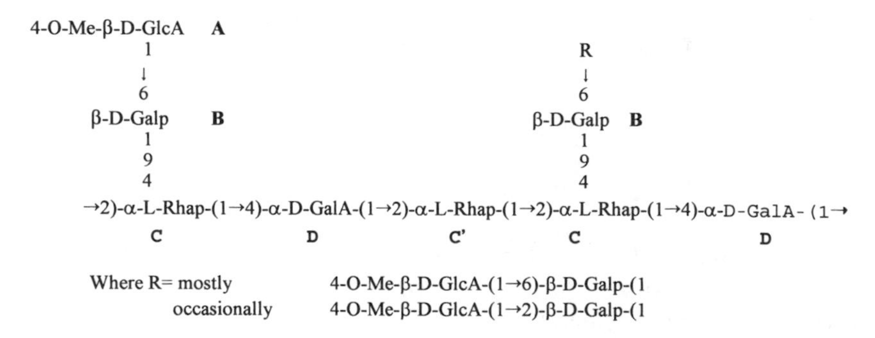

Figure 7.4 Average repeating unit of WSCP-III. (Reprinted from Reference [23], with kind permission from Elsevier Science Ltd, The Boulevard, Langford Lane, Kidlington OX5 1GB, UK).

cal properties similar to xanthan gum. It exhibits shear thinning flow behaviour at concentrations above 0.3%, weak-gel properties, and interacts synergistically with galactomannans.

The flow profiles and mechanical spectra of yellow mustard mucilage and its fractions are shown in Figures 7.5 and 7.6. Because of charged groups on the polysaccharide chains, the effects of pH and salt on viscosity are significant (Figure 7.7). When YMM is mixed with locust bean gum (LBG) and guar gum, the viscosity of the mixed systems increases significantly [15]. At a total polymer concentration of 0.5% (w/w), significant synergistic interactions are evident in 1 : 1 and 1 : 9 (LBG:YMM) blends. The dynamic viscosity of the 9:1 (LBG: YMM) blend is lower than pure LBG but slightly higher than YMM. In contrast, the dynamic viscosity of the 1:1 and 1:9 LBG:YMM blends is significantly enhanced. Maximising the synergistic interaction between LBG and YMM, Cui and Eskin [25] added a small amount of LBG to YMM to a salad cream product. The emulsion stability of the salad cream products made with an LBG:YMM (1:9) 0.3% blend compared favourably with commercial products made with xanthan gum with or without alginates.

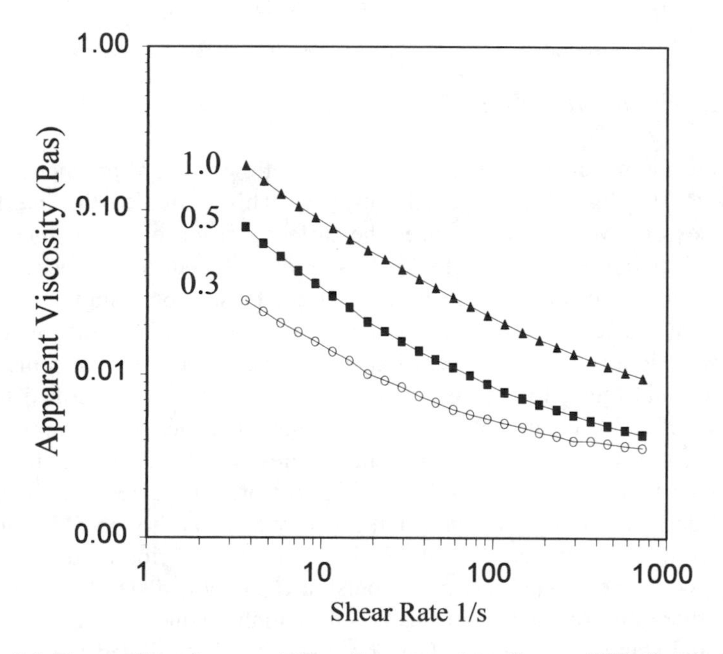

Figure 7.5 Flow profiles of water-soluble yellow mustard mucilage at 22°C. (Reprinted from Reference [13], with kind permission from Elsevier Science Ltd, The Boulevard, Langford Lane, Kidlington OX5 1GB, UK.)

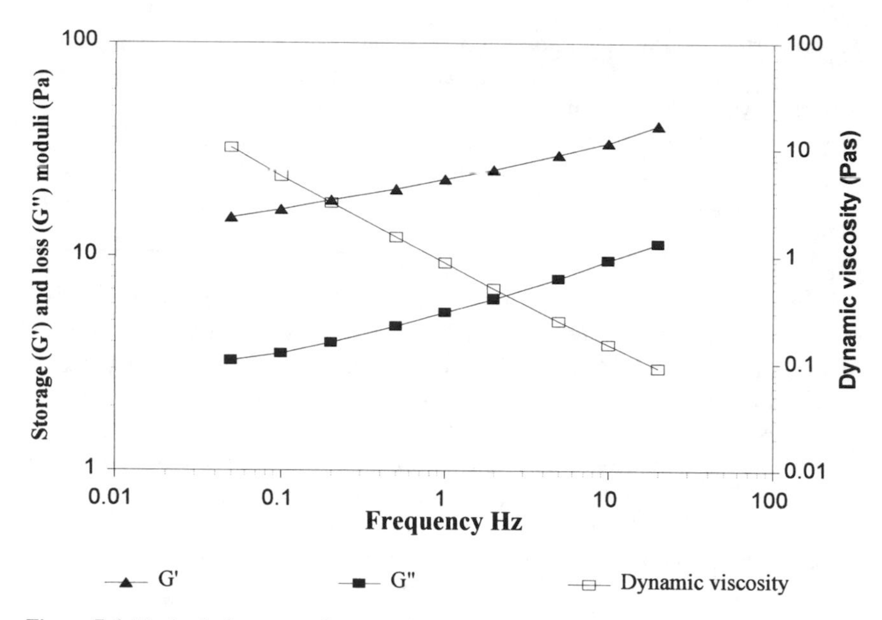

Figure 7.6 Mechanical spectra of water-soluble yellow mustard mucilage at 22°C, 2.0% polymer concentration (w/w). (Reprinted from Reference [19], with kind permission from Elsevier Science Ltd, The Boulevard, Langford Lane, Kidlington OX5 1GB, UK.)

3.3.4.2. Emulsion Stability Capacity

One of the major functional properties of yellow mustard products is their ability to stabilise oil/water emulsions [13]. This is due to the interfacial properties of YMM, which reduces the surface tension of water. Increasing the mucilage concentration up to 0.05% substantially reduced surface tension. Further addition of mucilage decreased surface tension only slightly. WS exhibited the greatest reduction in surface tension compared to crude mucilage or its WI fraction. The surface tension and interfacial activities of some plant hydrocolloids (guar, locust bean gums, etc.) were recently ascribed to the presence of residual surface active constituents/impurities. For example, protein present in YMM and its fractions may contribute to surface activity of the polysaccharides; however, WS with the lowest protein content exhibited the highest surface activity. The emulsion capacity and stability of YMM and its fractions were compared to commercial gums [13]. Prior to dialysis, the crude mucilage exhibited the most emulsion capacity and stability compared to the other gums or fractions. Dialysis substantially reduced the emulsion capacity and stability of the mucilage; however, it still exhibited higher emulsion capacity and stability than xanthan, guar and gum arabic.

A separate stability study compared YMM with commonly used gums including locust bean gum, guar gum, CMC, xanthan, tracacanth and propylene

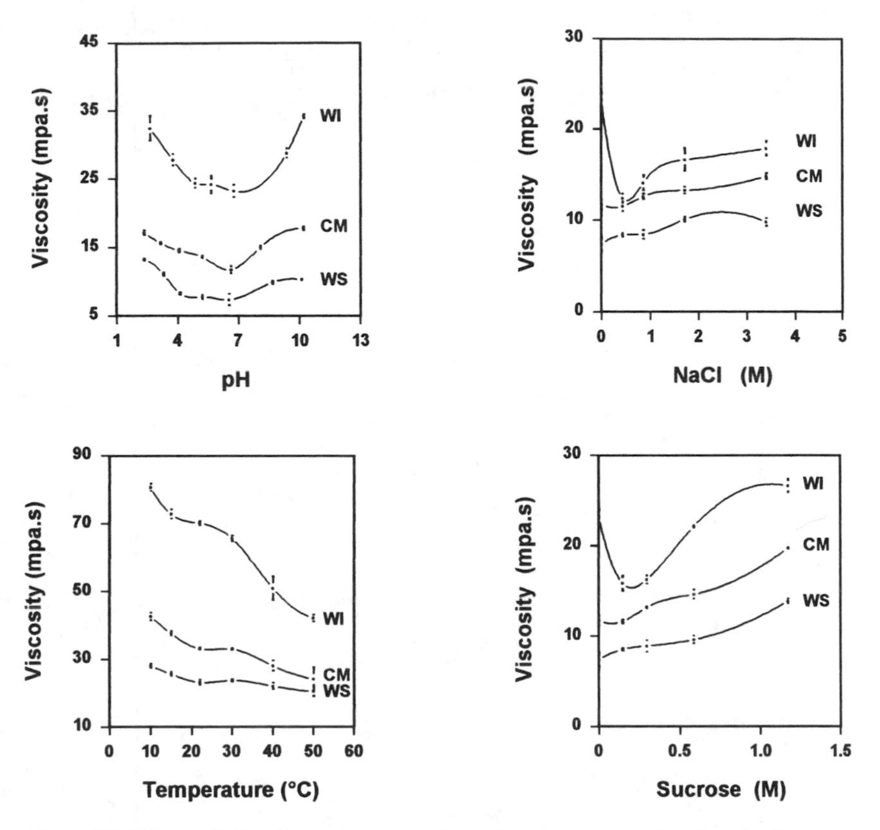

Figure 7.7 Effects of pH, salt, temperature, and sugar on the apparent viscosity of yellow mustard mucilage (CM) and its water-soluble (WS) and water-insoluble (WI) fraction at 22.0°C, 0.5% polymer concentration (w/w). (Reprinted from Reference [13], with kind permission from Elsevier Science Ltd, The Boulevard, Langford Lane, Kidlington OX5 1GB, UK.)

glycol alginate. A favourable comparison was observed between 0.25% YMM, 0.5% guar gum and 0.5% CMC (Table 7.5). In addition, 0.75% YMM compared favourably with both 0.5% CMC and xanthan gum. It is apparent that the addition of a small amount of locust bean gum enhances the emulsion stability of YMM.

3.4. PROTEINS

The high content of protein of around 30% for whole mustard seeds and flours (Table 7.1) appears satisfactory for growth and development. The amino acid composition of protein-rich mustard meal is given in Table 7.6 [26]. Compared to other oilseeds, mustard protein is high in lysine and sulfur amino

TABLE 7.5. Emulsification of 40% Vegetable Oil and Water Produced by Hydrocolloids.

Concentration (%)	Gums Added	Viscosity (cps)	Droplet Range	Average Droplet Size	Emulsion Stability
0.25	Mustard mucilage	650	10–75	30	52
0.50	Mustard mucilage	1810	5–50	20	82
0.75	Mustard mucilage	3375	2–50	15	99
1.00	Mustard mucilage	5800	2–35	8	100
0.5	Locust bean	1615	15–90	45	63
0.5	(0.8 Locust bean/0.2 Mucilage)	2463	5–65	35	85
0.5	Guar	3600	20–150	90	62
0.5	(0.9 Guar/0.1 Mucilage)	3900	10–80	50	81
0.5	CMC	135	10–200	40	65
0.5	(0.6 CMC/0.4 Mucilage)	1725	5–130	20	99
0.5	Xanthan	3000	5–125	8	100
0.5	(0.8 Xanthan/0.2 Mucilage)	2350	2–80	10	100
0.5	Tragacanth	1110	10–135	45	75
	(0.7 Trag/0.3 Mucilage)	1515	5–80	15	89
0.5	Propylene glycol alginate	180	2–60	5	100

Source: Adapted from the "Product Data Sheet" of UFL Foods Inc., Mississauga, Ontario.

TABLE 7.6. Amino Acid Composition of Oilseed Meals (% of air dried meal).

Amino Acids (%)	Soybean	Cotton Seed	Sunflower (dehulled)	Mustard	Sesame
Arginine	3.8	4.5	3.7	2.1	4.7
Histidine	0.8	0.8	0.7	0.8	0.6
Cystine	1.2	1.1	0.9	1.0	1.1
Isoleucine	2.6	1.6	1.6	1.4	2.1
Leucine	3.8	2.5	2.5	2.7	3.4
Lysine	3.2	1.7	1.4	2.0	1.3
Methionine	0.7	0.6	0.6	0.9	1.4
Phenylalanine	2.7	2.2	2.0	1.5	1.3
Threonine	2.0	1.4	1.3	1.7	1.6
Tryptophan	0.6	0.5	0.6	0.4	0.8
Tyrosine	2.0	0.7	—	1.3	2.0
Valine	2.7	0.7	2.2	1.8	2.4

Source: Adapted from Reference [26].

acids. Manufacturing protein concentrates from mustard seeds requires inactivation of the enzyme myrosinase to prevent formation of isothiocyanates and development of the hot mustard flavor. Presently, yellow mustard seeds are processed to produce a deheated ground mustard flour that is used extensively in processed meats such as sausages. The maximum amount of ground mustard allowed in processed meat products prior to the early 1990s was 1%. Recently the permitted levels in sausages and other processed meats have been increased to 5%; the product is still labelled as "spice" or "mustard." It is the water-soluble portion of the protein-rich mustard seed meal that contributes to the emulsification properties of mustard products [27].

Niazi and co-workers [28] prepared a mustard protein concentrate by enzymic treatment of mustard meal followed by steeping in 4% NaCl solution at pH 5. This method eliminated glucosinolates as well as 85.7% of phytate, with the resulting concentrate containing 53.1% protein, 6.1% crude fibre, 5.8% ash, and 0.4% phytate. Nutritional assessment of the mustard protein concentrate by rat bioassay showed that it compared favourably with casein with a PER (Protein Efficiency Ratio) of 2.4, NPU (Net Protein Utilization) of 68.5%, TD (Total Digestibility) of 87.0%, and a BV (Biological Value) of 78.4%.

3.5. PHENOLICS

Concern over the safety of synthetic antioxidants has given a strong impetus to research on natural antioxidants such as phenolic compounds, toco-

TABLE 7.7. TBA Values of Cooked Ground Pork Treated with 0–2% LPGMS Compared with BHT and TBHQ.[a]

	Storage Period (days)		
Additive	0	10	20
None	6.1	8.6	10.3
LPGMS 0.5%	3.4	6.6	6.8
LPGMS 1.0%	1.1	2.7	2.5
LPGMS 1.5%	0.6	0.8	0.7
LPGMS 2.0%	0.3	0.4	0.4
BHT 30 ppm	1.6	4.7	4.3
BHT 200 ppm	0.5	1.0	1.0
TBHQ 30 ppm	0.1	0.5	0.4
TBHQ 200 ppm	0.1	0.4	0.5

[a]TBA expressed as milligrams of malondialdehyde equivalents/100 g sample.
Source: Adapted from Reference [32].

pherols, phospholipids, and amino acids [29,30]. Oilseeds in general are rich in phenolic compounds that retard oxidation of the oil. Koslowska and co-workers [31] reported the presence of phenolic acids in rapeseed and mustard in which sinapic acid isomers were the predominant forms present. Recent research by Saleemi et al. [32] compared the antioxidant properties of low-pungency ground mustard seed (LPGMS) with synthetic antioxidants butylated hydroxytoluene (BHT) and tertiary-butyl hydroquinone (TBHQ) on the stability of comminuted pork. Table 7.7 shows that the addition of 1.5% and 2.0% LPGMS was as effective as 200 ppm of BHT or 30 ppm of TBHQ in controlling oxidative rancidity as measured by TBA. Further work by these researchers [33] showed that an 85% methanolic extract from LPGMS exhibited the strongest antioxidant activity due to the presence of much higher levels of phenolics compared to either water or 10% methanolic extracts. In addition to antioxidant activity, LPGMS also enhanced cook yield without exerting a detrimental effect on the color quality of the treated meat samples [32].

3.6. PHYTIN

Phytin or phytate accounts for approximately 2–3% of mustard seeds. It is generally considered an antinutrient because its structure confers strong chelation properties. In recent years, however, it has found wide industrial applications particularly outside the United States [34]. Labelled phytates, for example, have been used in medicine as imaging agents for organ scintigraphy [35–38]. The cariostatic properties of phytate have led to a number of patents that describe its use in oral care products such as dentifrices, mouth rinses, dental cements and cleaning agents for dentures [34]. The very chelating properties associated with phytate are also responsible for its strong anti-corrosive properties. The patent literature is filled with phytate-containing coating materials for metals and alloys, which not only inhibit corrosion but also improve paint adhesion [34]. The industrial and medical applications of phytate suggest mustard could be a good source of this compound.

3.7. MINERALS

Mustard seeds are rich in phosphorus, calcium, potassium and magnesium accounting for 0.56–0.76, 0.4–0.47, 0.68–0.76, and 0.28–0.29%, respectively. Other minerals identified include iron, sodium, zinc, manganese, copper, barium, aluminum, and strontium. Sodium has been found to be present at only 15 ppm in *Sinapis alba* seeds and has not been detected in *Brassica juncea* seeds.

4. PHYSIOLOGICAL PROPERTIES OF MUSTARD COMPONENTS

The most important components of mustard seed and products that have desirable functional properties and exhibit beneficial physiological effects are isothiocyanates, dithiolthiones and mucilage.

4.1. ISOTHIOCYANATES

4.1.1. Antimicrobial Properties

The antimicrobial properties of isothiocyanates (ITCs) from plant sources have been reviewed [39]. Mustard oil was reported over half a century ago to exhibit antifungal activity [40,41]. As described in Section 3.1, two isothiocyanates are released from mustard by enzymic hydrolysis of their respective glucosinolates, allyl isothiocyanate (AIT, from *Brassica juncea* seeds) and 4-hydroxybenzyl isothiocyanate (PHBIT, from *Sinapis alba* seeds). The more aromatic PHBIT appears to be far more fungiotoxic than the aliphatic ITs. The antifungal activity of AIT has been demonstrated by several authors, including Zsolnai [42], Hejrnanskowa [43] and Tsunoda [44]. Evidence accrued to date points to AIT and other volatile isothiocyanates as being particularly effective against the germination and growth of several plant pathogens [45]. In the vapor phase, AIT from brown mustard has been found to be a potent antifungal agent when included in modified atmosphere packaging of food products [46].

AIT appears to be especially effective against mycotoxin-producing molds such as *Aspergillus flavus*, *Penicillium citrinum* and *Fusarium graminearum*.

Mustard oil has been shown to inhibit the growth of several yeasts including *Neurospora* yeast [47]. AIT also inhibited the growth of yeast when added to fruit juices at a concentration of 1%, which may explain why the Romans used mustard oil to prevent fermentation of fruit juices or finished wines [48].

The antibacterial activity of ITCs differs substantially. For example, benzyl (BIT), β-phenylethyl (PEIT), *m*-methoxylbenzyl (MTBIT) and *p*-methoxybenzyl (PMBIT) isothiocyanates were all found to be more effective against *Staphylococcus aureus* than aliphatic ITCs. AIT and phenyl isothiocyanate (PIT), however, were both found to be ineffective against *Streptococcus pyrogenes, Staphylococcus aureus* or three gram-negative bacteria at levels that severely inhibited the growth of yeasts and fungi [42]. A recent study on food-borne pathogens by Delaquis and Mazza [49] showed that the effect of gaseous AIT was dose dependent (Figure 7.8). The growth of microorganisms was inhibited at concentrations above 500 ng/ml. The log number of killed bacteria was proportional to the AIT concentration for *Salmonella typhimurium* and *Listeria monocytogenes*, but almost unchanged for *Escherichia coli*. Some ITCs, such as BIT, exhibit antibiotic activity *in vitro*, and are sold as pharmaceuticals for treatment of infections of the respiratory and urinary tracts [50–53].

4.1.2. Anticarcinogenic Properties

The ability of ITCs to block carcinogenesis was recognized over 35 years ago [54,55]. In long-term feeding studies, α-naphthyl-ITC significantly reduced (in a dose-dependent manner) formation of liver tumors in male Wistar rats. β-Napthyl-IT also blocked hepatic tumor formation in rats fed the carcinogen 4-dimethylaminobenzene. Both of these ITCs had profound effects on hepatic enzymes that metabolize xenobiotics [56,57]. These findings laid the groundwork for subsequent studies on the tumor-blocking activities of ITCs, which were usually administered for only short periods of time.

Aromatic ITCs appear to exert anticarcinogenic activities against a variety of animal cancers including mammary, forestomach and lung tumors, as well as tumors of the esophagus [58,59]. Single doses of PIT, PEIT and BIT markedly reduced the incidence and mulitiplicity of mammary tumors in female Sprague Dawley rats. When BIT was administered by gavage 2 hr prior to a single dose of carcinogen, the average number of rats bearing tumors was reduced from 77% to 8%, while the number of tumors per animal dropped from 1.6 to 0.08 [60]. BIT inhibited benzo(a)pyrene-induced tumor develop-

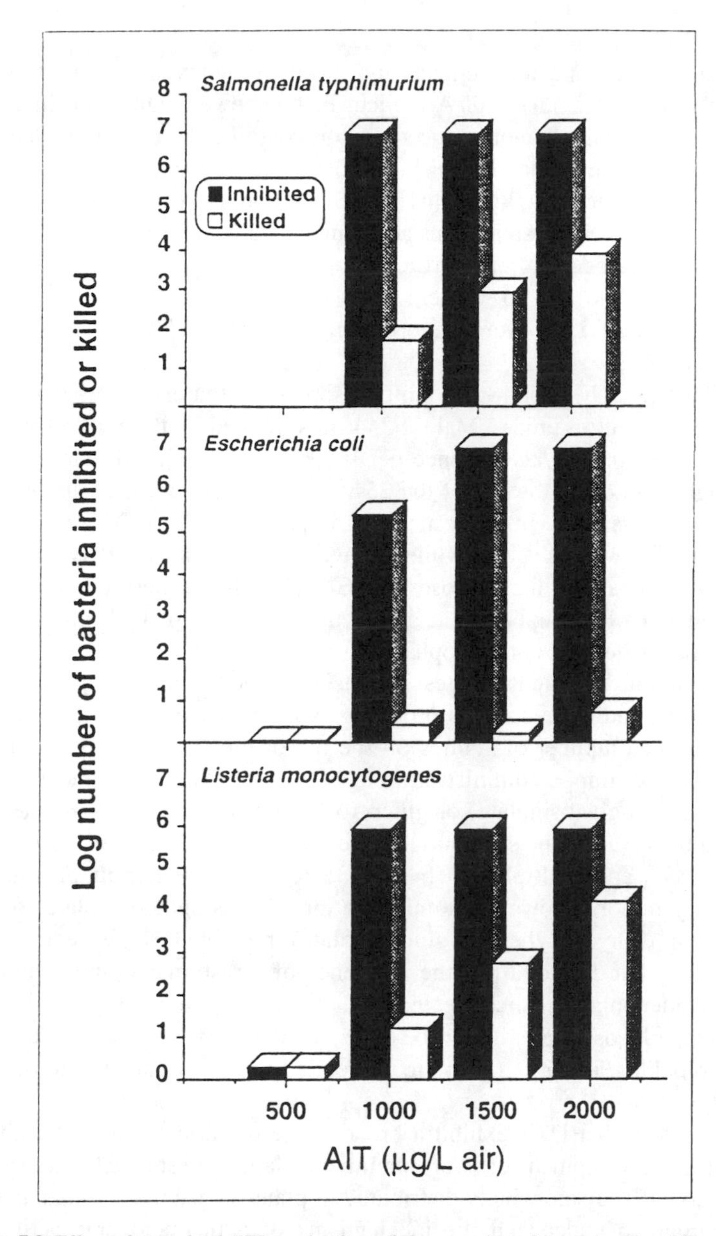

Figure 7.8 Effect of vaporized AIT on the fate of three strains of bacteria. The difference between the number of colonies on control disks (incubated without AIT) and tests provided the number of bacteria inhibited by the compound. Agar disks without evidence of growth were incubated a further 2 days in air at 35°C to estimate the number of bacteria killed by AIT. The limit of detection for the inhibition assay was 100 colony forming units. (Reprinted from Reference [39], with permission from *Food Technology*.)

ment in the lung and forestomach and N-nitrosodiethylamine-induced neoplasms in the forestomach of A/J mice. PEIT showed significant inhibitory effects against lung tumor induced by nitrosamine 4-(methylnitrosamino)-1-(3-pyridyl)-1-butanone (NNK) but had no effect against benzo(a)pyrene-induced lung tumor in A/J mice [61,62]. Since both NNK and benzo(a)pyrene are important tobacco carcinogens and lung cancer is attributed to tobacco usage, ITCs may be more effective chemoprotective agents for prevention of lung cancers. Jiao and co-workers [63] suggested that the lipophilicity and low reactivity of ITCs were important factors for inhibiting NNK-induced lung cancers.

PEIT has also been shown to inhibit esophageal tumors in rats induced by asymmetrical nitrosamine. Male F344 rats treated with N-nitrosobenzylmethylamine (0.5 mg/kg s.c. once per week for 15 weeks) developed 100% esophageal tumors at the end of the 25-week assay period, with tumor multiplicity of 11.5/animal. In experimental groups fed PEIT (3 μM/g of diet), tumor incidence was only 13% while the average tumor multiplicity was negligible (0.1/animal). At higher doses of PEIT (6 μM/g of diet) no tumors were observed [64]. PEIT appeared to block the formation of both preneoplastic and neoplastic lesions in the esophagus.

The amount of glucosinolates in mustard seeds is much higher than in their corresponding hydrolysis products, isothiocyanates. However, there is only a limited number of studies on the tumor-blocking effects of glucosinolates. For example, administration of large single doses of glucobrassicin (indoylmethyl glucosinolate) or glucotropaeolin (benzyl glucosinolate) 4 hr prior to benzo(a)pyrene substantially reduced both the incidence (from 75% to 25–38%) and multiplicity (from 1.35 to 0.5–0.69 tumours/animal) of mammary tumors. However, administration of these glucosinolates or glucosinalbin (4-hydroxybenzyl glucosinolate) produced some reduction in multiplicity but did not affect the incidence of forestomach tumors and pulmonary adenomas in mice treated with benzo(a)pyrene [65]. The overall effect of glucosinolates may be due to their hydrolysis products, as tumor-blocking activity appears to be related to the extent of glucosinolate hydrolysis.

It is evident that ITCs exhibit a broad range of anticarcinogenic activities against the development of liver, mammary gland, forestomach and esophagus tumours. They are widely distributed in plants consumed by man, making it important to understand the mechanisms of anticarcinogenic activity to maximise the benefits from these compounds. ITCs may inhibit carcinogenesis by neutralization of carcinogens or by suppressing proliferation activity of neoplastic cells. These compounds could prevent carcinogens from reaching their target site or weaken the effects of genetic modification that occur during the early stages of neoplastic transformations as well as inhibit key enzymes involved in the regulation of cell division [59].

4.2. DITHIOLTHIONES

Many spices used in foods are also recognized for their medicinal properties [66]. Brown mustard seeds or *Brassica nigra,* a common condiment used in India, was recently examined for its antimutagenic properties by Polassa and co-workers [67] using the carcinogen benzo(a)pyrene. Rats injected with the carcinogen were fed diets containing 1 to 10% mustard seeds for up to one month with 24 hr urine samples collected for examination of mutagens. A diet containing 1% mustard exhibited a strong antimutagenic effect, which did not change in diets containing up to 10% mustard seeds (Figure 7.9). These researchers attributed this effect to the presence of sulfur-containing compounds, dithiolthiones, in mustard. These compounds were thought to be partly responsible for the anticarcinogenic properties of diets high in vegetables [68]. Dithiolthiones exert their effect by increasing tissue levels of glutathione and detoxifying enzymes such as glutathione transferase [69]. A diet containing 10% mustard was shown by Polassa et al. [67] to elevate glutathione-*S*-transferase in rat liver. The ability of 1% mustard diets to significantly inhibit the mutagenicity of benzo(a)pyrene *in vivo* is important, as mustard is only consumed in small quantities in our diet. Dithiolthiones, the active principle of mustard and other *Brassica,* are used as antichistomal drugs for humans [70]. The structure of oltipraz, a typical dithiolthione, is shown below:

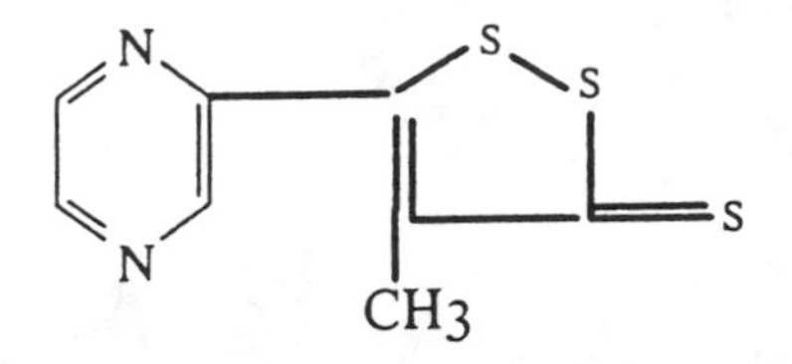

Structure of oltipraz

The specific levels of dithiolthiones in mustard, however, are unknown and require further examination.

4.3. YELLOW MUSTARD MUCILAGE

Dietary fibre is defined as "endogenous components of plant material in the diet which are resistant to digestion by enzymes produced by man. They are predominantly non-starch polysaccharides and lignin and may include associated substances." YMM appears to fall in this category so that it is reasonable to expect physiological effects such as regularizing colonic function, normalising serum lipid levels, attenuating the postprandial glucose response and possibly appetite suppression. A study by Begin and co-workers [71] examined the effect of YMM and other soluble fibres on glycemia, insulinaemia and gastroin-

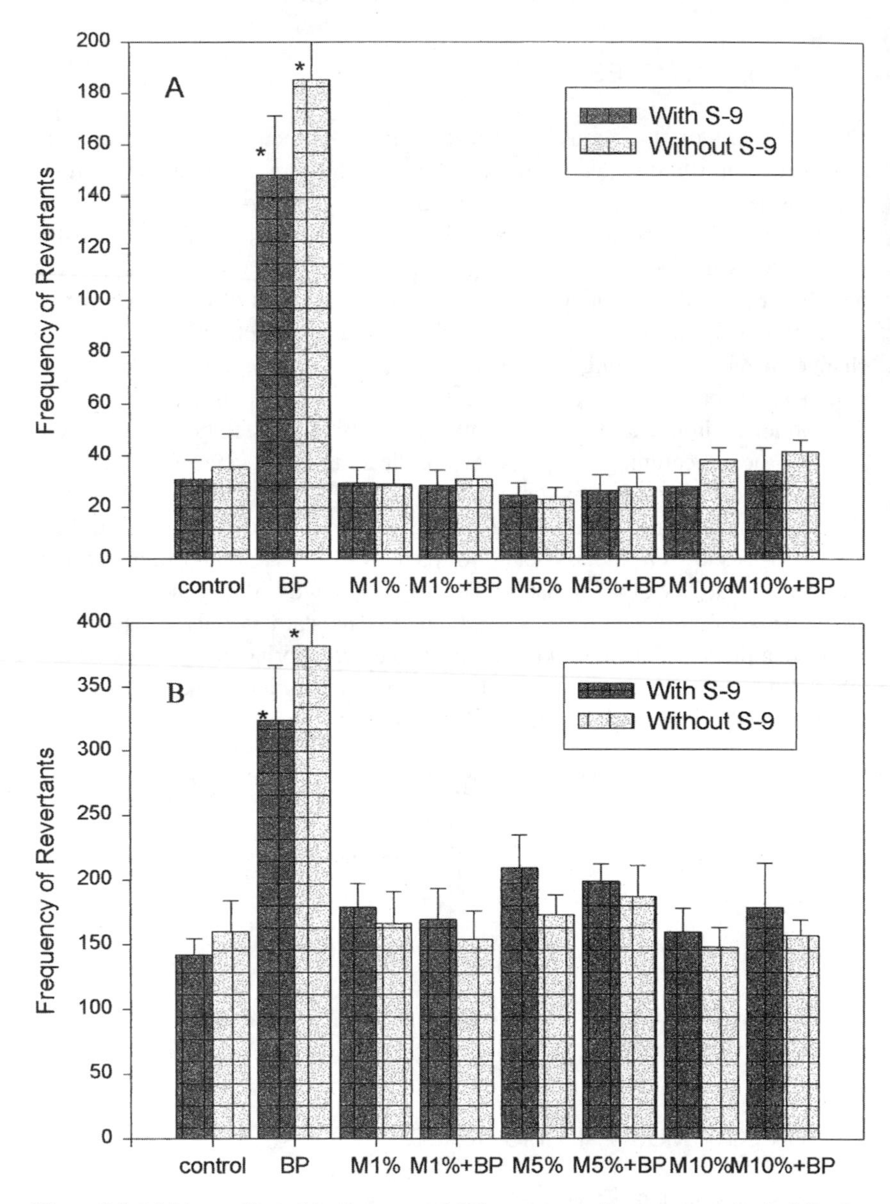

Figure 7.9 Inhibitory effect of feeding mustard (M) to rats on urinary mutagen levels following treatment with 1 mg benzo(a)pyrene (BP). Mutagenicity was tested with *Salmonella typhimurium* (a) TA98 and (b) TA100 with and without S-9 mix. Those groups marked with asterisks differ significantly (Duncan's multiple range test) from the values for the other corresponding groups ($p < 0.001$). Range bars indicate standard deviation. (Reprinted from Reference [67], with kind permission from Elsevier Science Ltd, The Boulevard, Langford Lane, Kidlington OX5 1GB, UK.)

testinal function in the rat. They found that YMM, guar gum, oat β-glucan and carboxymethylcellulose all significantly decreased postprandial insulin levels, indicating a reduction in glucose absorption. As a result, they suggested that YMM decreased insulinemia primarily by delaying gastric emptying, while the other fibres increased intestinal contents and consequently decreased absorption. Viscosity was considered a major contributory factor to the improved insulin status at peak time. Since viscosity of YMM increases at acid pH (Figure 7.7), it exerts a stronger gastric effect than the other fibres examined. Incorporating mustard fibre into white bread at levels not affecting palatability had a modest but significant effect in reducing the glycemic index of the bread in both normal and diabetic human volunteers [72]. A significant reduction in percent peak rise in postprandial blood glucose was also observed (Figure 7.10).

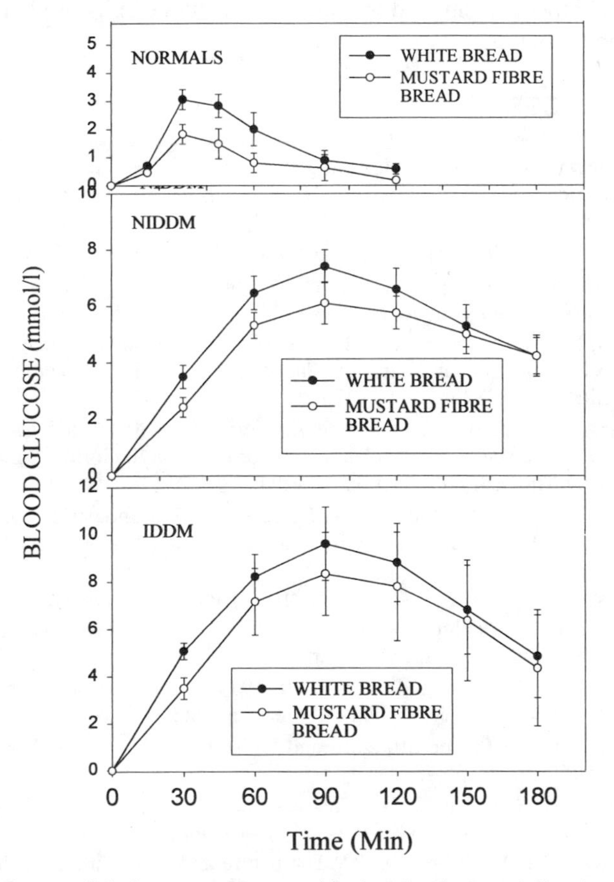

Figure 7.10 Postprandial glucose response to white bread and mustard fibre bread in normal volunteers (NORMALS), noninsulin-dependent (NIDDM) and insulin-dependent (IDDM) diabetics. (Replotted from Jenkins et al. [73].)

While no research on the effect of YMM on blood cholesterol has been reported, a positive response is anticipated.

5. CONCLUSION

Although the primary use of mustard seeds is as condiments, important new food applications are regularly being found. Commercially available mustard products include mustard oil, mustard flour, ground and prepared mustards, and mustard bran. Mustard mucilage has rheological and interfacial properties that should find a wide range of applications in the food and nonfood industries. Many of the components of mustard have beneficial physiological effects. These include isothiocyanates for possible effects on cancer prevention and antimicrobial activity; the viscous fibre and its effects on glucose and lipid metabolism; and the potential health benefits of phytates, dithiolthiones and proteins.

6. REFERENCES

1. Hemmingway, J. S. 1993. "Mustard and condiment products," Encyclopedia of Food Science and Technology and Nutrition, New York: Academic Press. pp. 3178–3182.
2. Vaughan, J. G. 1959. "The utilization of mustards." Econ. Bot. 13:196–204.
3. Farrell, K. T. 1990. "Spices, Condiments and Seasonings," 2nd Edition. New York: Van Nostrand Reinhold. pp. 138–148.
4. Johnston, P. V. 1995. "Flaxseed oil and cancer: α-linolenic acid and carcinogenesis," Flaxseed and Human Nutrition, Cunnane, S. C. and L. U. Thompson. Champaign, Illinois: AOCS Press. pp. 207–218.
5. Nieschlag, H. J., J. W. Hagemann, I. A. Wolff, W. E. Palm and L. P. Witnauer. 1967. "Brassylic acid esters as plasticizers for poly(vinylchloride)." Industrial and Engineering Chemistry, Product 6:201–204.
6. Van Dyne, D. L., M. G. Blase and K. D. Carlson. 1990. Industrial Feedstocks and Products from High Erucic Acid Oil: Crambe and Industrial Rapeseed, University of Missouri, Columbia.
7. Chang, S. P., T. K. Miwa and W. H. Tallent. 1969. "Reactivity ratios for copolymerization of vinyl chloride with 2-methylpentyl vinyl brassylate by computerized linearization." J. Polymer Sci. Part A-1 7:471–477.
8. Chang, S. P., T. K. Miwa and L. A. Wolff. 1974. "Allylic prepolymers from brassylic and azelaic acids." J. Applied Polymer Sci. 18:319–334.
9. Vaughan, J. G. 1970. The Structure and Utilization of Oilseeds. London: Chapman and Hall Ltd. pp. 55–57.
10. Siddiqui, I. R., S. H. Yiu, J. D. Jones and M. Kalab. 1986. "Mucilage in yellow mustard (*Brassica hirta*) seeds." Food Microstructure 5:157–162.
11. Bailey, K. and F. W. Norris. 1932. "The nature and composition of the mucilage from seeds of white mustard (*Brassica alba*)." Biochem. J. 26:1609–1623.

12. Woods, D. L. and R. K. Downey. 1980. "Mucilage from yellow mustard." Can. J. Plant Sci. 60:1031–1033.
13. Cui, W., N. A. M. Eskin and C. G. Biliaderis. 1993. "Chemical and physical properties of yellow mustard (*Sinapis alba*) mucilage." Food Chem. 46:169–176.
14. Hirst, E. L., D. A. Rees and N. G. Richardson. 1965. "Seed polysaccharides and their role in germination." Biochem. J. 95:453–458.
15. Weber, F. E., S. A. Taillie and K. R. Stauffer. 1974. "Functional characteristics of mustard mucilage." J. Food Sci. 39:461–466.
16. Vose, J. R. 1974. "Chemical and physical studies of mustard and rapeseed coats." Cereal Chem. 51:658–665.
17. Cui, W. and N. A. M. Eskin. 1997. "Yellow mustard gum. 1. Optimization of extraction process and rheological properties." Food Hydrocolloids (submitted).
18. Theander, O., P. Aman, G. E. Miksche and S. Yasuda. 1977. "Carbohydrates, polyphenols and lignin in seed hulls of different colors from turnip rapeseed." J. Agric. Food Chem. 25:270–273.
19. Cui, W., N. A. M. Eskin and C. G. Biliaderis. 1993. "Water-soluble yellow mustard (*Sinapis alba* L.) polysaccharides: partial characterization, molecular size distribution and rheological properties." Carbohydr. Polym. 20:215–225.
20. Cui, W., N. A. M. Eskin and C. G. Biliaderis. 1994. "Fractionation, structural analysis and rheological properties of water-soluble yellow mustard (*Sinapis alba* L.) polysaccharides." J. Agric. Food Chem. 42:657–664.
21. Cui, W., N. A. M. Eskin and C. G. Biliaderis. 1994. "Yellow mustard mucilage: chemical structure and rheological properties." Food Hydrocolloids. 8:203–214.
22. Cui, W., N. A. M. Eskin and C. G. Biliaderis. 1995. "NMR characterization of a 1,4-linked β-D-glucan having ether groups from yellow mustard (*Sinapis alba* L.) mucilage." Carbohydr. Polym. 27:117–122.
23. Cui, W., N. A. M. Eskin, C. G. Biliaderis and K. Marat. 1996. "NMR characterization of a 4-*O*-methyl-β-D-glucuronic acid containing rhamno-galacturonan from yellow mustard (*Sinapis alba* L.) mucilage." Carbohydr. Res. 292:173–183.
24. Cui, W. , N. A. M. Eskin, C. G. Biliaderis and G. Mazza. 1995. "Synergistic interactions between yellow mustard polysaccharides and galactomannans." Carbohydr. Polym. 27:123–127.
25. Cui, W. and N. A. M. Eskin. 1996. "Interaction between yellow mustard gum and locust bean gum: impact on a salad cream product." Gums and Stabilisers for the Food Industry 8, Phillips, G. O., P. A. Williams and D. J. Wedlock. IRL Press at Oxford University. pp. 161–170.
26. Bell, J. M. 1989. "Nutritional characteristics and protein uses of oilseed meals," Oil Crops of the World, Robbelen, G., R. K. Downey and A. Ashri. McGraw Hill Publishing Company. pp. 192–195.
27. R. J. French Company. 1990. Product portfolio. pp. 2–11.
28. Niazi, A. H. K., A. D. Khan and F. H. Shah. 1989. "Nutritional quality of mustard protein concentrate." Pakistan J. Scientific and Industrial Res. 32:546–548.
29. Barlow, S. M. 1990. "Technological aspects of antioxidants used as food additives," Food Antioxidants, Hudson, B. J. F. London: Elsevier. pp. 253–307.
30. Dugan, L. R. 1980. "Natural antioxidants," Autoxidation in Food and Biological Systems, Simic, M. G. and M. Karel. New York: Plenum Press. pp. 261–282.

31. Kozlowska, K., D. A. Rotkiewicz and R. Zadernowski. 1983. "Phenolic acids in rapeseed and mustard." J. Amer. Oil Chem. Soc. 60:1119–1123.
32. Saleemi, Z. O., P. K. Janitha, P. D. Wanasundara, and F. Shahidi. 1993. "Effects of low pungency ground mustard seed on oxidative stability, cooking yield and color characteristics of comminuted pork." J. Agric. Food Chem. 60:1861–1867.
33. Shahidi, F., P. D. Wanasundara and R. Amarowiczy. 1996. "Natural antioxidants from low-pungency mustard flour. Food Res. Internat. 27:489–493.
34. Graf, E. 1983. "Application of phytic acid." J. Amer. Oil Chem. Soc. 60:1861–1867.
35. Alavi, A., M. M. Staum, B. F. Shesol and P. H. Bloch. 1978. "Technetium-99m stannous phytate as an imaging agent for lymph nodes. J. Nucl. Med. 19:422–426.
36. Campbell, J., J. C. Bellen, R. J. Baker and D. J. Cook. 1981. "Technetium-99m calcium phytate: optimization of calcium content for liver and spleen scintography." J. Nucl. Med. 22:157–160.
37. Isitman, A. T., M. Manoli, G. H. Schmidt and R. A. Holmes. 1974. "Assessment of alveolar deposition and pulmonary clearance of radiopharmaceuticals after nebulization." Amer. J. Roentgenol. Radium Ther. Nucl. Med. 120: 776–781.
38. Sewatkar, A. B., O. P. D. Noronha, R. D. Ganstra and H. Glenn. 1975. "Radiopharmaceutics of technetium-99m labeled phytate." J. Nucl. Med. 14:46–51.
39. Delaquis, P. J. and G. Mazza. 1995. "Antimicrobial properties of isothiocyanates in food preservation." Food Technol. 49(11):73–84.
40. Hoffman, C. and A. C. Evans. 1911. "The use of spices as preservatives." J. Ind. Eng. Chem., 3:835–838.
41. Blum, H. B. and F. W. Fabian. 1943. "Spice oils and their components for controlling microbial surface growth." Fruit Prod. J. 22:326–329.
42. Zsolnai, T. 1966. "Die antimikrobielle Wirkung von Thiocyanatee und Isothiocyanates." Arzneimittel Forschung. 16:870–876.
43. Hejmankova, N., L. Leiferlova and M. Lisa. 1979. "Study on antifungal effects of allylisothiocyanate." Acta Univer. Palackianan Olomucensis (Fac. Med.) 89:9–16.
44. Tsunoda, K. 1994. "Effect of gaseous treatment with allylisothiocyanate on the control of microbial growth on a wood surface." J. Antibact. Antifung. Agents, 22:145–148.
45. Mari, M., R. Iori, O. Leoni and A. Marchi. 1993. "In vitro activity of glucosinolate derived isothiocyanates against postharvest fruit pathogens." Ann. Appl. Bio. 123:155–164.
46. Isshiki, K., K. Tokuora, R. Mori and S. Chiba. 1992. "Preliminary examination of allylisothiocyanate vapor for food preservation." Biosci. Biotech. Biochem., 55:1476–1477.
47. Webb, A. H. and F. W. Tanner. 1946. "Effect of spices and flavoring materials on growth of yeasts." Food Res. 10:273–282.
48. Tressler, K. D. and M. A. Joslyn. 1954. The Chemistry and Technology of Fruits and Vegetable Juice Production. New York: Avi Pub. Co. Inc. pp. 204–205.
49. Delaquis, P. J. and G. Mazza. 1994. Unpublished data. Agriculture and Agri-Food Research Centre, Summerland, B.C.
50. Massier, J. 1964. "Uber Erfahrungen mit einem pflanzlichen Antibiotikum in der Urologie." Die Medizinische Welt:2390–2393.

51. Bergmann, M., H. Lipsky and F. Glawogger. 1996. "Ein Antibiotikum aus der Kapuzinerkresse bei Harnwegsinfektionen." Medizinische Klinik 61:1469–1472.
52. Borowski, J. 1966. "Infekt-Behandlung in der taglichen Praxis." Die Medizinische Welt 17(N.F.):2431–2433.
53. Ebbinghaus, K. D. 1966. "Zur Langzeithandlung der Pyelonphritis." Die Medizinische Welt 17(N.F.):58–61.
54. Sassaki, S. 1963. "Inhibitory effects by naphthyl-isothiocyanate on development of hepatoma in rats treated with 3′-methyl-4-dimethyl-aminobenzene." J. Nara Med. Assoc. 14:101–105.
55. Sidranksky, H., N. Ito and E. Verney. 1966. "Influence of naphthyl-isothiocyanate on development of hepatoma in rats treated with 3′-methyl-4-dimethyl-aminoazobenzene." J. Nara Med. Assoc. 37:677–686.
56. Leonard, T. B., J. A. Popp, M. E. Graichen and J. G. Dent. 1981. "Naphthyl-isothiocyanate induced alterations in hepatic drug metabolizing enzymes and liver morphology. Implications concerning anticarcinogenesis." Carcinogenesis (Lond.) 2:473–482.
57. Leonard, T. B., J. A. Popp, M. E. Graichen and J. G. Dent. 1981. Naphthyl-isothiocyanate induced alterations in hepatic drug metabolism and liver morphology." Toxicol. Appl. Pharmacol. 60:527–534.
58. Morse, M. A., C.-X. Wang, G. D. Stoner, S. Mandal, P. B. Conrad, S. G. Amin, S. S. Hecht and Chung, F-L. 1989. "Inhibition of 4-(methylnitrosamino)-1-(3-pyridyl)-1-butazone-induced DNA adduct formation and tumorigenicity in the lung of F344 rats by dietary phenethyl isothiocyanate." Cancer Res. 49:549–553.
59. Zhang, Y. and P. Talalay. 1994. "Anticarcinogenic activities of organic isothiocyanates: chemistry and mechanisms." Cancer Res. 54:1976–1981.
60. Wattenberg, L. W. 1981. "Inhibition of carcinogen-induced neoplasia by sodium cyanate, tert-butyl isothiocyanate and benzyl isothiocyanate administered subsequent to carcinogen exposure." Cancer Res. 41:2991–2994.
61. Wattenberg, L. W. 1978. "Inhibition of carcinogenic effects of polycyclic hydrocarbons by benzyl isothiocyanate and related compounds." J. Natl. Cancer Inst. 58:395–398.
62. Wattenberg, L. W. 1987. "Inhibitory effect of benzyl isothiocyanate administered shortly before diethylnitrosamines or benzo(a)pyrene on pulmonary and forestomach neoplasis in A/J mice." Carcinogenesis (Lond.) 8:1971–1973.
63. Jiano, D., K. I. Eklind, C. I. Choi, D. H. Desai, S. G. Amin and F. L. Chung. 1994. "Structure-activity relationships of isothiocyanates as mechanism-based inhibitors of 4-(methylnitrosamino)-1-(3-pyridyl)-1-butanone-induced lung tumorigenesis in A/J mice," Cancer Res. 54:4327–4333.
64. Stoner, G. D., D. T. Morissey, Y.-H. Heur, E.M. Daniel, A. J. Galati and S. A. Wagner. 1991. "Inhibitory effects of phenylethyl isothiocyanate on *N*-nitrosobenzyl-methylamine carcinogenesis in the rat esophagus." Cancer Res. 51: 2063–2068.
65. Wattenberg, L. W., A. B. Hanley, G. Barany, V. L. Sparmins, L. K. T. Lam and G. R. Fenwick. 1986. "Inhibition of carcinogenesis by some minor dietary constituents," Diet, Nutrition and Cancer, Y. Hayashi et al. Tokyo, Japan Science Society Press. pp. 193–203.
66. Pruthi, J. S. 1976. Spices and Condiments. National Book Trust, New Delhi.

67. Polasa, J. A., P. U. Kumar and K. Krishnaswamy. 1994. "Effect of Brassica nigra on benzo(a)pyrene mutagenicity." Food Chem. Toxic. 32:777–781.
68. Ansher, S. S., P. Dolan, and Bueding, E. 1983. "Chemoprotective effects of two dithiolthiones and of butylhydroxyanisole against CCl_4 and acetaminophen toxicity." Hepatology 3:932–935.
69. Ansher, S. S., P. Dolan and E. Bueding. 1986. "Biochemical effects of dithiolthiones," Food Chem. Toxic. 24:405–415.
70. Ansher, S. S. 1985. "The chemotherapy of schistomiasis." Ann. Rev. Pharmacol. and Toxicol. 25:485–508.
71. Begin, F., C. Vachon, J. Jones, P. J. Wood and L. Savoie. 1988. "Effect of dietary fibers on glycemia and insulinemia and on gastrointestinal function in rats." Can. J. Physiol. Pharmacol. 67:1265–1271.
72. Jenkins, A. L., D. J. A. Jenkins, F. Ferrari, G. Collier, A. V. Rao, S. Samuels, J. D. Jones, G. S. Wong and R. G. Josse. 1987. "Effect of mustard seed fiber on carbohydrate tolerance." J. Clin. Nutr. Gastrenterol. 2:81–86.

CHAPTER 8

Designer Vegetable Oils

B. E. McDONALD[1]
K. FITZPATRICK[2]

1. INTRODUCTION

FATS and oils, in particular vegetable oil sources, have been a topic of keen interest over the past 20 years. The role of dietary fats in human nutrition has created widespread interest in fats and oils among consumers, clinicians, researchers, health educators, food producers, and food processors and distributors. Of particular interest have been the health effects of level of intake and type of fats and oils. Much of the current interest stems from the implication of dietary fat in the etiology of chronic diseases such as coronary heart disease (CHD), cancer, diabetes, obesity, and hypertension. Concern with type of fat (viz., saturated fat) as an important dietary risk factor in CHD has been a major impetus for the development of specially modified fats and oils. Other factors that contributed to this interest in modified and specifically designed fats and oils include the demonstration that: (1) monounsaturated fatty acids were equally as effective as polyunsaturated fatty acids in lowering blood cholesterol levels, at least in diets providing 30–40% of energy as fat; (2) the *trans* fatty acids found in hydrogenated fats may have deleterious physiological effects; (3) omega-3 fatty acids play a role in early development; and (4) there is a relationship between specific fatty acids, such as γ-linolenic acid, and physiological responses in disease states.

[1]Department of Foods & Nutrition, University of Manitoba, Winnipeg, MB, Canada.
[2]Plant Biotechnology Institute, National Research Council, Saskatoon, SK, Canada.

This chapter will not cover all of the developments over the past decade with respect to dietary fats and oils but deal with specific examples of some of the major developments. Likewise, the chapter will not deal with changes to fats and oils intended primarily for industrial uses. The discussion will begin with examples of genetic manipulation of traditional vegetable oils to produce oils with different nutritional and functional properties and conclude with a discussion of lipid engineering in terms of modification of the lipid structure by interesterification. Although other techniques, such as hydrogenation and fractionation, are used to modify fats and oils for specific uses, these lipid modification strategies will not be discussed in this chapter. The chapter deals exclusively with vegetable oils except for Section 4, which discusses the blending of vegetable oils and animal fats aimed at optimizing the functional properties and the nutritional quality of the resulting fat.

2. MODIFIED OR PROPERTY-ENHANCED FATS AND OILS

2.1. SPECIFICALLY MODIFIED VEGETABLE OILS

Canola oil was one of the early arrivals among the modified or property-enhanced vegetable oils (i.e., vegetable oils with specific fatty acid composition). Canola oil, a low-erucic acid rapeseed oil, was developed because of nutritional concerns with erucic acid. The method plant breeders used to develop low-erucic rapeseed simply involved identifying low-erucic acid plants and introducing the gene or genes (one or two gene loci depending on the species) from these selections into adapted cultivars of rapeseed following traditional plant breeding techniques [1]. Canola, in addition to low levels of erucic acid, also contains low seed glucosinolate levels. Canola was developed by introducing the low glucosinolate trait into low-erucic acid rapeseed cultivars. The inheritance of the low glucosinolate trait, however, is much more complex than the low-erucic acid trait; several genes apparently are involved in the control of glucosinolate levels in the seed [1]. In canola oil, oleic acid replaced the erucic acid found in traditional rapeseed oil [2] (Table 8.1). The relatively high level of oleic acid (viz., 61% of total fatty acids) together with the low level of total saturated fatty acids (approx. 7%) probably account for the cholesterol-lowering effect of canola oil in humans [3]. Plant breeding efforts have resulted in further modification of the fatty acid profile of canola oil. Low α-linolenic acid (18:3n$-$3; $<$2% vs. traditional 10%) and high-oleic acid (up to 86%) cultivars have been developed during the past decade (Table 8.1). In these instances, however, chemical mutagenesis was used to produce the low-linolenic and high-oleic mutants [4]. In the case of the high-oleic cultivar, the high-oleic mutant was crossed with low-linolenic cultivars to produce the high-oleic line [4]. These modified canola oils have been developed in response to the demand for frying oils with low levels of

TABLE 8.1. Comparison of Major Fatty Acids in Traditional and Modified Vegetable Oils.

	Fatty Acids (% of total)[1]								
	12:0	14:0	16:0	18:0	18:1	18:2	18:3	20:1	22:1
Rapeseed	—	—	3.1	1.0	33.0	17.0	7.7	10.0	25.5
Canola									
Traditional	—	—	4.0	1.5	61.0	21.0	9.5	1.5	—
High-oleic	—	—	3.5	2.5	77.0	8.0	2.5	1.5	—
Low-linolenic	—	—	4.0	1.0	61.0	27.0	2.0	1.0	—
High-lauric	39.0	4.0	3.0	1.5	33.0	11.0	6.5	1.0	0.5
Sunflower									
Traditional	—	—	6.0	4.0	18.5	71.0	0.5	—	—
High-oleic	—	—	4.0	4.0	78.5	11.5	—	—	—
Flax									
Traditional	—	—	6.5	4.5	19.5	16.5	53.0	—	—
Low-linolenic (Linola™)	—	—	6.0	4.0	16.0	71.5	2.0	—	—

[1]All values adjusted to nearest 0.5% of total.
Source: Adapted from References [4–10].

saturated and *trans* fatty acids and relatively high stability to oxidative changes without having to be hydrogenated [11].

Another example of a modified vegetable oil is high-oleic acid sunflower oil (Table 8.1). As with the modified canola oils, it was developed in response to the need for a stable, low-saturated, non-hydrogenated frying oil. The original high-oleic sunflower appears to have originated in the Soviet Union where Russian scientists created the high-oleic variety through the use of chemical mutagenesis. This variety was brought to the United States and the trait was introduced into inbred lines of sunflower adapted to the growing conditions in north central United States [12]. Sunflower cultivars with oleic acid levels of 85% are currently in production in the United States and Canada and commercial lines, available under the trade name HO Sunola™, with oleic acid levels as high as 91%, are currently in field tests in Canada. Chemical mutagenesis also was used in the development of low-linolenic acid flax (Table 8.1). The latter, which is licensed in Canada under the trademark Linola™, is an alternative high linoleic acid (approx. 76%) vegetable oil source adapted to northern latitudes [13]. The specifications for Linola™ oil refers to oil derived from cultivars of flax containing less than 3% α-linolenic acid. The Flax Council of Canada has recently registered the name Solin as the generic term to describe flaxseed oil containing less than 5% α-linolenic acid. The United States Food and Drug Administration currently is reviewing a petition for GRAS (Generally Recognized As Safe) status for Solin.

A recent approach to the production of modified vegetable oils is the use of genetic engineering techniques. Scientists at Calgene Inc., Davis, California, have produced high-stearic acid and high-lauric acid canola cultivars using transgenic techniques. The high-stearic canola was produced by deliberately suppressing the gene activity associated with the conversion of stearic acid to oleic acid. The technique involved inserting the antisense gene construct for stearoyl-ACP desaturase into canola cultivars [14]. Insertion of the antisense construct resulted in a reduced level and activity of stearoyl desaturase activity in the developing seed and, in turn, significantly higher levels of stearic acid in the oil (up to 40% stearic acid vs. 2% in regular canola). The high-lauric canola (Table 8.1) was produced by transferring the lauroyl-ACP thioesterase gene from the California bay laurel plant into canola [15], presumably by a similar methodology to that described for the transfer of this gene into *Arabidopsis thaliana* [16]. The resulting cultivar produced oil containing over 40% lauric acid and, at least, initially will be used in "the soaps and detergent industry" [10]. In addition to canola, transgenic oilseed cultivars also have been reported for corn and soybean [17].

2.2. PROCESSING OF MODIFIED VEGETABLE OILS

All of the modified vegetable oil produced to date has been processed by the customary methods used in the extraction and processing of canola, soybean and sunflower oil for edible purposes [4,18–22]. The only difference lies in the effort that must be undertaken to segregate these higher-value seeds from the traditional crop. Speciality crops, such as low-linolenic canola, high-oleic sunflower, and high-lauric canola, are currently sold on the basis of specific quality and compositional parameters [23]. Identity-preserved (IP) oilseeds have recently been described as "Those types that are produced and marketed on the basis of specifications, i.e., a particular variety/hybrid or particular trait or set of traits, and that have a different pricing structure than commodity products" [24]. Quality assurance and product integrity are achieved by constant monitoring of the crop throughout all stages of production and processing. Del Vecchio [10] has outlined steps taken during commercial production of high-lauric canola to guarantee segregation from the traditional crop: all seed is grown under contract and growers must purchase new seed each year; the identity-preserved and traditional commodity crop may not be produced on the same farm; individual fields of the IP crop are routinely checked and the yields estimated to reduce the risk of growers adding commodity seed when delivering the specialty crop; separate elevators, unloading locations, and storage sites are used; and separate batch delivery, processing and storage are utilized at the crushing plants to prevent co-mingling with commodity seeds and product. An important determinant of the success of specialty oilseeds is whether or not the end-user will be willing to pay for the costs associated with the IP system.

Preparation of the seed and extraction of the oil may differ slightly depending on seed type. Sunflower seed, for example, may be dehulled before oil extraction. Likewise, a portion of the oil in canola and sunflower seeds usually is mechanically extracted by means of screw presses or expellers; a process termed "prepressing." Production of edible vegetable oil divides into two processes, namely, extraction and oil processing. The processes, except for minor differences, are similar for most vegetable oils produced from the seeds of the plants.

2.2.1. Extraction

The steps in the extraction process are summarized in Figure 8.1. The first step involves cleaning the seed to remove debris and foreign and damaged seeds. The next step is flaking. Sunflower seeds, however, often are dehulled (a process where about 75% of the seed hulls are removed) prior to flaking [22]. Flaking involves passing the seeds between rollers to produce flakes between 0.20 mm and 0.40 mm in thickness; a process that is necessary to ensure efficient extraction of the oil. Care must be taken throughout the flaking process to control the moisture content and temperature of the seed in order to optimize oil extraction. In the case of canola and sunflower, the flake is conditioned (i.e., heated or cooked) [4,18,22]. Conditioning serves several important functions, such as inactivation of enzymes that might adversely af-

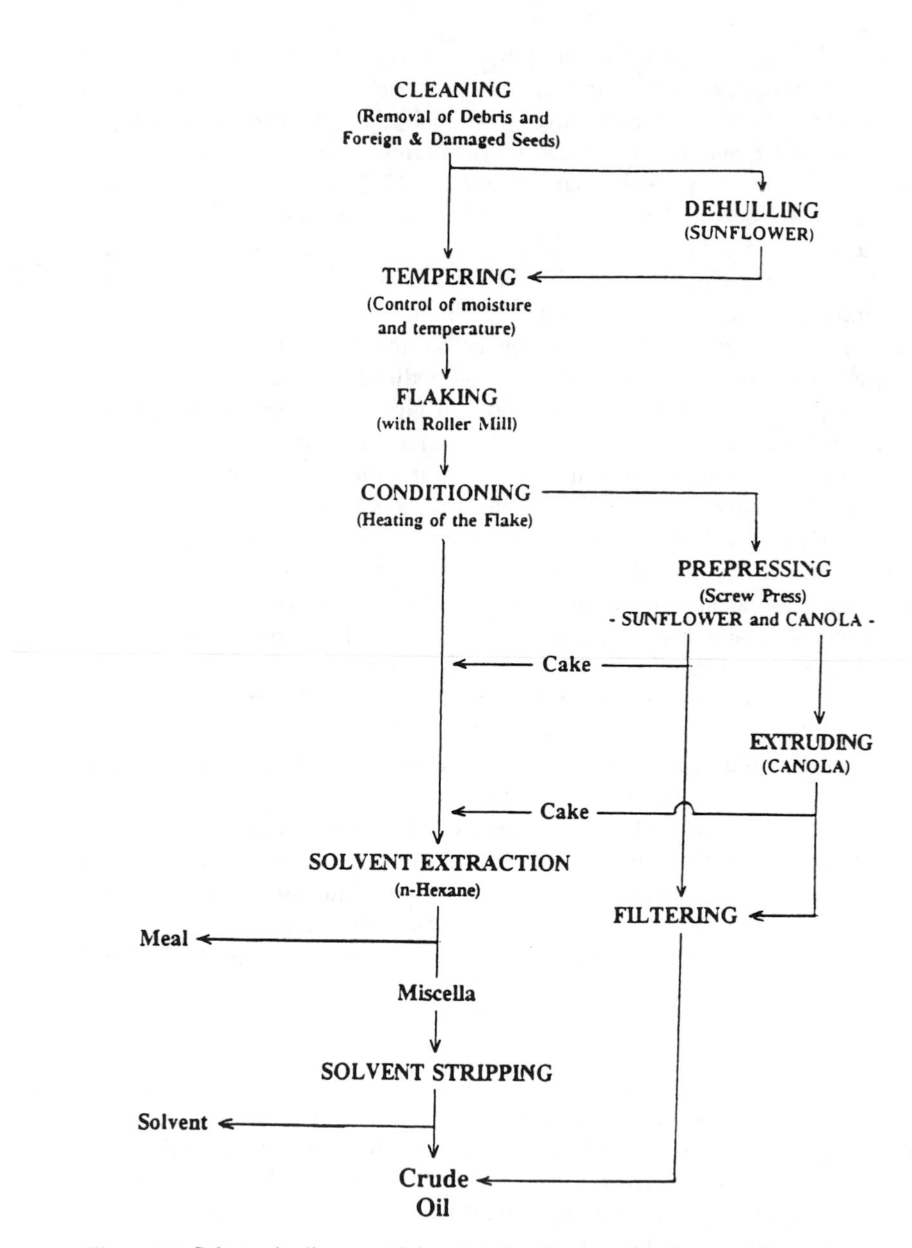

Figure 8.1 Schematic diagram of the steps in oil extraction from canola, soybean, and sunflower seeds. (Adapted from References [4,18,19,20,22].)

fect the quality of the oil and rupture of the cell wall, thereby facilitating separation of the oil from the solids. Canola and sunflower flakes, which contain relatively high levels of oil (40–50% by weight), are then passed through a screw press or expeller (prepressing) where about half of the oil is mechanically pressed from the seed [4,18,22]. The "cake" from the expeller is subsequently extracted, usually with *n*-hexane, to remove the remaining oil. In some canola processing plants, the cake is put through a mechanical extruder prior to solvent extraction [4,18] to improve the solvent extraction properties of the cake. With soybeans, the flake often goes directly to solvent extraction although some operations subject it to heat treatment [21].

Solvent extraction involves separation of the oil from the solids to form "miscella" (solvent plus oil). The miscella and solvent are allowed to percolate through the cake or flake in stages. The solids eventually leave the extractor, after a wash with fresh solvent, as meal containing less than 1% residual oil. The miscella coming from the extractor is a mixture of solvent, crude oil, moisture and very fine solid particles. The solvent is removed from the oil by evaporation and steam stripping. Most of the solvent is removed by multistage evaporation with the final traces being removed by steam stripping. The solvent is recovered for reuse and the crude oil is ready for refining.

2.2.2. Oil Processing

Crude oil from the extraction process contains small amounts of impurities, namely, phospholipids (phosphatides), mucilaginous gums, free fatty acids, pigments, fine meal particles, and dirt. The objective of oil processing is to remove these impurities while causing minimal damage to the quality of the resulting oil. Figure 8.2 summarizes the major steps used in processing vegetable oils.

2.2.2.1. Degumming

The crude oil from the prepress and solvent extraction steps usually is combined and degummed before further processing. Degumming removes phosphatides and mucilaginous gums, which become insoluble in the oil when hydrated. Degumming is done for two primary reasons: (1) in the case of soybean oil, in particular, to produce soybean lecithin [21]; and (2) to produce an oil suitable for long-term storage or transport (the presence of substantial amount of phospholipids lead to dark-colored and off-flavored oils). Degumming is carried out using two methods: (1) degumming with water; and (2) degumming with acid and water. Degumming with water involves mixing the oil with about 2% water at 60–80°C for about 30 min to hydrate

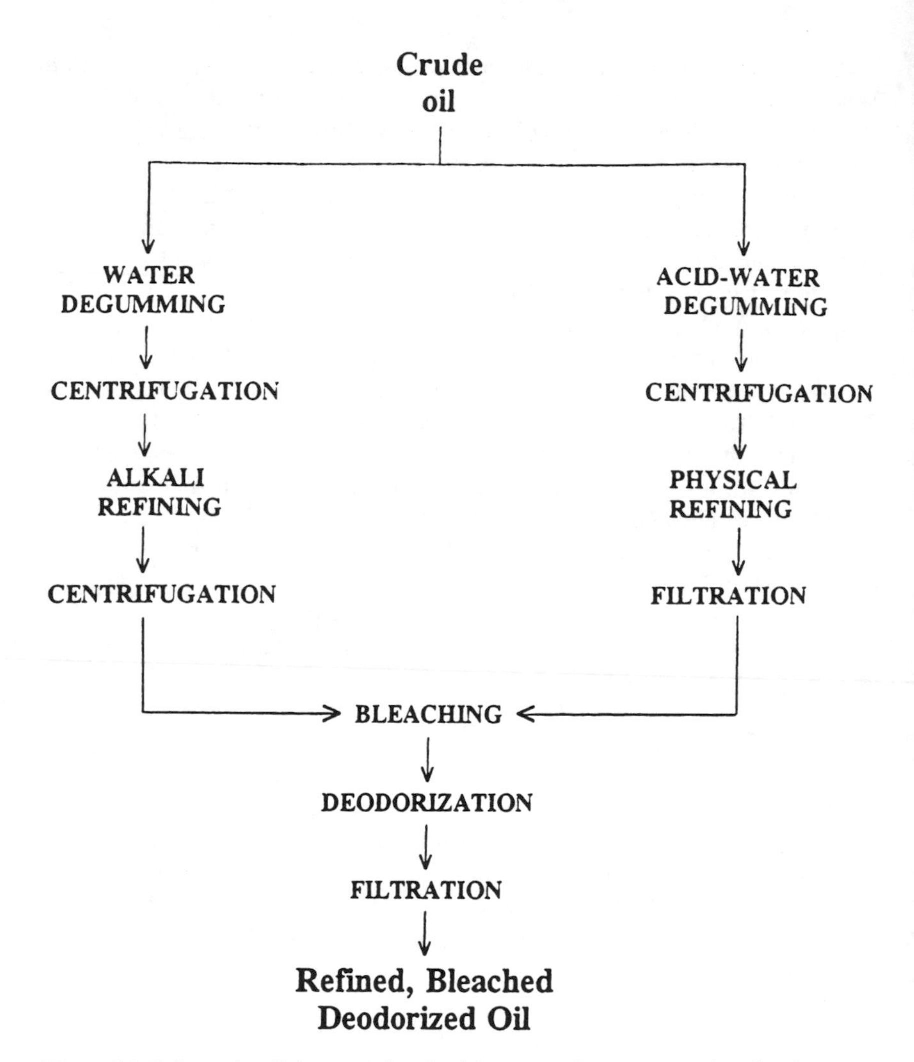

Figure 8.2 Schematic of the steps involved in processing prepressed and solvent-extracted vegetable oils. (Adapted from References [4,18,19,20].)

the phosphatides, thereby reducing their solubility in the oil. Degumming with acid and water follows a similar procedure, except the oil is first vigorously mixed with a 0.1–0.5% solution of 50% citric, malic or phosphoric acid and then mixed gently with 2% water [4,18,19]. Degumming with acid and water also removes the nonhydratable phosphatides. Following contact of the oil with water or acid and water, it is centrifuged to remove the precipitated material.

2.2.2.2. Alkali and Physical Refining

Degummed oil is further purified by refining. Again there are two methods: (1) alkali or caustic refining; and (2) physical or steam refining. Alkali refining is the more common process. In alkali refining the oil is mixed with 12% sodium hydroxide solution at 30–40°C. The oil/soap mixture is then heated to about 90°C and centrifuged to separate the aqueous soap phase from the oil. The oil is further washed with water and centrifuged to remove final traces of soap. The process removes free fatty acids and phosphatides. Physical refining can be substituted for alkali refining with acid-water degummed oils [4,18–20]. In physical refining, the degummed oil is first vigorously mixed with 0.05–0.10% of 85% phosphoric acid at 105–110°C in a vacuum. It is then mixed with 1–2% acid-activated bleaching clay for 10–15 min. The clay, precipitated phosphatides, chlorophyll, and carotenoids are then removed by filtration.

2.2.2.3. Bleaching

Alkali-refined oils must be bleached to remove pigments, metallic compounds, residual soaps, and traces of oxidation products. One of the most important effects of bleaching, especially with canola oil and soybean oil, is the removal of chlorophyll and chlorophyll derivatives [4,19]. Chlorophyll and its derivatives give the oil a greenish color and catalyze light-induced oxidation of the oil. Where chlorophyll is not the primary problem, the aim is removal of the primary and secondary oxidation products [21]. The exact process will vary depending on the equipment used in the bleaching process. The process generally involves mixing the oil with bleaching clay (an acid-treated bentonite clay) at about 100°C under vacuum for 5–30 min. The amount of activated bleaching clay used usually varies from 1–3%, depending on the level and type of chlorophyll compounds and residual phosphatides present in the oil. For optimum effectiveness, the clay should contain 10–15% moisture. The clay, absorbed compounds and precipitated materials are removed by filtration.

2.2.2.4. Deodorization

Deodorization is the final step in refining vegetable oils. The primary function of deodorization is removal of residual compounds characteristic of the taste and odor of the seed, odoriferous compounds formed during bleaching and traces of oxidation products. Deodorization is basically a high-temperature, high-vacuum, steam distillation process. The oil is heated to 225–260°C under vacuum (1.5–8.2 g/cm^2) and steam (1–3%) is blown through the oil to reduce odor and flavor constituents and other volatile compounds, such as free fatty acids, to very low levels. Steam increases the volatility of the compounds and improves the efficiency of the process. When vegetable oils are physically refined, deodorization serves to remove the small amounts of free fatty acids in the oil. It is important that the oil be free of chlorophyll, phosphatides and metallic compounds prior to deodorization.

3. SPECIALTY VEGETABLE OILS—HEALTH ASPECTS

3.1. BIOLOGICAL SIGNIFICANCE OF γ-LINOLENIC ACID

Increased attention to the possible role of specific fatty acids in health and disease has created an interest in specialty oils, in particular, sources of γ-linolenic acid (GLA; 18:3n-6). Research during the past decade, has indicated that γ-linolenic acid may play an important role in the etiology of a number of diseases. For example, treatment of rheumatoid arthritis patients with borage oil or a concentrate of γ-linoleic acid has been found to result in a reduction in the signs and symptoms of the disease [25]. The beneficial effect of γ-linolenic acid has been attributed to increased tissue levels of 1-series prostaglandinins, namely, PGE_1, which has been shown to suppress chronic inflammation. Likewise, γ-linolenic acid has been found effective in the treatment of diabetic neuropathy [26,27], a common complication of both insulin-dependent and noninsulin-dependent diabetes mellitus. There also is increasing evidence that γ-linolenic acid and its metabolites play an important role in the integrity of the epidermis [28] and thus in skin disorders such as atopic eczema [29]. In addition, γ-linolenic acid has been found particularly effective as an anti-tumor agent in experimental models [30] and in the treatment of certain cancers such as human brain malignant glioma [31]. Its ability to kill tumor cells appears to be related to lipid peroxidation and induced free radical production. Nonetheless, it appears to be a safe anti-cancer agent, as injection of γ-linolenic acid into the brain of dogs found that it is not cytotoxic to normal brain cells [32].

3.2. SOURCES OF γ-LINOLENIC ACID

In animals, γ-linolenic acid is formed from linoleic acid by the Δ6-desaturase enzyme (Figure 8.3). However, very little accumulates in the tissue lipids of animals because it is rapidly elongated to dihomo-γ-linolenic acid which, in turn, is converted to arachidonic acid. The absence of accumulation of γ-linolenic acid is believed to be related to the fact that the Δ6-desaturase enzyme is the rate-limiting step in this conversion. Hence, there has been a move to seek out dietary sources of γ-linolenic acid. The primary sources are plant oils, namely, borage, evening primrose, and black currant seeds. These sources vary somewhat in γ-linolenic acid content, with borage oil containing

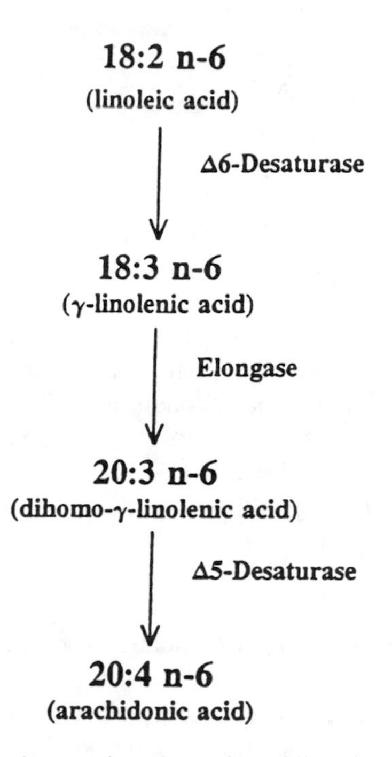

Figure 8.3 Pathway for the desaturation-elongation of linoleic acid in mammalian systems.

the highest level (22–25%), evening primrose oil the lowest (8–10%), and black currant oil intermediate (ca. 15%) between borage and evening primrose oils (Table 8.2). Borage seed also contains the highest level of fat (29–35% by wt) and evening primrose seed the lowest level (ca. 23%), with black currant seeds again intermediate (ca. 30%) [33,34].

TABLE 8.2. Fatty Acid Composition of Borage, Black Currant and Evening Primrose Seeds.

	Fatty Acids (% of total)[1]								
	16:0	18:0	18:1 n-9	18:2 n-6	18:3 n-6	18:3 n-3	18:4 n-3	20:1 n-9	22:1 n-9
Borage	10.5	3.5	16.0	37.5	23.5	—	—	4.0	2.0
Black currant	6.5	1.5	10.5	46.5	17.0	13.0	3.0	0.5	—
Evening primrose	6.0	2.0	9.0	72.0	9.0	—	—	—	—

[1]All values adjusted to nearest 0.5% of total.
Source: Adapted from References [33–38].

3.3. PROCESSING BORAGE, EVENING PRIMROSE AND BLACK CURRANT SEEDS

3.3.1. Hexane Extraction

Oil is extracted from the seeds of borage, evening primrose and black currant essentially as described in Section 2.2 for modified vegetable oils that go into the regular food supply (Figure 8.1). The only difference is the scale of operation; with borage, evening primrose and black currant, the scale of operation is equivalent to a large pilot plant. As described in Section 2.2.1, the seed is cleaned of foreign materials, conditioned, flaked, and prepressed. The resulting press cake is solvent extracted with *n*-hexane, the solvent is removed from the miscella as described in Section 2.2.1 and the crude oil is combined with the crude oil resulting from the prepressing operation.

3.3.2. Cold Pressing

Since γ-linolenic acid is prone to oxidation and thermal rearrangement, an alternative to prepressing and solvent extraction is the production of cold press oil. In the production of cold press oil, the solvent extraction step is omitted. In addition, the temperature of the cake during mechanical pressing of oil from the seed is controlled at less than 60°C by water cooling the screw press. The primary drawback to this process is the low recovery of oil due to the inefficiency of mechanical pressing at low temperatures and the relatively low oil content of the seeds of borage, evening primrose and black currant. Hence, alternative methods have been investigated, such as supercritical fluid extraction with carbon dioxide. Favati et al. [39] reported oil recoveries of over 95% in the supercritical carbon dioxide extraction of evening primrose at extraction pressures between 30 and 70 MPa and temperatures between 40 and 60°C. The primary drawback to supercritical fluid extraction is the relatively high cost of the process.

The crude oil from borage oil, evening primrose oil and black currant oil can be further processed as described for modified vegetable oils in Section 2.2.2. However, care must be taken to avoid destruction of the γ-linolenic acid by carefully controlling the temperatures of the processes and protecting the oil from oxygen. Wolff and Sebedio [40], for example, found that the degree of isomerization of γ-linolenic acid to *trans* isomers was less than one percent when borage oil was vacuum-steam deodorized (0.1–0.7 kg/cm^2 pressure; 3–5% steam by wt/hr) at 200°C for 2 hours. By contrast, the degree of isomerization of γ-linolenic acid increased to approximately 16% during vacuum-deodorization at 240°C. Since the purpose of deodorization is to remove components such as aldehydes and free fatty acids, the higher the temperature the better the quality of the oil in this respect. However, to preserve the quality of borage, evening primrose and black currant oils, deodorization should be carried out at temperatures less than 200°C. These oils generally are packaged in soft-gelatin capsules and sold as essential fatty acid supplements in the health and functional food markets [37].

The fact that borage oil, evening primrose oil and black currant oil are usually sold as soft-gelatin capsules [37] to protect the oil from oxidation, and that these natural oil sources contain relatively low levels of γ-linolenic acid, has stimulated interest in producing concentrates of γ-linolenic acid for therapeutic and pharmaceutical applications. Gunstone [33] described several methods that have been reported for upgrading the natural glyceride mixtures of γ-linolenic acid and for the production of concentrates of the fatty acid. Other methods that have been investigated for the enrichment of γ-linolenic acid from borage oil and evening primrose oil include lipase-catalyzed hydrolysis [41,42] or lipase-catalyzed esterification [38,42] of the oils. However, all of these enrichment methods add substantially to the cost of the γ-linolenic acid.

4. SPECIALLY PROCESSED AND FORMULATED FATS

4.1. RATIONALE FOR PRODUCTION OF SPECIALLY FORMULATED FATS

Saturated fats have been recognized to exert major effects on plasma cholesterol concentration since the 1950s. The work of Keys et al. [43] and Hegsted et al. [44] found that saturated fatty acids (SFA) were twice as effective in raising the level of plasma total cholesterol as polyunsaturated fatty acids (PUFA) were in lowering it. Concerns over dietary SFA resulted in a switch by the food industry to partially hydrogenated vegetable oils (PHVO). In the United States, this trend eventually culminated in a nearly complete switch to PHVO by the "fast" food industry in the early 1990s. The conversion from animal to PHVO shortenings, however, brought with it concerns over the loss of functional properties imparted by animal fats, such as the taste and texture of fried foods and the flakiness of baked goods. As a result, several companies sought to develop fats that retained the advantages of the animal fats while avoiding the health concerns with these fats.

Appetize®, which is specific blends of vegetable oils and animal fats from which cholesterol has been removed, is an example of one such product [45]. It is the result of collaborative research between Source Food Technology of Minnesota and Brandeis University of Massachusetts and was commercialized by Bunge Foods USA in the spring of 1996. The fatty acid composition of Appetize® is designed to give a balance that offsets the cholesterol-raising effect of the SFA in the animal fats. Three things were considered in the design of Appetize®: (1) removal of cholesterol from the animal fats; (2) avoidance of *trans* fatty acids from products such as PHVO; and (3) provision of a balance between linoleic acid and myristic acid that will lower plasma total and LDL cholesterol. The scientific basis for these conditions have been summarized by Hayes [46]. Of paramount importance was the recognition that SFA are not equally hypercholesterolemic. Stearic acid is generally thought to be neutral or hypocholesterolemic in its effect on plasma cholesterol [47,48]. By contrast, the situation with respect to palmitic acid is somewhat controversial. Hayes [46] took the stance in the development of Appetize® that palmitic acid becomes increasingly hypercholesterolemic as the level of dietary cholesterol increases [49]. Hence, the aim was to reduce dietary cholesterol intake as much as possible in order to minimize the effect of saturated fatty acids on serum cholesterol.

4.2. PRODUCTION OF APPETIZE®

The cholesterol in the animal fats used in the formulation of Appetize® is removed by steam stripping. The process (U.S. Patent 5,436,018), originally designed for the removal of cholesterol from fish oils, has been adapted for removal of cholesterol from tallow, lard and butterfat. In brief, the process involves first liquefying the fat by heating and then deaerated in a feed tank using a vacuum of 25 mm Hg (34 g/cm^2) pressure and a subsequent sparge with nitrogen. The deaerated fat is then introduced at an upper portion of a countercurrent thin-film steam stripper while simultaneously introducing steam at a lower portion of the device. The pressure of the stripper is continuously maintained at 1 mm Hg (1.4 g/cm^2) and the temperature at 400°F at least (205°C). The steam: fat ratio is varied, depending on the fat source and other processing conditions, from 1 to 15% by weight dry steam. A conventional tube and disc-type evaporator, commonly used for a variety of purposes, such as removal of hexane from vegetable oil in solvent extraction systems, serves as a stripper. The feed rate of the oil to the stripper is appreciably lower than that recommended by the manufacturer for this type of equipment when used for other purposes (viz., ⅕ to ⅒ the recommended rate). The thickness of the oil film, preferably 1 to 5 mm, which is a distinguishing feature of the process, varies with feed rate. Steam stripping removes essentially all of the non-esterified cholesterol. When operated under optimum conditions, the countercurrent thin-film steam stripper removes from 90 to 95% of the cholesterol in animal fats.

4.3. NUTRITIONAL AND FUNCTIONAL PROPERTIES

In addition to cholesterol removal from the animal fat portion, the other important feature of Appetize® is the ratio of linoleic acid to myristic acid in the product. When butterfat-safflower oil or tallow-safflower oil blends were tested with gerbils, elevated blood cholesterol levels on saturated fat diets declined to normal levels when the ratio of linoleic acid-to-myristic acid reached a range of 6–8 [46]. These results have been confirmed in a clinical study with humans [50]. Hassel et al. [50] found that substitution of Appetize® for animal fats in baked products and in the preparation of foods in the diets of postmenopausal nuns resulted in a 7% lower mean blood cholesterol level. The lower total blood cholesterol level on the Appetize® diet was due primarily to a 9% lower LDL-cholesterol level. Appetize® accounted for between 40 and 50% of the total fat in the subjects' diets.

Appetize® also was found to perform the same as traditional animal-based shortenings during deep-fat frying operations. For example, French fried potatoes prepared in Appetize® were similar to those fried in an animal-based shortening [45]. Another benefit reported for Appetize® is greater oxidative stability than either of the fats used in the blend [45,46]. Comparison of the stability of Appetize® with commercial corn oil or low-cholesterol tallow by the active oxygen method (AOM) found an appreciably greater stability for the blend (64, 25 and 13 hr., respectively). Likewise, production of oxidation decomposition compounds (viz., *trans*-2-alkenals and n-alkanals) during heating to frying temperatures was appreciably lower for Appetize® than for corn oil and low-cholesterol tallow. Appetize® also performed well in the preparation of baked products [45]. It resulted in taste and texture characteristics similar to those of products prepared with lard or partially hydrogenated soybean oil. In cases where flakiness is particularly important, such as pie crusts, its performance was superior to a PHVO shortening.

5. ENGINEERED LIPIDS—MODIFICATION OF TRIACYLGLYCERIDE STRUCTURE

5.1. INTRODUCTION

Food fats consist primarily of triacylglycerides, in other words, fatty acid esters of glycerol (Figure 8.4). The physical properties of triacylglycerides, commonly referred to as triglycerides, depend not only on their fatty acid composition but also on the positional distribution of the fatty acids in the glycerol structure. The use of fats and oils in food products is dependent on specific properties such as melting temperature, solids content, and crystallization characteristics. Cocoa butter, for example, which is used in the manufacture of chocolates and confectionary products, contains approximately two-thirds saturated and one-third monounsaturated fatty acids. In addition, the unsaturated fatty acid, namely, oleic acid, is esterified at the *sn*-2 position and the saturated fatty acids, primarily palmitic acid and stearic acid, at the *sn*-1 and *sn*-3 positions of the triacylglycerides. The fatty acid composition and the position of the fatty acids on the glycerol backbone also affect the digestion and metabolism of triacylglycerides. Since pancreatic lipase specifically hydrolyzes the fatty acids at the *sn*-1 and *sn*-3 positions of triacylglycerides, fats are absorbed as 2-monoglycerides and free fatty acids (Figure 8.4).

To obtain fats with specific properties, it is often necessary to modify them. The three techniques used by the food industry to alter fats and oils are hydrogenation [51,52], fractionation [53,54], and interesterification [55,56]. Hydrogenation is the application of choice by industry; approximately one-third of all edible fats and oils are hydrogenated whereas only 10% are fractionated or interesterified [57]. The U.S. industry, in particular, uses predominantly hydrogenation; interestification is used more widely in Europe. Although each has its own particular application, interesterification, particularly lipase-mediated interesterification, has the greatest potential for tailoring food fats to specific purposes.

5.2. INTERESTERIFICATION

Interesterification is a catalytical process involving the breaking of existing ester bonds and the simultaneous formation of new ester bonds. There are two types of interesterification, chemical and enzymatic. In addition, enzyme-mediated interesterification can be either random, as is the case with chemical catalysts, or position-specific, namely for the *sn*-1 and *sn*-3 positions [55,56]. In chemical interesterification, where the reaction is carried out at temperatures above the melting point of the highest-melting triacylglyceride, the reaction proceeds to equilibrium and the formation of a completely randomized mixture of all possible triacylglycerides. By contrast, lipase-catalyzed interesterification offers the possibility of producing structured triacylglycerides. Depending on the source of the lipase used in the reaction, the resulting triacylglycerides can vary in the *sn*-position of the fatty acids and in the particular fatty acids incorporated into the structure [56].

5.2.1. Chemical Interesterification

Chemical interesterification holds two primary advantages over enzymatic interesterification: the existence of industrial procedures and equipment; and a lower price for the catalyst. In addition, the triacylglycerides are generally easier to separate from the reaction mixture. Chemical interesterification was introduced on the industrial level by Swift & Company in the United States over 40 years ago to modify the functional properties of the company's lard-base shortening [57]. Today, the process is used to produce specialty fats such as margarines without *trans* fatty acids (e.g., Uniliver's Becel margarine). Saturated fats, such as modified palm oil, palm kernel oils or babassu oil, are interesterified and blended with liquid oils such as canola oil, sunflower oil and Linola™ (low-linolenic flax) oil.

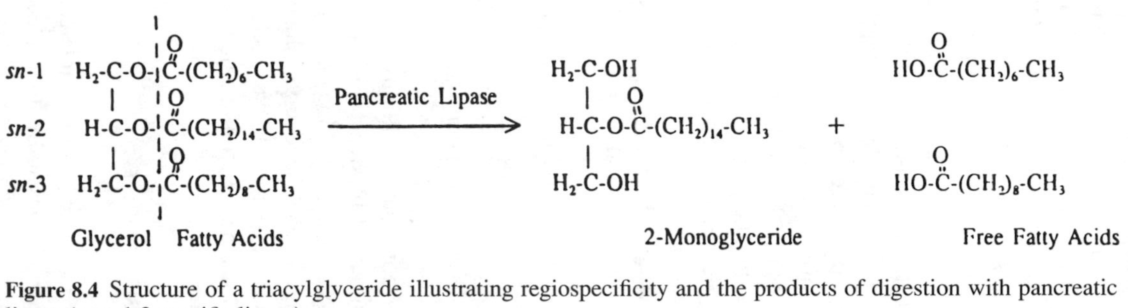

Figure 8.4 Structure of a triacylglyceride illustrating regiospecificity and the products of digestion with pancreatic lipase (a *sn*-1,3 specific lipase).

5.2.1.1. Chemical Catalysts

The most widely used catalysts are metallic sodium or sodium-potassium alloys and alkylates of sodium (e.g., Na methylate or Na ethylate). The sodium alkylates are easily dispersed in the fat to be interesterified and the reaction can be carried out at temperatures below 100°C and at atmospheric pressure [58]. Although the sodium alkylates are active at temperatures of 50–70°C, the catalytical activity of sodium methylate has been shown to be temperature sensitive [59]. Sodium metal requires special care in handling and it is more expensive than the sodium alkylates. All of these catalysts are easily inactivate by water and are sensitive to the quality of the oil. Thus it is necessary to pretreat the fats in an attempt to reduce: the water content to less than 0.01% by thoroughly drying the oil; the free fatty acid content to less than 0.1%; and the peroxides to a POV of less than 10 by bleaching [55,58].

Sodium alkylates must be handled with care because they are toxic and are highly reactive materials. Hence, it is important to protect these catalysts from moisture and air by storing them under dry, cool conditions in closed containers until just before use. The shelf life of sodium methylate is 3–6 months while the shelf life for sodium ethylate is 2–3 months [58].

5.2.1.2. Conditions in the Chemical Interesterification of Lipids

No special equipment is required for chemical interesterification. Conventional neutralizing and bleaching equipment is suitable together with facilities for drying the oil and for blending the catalyst into the oil. The process is a batch operation, and under optimum conditions the reaction is completed in less than 30 min. The endpoint of the reaction is usually based on measurement of the solid-fat content of the resulting product. Determination of the slip melting point or some standardized crystallization method is usually used. The reaction is stopped by destroying the catalyst by the addition of water. Frequently, some acid is added in combination with the water to reduce losses due to saponification.

5.2.2. Enzymatic Interesterification

The primary advantages of lipase-catalyzed interesterification over chemical interesterification include: the possibility to produce triacylglycerides with specific fatty acids at specific *sn*-positions; the ability to carry out the reaction at lower temperatures, thereby reducing energy cost and producing a higher-quality end product; and a lower sensitivity than the chemical catalysts to moisture and other contaminants in the starting material [56]. One of the most successful products of lipase-catalyzed interesterification is the production of cocoa butter substitutes [55,57]. Cocoa butter is not only one of the most expensive fats on the market but the price varies appreciably. In 1993, Loders Croklaan B.V. opened an enzymatic interesterification plant in The Netherlands for the production of fats for confectionary use. Interesterification of POP (palmityl-oleyl-palmitin), a rich fraction in palm oil, with stearic acid or ethyl stearate by *sn*-1,3-specific lipases results in the production of POS (palmityl-oleyl-stearin) and SOS (stearyl-oleyl-stearin) triacylglycerides [55].

5.2.2.1. Distinctive Features of Lipases

Lipases are an ubiquitous group of enzymes that exhibit maximum activity at an oil-water interphase where the primary reaction is hydrolysis of the ester bonds in triacylglycerides. However, under conditions of limited moisture, lipases catalyze the reverse reaction [60]. Lipases perform well in a wide variety of organic solvents as well as supercritical carbon dioxide. However, for optimum activity some water is necessary, usually at less than saturation, in a range of 0.75 to 4.0 (w/v) [61]. The use of immobilized lipases provides the added advantages of: eliminating the problems associated with distributing the enzyme uniformly ("solubilizing") in the fats; improved enzyme stability, thus increasing the lifespan of the enzyme and reducing its cost per unit of product; and the use of a continuous process [56,62].

A wide variety of lipases are available although only a small number are available commercially [55,56,63]. These lipases are the products of fermentation by selected microorganisms. Although both random and regiospecific (positional specific) lipases are available (Table 8.3), the nonspecific lipases, those that catalyze reactions at all positions in the triacylglyceride, offer few advantages over chemical catalysts. On the other hand, the regiospecific lipases, namely the *sn*-1,3 specific lipases, offer the greatest potential for industrial application in the production of structured lipids with special functional or physiological properties [62,64].

TABLE 8.3. Positional Selectivity of Some Lipases.

Source of Lipase	Selectivity
Candida rugosa	*sn*-nonspecific
Candida cylindracae	*sn*-nonspecific
Geotrichum candidum	*sn*-nonspecific
Mucor miehei	*sn*-1,3 specific
Aspergillus niger	*sn*-1,3 specific
Rhizopus arrhizius	*sn*-1,3 specific

Source: Adapted from References [55,56,62].

5.2.2.2. Conditions in Lipase-Mediated Interesterification

Lipases are proteins and thus can be denatured at temperatures above 40°C, especially in aqueous media. Immobilized enzymes, however, are more thermally stable and thus suitable for enzyme-catalyzed interesterification. A variety of support systems have been used to immobilize the lipases [61,62,65]. Usually some porous particulate material, such as ion exchange resins, silicas, clays, and so on, are used. The reaction can be carried out in either a batch reactor or continuously in a fixed-bed reactor [56,57,62]. The latter has the advantage of shortening the reaction time, thus limiting the isomerization of the *sn*-1,2 diglyceride, which is an intermediate in the *sn*-1,3 interesterification scheme, and thus limiting the formation of random triacylglycerides. In a fixed-bed reactor, three parameters affect the reaction: (1) the ratio of fatty acid or fatty acid ester to oil; (2) the water level in the feed stock; and (3) the flow rate through the reactor. The fatty acid-to-oil ratio, which determines the equilibrium composition of the reaction, is an economic balance between the cost of separation of the triacylglycerides versus the costs of the reaction and yields at each stage of the process where a multistage technique is used [62]. At a fixed ratio of oil-to-fatty acid, the flow rate is used to control product conversion. The progress of the reaction can be measured by determining the carbon number of the triacylglycerides by gas-liquid chromatography. However, measurement of catalytic activity often is simplified by estimating the conversion of free fatty acids into triacylglyceride, which is a first-order reaction, as measured by gas-liquid chromatography of fatty acid methyl esters [62]. Eventually, the activity of the lipase will deteriorate due to thermal destruction and poisoning by impurities in the feed stock. As activity drops, flow rate through the reactor must be decreased. When conversion drops below a predetermined point, the catalyst is replaced. Since the lipase catalyst is a major cost in the process, rate of catalyst decay is a major economic consideration. Hence, the temperature of the process and the quality (degree of refining) of the feed stock must be carefully controlled.

5.2.3. Current and Future Applications

Outside of the United States, interesterification is used in the production of plastic fats for use in the manufacture of margarines that are free of *trans* fatty acids, in addition to its use in the production of speciality fats. In Europe, interesterification of liquid oils with solid fats is a common practice in the manufacture of margarines. By contrast, interesterification in the United States is limited primarily to the production of high-value specialty fats such as confectionary fats and cocoa-butter substitutes. However, if consumer concern over *trans* fatty acids continues, chemical interesterification of liquid oils with appropriate solid fats in the production of zero-*trans* plastic fats will likely increase.

There is appreciable interest in the use of enzyme-mediated interesterification in the production of structured-triacylglycerides with improved physical and nutritional properties. Structured lipids are triacylglycerides with not only a specific fatty acid composition but a specific *sn*-positional distribution of the fatty acids (Figure 8.4). The use of immobilized lipases in the production of cocoa butter-like fats with the melting properties and unique consistency desired in the manufacture of chocolate and confectionary products is one of the best known examples of enzymatic interesterification.

Of increasing interest is the application of enzymatic interestification in the production of triacylglycerides with improved nutritional properties. Incorporation of Betapol, a structured fat designed to mimic human milk fat, into an infant formula improved the absorption of the long-chain saturated fatty acids and calcium over that of a conventional formula [66]. In Betapol, like human milk fat, a major portion of the predominant saturated fatty acid, palmitic acid, is esterified in the *sn*-2 position of the triacylglyceride. Structured triacylglycerides are currently being investigated for their use in specific clinical situations such as patients who have undergone surgery for cancer or patients with cystic fibrosis [67]. Structured triacylglycerides with essential fatty acids, such as linoleic acid, eicosapentaenoic or docosahexaenoic acid in the *sn*-2 position and medium-chain fatty acids (viz., C8:0 and C10:0) in the *sn*-1,3 positions, have been the fats of choice in these studies. The medium-chain fatty acids are the preferred energy substrate while the *sn*-2 monoglyceride provides the template for synthesis of functional lipids. The use of structured lipids in enteral and parenteral emulsions offers appreciable promise in the nourishment of premature infants or the treatment of patients with specific conditions. However, cost remains a major deterrent until clinical studies demonstrate a definite advantage to the use of structured lipids.

6. SUMMARY

Recognition of the importance of fats in human health coupled with an increased understanding of the metabolic importance of individual fatty acids has prompted a keen interest in the identification and production of dietary fats with specific functional and nutritional properties. One of the early developments in the production of designer vegetable oils was the introduction of modified or property-enhanced oils through the use of traditional plant breeding techniques. Canola oil was the first modified vegetable oil to come into large-scale commercial production. Other examples of modified vegetable oils include: low-linolenic acid canola oil; high-oleic acid canola oil; high-oleic acid sunflower oil; and low-linolenic acid flaxseed oil. In all of the latter group, chemical mutagenesis was used to produce the high-oleic or low-linolenic mutants. A recent approach in the production of modified vegetable oils is the use genetic engineering techniques. A high-lauric acid canola cultivar, produced using transgenic techniques, was introduced into commercial production in the United States in 1995. The seed from cultivars with modified oil composition has been processed using tradition methods for vegetable oil production. However, special care is taken in the growing and handling of many of these higher-value, modified vegetable oil crops, such as high-oleic sunflower or high-lauric canola, to prevent contamination with seed from traditional cultivars.

Interest in the possible role of specific fatty acids in health and disease has focused attention on specialty oils. γ-Linolenic acid has been of particular interest because of its possible role in the etiology of a number of chronic diseases. Hence, there has been a search for dietary sources of γ-linolenic acid. The primary plant sources of γ-linolenic acid are borage, evening primrose and black currant seed oils. The seeds from these crops are processed in essentially the same way as the seeds of traditional oilseed crops, except that the scale of operation is much smaller. In general, specialty oil crops, such as borage, evening primrose and black currant, are processed in plants equivalent in size to a large pilot plant. An alternative to traditional processing methods is the production of cold press oil from these specialty oil sources. The substitution of cold pressing for traditional processing methods stems from the susceptibility of γ-linolenic acid to oxidative and thermal destruction.

Concern with saturated fats, in particular animal fats, and partially hydrogenated vegetable oils (i.e., *trans* fatty acids) has led to an interest in the formulation of fat blends that preserve the functional properties imparted by animal shortenings while avoiding the health concerns of these fats. Specific blends of vegetable oils and animal fats from which cholesterol has been removed, marketed under the tradename Appetize®, is an example of such a product. Cholesterol is removed from the animal fats by steam stripping and the fat sources are blended to provide a fatty acid balance that has been found to lower blood cholesterol level.

One of the more exciting developments in the area of designer vegetable oils has been the engineering of structured lipids. The application of enzyme-mediated interesterification in the production of triacylglycerides with specific fatty acids at specific *sn*-positions in the molecule has enabled the production of fats with unique functional and nutritional properties. The current interest in structured lipids is restricted primarily to the production of particular fats, such as cocoa butter substitutes, for use in the manufacture of chocolates and confectionary products, and dietary fats with special nutritional properties, for patients with cystic fibrosis or for use in enteral and parenteral emulsions for premature infants. The cost of structured lipids is currently a major deterrent to the use of these products but this situation is likely to ease as development continues in this area.

7. REFERENCES

1. Buzza, G. C. 1995. "Plant breeding," Brassica Oilseeds: Production and Utilization, Kimber, D. and McGregor, D. I., eds. Wallingford, UK: CAB International, pp. 153–175.
2. Stefansson, B. R., F. W. Hougen and R. K. Downey. 1961. "Note on the isolation of rape plants with seed oil free from erucic acid," Canadian J. Plant Sci., 41:218–219.
3. McDonald, B. E. 1995. "Oil properties of importance in human nutrition," Brassica Oilseeds: Production and Utilization, Kimber, D. and McGregor, D. I., eds. Wallingford, UK: CAB International, pp. 291–299.
4. Eskin, N. A. M., B. E. McDonald, R. Przybylski, L. J. Malcolmson, R. Scarth, T. Mag, D. Ward and D. Adolphe. 1996. "Canola oil," Bailey's Industrial Oil and Fat Products, 5th ed., Hui, Y. H., ed. New York, NY: John Wiley & Sons, pp. 1–95.
5. Ackman, R. G. 1983. "Chemical composition of rapeseed oil," High and Low Erucic Acid Rapeseed Oils: Production, Usage, Chemistry, and Toxicological Evaluation, Kramer, J. K. G., Sauer, F. D. and Pigden W. J., eds. New York, NY: Academic Press, pp. 85–129.
6. Uppström, B. 1995. "Seed chemistry," Brassica Oilseeds: Production and Utilization, Kimber, D. and McGregor, D. I., eds. Wallingford, UK: CAB International, pp. 217–242.
7. Kolodziejczyk, P. and P. Fedec. 1995. "Processing flaxseed for human consumption," Flaxseed in Human Nutrition, Cunnane, S. C. and Thompson, L. U., eds. Champaign, IL: AOCS Press, pp. 261–280.
8. Keller, W. A. 1995. "Sources of oilseeds with specific fatty acid profiles," Development and Processing of Vegetable Oils for Human Nutrition, Przybylski, R. and McDonald, B. E., ed. Champaign, IL: AOCS Press, pp. 87–96.
9. Perez-Jimeney, F., A. Espino, F. Lopez-Segura, J. Blanco, V. Ruis-Gutierrez and J. L. Prada. 1995. "Lipoprotein concentrations in normolipidemic males consuming oleic-rich diets from two different sources: olive oil and oleic acid-rich sunflower oil," Am. J. Clin. Nutr., 62:769–775.
10. Del Vecchio, A. J. 1996. "High laurate canola," INFORM, 7:230–242.
11. Haumann, B. F. 1996. "The goal: tastier and 'healthier' fried foods," INFORM, 7:320–334.
12. Miller, J. F., D. C. Zimmerman and B. A. Vick. 1987. "Genetic control of high oleic acid content in sunflower oil," Crop Science, 27:923–926.
13. Dribnenki, J. C. P. and A. G. Green. 1995. "Linola™ '947' low linolenic flax," Canadian J. Plant Sci., 75:201–202.
14. Knutzon, D. S., G. A. Thompson, S. E. Radke, W. B. Johnson, V. C. Knauf and J. C. Kridl. 1992. "Modification of Brassica seed oil by antisense expression of a stearyol-acyl carrier protein desaturase gene," Proc. Natl. Acad. Sci., 89:2624–2628.
15. Anonymous. 1994. "Calgene seeks approval for modified canola," INFORM, 5:716.

16. Voelker, T. A., A. C. Worrell, L. Anderson, J. Bleibaum, C. Fan and D. J. Hawkins. 1992. "Fatty acid biosynthesis redirected to medium chains in transgenic oilseed plants," Science, 257:72–74.
17. Anonymous. 1995. "Transgenic oilseed harvests to begin in May," INFORM, 6:152–157.
18. Carr, R. A. 1995. "Processing the seed and oil," Brassica Oilseeds: Production and Utilization, Kimber, D. and McGregor, D. I., eds. Wallingford, UK: CAB International, pp. 267–290.
19. Sipos, E. F. and B. F. Szuhaj. 1996. "Soybean oil," Bailey's Industrial Oil and Fat Products, 5th ed., Hui, Y. H., ed. New York, NY: John Wiley & Sons, pp. 497–601.
20. Davidson, H. F., E. J. Campbell, R. J. Bell and R. A. Pritchard. 1996. "Sunflower oil," Bailey's Industrial Oil and Fat Products, 5th ed., Hui, Y. H., ed. New York, NY: John Wiley & Sons, pp. 603–689.
21. Erickson, D. R. and L. H. Wiedermann. 1990. "Soybean oil method processing and utilization," Edible Fats and Oils Processing: Basic Principles and Modern Practices, Erickson, D. R., ed. Champaign, IL: American Oil Chemists' Society, pp. 275–283.
22. Veldstra, J. and J. Klère. 1990. "Sunflower seed oil," Edible Fats and Oils Processing: Basic Principles and Modern Practices, Erickson, D. R., ed. Champaign, IL: American Oil Chemists' Society, pp. 284–288.
23. Del Vecchio, A. J. 1997. "Non-edible specific quality and compositional parameters," Joint Symp. of the Am. Oil Chemists' Soc./Instit. Food Technol., Seattle, WA, May 9–10, 1997.
24. Miller, J. E. and N. Frey. 1997. "Evolution of IP oilseed technology," Joint Symp. of the Am. Oil Chemists' Soc./Instit. Food Technol., Seattle, WA, May 9–10, 1997.
25. Zurier, R. B., P. DeLuca and D. Rothman. 1995. "γ-Linolenic, inflammation, immune responses, and rheumatoid arthritis," γ-Linolenic Acid: Metabolism and Its Roles in Nutrition and Medicine, Huang, Y. S. and Mills D. E. ed. Champaign, IL: American Oil Chemists' Society, pp. 129–136.
26. Jamal, G. A. 1994. "The use of gamma linolenic acid in the prevention and treatment of diabetic neuropathy," Diabetic Med., 11:145–149.
27. Keen, H., J. Payan, J. Allawi, J. Walker, G. A. Jamal and A. I. Weir. 1993. "Treatment of diabetic neuropathy with γ-linolenic acid," Diabetes Care, 14:8–15.
28. Ziboh, V. A. 1995. "The biological/nutritional significance of γ-linolenic acid in the epidermis: metabolism and generation of potent biological modulators," γ-Linolenic Acid: Metabolism and Its Roles in Nutrition and Medicine, Huang, Y. S. and Mills D. E. ed. Champaign, IL: American Oil Chemists' Society, pp. 118–128.
29. Wright, S. and J. L. Burton. 1982. "Oral evening primrose oil improves atopic eczema," Nature, ii:1120–1122.
30. de Antueno, R. J., M. Elliot, K. Jenkins, G. W. Ells and D. F. Horrobin. 1995. "Metabolism of Li-γ-linolenate (LiGLA) in human prostate, ovarian, and pancreatic carcinomas grown in nude mice," γ-Linolenic Acid: Metabolism and Its Roles in Nutrition and Medicine, Huang, Y. S. and Mills D. E. ed. Champaign, IL: American Oil Chemists' Society, pp. 293–303.

31. Das, U. N. 1995. "Anti-cancer actions of γ-linolenic acid with particular reference to the human brain malignant glioma," γ-Linolenic Acid: Metabolism and Its Roles in Nutrition and Medicine, Huang, Y. S. and Mills D. E. ed. Champaign, IL: American Oil Chemists' Society, pp. 282–292.
32. Das, U. N., V. V. S. K. Prasad and D. Raia Reddy. 1995. "Local application of gamma-linolenic acid in the treatment of human gliomas," Cancer Lett., 94:147–155.
33. Gunstone, F. D. 1992. "Gamma-linolenic acid—occurrence and physical and chemical properties," Prog. Lip. Res., 31:145–161.
34. Phillips, J. C. and Y. S. Huang. 1995. "Natural sources and biosynthesis of γ-linolenic acid: an overview," γ-Linolenic Acid: Metabolism and Its Roles in Nutrition and Medicine, Huang, Y. S. and Mills, D. E. eds. Champaign, IL: American Oil Chemists' Society, pp. 1–13.
35. Wolf, R. B., R. Kleiman and R. E. England. 1983. "New sources of γ-linolenic acid," J. Am. Oil Chemists' Soc., 60:1858–1860.
36. Barre, D. E. and B. J. Holub. 1992. "The effect of borage oil consumption on the composition of individual phospholipids in human platelets," Lipids, 27:315–320.
37. Gibson, R. A., D. R. Lines and M. A. Neuman. 1992. "Gamma linolenic acid (GLA) content of encapsulated evening primrose oil products," Lipids, 27:82–84.
38. Rahmatullah, M. S. K. S., V. K. S. Shukla and K. D. Mukherjee. 1994. "γ-Linolenic acid concentrates from borage and evening primrose oil fatty acids *via* lipase-catalyzed esterification," J. Am. Oil Chemists' Soc., 71:563–567.
39. Favati, F., J. W. King and M. Mazzanti. 1991. "Supercritical carbon dioxide extraction of evening primrose oil," J. Am. Oil Chemists' Soc., 68:422–427.
40. Wolff, R. L. and J. L. Sebedio. 1994. "Characterization of gamma-linolenic acid geometrical isomers in borage oil subjected to heat treatments (deodorization)," J. Am. Oil Chemists' Soc., 71:117–126.
41. Rahmatullah, M. S. K. S., V. K. S. Shukla and K. D. Mukherjee. 1994. "Enrichment of γ-linolenic acid from evening primrose oil and borage oil *via* lipase-catalyzed hydrolysis," J. Am. Oil Chemists' Soc., 71:569–573.
42. Foglia, T. A. and P. E. Sonnet. 1995. "Fatty acid selectivity of lipases: γ-linolenic acid from borage oil," J. Am. Oil Chemists' Soc., 72:417–420.
43. Keys, A., J. T. Anderson and F. Grande. 1965. "Serum cholesterol response to changes in diet. IV. Particular saturated fatty acids in the diet," Metabolism, 14:776–787.
44. Hegsted., D. M., R. B. McGandy, M. L. Meyers and F. J. Stare. 1965. "Quantitative effects of dietary fat on serum cholesterol in man," Am. J. Clin. Nutr., 57:875–883.
45. Kiley, R. D., C. T. Massie, A. L. Bachman and V. P. Wagher. 1996. "Advances in structured fats: Appetize shortening," Lipid Technology, 8(1):5–10.
46. Hayes, K. C. 1996. "Designing a cholesterol-removed fat blend for frying and baking," Food Technology 50(4):92–97.
47. Bonanome, A. and S. M. Grundy. 1988. "Effect of dietary stearic acid on plasma cholesterol and lipoprotein levels," N. Engl. J. Med., 319:1244–1248.
48. Tholstrup, T., P. Marckmann, J. Jespersen and B. Sandström. 1994. "Fat high in stearic acid favorably affects blood lipids and factor VII coagulant activity in

comparison with fats high in palmitic acid and high in myristic and lauric acids," Am. J. Clin. Nutr., 59:371–377.
49. Hayes, K. C. 1995. "Saturated fats and blood lipids: new slant on an old story," Can. J. Cardiology, 11(Suppl. G):39G–46G.
50. Hassel, C., M. Martini, J. Labat, T. Carr, B. Elhard, A. Olson, S. Bergmann and J. Slavin. 1995. "Cholesterolemic effects of modified animal fats in postmenopausal women," Fed. Am. Soc. Expt. Biol. J., 9:A979 (Abstract).
51. Hastert, R. C. 1990. "Cost/quality/health: the three pillars of hydrogenation," Edible Fats and Oils Processing: Basic Principles and Modern Practices, Erickson, D. R. ed. Champaign, IL: American Oil Chemists' Society, pp. 142–151.
52. Hastert, R. C. and R. F. Ariaansz. 1995. "Hydrogenation: a useful piece in solving the nutrition puzzle," Development and Processing of Vegetable Oils for Human Nutrition, Przybylski, R. and McDonald, B. E. ed. Champaign, IL: AOCS Press, pp. 47–61.
53. Willner, T., W. Sitzmann and E. W. Munch. 1990. "Production of cocoa butter replacers by fractionation of edible oils and fats," Edible Fats and Oils Processing: Basic Principles and Modern Practices, Erickson, D. R. ed. Champaign, IL: American Oil Chemists' Society, pp. 239–245.
54. Hamm, W. 1995. "Trends in edible oil fractionation," Food Sci. Technol., 4:121–126.
55. Marangoni, A. G. and D. Rousseau. 1995. "Engineering triacylglycerols: the role of interesterification," Trends Food Sci. Technol., 6:329–335.
56. Ramamurthi, S. and A. R. McCurdy. 1995. "Interesterification—current status and future prospects," Development and Processing of Vegetable Oils for Human Nutrition, Przybylski, R. and McDonald, B. E. eds. Champaign, IL: AOCS Press, pp. 62–86.
57. Haumann, B. F. 1994. "Tools: hydrogenation, interesterification," INFORM, 5:668–678.
58. Rozendaal, A. 1990. "Interesterification of oils and fats," Edible Fats and Oils Processing: Basic Principles and Modern Practices, Erickson, D. R. ed. Champaign, IL: American Oil Chemists' Society, pp. 152–157.
59. Konishi, H., W. E. Neff and T. L. Mounts. 1993. "Chemical interesterification with regioselectivity for edible oils," J. Am. Oil Chemists' Soc., 70:411–415.
60. Miller, C., H. Austin, L. Posorske and J. Gonzalez. 1988. "Characteristics of an immobilized lipase for the commercial synthesis of esters," J. Am. Oil Chemists' Soc., 68:927–931.
61. Quinlan, P. and S. Moore. 1993. "Modification of triglycerides by lipases: process technology and its application to the production of nutritionally improved fats," INFORM, 4:580–585.
62. Sonnet, P. E. 1995. "Lipase selectivities," J. Am. Oil Chemists' Soc., 65:900–904.
63. Kennedy, J. P. 1991. "Structured lipids: fats of the future," Food Technol., 45(11):76–83.
64. Malcata, F. X., H. R. Reyes, H. S. Garcia, G. H. Hill, Jr. and C. H. Amundson. 1990. "Immobilized lipase reactors for modification of fats and oils—a review," J. Am. Oil Chemists' Soc., 67:890–910.
65. Rucka, M., B. Turklewicz and J. S. Żuk. 1990. "Polymeric membranes for lipase immobilization," J. Am. Oil Chemists' Soc., 67:887–889.

66. Carnielli, V. P., I. H. T. Luijendijk, J. B. van Goudoever, E. J. Sulkers, A. A. Boerlage, H. J. Degenhart and P. J. J. Sauer. 1995. "Feeding premature newborn infants palmitic acid in amounts and stereoisomeric position similar to that of human milk: effects on fat and mineral balance," Am. J. Clin. Nutr., 61:1037–1042.
67. Bell, S. J., D. Bradley and R. A. Forse. 1997. "The new dietary fats in health and disease," J. Am. Diet. Assoc., 97:280–286.

CHAPTER 9

Functional Products of Plants Indigenous to Latin America: Amaranth, Quinoa, Common Beans, and Botanicals

S. H. GUZMÁN-MALDONADO[1]
O. PAREDES-LÓPEZ[1]

1. INTRODUCTION

IN addition to the nutrients that are involved in normal metabolic activity, plant foods contain components that may provide additional health benefits. These food components, generally referred to as phytochemicals and/or health-promoting elements, are present in a number of frequently consumed foods, such as cereals, legumes and fruits. In recent years, the number of food components shown to have potential benefits for human health has grown tremendously. Scientific evidence is accumulating to support the role of phytochemicals and functional foods in the prevention and treatment of diseases.

The Aztecs and Incas credited amaranth and quinoa with medicinal and sometimes magical properties. In recent years, scientific information has accumulated supporting the health benefits of these grains. Common beans have also been credited with numerous health benefits including lowering blood cholesterol, improving glucose tolerance and reducing insulin requirements. Despite these advantages, however, common beans present some undesirable characteristics that limit their acceptability. Various fruits that have traditionally been consumed for their sugars and/or vitamins have become potential functional foods, while herbs have been used since ancient times as alternative medicine.

[1]Depto. de Biotecnología y Bioquímica, Centro de Investigación y de Estudios Avanzados, Unidad Irapuato, Irapuato, GTO, México.

Processing of amaranth, quinoa, beans, and other traditional plants from Latin America into products that deliver nutritive as well as physiologically active nonnutritive components represents a major opportunity for food processors catering to the health-conscious market. This chapter will deal with the nature, distribution, and health-related effects of major and minor components of amaranth, quinoa, common beans, and selected vegetables and botanicals. The processing aspects of some of these crops will also be discussed.

2. PSEUDOCEREALS—AMARANTH AND QUINOA

2.1. COMPONENTS AND THEIR PHYSIOLOGICAL EFFECTS

2.1.1. Lipids, Proteins, and Carbohydrates

One of the attractive features of amaranth seeds (*Amarantus hypochondriacus*) is their protein content which, at 14–18%, is higher than that of most grains including quinoa (*Chenopodium quinoa*) (Table 9.1). It has been reported that the greater part of amaranth grain protein is found in the embryo, a ring surrounding a diploid starchy perisperm [1,2]. This distribution may be responsible for the high protein content [3]. Different studies have indicated that amaranth protein is adequate in lysine (4.8–6.4 g/100 g protein), tryptophan (1.0–4.0 g/100 g protein), and sulphur amino acids (3.7–5.5 g/100 g protein) compared with the FAO/WHO/UNU reference pattern [1,3–6]. In contrast, cereal grains are deficient in lysine, maize is deficient in tryptophan, while rice and wheat proteins are limited in lysine and threonine [1]. Consequently, the essential amino acid balance of amaranth grain protein is significantly better than that of many if not all other proteins of vegetable origin.

One health food niche for amaranth protein has been as a gluten- or prolamin-free protein. Celiac disease is characterized by sensitivity to the prolamin fraction of cereals, particularly hypersensitivity to the alcohol-soluble gliadins from wheat [7]. Total avoidance of gliadin is the lifelong treatment for such patients. Celiac patients may also be sensitive to the prolamin fraction of amaranth. Prolamins are present in amaranth in the range of 0.7–11.0% depending on specific extraction method and variety [5].

Another functional aspect of amaranth proteins is their globulins subunits, 7S and 11S. Protein isolation studies show that amaranth globulins and amarantin, the 11S fraction of globulins, represent 20.5 and 18.6% of the total seed protein, respectively [8–10]. Thus, globulins are composed principally of amarantin. It has been suggested that soy globulins 7S and 11S exert a cholesterol-lowering effect [11,12]. Thus, amaranth varieties with markedly modified protein composition, ranging from extremely high to extremely low

TABLE 9.1. Chemical Composition and Amino Acid Content of Amaranth and Quinoa Seeds.

Component	Amaranth	Quinoa	FAO/WHO/UNU Ref. Pattern	
			Adult	Child
Chemical composition (%, dry basis)				
Crude protein[1]	14.0–18.0	11.0–15.0	NA	NA
Crude fat	6.5–12.5	3.2–10.7	NA	NA
Crude fibre	3.9–17.8	1.1–10.7	NA	NA
Ash	3.2–3.9	2.1–10.7	NA	NA
Starch	56.0–78.0	53.0–85.7	NA	NA
Amino acid (g/100 g protein)				
Essential				
Hystidine	2.4–3.2	2.4–2.7	1.6	1.9
Isoleucine	3.5–4.1	3.6–6.4	1.3	2.8
Leucine	5.0–6.3	5.8–7.1	1.9	6.6
Lysine	4.8–6.4	5.5–6.6	1.6	5.8
Methionine + Cys	3.7–5.5	3.6–4.5	1.7	2.5
Phenylalanine + Tyr	7.1–9.1	6.2–7.4	1.9	6.3
Threonine	3.3–4.6	3.4–4.8	0.9	3.4
Tryptophan	1.0–4.0	0.9–1.1	0.5	1.1
Valine	3.2–4.8	4.0–5.0	1.3	3.5
Nonessential				
Alanine	3.4–3.9	4.0–4.7		
Arginine	6.9–9.2	7.0–8.7		
Aspartic acid	7.9–8.6	7.3–8.5		
Glutamic acid	13.9–17.1	11.9–15.9		
Glycine	6.4–8.6	5.0–6.6		
Proline	3.6–4.6	3.1–3.9		
Serine	4.2–8.7	3.7–5.9		

[1]Protein conversion factors (factor × %N) were: amaranth, 5.85; quinoa, 5.96; NA = not applicable.
Source: Data from References [4, 5].

7S: 11S ratio, may have an improved economic value. Such varieties would not only display improved nutritional qualities but also modify the potential medicinal effects of amaranth.

The lipid content of amaranth seeds is relatively high (6.5–12.5%) compared with maize (4.5%) or wheat (2.1) [4,13]. Amaranth oil contains a high degree of unsaturation with about 53–95% linoleic and oleic, 0.3–1.3% linolenic, and 2.2–5.4% stearic acid based on total oil [4]. It is well established that essential fatty acid deficiency results in lymphoid atrophy and depressed antibody responses. Small amounts of linoleic acid are required for the normal propagation and maturation of cell-mediated immune responses.

Furthermore, oil enriched in γ-linolenic acid (GLA) has been shown to suppress inflammation and joint tissue injury in a limited number of placebo-controlled studies [14]. Moreover, it has been suggested that GLA could effectively replace the nonsteroidal anti-inflammatory drugs [15,16].

Crude fibre values of amaranth range from 3.9–17.8% [17]. Starch is the major component of amaranth grain, constituting 56–78% of the total dry weight [4,5,18]. The recent consensus on healthy eating habits favors an increase in the proportion of polymeric plant carbohydrates in the daily diet, with a proportionately reduced intake of "refined" sugars [19]. However, in the western world the main purpose of starch inclusion in foods remains aesthetic rather than nutritional. Nevertheless, it is well known that starches have other uses, including serving as fat substitutes, which add organoleptic and textural characteristics to food, but at a lower energy density than fat [20]. Guzmán-Maldonado and Paredes-López [21] established the conditions to produce maltodextrins to be used as fat substitutes from amaranth grain.

The total protein content in quinoa seeds (11.0–15.0%) is higher than that of rice (8.5%) and maize (10.3%), and very close to that of barley (11.9%) and wheat (12.3) [5,22]. Furthermore, quinoa protein contains high levels of lysine (5.5–6.6 g/100 g protein) and sulphur amino acids (3.6–4.5 g/100 g protein) and adequate levels of tryptophan (0.9–1.1 g/100 g protein), compared with the FAO/WHO/UNU reference pattern (Table 9.1) [4,6,23].

Recently, an effort has been made to isolate and characterize one of the major seed-storage proteins of quinoa [24]. As a result, an 11S-type seed storage protein called "chenopodin" has been identified. Under optimal extraction conditions, the yield of chenopodin averages approximately 60% of total protein. Since only four amino acids (leucine, isoleucine, and phenylalanine plus tyrosine) exceed the FAO standards, other proteins may contribute to the reported high nutritional protein quality of quinoa seed. Recently, a high-cysteine 2S seed-storage protein was also isolated from this seed [25].

The fatty acids of quinoa oils are dominated by linoleic and oleic acids (68–84 g/100 g oil); interestingly, this oil also contains 7.0–9.5 g of linolenic acid/100 g oil, which suggests that quinoa seeds have nutraceutical applications in the treatment of immune response, suppressing inflammation and joint tissue injury, and as substitutes for anti-inflammatory drugs used to treat rheumatoid arthritis patients [14–16].

2.1.2. Vitamins and Minerals

The vitamins and minerals in the grain of amaranth and quinoa species are listed in Table 9.2. Niacin and thiamin contents are lower than those found in cereal grains. Riboflavin and ascorbic acid levels in amaranth and quinoa exceed the levels in cereals [26,27]. For example, a 100 g portion of amaranth

TABLE 9.2. Vitamin and Mineral Content of Amaranth and Quinoa Seeds.

			FAO/WHO/UNU	
Component	Amaranth	Quinoa	Adult	Child
Vitamins (mg/100 g)				
Ascorbic acid	3.0–7.1	3.0–4.9	60	30–35
α-Tocopherol	1.57	2.0–5.4	9	3–4
Biotin	43–51	NA	0.3–1.0	NA
Folic acid	42–44	NA	0.18–0.20	0.03
Niacin	1.0–1.5	1.5	15–19	5–6
Retinol	NA	15	0.8–1.0	0.38
Riboflavin	0.19–0.32	0.39	1.3–1.7	0.4–0.5
Thiamin	0.10–0.14	0.31	1.1–1.5	0.3–0.4
Minerals (mg/g)				
Calcium	217–800	127–150		1000–1200
Copper	1–4	3.7		1.5–3.0 (μg)
Iron	21–104	12		12–15
Magnesium	319–344	270		280–400
Manganese	3–5	7.5		
Phosphorus	556–600	387		1200
Potassium	525–563	697		
Zinc	3–4	4.8		12–15

NA = not available.
Source: Data from References [26–28].

seed will provide about 12% of the ascorbic acid (vitamin C) requirements for optimal health for an adult and 22% of the vitamin C requirements for a child, whereas quinoa may contribute 8% of the recommended daily intake for adults and 15% of the RDI for children (Table 9.2) [28]. Vitamin C acts as an antioxidant and has at least two protective functions: (1) to regenerate some enzymes by reducing oxidized prosthetic groups, and (2) to scavenge oxidizers and free radicals [2,28]. Free radicals cause extensive damage to biological systems, and are suspected in the pathology of more than 70 medical conditions including atherosclerosis, cancer, diabetes, and cataracts [29,30,31].

It is interesting to note that 100 g of amaranth may contribute, on average, 17% of the recommended daily intake of α-tocopherol (vitamin E) for an adult, and may satisfy 45% of total requirements for a child. Some quinoa varieties provide as much as 60% of the daily intake of α-tocopherol for an adult and 154% for a child. Vitamin E is a highly effective antioxidant that readily donates the hydrogen atom from the hydroxyl group on the ring structure to free radicals, effectively neutralizing them. It also has a sparing effect on other antioxidant nutrients, such as vitamins C and A. Although α-tocopherol has the highest biological activity, some of the tocotrienols have been shown to be particularly effective antioxidants *in vitro* [28]. Amaranth seeds are also a good source of β-tocotrienol (0.59–1.15 mg/100 g) and γ-tocotrienol (0.10–0.87 mg/100 g) [32]. Tocotrienols have also been found to have cholesterol-lowering properties; moreover, a recent patent claims that amaranth contains new and potent cholesterol inhibitors, desmethyl-tocotrienol and didesmethyl-tocotrienol, in addition to the 8 vitamin E isomers [33].

An outstanding characteristic of amaranth seed is its biotin and folic acid content. The biotin content ranges from 43 to 51 mg/100 g seed whereas folic acid ranges from 42 to 44 mg/100 g seed; thus, amaranth can easily supply the current recommended levels for both biotin and folic acid. Biotin deficiency, caused by a diet rich in raw egg white, causes nausea, desquamation and anorexia with increased cholesterol and decreased hemoglobin in the blood [28]. A biotin deficiency may be corrected in a pediatric patient with administration of biotin at levels of 10 mg/day, which can be achieved with approximately 25 g of amaranth [34]. Biotin and folic acid have not been found to be toxic at megadose levels [28].

A 100 g portion of amaranth and quinoa may contribute as much as 71% and 87%, respectively, of the recommended daily intake of riboflavin for a child (Table 9.2). Additionally, when amaranth grain is run through a pearler, seed coat embryo and a perisperm flour fractions can be obtained [1,35]. The riboflavin content of the seed coat embryo flour reaches 0.43 mg/100 g, which may satisfy 100% of recommended daily allowances for infants and approximately 31% of RDIs for an adult. Moreover, the thiamin content in the coat embryo flour may reach 2.88 mg/100 g, fully satisfying the daily requirements of thiamin for humans (Table 9.2) [28,36].

The two most important minerals for human health are calcium and iron [37]. One gram of amaranth and quinoa seeds may contribute 46% and 13%, respectively, of the recommended daily intake of calcium. Both grains can fully satisfy the recommended dietary intake of iron (Table 9.2). This is particularly important in countries where vegetables are the main source of calcium and iron.

Dietary calcium deficiencies have been linked epidemiologically to several chronic diseases, including osteoporosis, hypertension, and colon cancer [38–40]. Iron deficiency is characterized by reduced red blood cell function and depressed function of numerous other cellular activities because of inadequate oxygen delivery [37]. However, several epidemiologic lines of evidence suggest that high intakes of iron by males and postmenopausal women may contribute to coronary heart disease.

2.1.3. Nutritional Characteristics of Proteins

Indexes used to evaluate protein quality include protein efficiency ratio (PER), net protein ratio (NPR), net protein utilization (NPU), true protein digestibility, and protein biological value [37]. Nutritional values of amaranth and quinoa seed meals are shown in Table 9.3. The PER, NPR and NPU values for raw amaranth are remarkably high compared to casein, whereas protein digestibility values are somewhat similar to those of casein. The biological value of raw amaranth comes closer than any other grain protein to the perfect balance of essential amino acids relative to maize (44), wheat (60), soybean (68) and cows' milk (72) [3,41].

When amaranth seeds are processed, the nutritional characteristics of the proteins increase. Thus, the NPR of raw amaranth may increase from 1.74–2.35 to 2.2–3.6 depending on processing treatment (Table 9.3). Specifically, wet cooking increases the NPR of amaranth to 3.4–3.6, a value similar to that of casein. Roasted amaranth shows true protein digestibility and protein biological values of 89.9% and 85.5%, respectively; these values are close to those of casein [42].

TABLE 9.3. Effect of Different Processes on Nutritional Characteristics of Amaranth and Quinoa Proteins.

Characteristic/Process	Amaranth	Quinoa	Casein
Protein efficiency ratio (PER)[1]			
Raw	1.6–2.5	1.95–2.33	2.5
Cooked		2.5	
Net protein ratio (NPR)			
Raw	1.74–2.35	2.91	3.65
Drum-dried	2.6		
Extruded	3.3–3.6		
Flaked	2.7–2.8		
Popped	3.2		
Roasted	2.2		
Wet cooked	3.4–3.6		
Net protein utilization (NPU) (%)			
Raw	73.8	75.7	94.7–96.0
Flaked	78.4		
Popped	76.0		
Roasted	76.8		
True protein digestibility (%)			
Raw	88.5	91.7–92.1	92.0
Flaked	89.5		
Popped	85.6		
Roasted	89.9		
Protein biological value (%)			
Raw	73.0	82.6	95.0–97.1
Flaked	87.6		
Popped	86.0		
Roasted	85.5		

[1]Adjusted.
Source: Data from References [4, 42].

PER values of raw quinoa seeds range from 1.95 to 2.33. When quinoa is cooked, the PER value reaches 100%, equivalent to that of casein [43]. Protein digestibility is remarkably high (91.7–92.1%), while net protein utilization and protein biological value appear to be moderate to high (75.7% and 82.6%, respectively). An insufficient number of studies have focused on relating the effect of processing of quinoa seeds to protein quality.

Processed amaranth and quinoa seeds can be used to provide humans with a more nutritionally balanced diet with a potential positive influence on optimal health. Some studies have investigated the protein quality of processed amaranth and its health effects in children and adults. For example, Morales et al. [42] tested toasted, popped, and flaked products from amaranth in convalescent, malnourished infants and young children. Their results indicated that apparent nitrogen retention from amaranth was superior to that from most cereals studied at isonitrogenous levels and was similar to that from rice or high-lysine maize.

2.1.4. Minor Components

Many studies suggest a variety of constituents of amaranth and quinoa that may possess positive or negative nutritional/health effects [43,44]. A summary of the best known minor components of amaranth and quinoa is presented in Table 9.4. The phytic acid values in amaranth (0.34–0.61%) are higher than those found in rice (0.10–0.14%), but lower than those reported for maize and wheat [26,44]; moreover, the concentration of polyphenols in amaranth (2.0 to 4.0 mg/g) is also higher than the levels of polyphenols found in soy (0.1–3.0 mg/g) [45].

Recently, four amaranth saponins were found in *A. hypochondriacus* [46]. However, to date, no studies have linked the saponins to the moist-heat, thermolabile antinutrients present in some amaranths [47]. Trypsin inhibitors (TI) are present at concentrations of 300 to 5,150 TI units/g; and chymotrypsin inhibitors are present at levels of 3,000 to 4,000 units/g. Quinoa seeds contain relatively low amounts of polyphenols and trypsin inhibitors (Table 9.4). Further, quinoa contains high levels of saponins including the aglycones, oleanolic acid and hederagenin [23,48,49].

There have been some efforts to determine the pharmaceutical effects of the minor components on different diseases. For example, phenolic compounds, especially flavonoids, have been reported to exhibit a wide range of biological effects, including anti-inflammatory, antibacterial, antiviral, antiallergenic, and vasodilatory actions [50,51]. In addition, flavonoids inhibit lipid peroxidation, platelet aggregation and the activity of enzymes such as lipoxygenase [52,53]. Polyphenols, which are widely distributed in the plant kingdom, occur at relatively high concentrations in legumes and in amaranth (Table 9.4).

TABLE 9.4. Minor Components of Amaranth and Quinoa.

Component	Amaranth	Quinoa
Chymotrysin inhibitors (U/g)	3000–4000	NA
Nitrates (mg/100 g)	29–62	NA
Oxalic acid (mg/100 g)	0–16	NA
Phytic acid (%)	0.34–0.61	NA
Polyphenols (mg/g)	2.0–4.0	0.2
Saponins (g/100 g)	NA	0.14–0.76
Trypsin inhibitors (TIU/g)	300–5150	1.36–5.04
Amaranthin (mg/g)	1.6–1.7	—
Amaranthine	Traces	—
Dietary fibre (g/100 g)	7.11–17.5	13.3–13.4

NA = not available.

Saponins can be partially removed by washing quinoa seeds vigorously in cold, running water, followed by drying overnight at 60°C [4,22,27,49]. Using this approach, saponin levels can be reduced to 0.67 g/100 g seeds [27]. Saponins are generally regarded as antinutrients; however, recent studies have indicated that some saponins have hypocholesterolemic, immunostimulatory and anticarcinogenic properties [54]. The proposed mechanisms for the anticarcinogenicity of saponins include an antioxidant effect, cytotoxicity to cancer cells, immune modulation, and regulation of cell proliferation [54]. The high levels of saponins found in some quinoa varieties make them an excellent source from which to extract saponins, which can be purified and used for medical purposes.

The fact that amaranth contains high levels of trypsin and chymotrypsin inhibitors indicates that there may be a need to further investigate this plant for medical applications. The Bowman-Birk trypsin- and chymotrypsin-inhibitor (BBI) has been under criticism, since studies have indicated that ingestion of raw soybean meal or soybean trypsin inhibitors can cause enlargement of the pancreas in mice and young guinea pigs but not in adult guinea pigs, dogs, calves or monkeys. Presumably there is no effect in humans, however [55]. Reports of the involvement of BBI in suppression or prevention of carcinogenesis in mice *in vivo* triggered a series of experiments leading to the cloning and expression of BBI in *E. coli* and yeast. Purified BBI was subsequently shown to significantly counteract nephrotoxicity induced by the antibiotic drug gentamicin [55].

Other minor components of amaranth that have known physiological effects are the lectins. These compounds have been isolated from different amaranth species [56–61], and the lectin amaranth isolated from *A. cruentus* has been extensively studied [57,61]; in amaranth, the concentration of amaranthin ranges from 1.6 to 1.7 mg/g (Table 9.4). Amaranthin also binds to the Thomsen-Friedenreich antigen (T-antigen), which has been proposed as a specific carcinoma marker [62–64]. Amaranthin has been used as a histochemical probe for proliferating cells in sections of human colonic tissues. Binding inhibitor studies showed that amaranthin binds to different sites on histological sections when compared to peanut agglutinin, which also recognizes the T-antigen. Amaranthin binds selectively to the cells at the base of the colonic crypt, which is the zone of proliferation in this tissue. A marked increase in histochemical labelling by amaranthin was seen in adenomatous polyps and denocarcinomas of the colon [63]. Experimental data suggest that amaranthin may be useful for identifying abnormal proliferation in colorectal cancer syndromes, and histochemical evidence indicates that amaranthin is a more specific anti-T reagent than peanut lectin [63,64].

The amaranth pigment betacyanin amaranthine has also been extracted from the leaves of amaranth [65,66]. Amaranthine is comparable in most respects to betanine, which is responsible for the red color of beets, and has been commercialized as a natural food color [67]. The pigment was designated amaranthine rather than amaranthin presumably to avoid confusion with the lectin amaranthin [60,61]. Amaranthine, if properly extracted, could be used as a natural coloring agent in food and other applications. Paredes-López and co-workers found that with germination, amaranth seeds synthesize a red pigment that may be related to amaranthine [68,69]. Further studies on this topic are pending.

An outstanding bioactive component of amaranth is its high dietary fibre content, ranging from 7.1 to 17.5% of the seed, depending on variety (Table 9.4). The crude fibre of amaranth is composed primarily of lignin and cellulose [17]. However, dietary fibre includes lignin and cellulose, as well as hemicellulose, pectic substances, gums, and certain other carbohydrates. There have been some discrepancies related to crude fibre contents in amaranth because of inadequacies of analytical methods for its determination [70–72]. It is necessary to develop a reliable method to obtain total dietary fibre (TDF) values for these high-crude fibre species. Dietary fibre can be separated into insoluble (IDF) and soluble (SDF) fractions; IDF includes cellulose, some hemicellulose, and lignin whereas SDF includes gums, pectins, and other hemicelluloses. The TDF fraction of *A. hypochondriacus* consisted of 75% IDF and 25% SDF, while that of *A. cruentus* was higher in insoluble fibre and, consequently, lower in soluble fibre (86% IDF and 14% SDF) [71].

The physiological effects of amaranth dietary fibre on rats have been studied [73]. Amaranth diets resulted in lower serum cholesterol values than those of fibre-free controls and lower liver cholesterol values than those of cellulose, a poorly fermented fibre. The hypocholesterolemic effect of amaranth seeds was also evaluated in male Wistar strain albino rats [74]. Liver weights were significantly higher in animals fed a hypercholesterolemia-induced diet than in rats fed with amaranth. The authors suggested that amaranth behaved like soluble fibres to lower serum cholesterol, but had an effect similar to that of insoluble fibre in its action in the colon. Since the cholesterol-lowering properties of oat bran and pectin are assumed to be due to the SDF fraction, and since amaranth in general is low in SDF, it appears that the hypocholesterolemic effects associated with amaranth are attributable to components other than those comprising SDF.

The relationship between dietary fibre and cancer has received widespread attention in recent years and several approaches have been used to address this relationship. Conflicting results regarding the association between cereal consumption and several types of cancer have been reported, although the majority have demonstrated a protective effect of fibre [41,75]. The possible action of fibre may be to reduce transit time in the bowel, thereby reducing the time the bowel is in contact with potential carcinogens. Other effects may include an alteration of the intestinal microflora, the binding of potentially carcinogenic agents, dilution of toxic compounds due to its hydrophilicity, and/or changing the biological behaviour of intestinal cells, including their response to gut hormones [41]. Dietary fibre has also been claimed to be useful in the control of obesity [20].

The total dietary fibre content (13.3–13.4%) of whole quinoa seeds is slightly lower than values reported for whole-grain wheat flour (14%) and whole-grain rye flour (17%) [76]. The IDF of quinoa accounts for 10 to 11% of seed, the SDF 2.4–3.3%. Cooked samples show significantly less total dietary fibre content (11.0%), while the SDF fraction is significantly less both in cooked (0.9%) and in autoclaved (1.0%) samples than in raw samples. Some soluble fibre from the cooked samples is obviously lost during cooking, while loss of soluble fibre during autoclaving may be due to depolymerization of fibre [77]. Quinoa seed is listed among the best natural sources of fibre [78].

2.2. PROCESSING ASPECTS

2.2.1. Enzymatic Hydrolysis

The use of amylolytic enzymes to produce a high-protein amaranth flour (HPAF) has been proposed. The enzymatic conditions for the hydrolysis of amaranth flour to HPAF and a carbohydrate-rich fraction (CRF) has been optimized (Figure 9.1) [21,79,80]. The CRF must be clarified to remove a major part of the color [81,82]. The protein content of amaranth increased from 15.6% (raw flour) to 40% (HPAF) following enzymatic hydrolysis. Moreover, fat and fibre contents were enhanced from 7.3% and 5.2% to 13.1% and 10.7%, respectively. *In vitro* protein digestibility and reactive lysine were

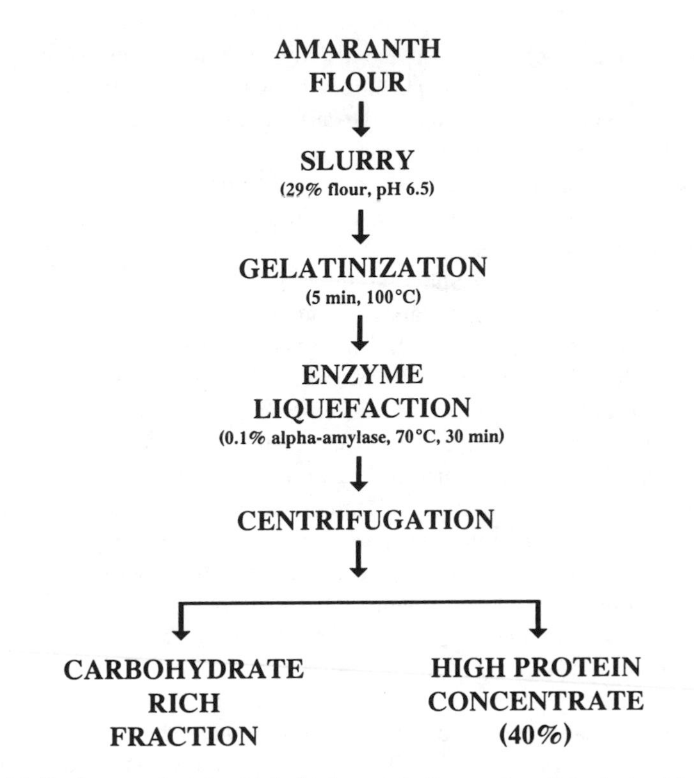

Figure 9.1 Basic procedure to obtain high-protein flour and carbohydrate-rich fraction from amaranth seeds. (Adapted from Reference [80].)

comparable to values for the raw seed. HPAF's protein qualities have not been evaluated in detail. Nevertheless, studies have evaluated the nutritional characteristics of high-protein amaranth concentrates. Sánchez-Marroquín et al. [83] and Del Valle and co-workers [84,85] tested two formulations incorporating amaranth proteins in nitrogen balance studies with children. These formulations were comparable to one containing both soybean flour and oats. No significant differences between the three formulations in nitrogen absorption or nitrogen retention were found. Moreover, Morales et al. [42] indicated that in isoenergetic amounts, the higher protein content of the amaranth should make it a superior source of dietary protein, compared to rice and high-lysine maize. The high protein content of amaranth and its products has led to their marketing as bodybuilding foods, as a vegetarian option, as dry milk extenders and as part of feeding programs for children [80,86,87].

Oligosaccharides of various types are found as natural components of many common foods including fruits, vegetables, milk, and honey. During the past decade, the popularity of oligosaccharides as food ingredients has grown rapidly, due largely to the possible health benefits associated with their consumption [88]. Oligosaccharide ingestion increases the numbers of indigenous bifidobacteria in the colon that antagonistically suppress the activity of putrefactive bacteria and reduce the formation of toxic fermentation products [88,89]. Bifidin, an antibiotic produced by *Bifidobacterium bifidum,* is effective against *Shigella dysenteriae, Salmonella typhosa, Staphylococcus aureus, E. coli,* and other bacteria [89,90]. Other benefits of oligosaccharide ingestion include reduction of levels of toxic metabolites and prevention of liver malfunction by the elimination of such toxic compounds. Oligosaccharides are also useful in the prevention of constipation and the reduction of serum cholesterol and blood pressure. In addition, they may have anti-cancer compounds [88,89,91,92]. It is important to note that these effects may be obtained through ingestion of 2–3 g/day of oligosaccharides [89,93]. The fear of flatulence seems to be unwarranted since it has been shown that daily ingestion of 100 ml of a carbonated soft drink containing 3 g of soybean oligosaccharides for 2 weeks caused neither increased flatulence nor diarrhea [92].

After sucrose, raffinose is the principal oligosaccharide in most amaranth species studied; stachyose is the other major oligosaccharide in amaranth [94]. The levels of raffinose and stachyose present in amaranth are low (1.65% and 0.15%, respectively) [37,95]. These oligosaccharides may be present in the carbohydrate-rich fraction obtained from enzymatic hydrolysis of amaranth flour (Figure 9.1), because in raffinose and stachyose, one or two molecules of galactose are bound to the glucose residue of sucrose by $\alpha(1-6)$ linkage and would not be cleaved by α-amylase, which hydrolyses only $\alpha(1-4)$ bonds [21,90]. Oligosaccharides present in the carbohydrate-rich fraction may be important in the prevention of the health problems cited above. Furthermore, the high carbohydrate content of CRF makes it useful as an ingredient in high-calorie drinks for athletes.

2.2.2. Germination

It has long been claimed that germination generally enhances the nutritive value of cereals and legumes [96–98]. Germination does not require a sophisticated infrastructure; the time for the treatment is short, and yields are fairly high [68]. The development of this kind of process for generating new products with desirable nutritional and functional properties could lead to increased production and consumption of crops such as amaranth.

The process of germination of amaranth for the purpose of producing value-added products was studied by Paredes-López et al. [68,69]. The optimal conditions for germination of amaranth seeds were surface sterilization by soaking for 2 h in distilled water containing 0.1% sodium hypochlorite at room temperature. After rinsing well with distilled water for 10 min, the seeds were evenly spread on pieces of dampened cloth placed in shallow plastic trays; the trays were incubated at 37°C and 90% relative humidity for 48 h in a germination chamber. The samples were then dried for 12 h in a forced-air oven 40°C. Finally, the dried seeds were milled and chemically analysed.

As a result of germination, protein and crude fibre increased, while fat content decreased from 8.0 to 4.5% (Table 9.5). Reactive lysine, net protein ratio value, and *in vitro* protein digestibility remained essentially unchanged after 48 h germination. Although prolamin content was reduced from 4.3% to 2.4%, riboflavin and ascorbic acid (vitamin C) levels increased significantly.

The reduction in prolamin content may be important from a nutraceutical viewpoint, especially for celiac-sprue sufferers who may be sensitive to the prolamin fraction of amaranth [2].

Increases in the levels of riboflavin and ascorbic acid in germinated amaranth increases the nutritional properties of amaranth. For example, a 100 g portion of germinated amaranth contributes 118% of recommended dietary allowance (RDA) of riboflavin for infants, 53% of the RDA for children age 11, and 35% of the RDA for adults. In addition, such a serving provides 38% of recommended daily allowance of vitamin C for infants and 20% of the RDA for adults (see Tables 9.2 and 9.5) [28,99]. Riboflavin deficiency symptoms include dermatitis around the nose, fatigued and sensitive eyes, and bloodshot and vascularized eyes. Symptoms of ascorbic acid deficiency are irritability, retardation of growth, anaemia and susceptibility to infections [28]. Riboflavin and ascorbic acid may also modify cancer development by inhibiting formation of carcinogens such as nitrosamines and altering the formation of endogenously formed mutagens or anticarcinogens [14,41].

2.3. PROSPECTIVES

The health benefits of amaranth and quinoa, including the prevention and treatment of diseases, have been known for a long time [48,78]. In this vein, Lehemann [78] advanced a ring hypothesis for grain amaranth and quinoa in which vitamin E, oil components, minerals, and high-quality protein are released from the ring embryo upon popping.

Bioavailability studies are needed on the effect of processing on the release of calcium and the physiological effects of dietary amaranth and quinoa consumption on humans. The hypocholesterolemic effects of amaranth might enhance its marketability; however, further studies to elucidate the nature and properties of the active ingredients are required. Pharmacological information on phytochemicals such as vitamin E isomers, saponins and squalene is limited, while more familiar agents such as dietary fibre or soluble fibre components might be more readily advanced as bioactives associated with amaranth and quinoa.

Food and pharmaceutical companies often express concern about how amaranth, quinoa, and their products will be treated by regulatory agencies

TABLE 9.5. Effect of Germination on the Proximate Composition and Nutritive Value of Amaranth.

Germination Time (h)	Chemical Composition (%, dry basis)				Reactive Lysine (g/100 g protein)	NPR	*In vitro* Protein Digestibility	Prolamins (%)	Vitamins (mg/100 g)	
	Protein[1]	Fat	Crude Fibre	Ash					Riboflavin	Ascorbic Acid
0	15.5	8.0	3.9	3.4	5.8	2.2	80.6	4.3	0.19	7.05
12	17.4	7.1	3.9	3.4	5.5	—	78.0	—	—	—
24	21.0	5.3	4.2	—	5.6	2.3	77.0	—	0.25	9.68
48	21.0	4.5	4.6	3.2	5.7	2.1	79.2	2.4	0.53	12.05

[1] $N \times 5.85$
NPR = net protein ratio.
Source: Data from References [68, 69].

such as the FDA. According to the Amaranth Institute, amaranth is a traditional food with a long history of use; therefore, amaranth products such as starch, oil, and squalene should be subjected to purity and diagnostic tests similar to those imposed on traditional foods [2].

For the food scientist, amaranth and quinoa remain premium-priced grains. Although they can be milled, pearled, and extruded into conventional cereal products, their unique seed structure suggests potential for novel and innovative processes and products for their oil and protein-laden embryo. These products will be of great interest as sources of moderate amounts (not megadoses) of dietary nutrients. Great promise lies in using amaranth and quinoa products to prevent or delay the development of diseases such as diabetes, arthritis, cancer, and atherosclerosis. However, consumption of these grains may not afford individuals relief from symptoms of pre-existing conditions.

3. COMMON BEANS

3.1. PROTEINS AND AMINO ACIDS

Archaeological, historical, linguistic, and botanical evidence all suggest that the common bean (*Phaseolus vulgaris*) originated on the American continent [100]. Common bean is one of the most important sources of protein, calories, B-complex vitamins, and minerals in Latin America [101]. Although the protein content of common commercial bean cultivars is relatively constant, values ranging from 16 to 33% have been reported for many diverse bean lines [102–105]. Common bean proteins are of poor nutritional value unless subjected to heat treatment. Table 9.6 shows the protein efficiency ratio (PER), biological value, and true protein digestibility of cooked common beans. PER values generally ranges from 0.9 to 1.7, while true protein digestibility values range from 72 to 92% depending on bean variety [101].

Legume protein intake has been associated with a variety of diseases. Soy protein administration reduced LDL cholesterol level in humans and rabbits [105]. In addition, when elite gymnasts were fed diets with and without soy protein supplementation, the metabolic-hormonal profile was lower [106]. Common beans are reportedly effective in lowering blood cholesterol levels [107,108]. The hypocholesterolemic effect of common bean has been related to its fibre content. The mechanism may be similar to that suggested for dietary fibre and protein of soy, which are believed to lower cholesterol through a synergistic relationship between these two components [109,110]. Several studies have suggested that excessive intake of animal protein can be calciuretic and that high protein intakes may be responsible for the high fracture rates in western nations [110]. Common bean and soybean proteins are excellent options for substituting or lowering the intake of animal proteins, and thereby perhaps reducing the risk of fractures.

TABLE 9.6. Components of Common Beans with Claimed Biological Effects.

Component	Content	Biological Effects
Protein content[1] (%, dry basis)	16–33	Building, maintaining, and repairing body tissues
Nutritional characteristics of cooked beans		
PER[2]	0.9–1.7	
Biological value (%)	77–92	
True protein digestibility (%)	77–92	
Methionine + cysteine (g/100 g protein)	2.24–2.53	
Lysine (g/100 g protein)	8.7	Carnitine synthesis
Dietary fibre (%, dry basis)	14–19	Lowering blood cholesterol, improving glucose tolerance, reducing insulin requirements
Raw bean		
Insoluble fibre	0.1–13.1	
Soluble fibre	3.3–7.6	
Cooked bean		
Insoluble fibre	13.4–22.9	
Soluble fibre	3.1–7.0	
Fatty acids (g/100 g free lipids)		Immunostimulant, substitute for rheumatoid drugs
Linoleic	21–28	
Linolenic	37–54	
Vitamins (mg/100 g)		
Folic acid	0.17–0.59	Megaloblastic anemia
Niacin	1.16–2.68	
Riboflavin	0.14–0.27	
Thiamin	0.9–1.2	Cardiovascular complications
Oligosaccharides (g/100 g)		Reduction of serum cholesterol levels and blood pressure, anticancer
Raffinose	0.19–0.22	
Stachyose	1.84–2.45	
Phytic acid (mg/g)	22–28	
Tannins (mg cat. eq./mg)	9.6–131.4	Lowering cancer risk
Trypsin inhibitors (TIU/g)	13–29	Anticarcinogenic

[1]$N \times 6.25$.
[2]PER, protein efficiency ratio.

The protein of the common bean is generally characterized by its deficiency in the sulphur amino acids and tryptophan. Studies have concentrated on these amino acids, especially methionine and cysteine, since they are the specific limiting essential amino acids [101]. The low availability of cysteine in colored cooked bean has been partially related to its high content of polyphenols; these compounds, especially during heat treatments, can react with the protein rendering the cysteine biologically unavailable [111].

Since lysine is the principal essential amino acid deficient in most plant proteins, the importance of legumes such as common bean in human nutrition may be grossly underestimated [112]. Although cereals supply nearly 50% of the protein in the human diet worldwide, their unfavorable balance of amino acids requires a complementary protein for optimal nutrition [113]. One of the most important beneficial characteristics of protein from common bean may be its outstanding level of lysine. Thus, levels of lysine in common bean satisfy more than 500% of the current allowances for an adult and 150% of the allowances for children compared with the FAO/WHO/UNU reference pattern (see Tables 9.1 and 9.6) [6,114,115]. Moreover, lysine is an important factor in certain disease conditions. For example, when liver function is impaired, the synthesis of carnitine may also be impaired. Carnitine is synthesized in the liver from lysine and methionine [116]. All the long-chain fatty acids supplied in the diet must be transported to the mitocondria via the carnitine pathway before they can be oxidized to produce energy.

3.2. DIETARY FIBRE

Dietary fibre is another outstanding component of common bean. Numerous health benefits have been associated with the consumption of adequate amounts of fibre, including lower blood cholesterol levels, reduced risk of heart disease, increased fecal bulk, decreased intestinal transit time, reduced risk of colon cancer, and improved glucose tolerance, which is especially beneficial for individuals with diabetes [20,40,73–75,117–120]. Attention has been focused on common bean dietary fibre because of its effectiveness in lowering blood cholesterol, improving glucose tolerance, and reducing insulin requirements in diabetes patients [121–125]. The dietary fibre content of the common bean ranges from 14 to 19% in raw seeds [126,127]. Cooking slightly decreases the levels of soluble dietary and markedly increases the insoluble dietary fibre content (Table 9.6) [125].

3.3. FATTY ACIDS

Common beans contain from 1.0 to 3.0% lipids depending on variety [128,129]. Neutral lipids are the predominant class of lipids, consisting primarily of triglycerides, along with smaller portions of free fatty acids, sterols and sterol esters. Bean lipids contain substantial amounts of unsaturated fatty acids with a very high content of linoleic and linolenic acids (Table 9.6) [128–130]. These polyunsaturated fatty acids cannot be synthesized by animals or humans and are required for normal growth, cell structure, functions of all tissues, and prostaglandin synthesis [129]. They must be consumed in the diet. The hypocholesterolemic effect of common beans in rats has been attributed in part to the high levels of polyunsaturated fatty acids such as linoleic and linolenic [131]. These acids may also serve as substitutes for nonsteroidal anti-inflammatory drugs for the treatment of rheumatoid arthritis, and may also have immunostimulatory properties [14–16].

3.4. VITAMINS

Raw common beans are a relatively good source of water-soluble vitamins, especially thiamine (0.9–1.2 mg/100 g), riboflavin (0.14–0.27 mg/100 g), niacin (1.16–2.68 mg/100 g), and folic acid (0.17–0.59 mg/100 g). Nutrient retention values during cooking vary from 70.9 to 75.9% depending on the vitamin [101,132]. Folic acid has been suggested to be a potential nutraceutical. The common bean is an excellent source of folic acid; for example, a 100 g portion of common bean can satisfy the daily requirement for folic acid for both adults and children (see Tables 9.2 and 9.6). Deficiencies of B-complex vitamins lead to megaloblastic anaemia in which the proper maturation of red blood cells is impaired, resulting in fewer red blood cells and release of the large nucleated precursor cells. Folic acid deficiency during pregnancy may lead to neural tube defects, and severe deficiency causes megablastic anemia [28].

Common bean can contribute substantial amounts of thiamine to a diet, since a 100 g portion contains close to the recommended dietary allowance for adults and fully satisfies the daily intake for children. Thiamin deficiency symptoms include fatigue, irritability, weight loss, gastrointestinal disturbances, and cardiovascular complications [28].

3.5. OTHER COMPONENTS

Other components of common beans include oligosaccharides, tannins, trypsin inhibitors, and phytic acid (Table 9.6) [133–136]. The nutritional quality of beans can be improved by soaking, cooking, germination or irradiation [134,137]. The effects of such treatments vary with cultivar and treatment. In general, all treatments reduce the levels of oligosaccharides and so-called antinutritional factors in beans [138,139]. Nevertheless, flatulent activity associated with common bean consumption is often considered one of the factors that limit their consumption, especially in the developed Western nations.

Despite the negative aspects associated with the oligosaccharides raffinose and stachyose in common bean, these compounds can exert beneficial effects such as prevention of constipation, reduction of serum cholesterol and blood pressure, and anti-cancer effect [90–93]. Increased intakes of dietary fibre, which includes oligosaccharides, are being recommended in the North American daily diet. The presence of a large number of fibre-rich foods in supermarkets, as well as the media, is an indication of public awareness on the issue of dietary fibre. The bean flatus potential is but a small price to pay for the overwhelmingly large health benefits to the consumer of common bean [113].

Components of beans such as polyphenols and condensed tannins cannot be completely removed by processing [113]. High levels of polyphenols are present in coloured beans (yellow, beige, red, pinto, and black) [135,136]. Coloured bean varieties and types are the favoured legumes in several South and Latin American countries [113,140]. People in these countries have grown used to the sensory attributes of coloured beans, and generally consume only small amounts of other genotypes. In the past, tannins have been considered negatively; however, a number of recent reports have ascribed certain beneficial properties to these compounds [113]. Similarly, polyphenols have been touted as anticarcinogenic and as anti-atherosclerotic agents [50,52].

4. SELECTED FRUITS AND VEGETABLES INDIGENOUS TO LATIN AMERICA

Some of the most familiar food items consumed today by the inhabitants of most of the world are tropical and subtropical fruits, several of which are of Mexican origin (Table 9.7). For example, lemon has long shared space with papaya and avocado in modern supermarkets, while more recently guava and even prickly pear have become familiar to consumers. Other fruits are produced and consumed only in specific geographic regions. For example, capulin (*Prunus serotina*) is principally consumed in the central part of México. Pineapple (*Ananas sativus*), on the other hand, is an example of a South American fruit that has been transplanted to many other regions of the world.

Fruits have been always considered excellent sources of sugars and vitamins, but recently, they have became more important from a nutritional standpoint due to their content of biologically active components. The mode of action of these compounds is not fully understood; however, it appears that many are antioxidants, and as such, they scavenge free radicals formed either during the preparation of foods or by biological processes in the body [141]. Some of the compounds associated with tropical fruits and vegetables are listed in Table 9.7.

Guava ranks at the top of the chart of major sources of vitamin C with 180 mg/100 g, whereas avocado contains 17 mg/100 g, pineapple contains 30 mg/100 g, and tomato contains 20 mg/100 g [142,143]. Current recommended daily allowances for vitamin C in the United Kingdom and United States are 30 and 60 mg/day, respectively, although 100–150 mg/day has been suggested as an optimum intake [144]. Vitamin C, which is synthesized by most animals

TABLE 9.7. Major Mexican and South American Fruits with Biologically Active Ingredients and Properties.

Fruit/Vegetable	Botanical Name	Active Ingredient	Reported Disease Prevention/Treatment
Avocado	*Persea americana*	α-Tocopherol	Cardiovascular disease (CVD) and cancer prevention, antiparasitic action (intestine)
Capulín	*Prunus serotina*	Unknown	Antitussive, antiinflammatory, bactericidal, bacteriostatic, antidiarrhetic, fever, cold and flu, cough, urinary tract cleaning.
Chili pepper	*Capsicum annum*	Capsaicin, citric acid	Chemopreventive
Guava	*Psidium guajava*	Ascorbic acid, phenolics	CVD and cancer prevention, cold and flu
Lemon	*Citrus aurantiifolia*	Unknown	Cold and flu, throat infection, urinary tract
Papaya	*Carica papaya*	Unknown	Laxative, digestive aid, antiamibiatic?
Pineapple	*Ananas sativus*	α-Tocopherol, retinol	Diuretic, kidney stones, antiinflammatory, ulcer
Pumpkin	*Cucurbita pepo*	Unknown	Urinary complaints, kidney stones, antirheumatic
Tomato	*Licopersicum esculentum*	Lycopene	Anticarcinogenic agent
Vanilla	*Vanilla planifolia*	Unknown	Fever, sore stomach, diuretic
Zapote blanco	*Casimiroa edulis*	Unknown	Lowering blood pressure, diuretic

CVD = cardiovascular diseases.
Source: Adapted from Reference [148].

but not by humans, is one of the most important water-soluble antioxidants. It efficiently scavenges hydroxyl, peroxy radicals and singlet oxygen, and may also be involved in the regeneration of vitamin E. By trapping peroxy radicals in the aqueous phase of the plasma or cytosol, vitamin C protects biomembranes and LDL from peroxidative damage [142,145].

A 100 g food portion of avocado contains 3.5 mg of α-tocopherol. In comparison, tomato contains only about half as much vitamin E content as does avocado. The current U.S. recommended daily allowance for vitamin E is 8–10 mg/day [142]. Possible protection against cancer has been ascribed to vitamins C and E for over 50 years. Epidemiologic studies have shown that consumption of foods containing high concentrations of these vitamins correlates with a reduction in cancer incidence. Vitamin C is effective especially in prevention of cancer of the stomach and esophagus, while vitamin E reduces fecal mutagenicity [40]. Other studies involving different species of experimental animals and using deficient as well as high dietary levels of these vitamins indicate that ascorbic acid and α-tocopherol are involved in the maintenance of normal immune function [14].

A non-enzymatic scavenger for superoxide radicals (O_2^-) was found in the leaves of guava [146]. Heat treatment of the leaves did not reduce the scavenging effect of the active components. In México, guava leaves are used to make tea, which is used as a remedy for diarrhea, cold and flu, and stomach cramps (Table 9.7) [147,148]. Similarly, in Cameroon, a multi-component herbal mixture consisting of the leaves of *Carica papaya* and guava was developed for the treatment of the side effects of malaria, such as kidney damage [149].

Capulin (*Prunus serotina*) is widely believed to exert antitussive, anti-inflammatory, bactericidal, and bacteriostatic effects (Table 9.7) [150]. In México, cooked capulin fruit is used as medicine against urinary problems as well as cold and flu, while the leaves and roots are used to alleviate coughs, diarrhea, and fever. Some aborigines of Central America also use capulin fruit for the treatment of dysentery and other gastrointestinal diseases [147,148].

Chili pepper is eaten as a vegetable when green or red, raw or cooked, alone or in combination with other vegetables. Varieties of chili contain capsaicin, which is a pungent and irritating compound. *Capsicum* preparations are used for the treatment of lumbago, neuralgia, and rheumatic disorders. Peppers also contain high levels of vitamins A and C, which have been implicated as anticarcinogenic nutrients [151]. A recent study suggests that capsaicin acts as a chemoprotective and can reduce the potency of some chemical carcinogens and mutagenic agents [152].

Pineapple is used fresh, canned, or made into juices. Pineapple bran, the residue remaining after juicing, is high in vitamin A, and is used in livestock feed [151]. The fruit, peel and juice are used in folk remedies for the treatment of kidney stones and warts. Many pharmacological effects are attributed to the enzyme bromelin which is generally prepared from pineapple wastes. Bromelin is claimed to be useful as an anti-inflammatory, in ulcer prevention, and as a sinusitis relief agent [151]. Ripe pineapple has a diuretic action, and in large doses may cause uterine contractions (Table 9.7).

A variety of other fruits are used in folk medicine for different diseases. For example, lemon is recommended for treating cold, flu, and throat infections and to clean the urinary system. Pumpkin is used by indigenous medical workers to treat urinary complaints, kidney stones and as an antirheumatic agent, while tomato is recommended for reducing the risk of cardiovascular diseases and for prevention of prostate cancer [142]. The medicinal properties of tomato may be due to its high lycopene content. Finally, vanilla and zapote blanco fruits are used to treat fever, stomachache and as a diuretic and for lowering blood pressure.

5. HERBS AND BOTANICALS

Herbal medicines, also known as botanicals, have been used as alternative medicines in México since ancient times and have also been known as traditional Chinese herbals, East Indian preparations, African and European preparations and herbs. Though not always supported by scientific evidence, the use of herbal medicines by *curanderos* (indigenous Mexican doctors) has been stimulated by such factors as a general presumption of safety, limited side effects, remedy for chronic conditions often associated with aging, low cost and emphasis on prevention of diseases [154].

From a pharmaceutical point of view, at least two Mexican herbals are claimed to have cancer-curing properties: cempasúchil (*Tagetes erecta*) and cuachalalate (*Amphypteryngium adstingens*) (Table 9.8) [148]. It is recommended that the whole plant of cempasúchil be boiled in water and used as a tea, while the cuachalalate bark is soaked until the soaking water becomes colored. The patient with stomach cancer or ulcer drinks the cuachalalate preparation as a cold tea.

At least three Mexican indigenous plants are used for treating kidney stones: dry corn silks (*Zea mays*), cardo santo (*Cirsium mexicanum*), and gobernadora (*Larrea tridentata*) (Table 9.8). The most accepted herb in Mexican folk medicine for the treatment of kidney stones is the cooking water of *L. tridentata*. Tinctures prepared from arnica (*Heterotheca inuloides*) are used medicinally as anti-inflammatory and antiseptic agents [155]; and arnica polysaccharides have been found to have immunological activity [156]. One of the most common herbals used against *Ascaris lumbricoides* in Madagascar is epazote (*Chenopodium ambrosioides*), an herb that originated in México [157].

The nopal (*Opuntia* spp.) is a succulent plant native to the American continent. It belongs to the Cactus family, *Opuntia* genus, Plantyopuntia subgenus,

TABLE 9.8. Major Pharmaceutical Herbals.

Common Name	Botanical Name	Reported Biological Effects	Active Ingredients
Herbals indigenous to México			
Arnica	*Heterotheca inuloides*	Stomach, lung and chest pain, analgesic, ulcer, antiinflammatory	
Cabello de elote	*Zea mays*	Urinary complaints, kidney stones, diuretic, antispasmodic	
Cardo santo	*Cirsium mexicanum*	Fever, diabetes, laxative, diuretic, kidney stones, headache	
Cempasúchil	*Tagetes erecta*	Stomach cramps, antidiarrhetic, intestinal parasites, digestive aid, digestive system cleaning, cold and flu, fever, anticarcinogenic	
Epazote	*Chenopodium ambrosioides*	Sore stomatch, colic, intestinal parasites, antidiarrhetic, analgesic, menstrual cramps	
Gobernadora	*Larrea tridentata*	Kidney stones, female sterility, menstrual disorders, cicatrizing	
Other herbals			
Aloe	*Aloe* spp.	Laxative, burns, sunburn, wound healing, gastrointestinal cleaning	Anthraquinone, mannans, acemannan (complex carbohydrate)
Astragalus	*Astaragalus membranaceus*	Immunostimulant, cold and flu, antitumor, adjunct therapy for chemotherapy and AIDS	Polysaccharide, cycloastragenol, astragenol
Capsium	*Cayenne-capsicum* spp.	Cardiovascular therapy, sore muscles and arthritic pain	Oleoresin
Cascara sagrada	*Rhamnus purshiana*	Stimulant, laxative	Anthraquinone (cascarosdes)
Chamomile	*Chamomille recutita*	Antiinflammatory and antispasmodic	Undetermined

(continued)

TABLE 9.8. (continued)

Common Name	Botanical Name	Reported Biological Effects	Active Ingredients
Dong quai	*Angelica sinensis*	Genito-urinary complaints of women, analgesic, antispasmodic, antiinflammatory dysmenorrhea	Psoralen, angelicin
Echinacea	*Echinaceae purpurea*	Anti-inflammatory, antiviral, medicine for cold and infection, healing sores and wounds, immunostimulant	Undetermined
Feverfew	*Tanacetum parthenium*	Migraine headache, antimalarial, analgesic for menstrual cramps	Parthenolide
Garlic	*Zingiber officinale*	Prevent motion sickness	Gingerol, zingerone
Ginseng	*Panax ginseng*	Tonic	Ginsinoside-soponins
Goldenseal	*Hydrastis canadensis*	Cold and flu, masking illicit drugs in urine	Undetermined
Hawthorne	*Crateagus* spp.	Cardiotonic and hypotensive arrhythmias and angina	Flavonoids
Licorice	*Glycyrrhiza* spp.	Demulcent action in chest, stimulant/tonic	Glycyrrhizin, glycyrrhetic acid
Mahuang	*Ephedra sinica*	Stimulant central nervous system and supplement appetite	Ephedra alkaloids-ephedrine
Milk thistle	*Silybum marianum*	Restore liver function after exposure to pollutant, alcohol, and drugs; liver cirrhosis	Flavonolignans
Peppermint	*Mebtha peperita*	Digestion-enhancing, carminative action	Undetermined
Sarsaparilla	*Smilax* spp.	Diuretic, tonic	Steroidal saponins
Saw palmetto	*Serenoa repen*	Benign prostate hypertrophy, antiandrogenic and antiinflammatory	Undetermined
Siberian ginseng	*Eleutherococcus senticosus*	Stress tonic	Eleutheroside E
Slippery elm	*Ulmus rubra*	Demulcent for throat and gastrointestinal irritation	Undetermined
Valerian	*Valeruaba officubakus*	Sedative and sleep aid	Sequiterpenes, valerenic acid

Source: Adapted from References [148, 149, 154].

and grows abundantly in arid and semiarid areas of México. The shape of the nopal plant is unusual, in that the so-called leaves (cladodes) are actually stems that grow on top of each other in an irregular manner [158]. The fruit of the nopal, the prickly pear, is consumed raw after being peeled, and the fermented juice (without the seeds) is consumed as a beer called *colonche*. The fruit is also used in various other food products [159]. Some of the diseases and ailments against which nopal products are claimed to be effective include: gastritis and peptic ulcers, fatigue and dyspnea, glaucoma, liver congestion and hypertrophy resulting from alcohol abuse. Warm cladodes are used as a topical treatment for rheumatic pain, fresh wounds, burns and chronic skin ulcers [158].

Besides the traditional uses of nopal, some new applications based on scientific data are now being tried, such as the consumption of nopal cladodes for the prevention or treatment of hyperglycemia, gastric acidity and atherosclerosis. In addition, nopal cladodes are used widely throughout México for the treatment of diabetes [160].

A few studies have been conducted to evaluate the different chemical compounds of nopal such as the tannins, the reducing and non-reducing sugars, the flavonoids, and some of its alkaloids, but none of these components seems to be responsible for the hypoglycemic effect found in the complete cladode. The possible mechanisms of action of active hypoglycemic or hypolipidemic factors are not known; however, they may be due to the high content of soluble fibre.

Prickly pear consumption reduces plasma and liver LDL cholesterol levels in guinea pigs with induced hypercholesterolemia. It is possible that prickly pear acts as mechanical bile-acid-sequestering factor [161]. Other interesting components of the nopal cladodes include retinol, calcium and potassium.

In spite of the many claimed health benefits attributed to botanicals, consumers of these products must be aware of the potential toxicity of herbal remedies. An independent quality assurance program aimed at monitoring herbal medicines for contaminants such as heavy metals [162,163], natural toxicants [164] and allergens [164,165] is required. Also, well-designed studies aimed at achieving a better understanding of the nature and properties of the active ingredients and their medicinal values of these fascinating plants are urgently required.

6. REFERENCES

1. Betschart, A. A., D. W. Irving, A. D. Shepherd and M. R. Saunders. 1981. "*Amaranthus cruentus:* milling characteristics, distribution of nutrients within seed components, and the effect of temperature on nutritional quality," J. Food Sci. 46:1181–1186.

2. Lehmann, J. W. 1996. "Case of history of grain amaranth as an alternative crop," Cereal Foods World 41:399–411.
3. Bressani, R. 1989. "The proteins of grain amaranth," Food Rev. Int. 5:13–38.
4. Paredes-López, O., H. Guzmán-Maldonado and C. Ordorica-Falomir. 1994. "Food proteins from emerging seed sources," New and Developing Sources of Food Proteins, Hudson, B. J. F., London, UK: Chapman & Hall. pp. 241–279.
5. Segura-Nieto, M., A. P. Barba de la Rosa and O. Paredes-López. 1994. "Biochemistry of amaranth proteins," Amaranth Biology, Chemistry and Technology, Paredes-López, O., Boca Raton, FL: CRC Press. pp. 75–106.
6. FAO/WHO/UNU. 1985. Energy and Protein Requirements. Report of a Joint FAO/WHO/UNU Meeting. WHO, Geneva.
7. Miletic, I. D., V. D. Miletic, E. A. Sattely-Miller and S. S. Schiffman. 1994. "Identification of gliadin presence in pharmaceutical products," J. Pediatric Gastroenterol. Nut. 19:27–33.
8. Barba de la Rosa, A. P., J. Gueguen, O. Paredes-López and G. Viroben. 1992. "Fractionation procedures, electrophoretic characterization, and amino acid composition of amaranth seed protein," J. Agric. Food Chem. 40:931–935.
9. Romero-Zepeda, H. and O. Paredes-López. 1996. "Isolation and characterization of amarantin, the 11S amaranth seed globulin," J. Food Biochem. 19:329–339.
10. Barba de la Rosa, A. P., O. Paredes-López and J. Gueguen. 1992. "Characterization of amaranth globulins by ultracentrifugation and chromatographic techniques," J. Agric. Food Chem. 40:937–942.
11. Sirtori, C. R., C. Manzoni, E. Gianazza and M. R. Lovati. 1996. "Soy and cholesterol reduction: clinical experience and molecular mechanisms," Second International Symposium on the Role of Soy in Preventing and Treating Chronic Disease, September 15–18, 1996, Brussels, Belgium. pp. 21.
12. Kitamura, K. 1996. "Genetic modification of seed storage proteins in soybean," Second International Symposium on the Role of Soy in Preventing and Treating Chronic Disease, September 15–18, 1996, Brussels, Belgium. pp. 48.
13. Becker, R. 1994. "Amaranth oil: composition, processing, and nutritional qualities," Amaranth Biology, Chemistry and Technology, Paredes-López, O., Boca Raton, FL: CRC Press. pp. 133–141.
14. Blumberg, J. B. 1994. "Nutrient control of immune function," Functional Foods Designer Foods, Pharmafoods, and Nutraceuticals, Goldberg, I., London, UK: Chapman & Hall. pp. 87–108.
15. Hansen, T. M., A. Lech, V. Kassis, I. Lorenzen and J. Sondergard. 1983. "Treatment of rheumatoid arthritis with PGE_1 precursors CIS-linoleic acid and gamma linolenic acid," Scand. J. Rheumatol. 12:85–89.
16. Belch, J. J. F., D. Ansel, R. Madhok and A. O'Dowd. 1988. "Effects of altering dietary essential fatty acids on requirements for nonsteroidal anti-inflammatory drugs in patients with rheumatoid arthritis: a double blind placebo controlled study." Ann. Rheum. Dis. 47:96–102.
17. Pedersen, B., K. E. Bach Knudsen and B. O. Eggum. 1990. "The nutritive value of amaranth grain (*Amaranthus caudatus*). III. Energy and fibre of raw and processed grain," Plant Food Hum. Nutr. 40:61–64.
18. Teutonico, R. A., and D. Knorr. 1985. "Amaranth: composition, properties and applications of a rediscovered food crop," Food Technol. 39(4):49–52.
19. Expert Panel on Detection, Evaluation, and Treatment of High Blood Choles-

terol in Adults. 1993. Summary of the second report of the National Cholesterol Education Program. JAMA 269:3015–3023.

20. Wahlqvist, M. L. 1994. "Functional foods in the control of obesity," Functional Foods, Designer Foods, Pharmafoods and Nutraceuticals. Goldberg, I., London, UK: Chapman & Hall. pp. 71–86.
21. Guzmán-Maldonado, H., O. Paredes-López and J. Domínguez. 1993. "Optimization of an enzymatic procedure for the hydrolytic depolymerization of starch by response surface methodology," Food Sci. Technol. (Lebensm. Wiss. Technol.) 26:28–33.
22. Coulter, L. and K. Lorenz. 1990. "Quinoa—composition, nutritional value, and food applications," Food Sci. Technol. (Lebensm. Wiss. Technol.) 23:203–207.
23. Becker, R. and G. D. Hanners. 1990. "Composition and nutritional evaluation of quinoa whole grain flour and mill fractions," Food Sci. Technol. 23:445–450.
24. Brinegar, C. and S. Goundan. 1993. "Isolation and characterization of chenopodin, the 11S seed storage protein of quinoa (*Chenopodium quinoa*)," J. Agric. Food Chem. 41:182–185.
25. Brinegar, C., B. Sine and L. Nwokocha. 1996. "High-cysteine 2S seed storage proteins from quinoa (*Chenopodium quinoa*)," J. Agric. Food Chem. 44:1621–1623.
26. Bressani, R. 1994. "Composition and nutritional properties of amaranth," Amaranth Biology, Chemistry and Technology, Paredes-López, O., Boca Raton, FL: CRC Press. pp. 185–205.
27. Kozoi, M. J. 1990. "Composición química," Quinoa-Hacia su Cultivo Comercial, Wahli, C., Latinreco, S. A., Quito Ecuador. pp. 137–160.
28. Padh, H. 1994. "Vitamins for optimal health," Functional Foods, Designer Foods, Pharmafoods and Nutraceuticals, Goldberg, I., London, UK: Chapman & Hall. pp. 261–293.
29. Witters, R. E. 1985. "Vitamin C and cancer," N. Engl. J. Med. 312:178–179.
30. Pecorano, R. E. and M. S. Chen. 1987. "Ascorbic acid metabolism in diabetes mellitus," Ann. N.Y. Acad. Sci. 498:248–258.
31. Gerster. H. 1989. "Antioxidant vitamins in cataract prevention," Z. Ernahrugswissenschaft 28:56–75.
32. Lehmann, J. W., D. H. Putnam and A. A. Qureshi. 1994. "Vitamin E isomers in grain amaranth (*Amaranthus* spp.)," Lipids 29:177–181.
33. Queshi, A. A., R. Lane and A. W. Salsers. 1995. U.S. Patent 91 U.S. 5,591,772.
34. Fisher, A., A. Munnich, J. M. Saudubray, S. Mamas, F. X. Coudie, C. Charpentier, F. Dray, J. Friezal and C. Gridcelli. 1982. "Biotin-responsive immunoregulatory dysfunction in multiple carboxylase deficiency," J. Clin. Immunol. 2: 35–38.
35. Becker, R., S. W. Irving and R. M. Saunders. 1986. "Production of debranned amaranth flour by stone milling," Lebensm. Wiss. Technol. 19:372–375.
36. Paredes-López, O., A. P. Barba de la Rosa, D. Hernáudez-López and A. Cárabez-Trejo. 1990. "Amaranto-características alimentarias y aprovechamiento agroindustrial." Secretaría General de la Organización de los Estados Americanos, Programa Regional de Desarrollo Científico y Tecnológico, Washington, DC.
37. Allen, J. C. 1994. "Nutrition of macrominerals and trace elements," Functional Foods, Designer Foods, Pharmafoods and Nutraceuticals, Goldberg, I., London, UK: Chapman & Hall. pp. 323–354.

38. Weaver, C. M. 1992. "Calcium bioavailability and its relation to osteoporosis," Proc. Soc. Exp. Biol. Med. 200:157–160.
39. Wargovich, M. J., G. Isbell, M. Shabot, R. Winn, F. Lanza, L. Hochman, E. Larson, P. Lynch, L. Rouben and B. Levin. 1992. "Calcium supplementation decreases rectal epithelial cell proliferation in subjects with sporadic adenoma," Gastroenterol 103:92–97.
40. Milner, J. A. 1994. "Reducing the risk of cancer," Functional Foods Designer Foods, Pharmafoods, Nutraceuticals, Goldberg, I., London, UK: Chapman & Hall. pp. 39–70.
41. National Research Council. 1984. Amaranth: Modern Prospects for an Ancient Crop, Washington, DC: National Academy Press.
42. Morales, E., J. Lembcke and G.G. Graham. 1988. "Nutritional value for young children of grain amaranth and maize-amaranth mixtures: effect of processing," J. Nutr. 118:78–83.
43. Koziol, M. J. 1992. "Chemical composition and nutrient evaluation of quinoa (*Chenopodium quinoa* Willd.)," J. Food Comp. Analysis 5:35–68.
44. Lorenz, K. and White, B. 1984. "Phytate and tannin content of amaranth," Food Chem. 14:27–32.
45. Setchell, K. D. 1996. "Overview of isoflavone structure, metabolism and pharmacokinetics," Second International Symposium on the Role of Soy in Preventing and Treating Chronic Disease, September 15–18, 1996, Brussels, Belgium. pp. 15.
46. Kohda, H., S. Tanaka, Y. Yamaoka and Y. Ohara. 1991. "Saponins from *Amaranthus hypochondriacus,*" Chem. Pharm. Bull. 39:2609–2613.
47. García, L. A., M. A. Alfaro and R. Bressanin. 1987. "Digestibility and protein quality of raw and heat-processed defatted and non-defatted flours prepared with three amaranth species," J. Agric. Food Chem. 35:604–609.
48. González, J. A., A. Roldán, M. Gallardo, T. Escudero and F. E. Prado. 1989. "Quantitative determination of chemical compounds with nutritional value from inca crops: *Chenopodium quioa* ('quinoa')," Plant Foods Hum. Nutr. 39:331–337.
49. Ridout, C. L., K. R. Price, M. S. DuPont, M. L. Parker and G. R. Fenwick. 1991. "Quinoa saponins—analysis and preliminary investigations into the effects of reduction by processing," J. Sci. Food Agric. 54:165–169.
50. Hanasaki, Y., S. Ogawa and S. Fukui. 1994. The correlation between active oxygens scavenging and antioxidative effects of flavonoids. Free Radical Biol. Med. 16:845–850.
51. Stavric, B. and T. I. Matula. 1992. "Flavonoids in foods: their significance for nutrition and health," Lipid-Soluble Antioxidants, Augustine et al., Basel, Switzerland: Birkhäuser Verlag. pp. 274–294.
52. Cook, N. C. and S. Samman. 1996. "Flavonoids—chemistry, metabolism, cardioprotective effects, and dietary source," J. Nutr. Biochem. 7:66–76.
53. Wang, W., A. Franke, L. J. Custer and L. L. Marchand. 1996. "Antioxidant properties of dietary phenolic agents in a human LDL-oxidation *ex-vivo* model," Second International Symposium on the Role of Soy in Preventing and Treating Chronic Disease, September 15–18, 1996, Brussels, Belgium. pp. 28.
54. Rao, A. V. 1996. "Anticarcinogenic properties of plant saponins," Second International Symposium on the Role of Soy in Preventing and Treating Chronic Disease, September 15–18, 1996, Brussels, Belgium. pp. 33.

55. Birk, Y. 1996. "BBI—the trypsin- and chymo-trypsin-inhibitor from soybean: friend or foe?" Second International Symposium on the Role of Soy in Preventing and Treating Chronic Disease, September 15–18, 1996, Brussels, Belgium. pp. 32.
56. Zenteno, E. and J. L. Ochoa. 1988. "Purification of a lectin from *Amaranthus leucocarpus* by affinity chromatography," Phytochemistry 27(2):313–315.
57. Koeppe, S. J. and J. H. Rupnow. 1988. "Purification and characterization of a lectin from the seeds of amaranth (*Amaranthus cruentus*)," J. Food Sci. 53:1412–1416.
58. Rinderle, S. J., I. J. Goldstein and E. E. Remsen. 1990. "Physicochemical properties of amaranthin, the lectin from *Amaranthus caudatus* seeds," Biochem. 29:10555–10558.
59. Rinderle, S. J., I. J. Goldstein, K. L. Matta and R. M. Ratclliffe. 1989. "Isolation and characterization of amaranthin, a lectin present in the seeds of *Amaranthus caudatus,* that recognizes the T- (or cryptic T)- antigen," J. Biol. Chem. 264:16123–16131.
60. Sharon, N. and H. Lis. 1982. "Glycoproteins: research booming on long ignored ubiquitous compounds," Mol. Cell Biochem. 42:167–171.
61. Goldstein, I. J., R. C. Hughes, M. Monsigni, T. Osawa and N. Sharon. 1980. "What should we call a lectin," Nature 285:66–68.
62. Springer, G. F. 1984. "T and Tn, general carcinoma autoantigens," Science 224:1198–1206.
63. Boland, C. R., V. F. Chen, S. J. Rinderle, J. H. Resau, G. D. Luk, H. T. Lynch and I. J. Goldstein. 1991. "Use of the lectin from *Amaranthus caudatus* as a histochemical probe of proliferating colonic epithelial cells," Cancer Res. 51:657–665.
64. Sata, T., C. Zuber, S. J. Rinderle, I. J. Goldstein and J. Roth. 1990. "Expression patterns of the T-antigen and the cryptic T-antigen in rat fetuses: detection with the lectin amaranthin," J. Histochem. Cytochem. 38:763–774.
65. Huang, A. S. and J. H. Von Elbe. 1986. "Stability comparison of two betacyanine pigments—amaranthine and betanine," J. Food Sci. 51:670–675.
66. Curran, P. J., J. L. Dungan, B. A. Macler, S. E. Plummer and D. L. Peterson. 1992. "Reflectance spectroscopy of fresh whole leaves for the estimation of chemical concentration," Remote Sensing Environ. 39:153–166.
67. Schnetzler, K. A. and W. M. Breene. 1994. "Food uses and amaranth product research: a comprehensive review," Amaranth Biology, Chemistry and Technology, Paredes-López, O., Boca Raton, FL.: CRC Press. pp. 155–185.
68. Paredes-López, O., A. Cárabez-Trejo, S. Pérez-Herrera and J. González-Castañeda. 1988. "Influence of germination on physico-chemical properties of amaranth flour and starch microscopic structure," Starch/Stärke 40:290–294.
69. Paredes-López, O. and R. Mora-Escobedo. 1989. "Germination of amaranth seeds: effects on nutrition composition and color," J. Food Sci. 54:761–762.
70. Bressani, R., L. G. Elias, J. M. González and R. Gómez-Brenes. 1987. "The chemical composition and protein quality of amaranth grain germplasm in Guatemala," Arch. Latinoam. Nutr. 37:364–369.
71. Schnetzler, K. A. 1992. "Twin-screw extrusion processing of amaranth," M. S. Thesis, University of Minnesota, MN.

72. Singhal, R. S. and P. R. Kulkarni. 1988. "Composition of the seeds of some *Amaranthus* species," J. Sci. Food Agric. 42:325–331.
73. Danz, R. A. and J. R. Lupton. 1992. "Physiological effects of dietary fiber of amaranth (*Amaranthus cruentus*) on rats," Cereal Foods World 37:489–495.
74. Chaturvedi, A., G. Sarojini and N. L. Devi. 1993. "Hypocholesterolemic effect of amaranth seeds (*Amaranthus esculentus*)," Plant Foods Hum. Nutr. 44: 63–70.
75. Klurfeld, D. M. 1992. "Dietary fiber-mediated mechanisms in carcinogenesis," Cancer Res. 52:2055–2059.
76. Liebman, B. 1993. "In search of the whole grain," Nutr. Action 20:10–15.
77. Ruales, J. and B. M. Nair. 1994. "Properties of starch and dietary fibre in raw and processed quinoa (*Chenopodium quinoa,* Willd) seeds," Plant Foods Human Nutr. 45:223–246.
78. Lehmann, J. W. 1994. "Amaranth: commercialization and industrialization," Amaranth Biology, Chemistry and Technology, Paredes-López, O., Boca Raton, FL: CRC Press. pp. 207–217.
79. Paredes-López, O., A. P. Barba de la Rosa and A. Cárabez-Trejo. 1990. "Enzymatic production of high-protein amaranth flour and carbohydrate rich fraction," J. Food Sci. 55:1157–1161.
80. Guzmán-Maldonado, H., and O. Paredes-López. 1994. "Production of high-protein flour and maltodextrins from amaranth grain," Process Biochem. 29: 289–293.
81. Guzmán-Maldonado, H. 1992. "Optimización de un procedimiento enzimático para la licuefacción y sacarificación del almidón mediante la metodología de superficie de respuesta. MSc. thesis, CINVESTAV-IPN, Unidad Irapuato, México, pp. 72–73.
82. Berghofer, E. and S. Sarhaddar. 1988. "Production of glucose and high fructose by enzymatic direct hydrolysis of cassava roots," Process Biochem. 23: 188–194.
83. Sánchez-Marroquín, A., R. F. Del Valle, M. Escobedo, R. Avitia, S. Maya and M. Vega. 1986. "Evaluation of whole amaranth (*Amaranthus cruentus*) flour, its air-classified fractions and blends of these with wheat and oats as possible components for infant formulas," J. Food Sci. 5:1231–1237.
84. Del Valle, F. R., M. Escobedo, A. Sánchez-Marroquín, H. Bourges, M. A. Bock and P. Biemer. 1992. "Nitrogen balance in infants fed formulas containing amaranth or a soy-oat formula," Cereal Chem. 69:156–162.
85. Del Valle, F. R., M. Escobedo, A. Sánchez-Marroquín, H. Bourges, M. A. Bock and P. Biemer. 1993. "Chemical and nutritional evaluation of two amaranth (*Amaranthus caudatus*) based infant formulas," Plant Foods Hum. Nutr. 43:145–151.
86. Mitchell, D. T. 1993. "Two new bodybuilding grains from the Aztecs and Incas," Muscle and Fitness 54:46–50.
87. Ley, B. M. 1992. "The right combination: new vegetarian diet reveals protein sources to pack on the beef without eating it," Muscle and Fitness 53:152–155.
88. Crittenden, R. G. and M. J. Playne. 1996. "Production, properties and applications of food-grade oligosaccharides," Trends Food Sci. Technol. 7:353–361.

89. Tomomatsu, H. 1994. "Health effects of oligosaccharides," Food Technol. 48(10): 61–65.
90. Oku, T. 1994. "Special physiological functions of newly developed mono- and oligosaccharides," Functional Foods, Designer Foods, Pharmafoods and Nutraceuticals, Goldberg, I., London, UK: Chapman & Hall. pp. 202–218.
91. Saito, Y., T. Takano and I. Rowland. 1992. "Effects of soybean oligosaccharides on the human gut microflora in *in vitro* culture," Microbial Ecol. Health Dis. 5:105–111.
92. Hata, Y., T. Hara, T. Oikawa, M. Yamamoto, N. Hirose, T. Nagashima, N. Torihama, K. Nakajima, A. Watabe and M. Yamashita. 1983. "The effects of fructo-oligosaccharides against hyperlipidemia," Geriatr. Med. 21:156–167.
93. Hata, Y., K. Nakajima, Y. Hosono and M. Yamamoto. 1989. "Effects of soybean oligosaccharides on human digestive organs," J. Japan. Soc. Clin. Nutr. 11:42–46.
94. Saunders, R. M. and R. Becker. 1984. "*Amaranthus:* a potential food and feed resource," Advances in Cereal Science and Technology, Pomeranz, Y., St. Paul, MN: American Association of Cereal Chemists. pp. 357–396.
95. Lorenz, K. and M. Gross. 1984. "Saccharides of amaranth," Nutr. Rep. Int. 29:721–724.
96. Fernández, M. L. and J. W. Berry. 1988. "Nutritional evaluation of chickpea and germinated chickpea flours," Plant Foods Hum. Nutr. 38:127–132.
97. Price, T. V. 1988. "Seed sprout production for human consumption—a review," Can. Inst. Food Sci. Technol. J. 21:57–85.
98. Lorenz, K. 1980. "Cereal sprouts: composition, nutritive value and food applications," CRC Crit. Rev. Food Sci. Nutr. 13:353–380.
99. Colmenares de Ruiz, A. S. and R. Bressani. 1990. "Effect of germination on the chemical composition and nutritive value of amaranth grain," Cereal Chem. 67: 519–522.
100. Gepts, P. and D. Dobouck. 1991. "Origin, domestication, and evolution of the common bean (*Phaseolus vulgaris* L.)," Common Beans: Research for Crop Improvement, Van Schoonhoven, A. and Voysest, O., Wallingford, England: CAB International. pp. 7–53.
101. Reyes-Moreno, C. and O. Paredes-López. 1993. "Hard-to-cook phenomenon in common beans—a review," CRC Crit. Rev. Food Sci. Nutr. 33:227–286.
102. Deshpande, S. S., S. K. Sathe and D. K. Salunkhe. 1984. "Interrelationship between certain physical and chemical properties of dry beans (*Phaseolus vulgaris* L.)," Plant. Foods Hum. Nutr. 34:53–59.
103. Osborn, T. C. 1988. "Genetic control of bean seed protein," CRC Crit. Rev. Plant. Sci. 7:93–145.
104. Chang, K. C. and L. D. Satterlee. 1982. "Chemistry of dry bean proteins," J. Food Proc. Preserv. 6:203–210.
105. Kanazawa, T. 1996. "Anti-atherogenic effects of soybean protein. Viewpoints from peroxidizability and molecular size of LDL and from anti-platelet aggregation," Second International Symposium on the Role of Soy in Preventing and Treating Chronic Disease, September 15–18, 1996, Brussels, Belgium. pp. 27.
106. Stroescul, V., I. Sragan, L. Simionescu and O. V. Stroescu. 1996. "Hormonal effects of soy," Second International Symposium on the Role of Soy in Preventing and Treating Chronic Disease, September 15–18, 1996, Brussels, Belgium. pp. 38.

107. Hughes, J. S. 1991. "Potential contribution of dry bean dietary fiber to health," Food Technol. 45(2):122–126.
108. Morrow, B. 1991. "The rebirth of legumes," Food Technol. 45(4):96–101.
109. Moundras, C., C. Rémésy, M. A. Levrat, S. R. Behr and C. Demigné. 1996. "Interactions between soy protein and soy fiber on lipid metabolism in the rat," Second International Symposium on the Role of Soy in Preventing and Treating Chronic Disease. September 15–18, 1996, Brussels, Belgium. pp. 53.
110. Anderson, J. J. B., and J. C. Allen. 1994. "Nutrition of macrominerals and trace elements," Functional Foods Designer Foods, Pharmafoods, Nutraceuticals, Goldberg, I., London, UK: Chapman & Hall. pp. 323–354.
111. Marletta, L., M. Carbonaro and E. Carnovale. 1992. "In-vitro protein and sulphur amino acid availability as a measure of bean protein quality," J. Sci. Food Agric. 59:497–504.
112. Deshpande, S. S. and S. Damodaran. 1990. "Food legumes: chemistry and technology," Adv. Cereal Sci. Technol. 10:147–153.
113. Deshpande, S. S. 1992. "Food legumes in human nutrition: a personal perspective," CRC Crit. Rev. Food Sci. Nutr. 32:333–363.
114. Blanco, A. and R. Bressani. 1991. "Biodisponibilidad de amino ácidos en el frijol," Arch. Latinoam. Nutr. 41:38–52.
115. Tezoto, S. S. and V. C. Sgarbieri. 1990. "Protein nutritive value of a new cultivar of bean (*Phaseolus vulgaris* L.)," J. Agric. Food Chem. 38:1152–1156.
116. Schmidl, M. K. and T. P. Labuza. 1994. "Medical foods," Functional Foods, Designer Foods, Pharmafoods and Nutraceuticals, Goldberg, I., London, UK: Chapman & Hall. pp. 151–179.
117. NRC. 1989. "Dietary fiber," Diet and Health: Implications for Reducing Chronic Diseases Risk, Natl. Res. Council, Washington, DC: National Academy Press.
118. Schneeman, B. O. 1986. "Dietary fiber: physical and chemical properties, methods of analysis and physiological effects," Food Technol. 40(5):104–109.
119. Toma, R. B. and D. J. Curtis. 1986. "Dietary fiber: its role for diabetics," Food Technol. 40(5):118–122.
120. Roberfroid, M. 1993. "Dietary fiber, inulin, and oligofructose: a review comparing their physiological effects," CRC Crit. Rev. Food Sci. Nutr. 33:103–148.
121. Anderson, J. W., L. Story, B. Sieling, W. J. Chen, M. S. Petro and J. Story. 1984. "Hypocholesterolemic effects of oat-bran or bean intake for hypocholesterolemic men," Am. J. Clin. Nutr. 40:1146–1151.
122. Shutler, S. M., G. M. Bircher, J. A. Tredger, L. A. Morgan, A. F. Wakerand and A. G. Low. 1989. "The effect of daily baked bean (*Phaseolus vulgaris*) consumption on the plasma lipid levels of young, normo-cholesterolemic men," Br. J. Nutr. 61:257–263.
123. Jenkins, D. J. A., T. M. S. Wolever, R. H. Taylor, H. Barler and H. Dielden. 1980. "Exceptionally low blood glucose response to dried beans: comparisons with other carbohydrate foods," Br. Med. J. 2:578–583.
124. Potter, J. G., K. P. Coffman, R. L. Reid, J. M. Krall and M. J. Albrink. 1981. "Effect of test meals of varying dietary fiber content on plasma insulin and glucose response," Am. J. Clin. Nutr. 34:328–335.
125. Tappy, L., P. Wursch, J. P. Randin, J. P. Felber and E. Jéquier. 1986. "Metabolic effect of precooked instant preparation of bean and potato in normal and in diabetic subjects," Am. J. Clin. Nutr. 43:30–35.

126. Hughes, J. S. and B. G. Swanson. 1989. "Soluble and insoluble dietary fiber in cooked common beans (*Phaseolus vulgaris*) seeds," Food Microstruct. 8:15–19.
127. Pak, N., C. Ayala, G. Vera, I. Pannacchiotti and H. Araya. 1990. "Soluble and insoluble dietary fiber in cereals and legumes cultivated in chile," Arch. Latinoam. Nutr. 40:116–125.
128. Patte, H. E., D. K. Salunkhe, S. K. Sathe and N. R. Reddy. 1982. "Legume lipids," CRC Crit. Rev. Food Sci. Nutr. 17:97–140.
129. Sathe, S. K., S. S. Deshpande and D. K. Salunkhe. 1985. "Dry beans of *Phaseolus:* a review. II. Chemical composition: carbohydrates, fiber, minerals, vitamins and lipids," CRC Crit. Rev. Food Sci. Nutr. 46:1389–1414.
130. Hsieh, H. M., Y. Pomeranz and B. G. Swanson. 1992. "Composition, cooking time, and maturation of azuki (*Vigna angularis*) and common beans (*Phaseolus vulgaris*)," Cereal Chem. 69:244–248.
131. Mahadevappam V. G. and P. L. Raina. 1978. "Nature of some Indian legume lipids," J. Agric. Food. Chem. 26:1241–1246.
132. Agustin, J., C. B. Beck, G. Kalbfleish and L. C. Kagel. 1981. "Variation in the vitamin and mineral content of raw and cooked commercial *Phaseolus vulgaris* classes," Food Technol. 35(2):75–82.
133. Barampama, Z. and R. E. Simard. 1993. "Nutrient composition, protein quality and antinutritional factors of some varieties of dry beans (*Phaseolus vulgaris*) grown in Burundi," Food Chem. 42:159–167.
134. Barampama, Z. and R. E. Simard. 1994. "Oligosaccharides, antinutritional factors, and protein digestibility of dry beans as affected by processing," J. Food Sci. 59:833–838.
135. Guzmán-Maldonado, H., J. Castellanos and E. González de Mejía. 1996. "Relationship between theoretical and experimentally detected tannin content of common beans (*Phaseolus vulgaris* L.)," Food Chem. 55:333–335.
136. Guzmán-Maldonado, S. H., A. Marín-Jarillo, J. Z. Catellanos, E. González de Mejía and J. A. AcostaGallegos. 1996. "Relationship between physical and chemical characteristics and susceptibility to *Zabrotes subfasciatus* (Boh.) (Choleoptera: Bruchidae) and *Acanthoscelides obtectus* (Say) in common bean (*Phaseolus vulgaris* L.) varieties," J. Stored Prod. Res. 32:53–58.
137. Vishalakshi, I., D. K. Salunkhe, S. K. Sathe and L. B. Rockland. 1980. "Quick-cooking beans (*Phaseolus vulgaris*). II. Phytates, oligosaccharides and antienzymes," Qual. Plant. Pl. Food Hum. Nutr. 30:45–52.
138. Sathe, S. K., S. S. Deshpande, N. R. Reddy, D. E. Goll and D. K. Salunkhe. 1983. "Effect of germination of proteins, raffinose oligosaccharides, and antinutritional factors in the great northern beans (*Phaseolus vulgairs* L.)," J. Food Sci. 42: 1796–1800.
139. Desphande, S. S. and M. Cheryan. 1983. "Changes in phytic acid, tannins, and trypsin inhibitory activity on soaking of dry bean (*Phaseolus vulgaris*)," Nutr. Rep. Int. 27:371–377.
140. Kelly, J. D. and J. Castellanos. 1996. "Research pinpoints favorite bean flavors in México," Michigan Dry Bean Digest 20(3):17–21, 31.
141. Stavric, B. 1994. "Antimutagens and anticarcinogens in food," Food Chem. Toxic. 32:79–90.
142. Duthie, G. G. and K .M. Brown. 1994. "Reducing the risk of cardiovascular dis-

eases," Functional Foods, Designer Foods, Pharmafoods and Nutraceuticals, Goldberg, I., London, UK: Chapman & Hall. pp. 19–38.

143. Yusof, S. 1990. "Physico-chemical characteristics of some *Guava* varieties in Malasia," Acta Horticul. 269:301–305.

144. Esterbauer, H., F. K. Gey, J. Fuchs, M. R. Clemens and H. Seis. 1990. "Antioxidative Vitamine und degenerative Erkrankungen," Deutsch Arzteblatt 87:2620–2624.

145. Smith, C., M. J. Mitchison, O. I. Aruoma and B. Halliwell. 1992. "Stimulation of lipid peroxidation and hydroxyl-radical generation by the contents of human atherosclerotic lesions," Biochem. J. 286:901–905.

146. Luo, G. and A. Wang. 1994. "The scavenging effect of plant polyphenolics on superoxide radicals," J. Trop. Subtrop. Botany 2:95–99.

147. Martínez, M. 1981. "Las plantas medicinales en México," Martínes, M., México, D. F., Ediciones Botas. pp. 154.

148. Estrada-Lugo, E. I. J., A. Uribe and E. Estrada-Lugo. 1995. "Las plantas medicinales y los sistemas tradicionales de curación del municipio de Dr. Mora Gto," Plantas Medicinales de México, Estrada-Lugo, E., Texcoco, Edo. de México, Universidad Autónoma de Chapingo, pp. 299.

149. Kinyuy, W. C., D. Palevitch and E. Putievsky. 1993. "Through integrated biomedical/ethnomedical preparations and ethnotaxonomy, effective malaria and diabetic treatments have evolved," Acta Hort. 344:205–214.

150. Abigail, A. 1994. "Medicinal plants used for the treatment of respiratory diseases form ethnobotanical information of medical herbarium IMMSM," Abstracts of the Fourth International Congress of Ethnobiology, Uttar Pradesh, India. pp. 264.

151. Duke. J. 1985. Handbook of Medicinal Herbs, Duke, J., Boca Raton, FL: CRC Press. pp. 98–99.

152. Surh, S. 1995. "Capsaicin, a double-edged sword: toxicity, metabolism and chemopreventive potential," Life Sci. 56:1845–1855.

153. Van-Der-Beek, E. J., M. R. H. Lowik, K. F. A. M. Hulshof and C. Kistemaker. 1994. "Combination of low thiamin, riboflavin, vitamin B-6, and vitamin C intake among Dutch adults," J. Amer. College Nutr. 13:383–391.

154. Yuan, R. and M. Hsu. 1996. "Herbal medicines," Gen. Eng. News 6(12):29, 32.

155. Pietta, P. G., P. L. Mauri, A. Bruno and I. Merfort. 1994. "MERK as an improved method to detect falsification in the flowers of *Arnica montana* and *A. chamissonis*," Planta Medica 60:369–372.

156. Puhlmann, J., M. H. Zenk and H. Wagner. 1991. "Immunologically active polysaccharide of *Arnica montana* cell cultures," Phytochem. 30:1141–1145.

157. Kightlinger, L. K., J. R. Seed and M. B. Kightlinger. 1996. "*Ascaris lumbricoides* aggregation in relation of child growth status, delayed cutaneous hypersensitivity, and plant anthelmintic use in Madagascar," J. Parasitol. 82:25–33.

158. Muñoz de Chávez, M., A. Chávez, V. Valle and J. A. Roldán. 1995. "The nopal: a plant of manifold qualities," Plants Human Nutr. 77:109–134.

159. Paredes-López, O. and R. Rojo-Burgos. 1973. "Estudio para el envasado de jugo de tuna (Studies for the production of prickly pear juice)," Tecnol. Alimentos (Méx.) 8:237–240.

160. Fernández-Harp, J. A., A. C. Frati-Munari, A. Chávez-Negrete, H. De la Rive

and G. Marez-Gómez. 1984. "Estudios hormonales en la acción del nopal sobre la prueba de tolerancia a la glucosa," Informe Preeliminar, Rev. Med. IMMS 22:387.

161. Fernández, M. L., A. Trejo and C. McNamara. 1990. "Pectin isolated from prickly pear (*Opuntia* spp.) modifies low density lipoprotein metabolism of cholesterol in guinea pigs," New York: Publication of the American Institute of Nutrition. pp. 1283.
162. Smitherman, J. and P. Harber. 1992. "A case of mistaken identity: herbal medicine as a cause of lead toxicity," Amer. J. Indust. Med. 20:795–798.
163. Chan, T. Y. K. and J. A. J. H. Critchley. 1996. "Usage and adverse effects of chinese herbal medicines," Human Exper. Toxicol. 15:5–12.
164. Molyneux, R. J., T. A. Beek and H. Breteler. 1992. "Toxic range plants and their constituents," Phytochemistry and Agriculture, Proceedings of the Phytochemical Society of Europe 34:151–170.
165. Lewis, W. H. 1992. "Allergenic potential of commercial chamomile, *Chamaemelum nobile* (Asteraceae)," Econom. Botany 46:426–430.

CHAPTER 10

Physiological Components and Health Effects of Ginseng, *Echinacea*, and Sea Buckthorn

T. S. C. LI[1]
L. C. H. WANG[2]

1. GINSENG

Two of the most popular ginsengs on the market, Asian (*Panax ginseng* C. A. Meyer) and American ginseng (*P. quinquefolium* L.), are perennial semi-shade aromatic herbs belonging to the Araliaceae family, which are native to China and Canada, respectively [1,2]. Ginseng has been used for thousands of years by humans as an energy booster and general tonic [3]. Crude root extracts can decrease reactions to various noxious and stressful stimuli such as general hypoxia and cardiac ischemia and exert a stimulating effect on the metabolism by significantly altering lipid and carbohydrate mobilization and utilization [4,5,6]. In addition, it has been reported that ginseng also has health benefits such as insulin-like activity [7] and reduction of total cholesterol level [8]. Ginseng products have increased in popularity around the world in recent years, and a myriad manufactured forms are available in pharmacies and health food stores in North America. Fresh ginseng roots are also used in Asian delicacies.

There are nine species in the *Panax* genus. China is home to the greatest number of native species in the world [5], besides *P. ginseng*, *P. pseudoginseng* Wall, *P. notoginseng* (Burk.) F. H. Chen, *P. japonicum* C. A. Meyer, *P. zingiberensis* C. Y. Wu and K. M. Feng, and *P. stipuleanatus* H. T. Hsai and

[1]Agriculture and Agri-Food Canada, Pacific Agri-Food Research Centre, Summerland, BC, Canada.
[2]Department of Zoology, University of Alberta, Edmonton, AB, Canada.

K. M. Feng [9]. There are two native species in North America, *P. quinquefolium* L. and *P. trifolium* L. [10]. Recently, a new species, *P. vietnamensis* Ha et Grushv., was found in Vietnam [11].

Ginseng production is increasing rapidly around the world. For example, in China, yearly production of Asian ginseng increased from 1,600 tons in 1985 [12] to an estimated 8,000 tons in 1995. Ginseng production in North America has increased from 370 tons in 1983 [13] to an estimated 2,000 tons in 1995 with a farm-gate value of approximately 150–200 million (Canadian) dollars. The major production regions extend from Ontario and British Columbia [3] to central Alabama and from the east coast to just west of the Mississippi river [14]. Recently, ginseng production has expanded to Chile, Australia and New Zealand [15].

1.1. CULTIVATION

Ginseng is traditionally propagated by seeds. The embryo of newly harvested seeds are not fully developed and have to go through two lengthy development and stratification periods before germination [3,16]. Stratified seeds are planted in the fall on a raised bed, around 90 to 110 kg/ha, at a depth of 1–1.5 cm, and covered with 10 cm of straw immediately after seeding [3].

The earliest method of cultivation consisted of seeding or transplanting the young seedings in the forest; cultivation moved from mountainous to flat land and eventually to shaded. Ginseng is a shade-loving crop, traditionally grown under the shade of straw thatch with or without a layer of polyethylene [17], wooden lath or woven synthetic fabrics [18,19]. Ginseng can also be cultivated under natural shade [14].

Ginseng is a slow-growing root crop, best suited to well-drained sandy loam soil with a pH range of 5.0 to 6.5. It normally takes 6 years from seeding to harvest for Asian and 4 years for American ginseng. In British Columbia and Ontario, average yield is about 3000 kg/ha. After harvest, roots are washed and dried in forced-air dryers to a moisture content of around 8–10%. A recent review of the literature revealed that there are 65 fungal and eight bacterial pathogens infecting *Panax* species [20,21]. Most economically significant diseases are caused by fungal pathogens. They can infect every part of the plant and result in reduced growth, seed set and yield.

1.2. PHYSIOLOGICALLY ACTIVE COMPONENTS

Shibata et al. [22] identified ginseng saponin components by chromatography and named them ginsenosides Rx (x = o, a, b_1, b_2, c, d, e, f, g_1, g_2, g_3, h_1, h_2). In addition to saponins, ginseng contains many other phytochemicals including phytosterols, oils, acids, carbohydrates, flavonoids, nitrogen-containing compounds, vitamins, and inorganics [23].

There is considerable literature on the chemical components of ginseng [24]. The contents of polysaccharides in the roots of *P. ginseng* may change after processing. Han et al. [25] found that the total polysaccharide contents in processed *P. ginseng* (Korea red ginseng) was three times higher than in the nonprocessed form (451.4 vs. 152.7 units/g dry wt.). Smith et al. [26] claimed that ginsenosides in *P. quinquefolium* are located in the periderm, cortex, xylem, and pith regions of the root. This is somewhat different from the finding of Kubo et al. [27] and Tani et al. [28] who, using histochemical analysis, found that ginsenosides are localized in the periderm and cortex regions only. Ma et al. [29] analysed more than 60 commercial ginseng products, roots and tissue culture samples for ginsenoside content. They reported that ginseng samples contain a wide range of ginsenosides. Dried roots of *P. ginseng* and *P. quinquefolium* yielded the highest ginsenoside content, ranging from 1.2 to 8.6%.

The major active constituents of ginseng are now generally accepted as dammarane saponins, commonly referred to as ginsenosides [30,31,32]. A total of 28 ginsenosides have been extracted and identified in roots, stems, leaves, and flower buds [3]. Recently, a new ginsenoside, la, was isolated from leaves of *P. ginseng* [33]. The most abundant ginsenosides present in American ginseng are Rb_1, Rb_2, Rc, and Rd, which possess 20(S)-protopanaxadial as the aglycon (Figure 10.1); and Rg_1 and Re, which possess 20(S)-protopanaxatriol as the aglycon [34,35]. *P. quinquefolium* contains more Rb_1 and Re than *P. ginseng* but has no Rg_2 and Rf [29]. It has also been reported that the leaves and stems of *P. quinquefolium* contain mainly ginsenosides Rg_1, Re and Rd; the average total ginsenoside content is 2.84%. This is in agreement with the findings of Li et al. [35], who reported a total content of ginsenosides in leaves ranging from 1.86% to 4.18%, depending on the age of the leaves. A number of C_{17}-polyacetylenes have been isolated from the roots of *P. ginseng* [36]. F ujimoto et al. [37] reported that new C_{17}-and C_{14}-polyacetylenes and two known polyacetylenes, ginsenoyne G [38] and acetylpanaxydol [39], isolated from the dried roots of *P. quinquefolium,* exhibited cytotoxic activity against leukaemia cells in tissue culture. The polysaccharides isolated from *P. ginseng* have been reported to have immunological, anti-tumor, and hypoglycemic activities [40,41]. Recently, an anti-ulcer pectic polysaccharide extracted from leaves of *P. ginseng* was reported [42].

1.3. EFFECTS OF SOURCES, PARTS OF PLANT, ENVIRONMENTAL FACTORS, AND EXTRACTION METHODS ON THE CONTENT OF ACTIVE INGREDIENTS

Many factors affect the content and composition of ginsenosides. For example, maturity of leaves, age of roots, species, growing regions, and environmental factors all can play a role. Available information on how to maxi-

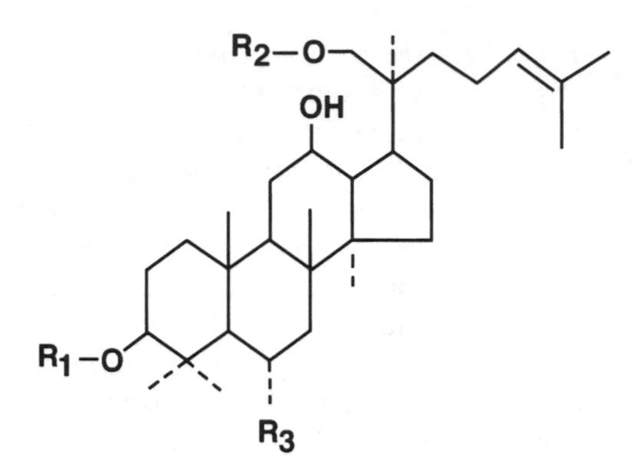

	R_1	R_2	R_3
R_{b1}	-glc[2→1]glc	-glc[6→1]glc	-H
R_{b2}	-glc[2→1]glc	-glc[6→1]ara(p)	-H
R_c	-glc[2→1]glc	-glc[6→1]ara(f)	-H
R_d	-glc[2→1]glc	-glc	-H
R_e	-H	-glc	-O-glc[2→1]rha
R_f	-H	-H	-O-glc[2→1]glc
R_{g1}	-H	-glc	-O-glc

glc : glucose ara(p) :α-Larabinopyranose ara(f) :α-Larabinofuranose rha : rhamnose

Figure 10.1 Structures of ginsenosides in ginseng.

mize the ginsenoside content for a particular ginseng species and/or cultivar is limited.

1.3.1. Genetics

The synthesis and accumulation of secondary metabolites in plants is highly variable between cultivars [43]. As a result, selection of cultivars is critical in ensuring a high-quality product [44]. Nonetheless, only a few genetic studies and breeding programs have been carried out with Asian ginseng in China and Korea [45,46], and there are no registered cultivars of American ginseng. Some evidence of genetic variability within *P. quinquefolium* populations has recently been observed in commercial ginseng gardens in British Columbia and Ontario (unpublished data). Selection and breeding of American ginseng will likely improve yield, disease resistance and the content of active ingredients [3].

Individual and total ginsenoside contents vary substantially among *Panax*

TABLE 10.1. Total Ginsenosides (g/100 g dry wt) in Different Parts of 6-Year-Old Plants of Three Ginseng Species.

	Species		
Sample	*P. ginseng*	*P. quinquefolium*	*P. pseudoginseng*
Main root	3.8	4.1	6.2
Side root	4.8	4.8	6.8
Root hair	9.0	8.4	10.0
Rhizome	7.3	8.4	10.3
Stem	2.3	2.2	nd
Leaf	10.1	11.0	8.2
Leaf petiole	1.0	2.2	nd
Flower bud	11.3	13.2	13.6
Seed pod	8.9	8.0	10.7
Seed	0.7	nd	nd

nd = not determined.
Source: Adapted from Reference [16].

species (Tables 10.1 and 10.4). Xiao et al. [16] reported that total ginsenosides extracted from the roots of *P. ginseng, P. quinquefolium,* and *P. pseudoginseng* were 3.8, 4.1 and 6.2%, respectively; levels in leaves were 10.1, 11.0 and 8.2%. In another study, Soldati and Sticher [47] reported that total ginsenosides (Rg_1, Re, Rf, Rg_2, Rb_1, Rc, Rb_2, and Rd) isolated from the roots of *P. ginseng* were 1.35%, and from *P. quinquefolium* (Rg_1, Re, Rb_1, Rc, and Rd) 1.71%. Ma et al. [29] found that total ginsenosides (Rg_1, Re, Rf, Rb_1, Rc, Rb_2, and Rd) extracted from the roots of *P. ginseng* ranged from 1.20 to 3.95%, and when extracted from *P. quinquefolium* (Rg_1, Re, Rb_1, Rc, Rd, and sometimes a trace of Rb_2) from 1.26 to 8.60%.

1.3.2. Age of the Plant

Content of ginsenosides varies with the age of the plant [48]. As shown in Table 10.2, total ginsenosides in roots of Asian ginseng from two different locations in China increased from 2.0% and 4.8% in 2-year-old to 4.4% and 6.4% in 6-year-old plants. On the other hand, 2- to 6-year-old roots from Japan contained less total ginsenosides in all ages and were around 2–3%. Furthermore, in roots of the same age ginsenoside contents may vary. For example, Smith et al. [26] reported that the ginsenoside levels of 20 samples of 4-year-old American ginseng collected from the same field ranged from 2.5 to 5.6%. This may be due to the size and physiological condition of the roots.

TABLE 10.2. Effects of Age and Sources of *P. ginseng* on Total Ginsenosides (g/100 g dry wt).

	Sample Source		
	China		
Age of the Roots	Ji-Lin Region	Tong-Hua Region	Japan
2	2.0	4.8	3.0
3	2.2	5.6	2.0
4	4.7	6.2	3.5
5	4.6	6.3	2.5
6	4.4	6.4	2.5

Source: Adapted from Reference [16].

1.3.3. Growing Region and Environmental Conditions

Growing region and environmental conditions significantly affect ginsenoside content. As shown in Table 10.2, total ginsenosides from 6-year-old Asian ginseng roots from the Ji-Lin and Tong-Hua regions of China were 4.4 and 6.4%, respectively, whereas roots grown in Japan contained 2.5% ginsenosides [16]. Li et al. [35] reported that total ginsenosides in 4-year-old American ginseng collected from nine locations in British Columbia ranged from 2.44 to 3.88% in roots and 4.14 to 5.58% in leaves (Table 10.3).

Ginseng production is influenced by environmental conditions such as soil texture, pH, fertility, and moisture; seasonal variations in temperature, humidity, photoperiod, and light intensity; amount of annual precipitation and its distribution pattern; and air movement. Recently, Li et al. [35] reported that in 4-year-old American ginseng plants, the content of total and of the individual ginsenosides Re, Rc, Rb_2, and Rd extracted from young leaves in early June

TABLE 10.3. Content of Total Ginsenosides (g/100 g dry wt) in Mature Leaves and Roots of 4-Year-Old Plants of American Ginseng Sampled from Nine Ginseng Gardens in British Columbia in 1995.

	Location								
Sample	1	2	3	4	5	6	7	8	9
Leaf	4.32	5.58	4.42	5.12	5.12	4.14	4.88	4.38	4.82
Root	2.69	2.79	2.44	3.29	3.88	3.56	2.65	2.52	3.16

Source: Adapted from Reference [35].

varied significantly among plants grown at different locations, while in mature leaves, collected in late August, only Rb_1 and Rb_2 showed significant differences between locations. However, in the roots, production site had a statistically significant effect on the level of Rb_1, Rc, Rd, and total ginsenosides [35].

Differences in total ginsenosides between wild and cultivated ginseng have been attributed to differences in growth caused by soil moisture and nutrition and physiological stresses associated with the rate of growth [49,50]. Soil fertility and root tissue nutrients affect the content of total and individual ginsenosides in leaf and in root [50]. Li et al. [35] found a low correlation between leaf and root ginsenosides of 4-year-old American ginseng plants.

1.3.4. Distribution of Ginsenosides within Ginseng Plant

Soldati and Sticher [47] reported that the total ginsenoside content and composition (Rg_1, Re, Rf, Rg_2, Rb_1, Rc, Rb_2, and Rd) of 4-year-old *P. ginseng* were different in leaves and roots. Specifically, the leaves contained mainly Rg_1, Re, and Rd and the root mainly Re, Rb_1 and Rc. The total ginsenoside content was 3.19, 1.35 and 3.53% in leaves, main roots and lateral roots, respectively. In *P. ginseng* (Table 10.1), Xiao et al. [16] reported that the highest content of total ginsenosides was extracted from flower buds and leaves, and the lowest from seeds. Han [51] claimed that saponins are present in all parts of the plant except seeds. In *P. quinquefolium*, Li et al. [35] reported that on a dry-weight basis, the total ginsenoside content in leaves (4.18%) is higher than that of roots (3.00%).

1.3.5. Extraction Methods

Active components of ginseng can be extracted with ether, methanol or water. Many factors affect differences in the extracts, including sample preparation, extraction procedure, and the solvent used. Ether extracts contain essential oils, polyacetylenes, phytosterols, and glycosides, whereas methanol extracts contain primarily low-molecular weight components but not starch, pectin, cellulose or protein. Methanol extraction followed by ether extraction yields mainly glycosides but may also include small molecule components such as sugars, amino acids, peptides and nucleotides. When ginseng is extracted with water, macromolecular substances as well as the ether- and alcohol-soluble components can be expected [23].

Han [51] reported that ether can only extract 0.7% of ginseng components while methanol can extract about 25.6%. Water is able to extract 47.6% of the components. This percentage can be increased up to 60% if water and ginseng are allowed to stand at 2–4°C for a period of time due to the enzymatic degradation of macromolecules such as starch into soluble smaller molecules.

Lui and Staba [34] compared three extraction methods, (a) water and *n*-butanol [52]; (b) chloroform, methanol, water and *n*-butanol [53]; and (c) mixture of chloroform, methanol, water and *n*-butanol [54], in extracting ginsenosides from the roots of American ginseng. The amount of ginsenosides extracted by Method b was considerably higher than the amounts obtained by using Methods a and c (4.7% vs. 2.2 and 4.0%).

1.4. VALUE-ADDED PROCESSED PRODUCTS

Value-added ginseng products presently being marketed include dried white and red roots, root slices, capsules, soft and hard gelatin capsules, tablets, extracts, wines, beverages, ice cream, cigarettes, soaps, cream lotions, and oil.

Lui and Staba [34] analysed Korean ginseng plants and products such as cigarettes and ginseng extracts (Table 10.4), and found very low levels of ginsenosides in processed products such as cigarettes. Liberti and Marderosian [52] tested ginseng tablets and teas and found that teas contained low concentrations of active ingredients. Soldati and Sticher [47] reported that there was

TABLE 10.4. Total Ginsenosides in Ginseng Plants and Products.

Material	Total Ginsenosides (g/100 g dry wt)
Plant roots	
P. quinquefolium (American)	5.9
P. quinquefolium (Canadian)	6.1
P. ginseng (Korean)	3.7
P. ginseng (China)	3.9
P. trifolium	0.8
P. japonicum	6.6
P. pseudoginseng	6.8
Plant leaves	
P. quinquefolium (American)	6.6
P. trifolium	3.3
Commercial products	
Korean ginseng cigarettes	None
P. ginseng capsules	2.5
P. ginseng soft gelatin	2.5
P. ginseng tablets	2.3
P. quinquefolium capsules	2.5
Extracts	
P. ginseng	21.9
P. quinquefolium	46.5

Source: Adapted from References [24, 29].

a wide range in the content of total ginsenosides in ginseng products such as extracts and hard gelatin capsules (Table 10.5). Ma et al. [29] tested over 60 commercial ginseng products and showed a wide range of total ginsenosides in *P. ginseng* tea, *P. quinquefolium* tea, *P. ginseng* tablets, *P. ginseng* capsules, *P. quinquefolium* capsules, and *P. ginseng* soft gelatin capsules (Table 10.5).

In the United States and Canada, no regulations require manufacturers to disclose or report types and amounts of active ingredients in ginseng products. In addition, there are no industry standards of quality control for these products. This is clearly an important issue that needs to be addressed in order to establish consumer confidence in value-added ginseng products.

1.5. MEDICINAL VALUES AND MECHANISMS OF ACTION

Ginseng is a very popular herb, used routinely by millions of healthy people to stimulate and maintain energy level and achieve a sense of well-being. Ginseng may be able to help maintain metabolic balance by eliciting a homeostatic effect [55]. Ginseng has been touted as an adaptogen [16], a substance that is harmless and ineffective in the absence of stress, but can return the body processes to normal when there is stress or damage irrespective of the source [56].

1.5.1. Effects on Stress and Fatigue

The effects of ginseng on stress and fatigue have long been expounded by Chinese herbalists. It is well known for its anti-stress and adaptogenic proper-

TABLE 10.5. Ginseng Value-Added Products and the Range of Their Total Ginsenosides.

Product	Total Ginsenosides (g/100 g dry wt)	Reference
Standardized ginseng extract	4.14–7.95	Soldati and Sticher [47]
Fluid ginseng extract	0.84–1.61	Soldati and Sticher [47]
Hard gelatin capsule	0–1.67	Soldati and Sticher [47]
P. ginseng tea	0.53–1.64	Ma et al. [29]
P. quinquefolium tea	0.25–9.05	Ma et al. [29]
P. ginseng tablets	0.62–5.88	Ma et al. [29]
P. ginseng capsules	2.45–2.63	Ma et al. [29]
P. quinquefolium capsules	2.53	Ma et al. [29]
P. ginseng soft gelatin capsules	2.00–6.71	Ma et al. [29]

ties, but only recently have these effects been scientifically examined. Various compounds in ginseng have been shown to increase nonspecific resistance to physical, chemical and biological stresses. Some of the manifestations include a decrease in body temperature, relaxing of muscle tone and analgesia [8,57]. In laboratory mice subjected to various stresses such as irradiation, bacterial infection and temperature extremes, survival rates are better in mice treated with ginseng than in those without. Further, rebound from behavioural and physiological stresses were found to be quicker in ginseng-treated animals than in nontreated controls. This anti-stress property has also been tested in humans. For example, hospital nurses treated with ginseng were able to stay awake and perform duties and not feel as fatigued as their nontreated counterparts [58]. This implies a more efficient use of body fuel reserves during physical activity and may be used to overcome the strain of exercise in humans. Indeed, it has been found that ginseng is able to reduce heart rate during strenuous exercise, reduce blood lactate, increase the efficiency of oxygen utilization, decrease reaction times, and increase pulmonary function [59].

In an experiment on the effect of *P. ginseng* on cold tolerance and recovery from acute hypothermia, Kumar et al. [60] found that laboratory rats fed an oil-based mixture of *P. ginseng* root extract and a multivitamin-mineral preparation at 0.5 ml/day was effective in developing resistance to cooling and in stimulating faster recovery from acute hypothermia. Wang and Lee [6] reported that rats receiving ginseng saponin at 10 and 20 mg/kg/day for 4 days significantly prolonged their aerobic endurance while exercising at approximately 70% VO_2 max. They concluded that both Rg_1 and Rb_1 can enhance aerobic endurance by altering fuel homeostasis during prolonged exercise, possibly through an increased free fatty acid utilization over that of glucose for cellular energy production.

1.5.2. Effects on Memory

Studies of patients with senile dementia of the Alzheimer type indicate that this disease is associated with degeneration of the cholinergic nerve tracts projecting from the medial forebrain complex to cortical and hippocampal regions [61]. In a laboratory study, Benishin et al. [62] found that the ginsenoside Rb_1 was able to improve memory deficits induced by anticholinergic drug treatment and facilitate acetylcholine release from rat brain hippocampal slices. The increase in acetylcholine release was associated with an increase in uptake of the precursor choline, and chronical administration of Rb_1 increased the maximum velocity of choline uptake in the hippocampus regions [63]. The specific effect of Rb_1 on cholinergic functions may warrant its further study for enhancing short-term memory acquisition and retention in senile dementia [64].

1.5.3. Effects on the Cardiovascular System

The effects of ginseng on the cardiovascular system have been extensively studied with contradictory results. After intensive exercise, heart rate in men was sustained at a lower level in a ginseng-treated group compared to non-treated controls [58]. Upon administration of ginseng, there is also increase in contraction force of heart and coronary blood flow [65]. It has been reported that ginseng is able to increase haemoglobin and erythrocyte counts in the blood of rats and mice [57], but these results have not been reproduced in humans.

Blood pressure can be affected by ginseng administration; however, the direction of effect is not agreed upon by all researchers. For example, some reports indicate decrease in blood pressure [56] while others report transient increases in blood pressure [57]. These discrepancies may be due to the different action of the individual ginsenosides. For instance, it has been reported that Rb_1 is capable of lowering blood pressure and acting as a depressant on the central nervous system with sedative and anti-stress properties, while Rg_1 has been shown to raise the blood pressure and stimulate central nervous system activity [8,66,67]. Lewis [55] indicated that the effects on blood pressure, either hypotension following vasodilation or hypertension subsequent to vasoconstriction, depended on the type of ginsenoside used or its preponderance in ginseng extracts. Kuku et al. [66] found that injection of Rg_1 (5–10 mg/kg) from *P. ginseng* caused a major fall in blood pressure and a decreased heart rate. However, with increased amount (30–100 mg/kg), blood pressure rose.

1.5.4. Effect on Immune System

You [68] reported that ginseng is able to act prophylactically as an anti-inflammatory agent in humans. It is also able to increase antibody levels, stimulate natural killer cells, and stimulate the release of the chemical messenger, interferon [69]. Interferon, in turn, can activate the immune system. Ginseng also possesses anti-complementary activity. The complement system is a complex set of proteins that acts as a defence against invading organisms or particles. A chemical from the leaves of *P. ginseng* that is considered anti-complementary of heteroglycans is able to alter the speed at which the complement system is able to recognize, attack and destroy pathogens [70].

1.5.5. Effect on Metabolism

Ginseng is able to lower cholesterol level in the blood either by stimulating cholesterol transport or stimulating an enzyme involved in cholesterol metabolism [71]. The decrease may also be due to an increased conversion of cholesterol into bile acids and/or the direct excretion of cholesterol [72]. Popov [73] also reported that ginseng has a beneficial effect on blood cholesterol, lowering the level from 280–310 mg% to less than 250 mg%, or adjusting the ratio between high-density lipoproteins (HDL) and low-density lipoproteins (LDL) [74]. Since LDL is linked to such conditions as atherosclerosis and heart disease, a reduction of LDL and a decrease in the HDL/LDL ratio favour maintenance of normal cardiovascular health.

Ginseng has also been studied for its effects on metabolism of nucleic acids, proteins and lipids; however, the results from these studies are highly contradictory [57]. More research is needed before general conclusions can be drawn.

1.5.6. Effect on reproductive system

Probably the most publicized effect of ginseng is its aphrodisiac effect. Although there is no evidence that sexual drive and performance are enhanced by taking ginseng [55], it has been believed for years that ginseng can be a stimulant for sexual activity. For example, several reports indicate that ginseng is able to promote spermatogenesis in rabbits, accelerate growth of ovaries and ovulation in frogs, stimulate egg laying in hens, and increase gonadal weight and testicular nucleic acid content in rats [75,76]. Research on ginseng and human reproductive systems has not been extensive; however, it has been tested as a treatment for impotence [77] and increasing sperm count [78] with positive results. Lewis [55] reported that ginseng may have a mild hormonal activity and pointed out that it should not be overlooked that many commercial aphrodisiac preparations contain modest amounts of ginseng.

1.5.7. Effect on Cancer

Recent potentially significant research has demonstrated that ginseng has an inhibitory effect on cancer development. You et al. [68] suggested that ginseng should be recognized as a functional food for cancer prevention. In a case-control study in the Korea Cancer Centre Hospital, Yun and Choi [79] reported, without mentioning the mechanisms involved, that the risk of oral pharyngal, stomach and liver cancers associated with smoking, was reduced with ginseng intake. Extract from ginseng root has also been found to inhibit active types of sarcoma, adenocarcinoma and leukemia. It is believed that ginseng exhibits a toxic effect against cancer cells by inhibiting the biosynthesis of macromolecules [57]. Mochizuki et al. [80] reported that in laboratory mice, ginsenoside Rg_1 displayed the ability to inhibit metastasis of lung tumour cells. You et al. [68] reported that three treatments, oral administration of ginseng extract, radiotherapy, and the combination of oral administration and radiotherapy, in combatting intrahepatic sarcoma-180 tumour cells in mice, increased life span by 15.4, 16.9 and 82.9%, respectively. Research on cancer inhibition by ginseng extracts is still in the early development stage. Results to date have been promising but more investigations are needed.

2. ECHINACEA

Echinacea is a North American native perennial plant of the Compositae family. It is indigenous to the prairies west of Ohio, from northern Texas to southern Canada, and occurs most abundantly in Nebraska and Kansas [81]. There are nine species in the genus *Echinacea* [82]. Among them, *E. purpurea* (L) Moench., *E. angustifolia* DC., and *E. pallida* Nutt. are the most popular and widely cultivated species [83]. *Echinacea* has been used for medicinal purpose for decades. It is used externally for snake bites [84] and internally for coughs, colds, infections, and inflammations [85]. Recently, laboratory and clinical research in Germany has confirmed its immunostimulatory, antiviral and antibacterial benefits to humans [86,87]. The consumption of *Echinacea* has increased rapidly in both Europe and North America in recent years and has become the best-selling medicinal health remedy in North America [88]. *Echinacea* is also widely planted as an ornamental [89] and is grown commercially for cut flowers [90].

Echinacea is winter hardy and drought resistant [91]. It produces a stout, hairy stem 30–100 cm in height. Leaves are 15–30 cm long, ovate to lanceolate, rough, hairy and contain 3–5 veins [82]. Roots are either in the form of a single taproot or fibrous [83]. Plants start to flower early summer to early fall in the second or third year, the color ranging from white or yellow to pink, rose or purple [92].

2.1. CULTIVATION

Echinacea can be propagated from seed, crown division and root sections [93]. In the wild, *Echinacea* grows in poor, rocky soil under full sun light. However, it thrives under cultivation in moderately rich and well-drained sandy loam soil with pH 6 to 7. Information on the nutrient requirements is very limited. A balanced fertilizer, low in nitrogen and with moderate levels of phosphorus and potassium, should be adequate [94].

Echinacea growers have commonly raised seedlings indoors which are transplanted to the field in the spring on flat beds, spaced at 30 cm apart in 120 cm wide beds [92]. It is not weed tolerant; thus, good weed control is an important factor to the success of cultivation. Thorough soil cultivation is essential for optimizing growth and yield. Normally, the roots do not reach desirable size until 3–4 years after sowing. Disease does not seem to be a problem with the *Echinacea* spp. [85], and very few cases of insect damage have been reported [95]. Nematodes are the potential pest in the soil and may cause a reduction of up to 10% in yield [96].

2.2. HARVEST AND VALUE-ADDED PRODUCTS

The best time to harvest flowers, leaves and roots for their maximum active ingredient content has yet to be determined. Normally, roots are harvested in the fall after the first frost has occurred, then washed and dried either in the air or in a forced-air dryer. Flowers can be harvested after pollination by cutting the stems 20 cm from the ground [94]. Leaves are claimed to represent a valuable source of active ingredients; however, there is no information on the best time to harvest the leaves, and on the effect of this operation on growth of the roots [92].

Many value-added health remedy products are available from North American health food stores and pharmacies in the forms of dry root, capsules, tablets, crude extracts, or tincture. Other forms, such as injectable preparations, are available in Germany [83]. *Echinacea* is also marketed in combination with other herbal products.

2.3. CHEMICAL COMPOSITION

Alkylamides [97], caffeic acid derivatives [98], polysaccharides [86] and polyacetylenes [99] are believed to represent the most important and valuable active ingredients of *Echinacea* (Figure 10.2). The contents of these active ingredients vary with species. The essential oil, representing 0.1% to 2% of the dry plant, and rich in borneol, and ∝-pinene [86], may find applications in the cosmetic industry [100]. Echinacein isolated from *E. angustifolia* and *E. pallida* is reported to have mosquito larvicidal effects [101].

2.4. MEDICINAL VALUES

Echinacea has been used as a health remedy more than any other herb since the beginning of the century [102]. Tinctures or crude extracts from *E. angustifolia* have been used for treating insect bites [103], snake bites [84] and wound healing [104].

From the medicinal perspective, the active ingredients of *Echinacea* include polysaccharides, flavonoids, caffeic acid derivatives, essential oils, polyacetylenes, and alkylamides. A number of water-soluble polysaccharides have been isolated with immunostimulatory and anti-inflammatory effects [86,105]. Caffeic acid derivatives are believed to be the most important pharmacologically effective compounds of *Echinacea*. Cichoric acid and chlorogenic acid were isolated and shown to have pharmaceutical properties [85]. Echinacin, an extract of *Echinacea purpurea*, has been used in veterinary

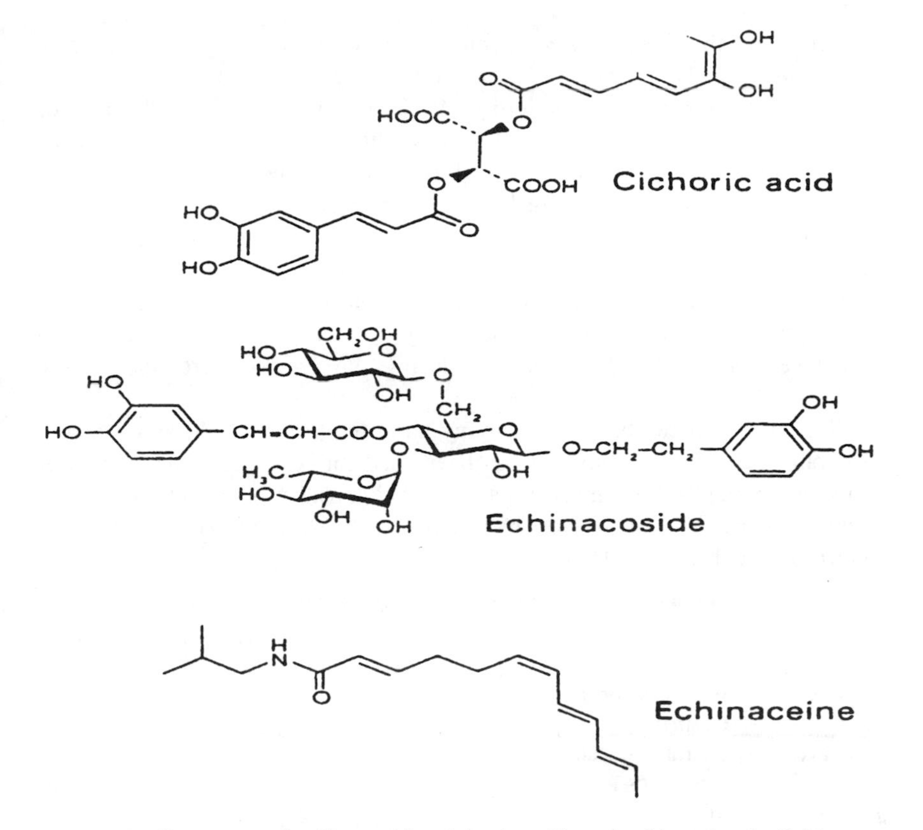

Figure 10.2 Structures of echinacoside, cichoric acid, and echinaceine in *Echinacea purpures*.

medicine to improve fertility [106] and puerperium [107] of heifers, and for the treatment of acute parenchymatous mastitis of cows [108].

3. SEA BUCKTHORN

Sea buckthorn (*Hippophae rhamnoides* L.) is a winter-hardy, deciduous shrub with yellow or orange berries [109]. It rapidly develops an extensive root system and is therefore an ideal plant for preventing soil erosion [110]. Sea buckthorn has also been used in land reclamation [111] for its ability to fix nitrogen and conserve other essential nutrients [112]. It can withstand temperatures from −43 to 40°C [113]. Although it is considered to be drought resistant [114], irrigation is needed in regions receiving <400 mm of rainfall per year for better growth [113].

There are three *Hippophae* species based on morphological variations: *H. rhamnoides* L., *H. salicifolia* D. Dom, and *H. tibetana* Schlecht [115]. A fourth species, *H. neurocarpa* Liu & He, was named in 1978 [116]. Sea buckthorn is distributed widely throughout the Himalayan regions in Asia [113] and on river banks and coastal dunes along the Baltic Coast and on the western coast along the Gulf of Bothnia in Europe [117].

Sea buckthorn is a deciduous, dioecious shrub, usually spinescent, reaching 2 to 4 m in height. It has brown or black rough bark and a thick grayish-green crown. Leaves are alternate, narrow, and lanceolate with a silver-grey color on the upper side [118]. Flower buds are formed mostly on 3-year-old wood, differentiated during the previous growing season [119].

Sea buckthorn can be used for many purposes (Figure 10.3) and has considerable economic potential. It has been used for centuries in its native Europe and Asia [109]. Recently, it has attracted considerable attention from researchers around the world, including North America, mainly for its nutritional and medicinal value.

Bark	→ Pharmaceuticals		
	→ Cosmetics		
Leaves	→ Pharmaceuticals		
	→ Cosmetics		
	→ Tea		
	→ Animal feeds		
Fruits	→ Volatile Oil	→ Pharmaceuticals	
		→ Drinks	
		→ Food Products	
		→ Cosmetics	
		→ Flavors and Fragrances	
	→ Juice	→ Sports drinks	
		→ Health drinks	
	→ Pulp	→ Ternary juice	→ Food
			→ Beverages
			→ Brewery
		→ Oil	→ Pharmaceuticals
			→ Cosmetics
		→ Residues	→ Animal feeds
Seeds	→ Oil	→ Pharmaceuticals	
		→ Cosmetics	
	→ Residues	→ Animal feeds	

Figure 10.3 Potential uses of components from different parts of sea buckthorn.

3.1. CULTIVATION

Sea buckthorn normally is transplanted or directly seeded in the spring. Best growth occurs in deep, well-drained, sandy loam soil with ample organic matter. In arid or semiarid areas, water must be supplied for establishment [109]. Soil acidity and alkalinity, except at extreme levels, are not limiting factors, although the shrub thrives best at pH 6 to 7. Sea buckthorn is sensitive to severe soil-moisture deficits, especially in spring when plants are flowering and young fruit are beginning to develop [113]. Like other crops, sea buckthorn requires adequate soil nutrients for a high yield of good-quality fruit. It responds well to phosphorus fertilizer. Nitrogen fertilization, on the other hand, can adversely affect root nodulation and delays the development of nodules after inoculation with *Frankia* [120].

Recommended plant spacing for sea buckthorn is 1 m within row and 4 m between rows to allow equipment access, with rows oriented in a north-south direction to provide maximum light [121]. High-density planting (1×1 m) is being considered in Europe to facilitate over-the-row harvesting equipment [122]. The ratio of male to female plants is important for maximizing the number of fruit-bearing trees. Recommendations for male:female ratio vary with plant density and region. For example, in British Columbia, with an orchard planting of 4000 trees per hectare, a 1:6 male:female ratio is considered adequate [123]. Moderate pruning of sea buckthorn increases the yield and fruiting of the plants. The crown should be pruned annually to remove overlapping branches, and long branches should be headed to encourage development of lateral shoots [109]. Weed control or vegetation management is very important in sea buckthorn plantings, especially for promoting growth of newly planted seedlings.

3.2. HARVESTING

Sea buckthorn berries persist on the branches all winter, due to the absence of abscission layer. This is undesirable for harvesting and became the major barrier to orchard production in Europe [122]. A number of methods for harvesting berries have been developed; most of them have both advantages and disadvantages. Some of the methods employed include: use of pneumatic shears to harvest entire fruiting shoots [124], a hand-picking device with two hinged jaws and teeth and brushes [125], and a pruning machine to trim sea buckthorn into a hedge suitable for mechanical harvesting [122]. In addition, Wolf and Wegert [121] described a method in which fruiting branches are removed and frozen overnight at $-36°C$ and frozen berries are removed by beating the branches. All of these methods are expensive and labour intensive. Therefore, development of a more economical method is considered a very high research priority and a limiting factor in the success of sea buckthorn as a viable cash crop [109].

3.3. CHEMICAL COMPONENTS

Sea buckthorn fruits are rich in carbohydrates, protein, organic acids, amino acids and vitamins [119]. The contents of these components vary with fruit maturity [126], fruit size [127], species [113] and geographic locations [128]. As shown in Table 10.6, the fruit contains 16 to 28 mg carotenoids/100 g of fruit [129], 310 to 2100 mg flavonoids/100 g dried leaf, and 120 to 1000 mg/100 g fruit, respectively [127]. The reported total volatile oil in the fruit is 36 mg/kg [130], dry matter is 24.6% to 33.8% [131], and oil extracted from seeds ranges from 8% to 12% (w/w) [113]. Saturated and unsaturated fatty acids are 47 to 53% of the fat from the fruit and 21% to 39% of the fat from the seed, respectively.

The vitamin C concentration (Table 10.7) ranges from 360 mg/100 g berry in European species [133,134] to 250 mg/100 g berry in Chinese species [110]. Thus, concentration of this vitamin in fruit of sea buckthorn is higher than in strawberry (64 mg) [135], kiwi (100–470 mg), orange (50 mg), tomato (12 mg), carrot (8 mg), and hawthorn (100–150 mg) [113]. As shown in Table 10.8, Lu [113] reported that vitamin E content in sea buckthorn (202.9 mg/100 g fruit) is also higher than wheat embryo (144.5 mg), safflower (3.3 mg), maize (34 mg) and soybean (7.5 mg).

TABLE 10.6. Chemical Components of Sea Buckthorn Fruits.

Component(s)	Content	Ref.
Carotene and carotenoid	16–28 mg/100 g fruit	Kudritskaya et al. [130]
Flavonoid (fruit)	120–2100 mg/100 g fruit	Chen et al. [128]
Flavonoid (leave)	310–2100 mg/100 g fruit	Chen et al. [128]
Volatile oil	3.6 mg/100 g fruit	Hisrvi and Honkanen [131]
Dry matter	24.6–33.8%	Igoshina et al. [132]
Oil (seed)	8.0–12.0%	Lu [113]
Saturated fatty acid (fruit)	47.0%	Franke and Muller [133]
Saturated fatty acid (seed)	21.0%	Franke and Muller [133]
Unsaturated fatty acid (fruit)	53.0%	Franke and Muller [133]
Unsaturated fatty acid (seed)	39.0%	Franke and Muller [133]

TABLE 10.7. Vitamin C Content (mg/100 g) of Sea Buckthorn (*H. rhamnoides*) and Other Fruits.

Fruit	Vitamin C (mg/100 g)	Reference
H. rhamnoides subsp. rhamnoides	360	Rousi and Aulin [134]; Yao et al. [135]
H. rhamnoides subsp. sinensis	250	Yao and Ticherstedt [110]
Strawberry	64	Gontea and Barduta [136]
Kiwi	100–470	Lu [113]
Orange	50	Lu [113]
Tomato	12	Lu [113]
Carrot	8	Lu [113]
Hawthorn	100–150	Lu [113]

Sea buckthorn is also high in protein, especially globulins and albumins [136], and fatty acids such as linoleic and linolenic acids [113].

3.4. MEDICINAL VALUES

Medicinal uses of sea buckthorn are well documented in Asia and Europe. Clinical tests on medicinal uses were first initiated in Russia during 1950s. Sea buckthorn oil was formally listed in the Pharmacopoeia in 1977 [137] and clinically tested in Russia and China. The most important pharmacological functions attributed to sea buckthorn oil include: anti-inflammatory, antimicrobial, pain relief and the promotion of tissue regeneration. Sea buck-

TABLE 10.8. Fatty Acids, Vitamin E, and β-Carotene in Sea Buckthorn and Other Plant Products.

Material	Linoleic and Linolenic Acid (%)	Vitamin E (mg/100 g)	β-Carotene (mg/100 g)
Sea buckthorn	64.6	202.9	248.9
Wheat embryo	—	144.5	—
Safflower	81.4	3.3	—
Maize	48.3	34.0	0.8
Soybean	62.8	7.5	0.1

Source: Adapted from Reference [113].

thorn oil is also recommended as a treatment for oral mucositis, rectum mucositis, vaginal mucositis, cervical erosion, radiation damage, burns, scalds, duodenal ulcers, gastric ulcers, chilblains, skin ulcers caused by malnutrition, and other skin damage [138,139,140]. According to an unconfirmed report from China, in a study with 350 patients, beauty cream made with sea buckthorn oil had positive therapeutic effects on melanosis, senile skin wrinkles and freckles [141].

3.5. VALUE-ADDED PRODUCTS

More than ten different drugs have been developed from sea buckthorn in Asia and Europe and are available in different forms, such as liquids, powders, plasters, films, pastes, pills, liniments, suppositories, and aerosols [109]. Sea buckthorn oil extracted from seeds is popular in cosmetic preparations, such as facial cream. Numerous products are made from sea buckthorn, including tea from leaves; beverages and jam from fruits; fermented products from pulp; and animal feeds from leaves, pulp and seed residues [109]. There is a very limited sea buckthorn industry in North America; however, unique products, especially those with superior nutritional quality, are gaining popularity. Development of a North American sea buckthorn industry presents a unique opportunity for production of a value-added crop on marginal land. A list of potential uses of components from different parts of sea buckthorn is given in Figure 10.3.

4. CONCLUSIONS

The herbal industry has expanded rapidly around the world. Thus, Asian and American ginseng and *Echinacea* are cultivated on a large scale and their products are used by millions of people for medicinal purposes. A full understanding of the nature of these fascinating crops is far from complete. More research is needed on improving cultural methods, better understanding of the active ingredients and their medicinal values, and the development of new value-added products for increased availability to consumers.

Sea buckthorn is a unique and valuable plant species currently being domesticated in various parts of the world. The plant has been used to a limited extent in North America for conservation plantings, but its use for food and nonfood application is only now beginning to be pursued.

There is an urgent need for a better understanding of the genetics, physiology, and biochemistry of ginseng, *Echinacea* and sea buckthorn, especially the biosynthetic pathways leading to the formation bio-active compounds such as ginsenosides. The physio-chemical properties, such as stability, reactivity, toxicity and mode of action both *in vitro* and *in vivo* of secondary metabolites used in the pharmaceutical industry, need to be understood. Improved methods of analysis for quality control of products also need to be developed and transferred to the industry. Herbal products need to be standardized with respect to composition of active ingredients, shelf life and dosage. Research is needed on how to minimize the content of fungicide residues, and to assist industry and regulatory agencies to set up standards for herbal products. Finally, further research on the pharmacological effects of ginseng, *Echinacea* and sea buckthorn are needed as available information is incomplete and often contradictory.

5. REFERENCES

1. Bae, H. W. 1978. "Introduction." Korean ginseng. 2nd ed. Bae, H. W., Korean Ginseng Res. Inst. Seoul, Republic of Korea. pp. 1–9.
2. Lewis, W. H. and V. E. Zenger. 1982. "Population dynamics of the American ginseng *Panax quinquefolium* (Araliacae)," Amer. J. Bot. 69:1483–1490.
3. Li, T. S. C. 1995. "Asian and American ginseng—a review," HortTechnology 5:27–34.
4. Hu, S. T. 1977. "A contribution to our knowledge of ginseng," Amer. J. Chinese Medicine. 5:1–23.
5. Liu, C. X. and P. G. Xiao. 1992. "Recent advances on ginseng research in China," J. Ethnopharmacol. 36:27–38.
6. Wang, L. C. H. and T. Lee. 1997. "Effect of ginseng saponins on exercise performance in non-trained rats," Appl. J. Physiology (in press).
7. Okuda, H. and R. Yoshida. 1980. Proc. 3rd Intl. Ginseng Symp. 1980. Seoul, Korea. pp. 53–57.
8. Muwalla, M. M. and N. M. Auirmeileh. 1990. "Suppression of avian hepatic cholesterogenesis by dietary ginseng," J. Nutr. Biochem. 1:518–21.
9. Baranov, A. 1966. "Recent advances in our knowledge of the morphology, cultivation and uses of ginseng (*Panax ginseng* C. A. Meyer)," Econ. Bot. 20:403–406.
10. Philbrick, C. Y. 1983. "Contributions to the reproductive biology of *Panax trifolium* L. (Araliaceae)," Rhodora 85:97–113.
11. Nguyen, T. N., V. D. Phan, C. L. Tran, M. D. Nguyen, S. Shibata, O. Tanaka and R. Kasai. 1995. "Pharmacognostical and chemical studies on Vietnamese ginseng, *Panax vietnamensis* Ha et Grushv. (Araliaceae)," J. Japanese Bot. 70:1–10.
12. Yu, Y. H. 1987. "Root rot diseases of *Panax ginseng* and their control in Korea," Korean J. Plant Pathol. 3:318–319.
13. Anonymous. 1990. An Industry Development Plan for British Columbia Ginseng Producers. British Columbia Ministry of Agriculture Fisheries and Food, The Associated Ginseng Growers of B.C., Simon Fraser Univ., and Agri. and Agri-Food Canada. 22 pp.
14. Persons, W. S., ed. 1994. American Ginseng Green Gold. Revised edition. Asheville, NC: Bright Mountain Books. 203 pp.
15. Smallfield, B. M., J. M. Follett, M. H. Douglas, J. A. Douglas, G. A. Pamenter, K. P. Svoboda, J. C. Laughlin and V. E. Brown. 1995. "Production of *Panax* spp. in New Zealand," Acta Hort. 390:83–91.

16. Xiao, P. G., Z. Y. Zhu, F. Q. Zhang, W. H. Zhu, J. T. Chen, G. D. Zhang and G. T. Liu. 1987. Ginseng Research and Cultivation. Beijing, China: Agri. Publ. House. 252 pp.
17. Kim, Y. H., Y. H. Yu, J. H. Lee, C. S. Park and S. H. Oh. 1990. "Effect of shading on the quality of raw, red and white ginseng and the contents of some minerals in ginseng roots," Korean J. Ginseng Sci. 14:36–43.
18. Bailey, W. G. 1990. "The adaptation of ginseng production of semi-arid environments: the example of British Columbia, Canada," Korean J. Ginseng Sci. 14: 297–309.
19. Oliver, A. 1996. Ginseng Production Guide for Commercial Growers. British Columbia Ministry of Agriculture, Fisheries and Food, 193 pp.
20. Li, T. S. C. and R. Utkhede. 1993. "Pathological and non-pathological diseases of ginseng and their control," Current Topics Bot. Res. 1:101–113.
21. Sholberg, P. L. and T. S. C. Li. 1996. "First report of powdery mildew on ginseng in North America," Plant Dis. 60:463.
22. Shibata S., O. Tanaka, T. Ando, M. Sado, S. Tsushima and T. Ohsawa. 1966. "Chemical studies on oriental plant drugs. XIV. Protopanaxadiol, a genuine sapogenins of ginseng saponins," Chem. Pharm. Bull. 14:595–600.
23. Choi, K. T. 1988. "Panax ginseng C. A. Meyer: Micropropagation and the in vitro production of saponins," Bajaj, Y. P. S., ed. Medicinal and Aromatic Plants I., Biotechnology in Agri. and Forestry 4. pp. 484–500.
24. Rashap, A. W., B. A. Braly and J. T. Stone. 1984. The Ginseng Research Institute's Indexed Bibliography. Rixbury, NY: Ginseng Res. Inst. 120 pp.
25. Han, Y. N., S. Y. Kim, H. Lee, W. I. Hwang and B. H. Han. 1992. "Pattern-analysis of *Panax ginseng* polysaccharide," Korean J. Ginseng Sci. 18:217–222.
26. Smith, R. G., D. Caswell, A. Carriere and B. Zielke. 1996. "Variation in the ginsenoside content of American ginseng, *Panax quinquefolius* L. roots," Can. J. Bot. 74:1616–1620.
27. Kubo, M., T. Tani, T. Katsuki, K. Ishizaki and S. Arichi. 1980. "Histochemistry. I. Ginsenosides in ginseng (*Panax ginseng* C. A. Meyer) root," J. Nat. Prod. (Lloydia) 43:278–283.
28. Tani, T., M. Kubo, T. Katsuki, M. Higashino, T. Hayashi and S. Arichi. 1981. "Histochemistry. II. Ginsenosides in ginseng (*Panax ginseng* C. A. Meyer) root," J. Nat. Prod. (Lloydia) 44:401–407.
29. Ma, Y. C., J. Zhu, L. Benkrima, M. Luo, L. Sun, S. Sain, K. Kont, and Y. Y. Plaut-Carcasson. 1995. "A comparative evaluation of ginsenosides in commercial ginseng products and tissue culture samples using HPLC," J. Herbs, Spices & Medicinal Plants 3:41–50.
30. Shibata, S., O.Tanaka, J. Shoji, and H. Saito. 1985. "Chemistry and pharmacology of *Panax*," Economic and Medicinal Plant Research. Wagner, H., H. Hikino and R. Norman, ed. Tokyo, Japan: Academic Press. pp. 217–284.
31. Tanaka, O. 1994. "Ginseng and its congeners," Food Phytochemicals for Cancer Prevention II. Ho, C. T., T. Osawa, M. T. Huang, and T. R. Rosen, ed. Washington, DC: Amer. Chem. Soc. pp. 335–341.
32. Schulten, H. R. and F. Soldati. 1980. "Identification of ginsenosides from *Panax ginseng* in fractions obtained by high-performance liquid chromatography by field desorption mass spectrometry, multiple internal reflection infrared spectroscopy and thin-layer chromatography," J. Chromatogr. 212:37–49.

33. Dou, D., H. Kawai, H. Fukushima, D. Q. Dou, Y. P. Pei, X. S. Yao, Y. J. Chen and Y. Wen. 1996. "Ginsenoside-la: a novel minor saponin from the leaves of *Panax ginseng*," Planta Medica. 62:179–181.
34. Lui, J. H. and E. J. Stara. 1980. "The ginsenosides of various ginseng plants and selected products," J. Natural Prod. 43:340–346.
35. Li, T. S. C., G. Mazza, A. C. Cottrell and L. Gao. 1996. "Ginsenosides in roots and leaves of American ginseng," J. Agri. Food Chem. 44:717–720.
36. Hansen, L. and P. M. Boll. 1986. "Polyacetylenes in araliaceae: Their chemistry, biosynthesis and biological significance," Phytochem. 25:285–293.
37. Fujimoto,Y., H. Wang, M. Satoh and N. Takeuchi. 1994. "Polyacetylenes from *Panax quinquefolium*," Phytochem. 35:1255–1257.
38. Hirakura, K., M. Morita, K. Nakajima, Y. Ikeya and H. Mitsuhashi. 1991. "Three acetylated polyacetylenes from the roots of *Panax ginseng*," Phytochem. 30:4053–4055.
39. Ahn, B. Z., S. I. Kim and Y. H. Lee. 1989. "Acetylpanaxydol and panaxydolchloroohydrin, two new poleyns from Korean ginseng with cytotoxic activity against L1210 cells," Archiv. der Pharmazie 322:223–226.
40. Konno, C., K. Sugiyama, M. Kano, M. Takahashi and H. Hikino. 1984. "Isolation and hypoglycaemic activity of panaxans A, B, C, D and E, glycans of *Panax ginseng* roots," J. Med. Plant Res. 50:434–436.
41. Konno, C. and H. Hikino. 1987. "Isolation and hypoglycemic activity of panaxans M, N, O and P, glycans of *Panax ginseng* roots," Internat. J. Crude Drug Res. 25:53–56.
42. Kiyohara, H., M. Hirano, X. G. Wen, T. Matsumoto, X. B. Sun and H. Yamada. 1994. "Characterisation of an anti-ulcer pectic polysaccharide from leaves of *Panax ginseng* C. A. Meyer," Carbohydr. Res. 263:89–101.
43. Gupta, R. 1991. "Agrotechnology of medicinal plants," Wijesekera, R. O. B. ed. The Medicinal Plant Industry. First edition. London, England: CRC Press. pp. 43–58.
44. Tetemnyi, P., ed. 1970. Intra-specific chemical taxa of medicinal plants. Budapest, Hungary: Akademia Kiado. 225 pp.
45. Zhao, S., R. Wang, Y. Liu and F. Li. 1992. "Studies on inheritance of major agronomic characters of *Panax ginseng*," Korean J. Ginseng Sci. 16:247.
46. Zhuang, W. G. 1990. "Prospects for ginseng breeding," J. Jinlin Agri. Univ. 12:98–101.
47. Soldati, F. and O. Sticher. 1980. "HPLC separation and quantitative determination of ginsenosides from *Panax ginseng, Panax quinquefolium* and from ginseng drug preparations," Planta Med. 38:348–357.
48. Soldati, F. and O. Tanaka. 1984. "*Panax ginseng:* relation between age of plant and content of ginsenosides," Planta Med. 50:351–352.
49. Betz, J. M., A. H. Der Morderosian and T. M. Lee. 1984. Proc. 6th N. Amer. Ginseng Conf. 1984, Guelph, Ontario. pp. 65–83.
50. Konsler, T. R., S. W. Zito, J. E. Shelton and E. J. Staba. 1990. "Lime and phosphorus effects on American ginseng II. Root and leaf ginsenoside content and their relationship," J. Amer. Soc. Hort. Sci. 115:575–580.
51. Han, B. H. 1978. "Chemical components of ginseng," Korean Ginseng. Bae, H. W. ed. Seoul, Korea: Korea Ginseng Research Inst. pp. 77–111.

52. Liberti, L. E. and A. Marderosian. 1978. "Evaluation of commercial ginseng products," J. Pharm. Sci. 67:1487–1489.
53. Chen, S. E. and E. J. Staba. 1978. "American ginseng. I. Large scale isolation of ginsenosides from leaves and stems," Lloydia 41:361–366.
54. Chung, N. J. 1978. Proc. 2nd Internat. Ginseng Symp. 1978, Seoul, Korea. pp. 115–134.
55. Lewis, W. H. 1988. "Ginseng: a medical enigma." Plants in Indigenous Medicine and Diet Biobehavioral Approaches. Etkin, N. L., ed., New York: Redgrave Publ. Co. pp. 290–305.
56. Fulder, S. 1977. "Ginseng: useless root or subtle medicine?" New Scientist 20:158–159.
57. Hikino, H. 1991. "Traditional remedies and modern assessment: the case of ginseng." The Medicinal Plant Industry. 1st edition. Wijesedera, R. O. B., ed., London, England, CRC Press. pp. 149–166.
58. Forgo, I. 1980. Proc. 3rd. Internat. Ginseng Symp. 1980, Seoul, Korea. pp. 11–14.
59. Tsung, S. I., C. Chen and S. Tang. 1964. "The sedative, fatigue relieving and temperature stress-combatting effects of Panax ginseng," Acta Physiol. Sinica 27:324–328.
60. Kumar, R., S. K. Grover, H. M. Divekar, A. K. Gupta, R. Shyam and K. K. Srivastave. 1996. "Enhanced thermogenesis in rats by *Panax ginseng,* multivitamins and minerals," Int. J. Biometeorol. 39:187–191.
61. Bartus, R. T., R. L. Dean, B. Beer and A. Lippa. 1982. "The cholinergic hypothesis of geriatric memory disfunction," Science 217:408.
62. Benishin, C. G., R. Lee, L. C. H. Wang and H. J. Liu. 1991. "Effects of ginsenoside Rb_1 on central cholinergic metabolism," Pharmacology 42:223–229.
63. Benishin, C. G. 1992. "Actions of ginsenoside Rb_1 on choline uptake in central cholinergic nerve endings," Neurochem. Internat. 21:1–5.
64. Wang, L. C. H. 1996. Proc. Prairie Medicinal and Aromatic Plants Conf., Olds, Alberta, Canada. Mar., 1996. pp. 103–106.
65. Kim, C. H., C. C. Choi, J. K. Kim, M. S. Kim, B. Y. Kim and H. J. Park. 1976. "Influence of ginseng on mating behaviour of male rats," Amer. J. Chinese Medicine 4:163–168.
66. Kuku, T., T. Miyata, T. Uruno, I. Saka and A. Kinoshita. 1975. "Chemicopharmacological studies on saponin of *Panax ginseng* C. A. Meyer. II. Pharmacological part," Arzneim.- Forsch. 25:539–547.
67. Bisset, N. G., ed. 1994. Herbal Drugs and Phytopharmaceuticals: A Handbook for Practice on a Scientific Basis, Boca Raton, FL:, CRC Press. 566 pp.
68. You, J. S., D. M. Hou, K. T. Chen and H. F. Huang. 1995. "Combined effects of ginseng and radiotherapy on experimental liver cancer," Phytotherapy Res. 9:331–335.
69. Wang, B. X., J. C. Cui and A. J. Liu. 1982. "The effect of polysaccharides of roots of *Panax ginseng* on the immune function," Yaoxue Xuebao 17:66–67.
70. Gao, Q. P., H. Kiyohara, J. C. Cyong and H. Yamada. 1991. "Chemical properties and anti-complementary activities of heteroglycans from the leaves of Panax ginseng," Planta Medica 57:132–136.

71. Koo, J. H. 1983. "The effect of ginseng saponin on the development of experimental atherosclerosis," Hanyang Uidae Haksulchi 3:273–276.
72. Yamamoto, M., T. Uemura, S. Nakama, M. Uemiya and A. Kumagai. 1983. "Serum HDL-cholesterol-increasing and fatty liver improving actions of Panax ginseng in high cholesterol diet-fed rats with clinical effect on hyperlipidemia in man," Amer. J. Clin. Med. 11:96–100.
73. Popov, I. M. 1975. Proc. Internat. Symp. Gerontology. Lugano-bioggio, Switzerland. pp. 121–127.
74. Schultz, J., F. H. Schultz Jr., R. Lowe and R. W. Woodley. 1981. Proc. 3rd Nat. Ginseng Conf. N. Carolina, U.S.A. pp. 45–50.
75. Rim, R. M. 1979. "Ultrastructural studies on the effects of Korean *Panax ginseng* on the cainterna of rat ovary," Amer. J. Chinese Med. 7:333–334.
76. Fahim, M. S., Z. Fahim, J. M. Harman, T. E. Clevenger, W. Mullins and E. S. E. Hafez. 1982. "Effect of *Panax ginseng* on testosterone level and prostate in male rats," Arch. Androl. 8:261–263.
77. McLeod, D. 1993. "The herbal treatment and management of impotence," Australian J. Medical Herbalism 5:41–44.
78. Shida, K., J. Shmazaki and E. Urano. 1970. "Clinical study on male infertility. II," Japanese J. Fertility and Sterility 15:113–118.
79. Yun, T. K. and S. Y. Choi. 1995. "Preventive effect of ginseng intake against various human cancers: a case-control study on 1987 pairs," Cancer, Epidemiology, Biomarkers & Prevention 4:401–408.
80. Mochizuki, M., K. Matsuzawa, Y. C. Yoo and I. Azuma. 1995. Proc. Korea-Japan Ginseng Symp. 1995. Seoul, Korea. pp. 41–44.
81. Stochberger, W. W. 1927. "Drug plants under cultivation," U.S.D.A. Farmers' Bull. 663. 38 pp.
82. McGregor, R. L. 1968. "The taxonomy of the genus *Echinacea* (Compositae)," The Univ. of Kansas Sci. Bull 48:113–142.
83. Awang, D. V. C. and D. G. Kindack. 1991. "Herbal medicine *Echinacea*," Can. Pharmaceutical J. 124:512–515.
84. Busing, K. 1952. "Hyaluronidasehemmung durch echinacin," Arzneim Forsh. 2:467–469.
85. Hobbs, C. R. 1989. The *Echinacea* handbook. Capitola: Botanica Press. 118 pp.
86. Bauer, R. and H. Wagner. 1991. "*Echinacea* species as potential immunostimulatory drugs," Economic and Medicinal Plant Research 5. Wagner, H. and N. R. Farnsworth, ed. pp. 253–321.
87. Parnham, M. J. 1996. "Benefit-risk assessment of squeezed sap of the purple coneflower (*Echinacea purpurea*) for long-term oral immunostimulation." Phytomedicine 3:95–102.
88. Rawls, R. 1996. "Europe's strong herbal brew," Chemical & Engineering News, Sept. 23, 1996, pp. 53–60.
89. Brown, E. 1986. "Some garden daisies and sunflowers," San Francisco: Pacific Hort. Foundation 47:24–28.
90. Starman, T. W., T. A. Cerny and A. J. MacKenzie. 1995. "Productivity and profitability of some field-grown specialty cut flowers," HortScience 30:1217–1220.
91. Chapman, D. S. and R. M. Auge. 1994. "Physiological mechanisms of drought

resistance in four native ornamental perennials," J. Amer. Soc. Hort. Sci. 119: 299–306.

92. Li, T. S. C. "*Echinacea:* Cultivation and medicinal value," HortTech. (in press).
93. Feghahati, S. M. J. and R. N. Reese. 1994. "Ethylene, light and pre-chill enhanced germination of *Echinacea angustifolia* seeds," J. Amer. Soc. Hort. Sci. 119:853–858.
94. Oliver, A., J. Price, T. S. C. Li and A. Gunner. 1995. "Echinacea: purple coneflower," British Columbia Min. Agri. Fisheries and Food Specialty Crops Infosheet. 8 p.
95. Williams, A. H. 1995. "New larval host plant and behaviour of *Chlosyne gorgone* (Lepidoptera: Nymphalidae)," Great Lakes Entomologist 28:93–94.
96. McKeown, A. W. and J. Potter. 1994. "Native wild grasses and flowers: new possibilities for nematodes," Agri-Food Res. in Ontario. Dec. pp. 20–25.
97. Schulthess, B. H., E. Giger and T. W. Baumann. 1991. "*Echinacea:* anatomy, phytochemical pattern, and germination of the achene," Planta Medica. 57:384–388.
98. Bauer, R. and S. Foster. 1991. "Analysis of alkamides and caffeic acid derivatives from *Echinacea simulata* and *E. paradoxa* roots," Planta Medica. 57:447–449.
99. Bauer, R., I. A. Khan and H. Wagner. 1988. "TLC and HPLC analysis of *Echinacea pallida* and *E. angustifolia* roots," Planta Medica. 54:426–430.
100. Delabays, N. and I. Slacanin. 1995. "Domestication and selection of new plant species of interest to the cosmetics industry," Revue Suisse de Viticulture, d'Arboricullture et d'Horticulture 27:143–147.
101. Jacobson, M. 1967. "The structure of Echinacein, the insecticidal component of American coneflower roots," J. Organic Chem. 32:1646–1647.
102. Gilmore, A. 1911. "Uses of plants by the Indians of the Missouri river region," Bur. Amer. 4th Ann. Rep. 33:368.
103. Hill, N., C. Stam, R. A. Van Haselen and R. A. Van-Haselen. 1996. "The efficacy of prikweg R. Gel in the treatment of insect bites: A double-blind, placebo-controlled clinical trial," Pharmacy World and Sci. 18:35–41.
104. Seidel, K. and H. Knobloch. 1957. "Nachweis und Vergleich der antiphlogistischen Wirkung antirheumatischer Medikamente Z," Für Rheum 16:231–238.
105. Tubaro, A. and E. Tragni. 1987. "Anti-inflammatory activity of a polysaccharide fraction of *Echinacea angustifolia,*" J. Pharm. Pharmacol. 39:567–569.
106. Fischer, K. D. 1976. "Experiments to improve the fertility results of heifers with Echinacin (extract of *Echinacea purpurea*)," Thesis. Tierarztliche Hochschule, Hannover. 44 pp.
107. Heimsoth, C. 1976. "Influence of prophylactic treatment with echinacin (extract from *Echinacea purpurea*) post partum in cows with reference to the puerperium and fertility," Thesis. Tierarztliche Hochschule, Hannover. 48 pp.
108. Otto, H. 1982. "Experiences with homeopathic treatment of acute parenchymatous mastitis in cows," Tierarztliche Umschau 37:732–734.
109. Li, T. S. C. 1996. "Sea buckthorn (*Hippophae rhamnoides* L.): a multipurpose plant," HortTech. 6:370–380.
110. Yao, Y. and P. M. A. Tigerstedt. 1994. "Genetic diversity in *Hippophae* L. and its use in plant breeding," Euphytica 77:165–169.

111. Schroeder, W. R. and Y. Yao. 1995. "Sea buckthorn: a promising multipurpose crop for Saskatchewan," Prairie Farm Rehabilitation Administration, Agriculture and Agri-Food Canada. 14 pp.
112. Akkermans, A. D. L., W. Roelofsen, J. Blom, K. Hussdanell and R. Harkink. 1983. "Utilization of carbon and nitrogen compounds by *Frankia* in synthetic media and in root nodules of *Alnus glutinosa, Hippophae rhamnoides* and *Datisca cannabina,*" Can. J. Bot. 61:2793–2800.
113. Lu, R. 1992. Sea Buckthorn: a Multipurpose Plant Species for Fragile Mountains. Intl. Ctr. Integrated Mountain Development, Karmandu, Nepal. 62 pp.
114. Heinze, M. and H. J. Fiedler. 1981. "Experimental planting of potash waste dumps. I. Communication: pot experiments with trees and shrubs under various water and nutrient conditions," Archiv für Acker- und Pflanzenbau und Bodenkunde 25:315–322.
115. Rousi, A. 1971. "The genus *Hippophae* L., a taxonomic study," Ann. Bot. Fennici 8:177–227.
116. Liu, S. W. and T. N. He. 1978. "The genus *Hippophae* from the Quin-Zing Plateau," Acta Phytotzxonomica 16:106–108.
117. Bidwas, M. R. and A. K. Biswas. 1980. "In desertification, control the deserts and create pastures," Environ. Sci. Applications 12:145–182.
118. Synge, P. M. 1974. Dictionary of Gardening: a Practical and Scientific Encyclopaedia of Horticulture. 2nd ed. Oxford: Clarendon Press. 235 pp.
119. Bernath, J. and D. Foldesi. 1992. "Sea buckthorn (*Hippophae rhamnoides* L.): A promising new medicinal and food crop," J. Herbs, Spices, Medicinal Plants 1:27–35.
120. MacKay, J., L. Simon and M. Laionde. 1987. "Effects of substrate on the performance of in vitro propagated *Alnus glutinosa* clones inoculated with Sp+ and Sp-*Frankia* strains," Plant and Soil 103:21–31.
121. Wolf, D. and F. Wegert. 1993. Experience Gained in the Harvesting and Utilization of Sea Buckthorn. Cultivation and Utilization of Wild Fruit Crops. Wolf, D., ed., Germany: Bernhard Thalacker Verlag Gmbh. & Co. pp. 23–29.
122. Olander, S. 1995. Proc. Intl. Sea Buckthorn Workshop 1995. Beijing, China. pp. 151–158.
123. Li, T. S. C. and C. McLoughlin. 1997. Sea Buckthorn Production Guide. Canada Seabuckthorn Enterprises Ltd. Peachland, British Columbia. pp. 18.
124. Koch, H. J. 1981. "Cultivation of sea buckthorn for fruit production for the fruit processing industry," Gartenbau 28:175–177.
125. Botenkov, V. P. and N. M. Kuchukov. 1984. "Device for collecting fruits of *Hippophae rhamnoides,*" Lesnoe Khozyaistvo 2:46–47.
126. Bounous, G. and E. Zanini. 1988. "The variability of some components and biometric characteristics of the fruits of six tree and shrub species," Hort. Abstr. 60:4153.
127. Chen, T. G., M. K. Ni, R. Li, F. Ji, and T. Chen. 1991. "Investigation of the biological properties of central Asian sea buckthorn growing in the province of Kansu, China," Chem. Natural Compounds 27:119–121.
128. Wang, S. 1990. "Studies on the chemical components in fruits of *Hippophae rhamnoides,*" Forest Res. 3:98–102.

129. Kudritskaya, S. E., L. M. Zagorodskaya and E. E. Shishkina. 1989. "Carotenoids of the sea buckthorn, variety Obil'naya," Chem. Natural Compounds 25:724–725.

130. Hirvi, T. and E. Honkancn. 1984. "The aroma of the fruit of sea buckthorn, *Hippophae rhamnoides* L," Zeitschrift fur Lebensmittel-Untersuchung und Forschung 179:387–388.

131. Igoshina, V. G., M. A. Korovina, V. E. Lobzhanidze and I. P. Eliscev. 1987. "Diversity of forms of *Hippophae rhamnoides* L. in Georgia," Rastitelnye Resursy 23:190–196.

132. Franke, W. and H. Muller. 1983. "A contribution to the biology of useful plants. 2. Quantity and composition of fatty acids in the fat of the fruit flesh and seed of sea buckthorn," Angewandre Botanik 57:77–83.

133. Rousi, A. and H. Aulin. 1977. "Ascorbic acid content in relation to ripeness in fruit of six *Hippophae rhamnoides* clones from Pyharanta, SW Finland," Ann. Agr. Fenn. 16:80–87.

134. Yao, Y., P. M. A. Tigerstdet and P. Joy. 1992. "Variation of vitamin C concentration and character correlation between and within natural sea buckthorn (*Hippophae rhamnoides* L.) Populations," Acta Agr. Scand. 42:12–17.

135. Gontea, I. and Z. Barduta. 1974. "The nutrient value of fruits from *Hippophae rhamnoides,*" Igiena 23:13–20.

136. Solonenko, L. P. and E. E. Shishkina. 1983. "Proteins and amino acids in sea buckthorn fruits," Biologiya, Khimiya i Farmakologiya Oblepikhi 1983, 67–82.

137. Xu, M. 1994. "The medical research and exploitation of sea buckthorn," Hippophae 7:32–84.

138. Abartene, D. Y. and A. I. Malakhovskis. 1975. "Combined action of a cytostatic preparation and sea buckthorn oil on biochemical indices. Part 2 hisphen," Lietuvos TSR Mokslu Akademijos Darbai Serija C. Biologijos Mokslai 1:167–171.

139. Buhatel, T., S. Vesa and R. Morar. 1991. "Data on the action of sea buckthorn oil extract in the cicatrization of wounds in animals," Buletinul Institutului Agronomic Cluj-Napoca Seria Zootechnie si Medicina Veterinara 45:129–133.

140. Chen, J. H. 1991. "Effect of the immunomodulating agent (BCG) and the juice of HRL on the activity of splenic NK cells and LAK cells from tumour bearing mice," Chinese J. Microbiol. Immunol. 11:105–108.

141. Zhong, C., X. Zhang and R. Shu. 1989. Proc. Intl. Symp. Sea buckthorn, Xian, China. pp. 322–324.

CHAPTER 11

Functional Milk and Dairy Products

P. JELEN[1]
S. LUTZ[2]

1. INTRODUCTION

MANY traditional products manufactured by the dairy industry can be considered foods with physiological functionality. Dairy products such as fluid milk, cheese, yogurt, and many others have been recognized for a long time as excellent sources of several important vitamins and minerals including riboflavin, phosphorus and calcium (Table 11.1). In various countries with a "western-type" diet, dairy products are the principal calcium source, providing about 60–75% of the total calcium intake [1]. Although calcium and calcium compounds are poorly soluble in aqueous systems, the principal milk protein, casein, has the ability to bind calcium in a nutritionally accessible state with phosphorus, creating one of nature's best physiologically functional food systems. Riboflavin is another important milk nutrient, as milk contains about 170 μg/100 g [2] and is the single most important source of this vitamin; about 30% of the human requirements for this vitamin is estimated to be supplied by milk and dairy products [3].

Similarly, fermented dairy products such as yogurt, kefir or various other types of sour milk have been the focus of health-related interests of scientists from the days of Metchnikoff [4]. In this case, the physiological functionality

[1]Department of Agricultural, Food and Nutritional Science, University of Alberta, Edmonton, AB, Canada.
[2]Food Processing Development Centre, Alberta Agriculture, Food and Rural Development, Leduc, AB, Canada.

TABLE 11.1. Milk and Dairy Products as Sources of Important Nutrients.

		Product				
Component	Unit	Whole Milk	Cheddar Cheese	Cottage Cheese	Yogurt[a]	Ice Cream
Protein	%	3.30	25.4	12.6	4.30	4.40
Calcium	%	0.12	0.72	0.08	0.16	0.15
Phosphorus	%	0.10	0.50	0.14	0.13	0.11
Riboflavin	mg%	0.17	0.45	0.24	0.21	0.25

[a]Milk fortified with 3% n. f. d. m..
Source: Reference [97].

is ascribed to the dairy bacteria and the metabolic products of their interaction with the milk medium. Metchnikoff's early studies have focused on longevity of life resulting from consumption of yogurt and other fermented dairy products, and this notion is still widely responsible for the popularity of yogurt as a consumer product with a healthful image. A new yogurt-like product, Gaio, was launched by the Danish MD Foods company in 1993 [5] capitalizing on the image of special healthful properties using bacterial cultures coming from the Caucassus region and claiming to reduce blood cholesterol. A recent review of the literature on the relationship between consumption of milk and fermented dairy products and blood cholesterol levels [6] showed that the effect may be hypocholesterolimic, especially for fermented dairy foods. The International Dairy Federation (IDF) Group of Experts F-20 has produced highly valuable information on various subjects related to fermented dairy products and human health [7].

Milk, intended as the first food for the mammalian neonate, contains various components with physiological functionality. The amounts and types of the physiologically active components in milk of various mammalian species vary, depending on the needs of the offspring, especially with respect to its immunological status. Cow's milk, the predominant raw material used for the manufacture of dairy products worldwide, contains a relatively high amount of immunoglobulins and other physiologically active compounds that are required for the protection of the newly born calf. In this context, bovine colostrum is especially important as it is the first food of the newly born calf, which will not have acquired the necessary immune responses *in utero* as is the case with human neonates. The calcium content of cow's milk (about 1120 mg/L) is much higher than that of the human milk (280 mg/L) due in part to the differences in the content of casein, the carrier of much of the milk calcium [1]. In Table 11.2, the composition of cow's, goat's and human milk is compared in general terms and more specifically with respect to their protein

TABLE 11.2. Proximate Composition and Protein Contents (%) of Cow's, Goat's and Human Milk.

	Cow	Goat	Human
Total solids	12.5	13.0	12.9
Fat	3.1	4.5	3.8
Lactose	4.8	4.1	7.1
Minerals	0.7	0.8	0.2
Protein	3.4	2.9	1.0
Casein	2.8	2.6	0.4
Total whey protein	0.6	0.6	0.5

fractions, containing several species of physiologically active compounds, especially physiologically active peptides (see Sections 5 and 6 below). This review is limited to cow's milk, its various biologically active components that are important for human applications and biological activity of dairy products related to technologies used by the contemporary dairy industry.

2. TECHNOLOGICAL PROCESSES FOR MAXIMUM PHYSIOLOGICAL FUNCTIONALITY

Traditional dairy processing techniques were developed largely before the focus on physiological functionality became an important determinant of nutritional quality. In many cases, the existing techniques serve the traditional needs of manufacturing dairy foods with optimal sensory qualities rather than optimal physiological functionality. For example, manufacture of cottage cheese, or in central Europe, quark, results in products that have high consumer appeal but poor calcium and poor vitamin B-2 (riboflavin) content. These physiologically valuable components are discarded in the whey which, until recently, has been largely unutilized. With the present interest in functional foods, new processing techniques (often based on membrane technology) will likely be utilized to produce modified products that better fit the current consumer expectations. The various membrane techniques available today [8] are capable of fractionating liquid systems such as milk or whey into streams containing components of varying molecular size or charge; this can be utilized to extract certain components of desired biological activity from the rest of the stream without altering its overall technological functionality. As the membrane processes operate on the principle of mechanical separations based on particle size selectivity, they can be used to execute fractionations of the desired liquid milk components. For example, the calcium content of acid-coagulated cheeses such as quark or cottage cheese may be increased by retaining the calcium-containing casein micelles before the subsequent acidification. While initial trials with quark produced by membrane technology [9] have shown that such optimization for maximum calcium retention may lead to serious sensory defects such as bitterness, the problem has been overcome as evidenced by the current industrial uses of ultrafiltration (UF) for production of quark and other fresh cheeses in Germany and several other countries. When the milk is preconcentrated by ultrafiltration to the desired final total solids concentration of a cheese before converting the "pre-cheese" stream into the final product [10], the result is the retention of the complete whey protein fraction in the cheese, thus increasing not only the yield of the operation, but also the potentially beneficial content of the various physiologically active components of the whey protein fraction (see Section 5 below). This approach is particularly suitable for fresh cheese production as widely practiced in France, while for the more traditional semi-hard cheeses, technological difficulties resulting from the inclusion of the whey protein fraction still need to be overcome.

One of the membrane techniques with rapidly increasing utilization in the dairy industry, the process of microfiltration (MF), can be advantageously used either to augment the traditional separation processes, such as centrifugation for fat removal, or to complement and/or replace the heating processes such as pasteurization for bacterial control [11]. Use of MF for removal of pathogenic or spoilage bacteria from liquid milk is now feasible [12] and may in principle be used to replace certain severe heating processes such as high-temperature pasteurization to protect heat–sensitive physiologically active compounds. As the sizes of the casein micelles are distinctly different from those of the whey protein molecules, the MF can be used to separate these two milk protein types. In a potentially important use of MF for processing of functional food products, the total milk protein fraction can be processed into casein-enriched, whey protein-reduced milk desirable for cheese production, whereas the resulting "native" whey can be utilized as an excellent source of several biologically active components [11]. Currently, the whey streams originating from traditional cheesemaking or casein processing have become an important raw material for production of functional food ingredients; however, as these wheys may contain additional components originating from some of the cheesemaking steps (e.g., chymosin action on the casein or the fermentation activities of the starter cultures), the nonuniformity of the raw material composition may cause technological complications that can be minimized by the microfiltration preprocessing of the milk.

Membrane separation processes are also likely to become the cornerstone of most novel technologies being developed for production of functional dairy products, such as bioactive peptides, based on enzymatic or microbial modifications of traditional dairy components. The downstream processing of functional food ingredients with increased physiological functionality often includes water removal by concentration followed by drying. Traditional processes such as vacuum evaporation or spray drying may need to be modified, as heat applied even under the most carefully controlled conditions is sometimes damaging to the biological functionality. Processes such as reverse osmosis, nanofiltration, freeze-concentration, or freeze-drying will likely find increased use in the production of these novel products.

Technological developments in the area of genetic engineering also may be expected to accelerate utilization of cow's milk as a major source of functional foods and ingredients. Techniques such as transgenesis [13], intramammary gene insertion [14], or immuno-induction [15] may lead to production of "natural" cow's milk with increased content of the specific physiologically functional components. As a result, development of new classes of traditional dairy products with added physiological functional value may be expected in the future and traditional technologies may have to be adapted to accommodate the "new" milk with modified technological properties.

Cultured dairy products such as buttermilk, kefir and other sour-milk types, and especially yogurt, have been the focus of many studies in terms of their alleged physiological functionality. In contrast to the biologically active components contained in the milk itself, the health-promoting effects of the cultured dairy products may be related to the biological activity of the bacteria used in the production of these foods and the metabolites generated during the fermentation processes. While in principle the processing of cultured dairy products is not complex (consisting primarily of incubation of the inoculated milk under controlled temperature conditions in batch tanks or in the retail packages as in the case of set yogurt), processing steps such as heat and membrane treatments, as well as product formulation, may need to be modified to accommodate growth conditions of new strains of bacteria capable of producing increased levels of the physiologically active compounds in these "traditional" products. Alternatively, as in the production of the probiotic yogurts, some of the desirable bacteria may be added as concentrated cultures after completion of the fermentation process. Survival of these probiotic bacteria (usually *Lactobacilus acidophilus* and the bifidobacteria) needs to be achieved in numbers high enough (typically above 10^6 cfu/ml) to be of physiological importance to the consumer [16]. The environment of the finished product including acidity or O_2 content has a major effect on the final viability of the added cultures [17]. This may also require reformulation, changes in the conduct of the fermentation process, use of adjuncts to stimulate the growth of the bacteria, new packaging materials, and perhaps other adjustments of the traditional processing technologies.

3. FERMENTED DAIRY PRODUCTS, PROBIOTICS, PREBIOTICS, AND SYNBIOTICS

Traditional fermented dairy products such as yogurt, kefir and kumis have been consumed for many generations in Europe, Asia and Africa. Identification of the micro-organisms responsible for the fermentation and our ability to prepare pure starter cultures have led to the development of more standardized commercial products including acidophilus milk (Lactobacilli), yogurt (Lactobacilli and Streptococci), and bifidus milk (Bifidobacteria). Since 1908, when Metchnikoff [4] theorized that fermented milk products provided health benefits, including longer life expectancy, these probiotic products have been viewed as "healthy" by consumers. The generally accepted definition of probiotics is that they are live microbial food or feed supplements that benefit humans and animals by improving the microbial balance in the intestine.

The major strains of bacteria used in probiotics, *Lactobacillus acidophilus* and various *Bifidobacterium* spp., are dominant organisms in human small and large intestines, respectively. These micro-organisms may play a role in inhibiting the growth of pathogenic organisms through production of organic acids and bacteriocins and by deconjugation of bile salts [18]. The prevalence of these organisms in the intestines may be reduced with age, dietary changes, antibiotic consumption, and/or stress, and their absence or low viability may cause varying degrees of digestive problems [19]. The effect of the consumption of active cultures to balance such losses has been under investigation for the past few decades.

Initial studies to substantiate the health benefits of consuming probiotics yielded many negative results. These reports need to be reviewed in light of our current knowledge of conditions required to achieve positive results, including: therapeutic cultures used must be highly acid and bile tolerant [20]; product must contain 10^6 viable organisms per ml [21]; product quantities greater than 100 ml should be consumed at least twice per week; and cultures should produce organic acids and other biologically active compounds in the gastrointestinal tract [22]. The test procedures that have been used to select organisms that meet these criteria have been reviewed by Kurmann and Rasic [16]. Commercial cultures of various species of *Lactobacillus acidophilus* and *Bifidobacterium* that meet these criteria are now available.

Yogurt is traditionally manufactured by fortifying whole or skimmed milk by evaporation or addition of skim milk powder, heating to 85–95°C for 10–30 minutes and inoculating with *Streptococcus thermophilus* and *Lactobacillus delbrueckii subsp. bulgaricus,* and then incubating at 42–45°C. Bifidus yogurts may be prepared by the addition of bifidobacteria, such as *B. bifidum* or *B. longum,* to the yogurt culture and incubating at 42°C for 3–4 hours. It is also possible to add bifidus cultures or bifidus milk to finished yogurt. Bifidus milk is prepared in a similar manner to yogurt, except it is cultured with approximately 10% of a starter culture of *B. bifidum* or *B. longum* and incubated at 37–42°C. *L. acidophilus* may be cultured to create acidophilus milk or may be used in combinations, such as with a yogurt culture to create an acidophilus yogurt. Additional blends are also being investigated such as *L. reuteri, L. plantarum* and *L. caseii* [23]. While yogurt is widely consumed in western diets, a wide variety of cultured products are now available worldwide such as Nu-Trish a/B, USA (acidophilus + bifidus); AB-yogurt, Denmark (acidophilus + bifidus + yogurt culture); Miru-Miru, Japan (acidophilus + *L. casei* + *B. breve*); Biogarde ice cream, Germany (acidophilus + *B. bifidum*); Real Active, United Kingdom (bifidus + yogurt culture); Cultura drink, Denmark (bifidus + acidophilus); and Bifighurt, Germany (*B. longum* + *S. thermophilus*) [16,24].

The amount of research being conducted in the area of probiotic dairy products, probiotic cultures and health benefits to humans or animals is vast and its review is beyond the scope of this work. In terms of the alleged health benefits, research studies available to date have demonstrated the following potential benefits: growth promotion in studies with rat and poultry [25,26]; production of riboflavin, niacin, thiamin, vitamin B_6, vitamin B_{12}, and folic acid [27,28]; increase in absorption of minerals [25]; increase in immune response through increased production of secretory immunoglobulin A [27,29]; decrease in populations of pathogens through the production of acetic and lactic acids as well as other bacteriocins [30–32]; reduction in lactose intolerance through consumption of *L. acidophilus*-containing products [33]; suppression of potentially harmful microbial enzymes associated with colon cancer in animals [27,34]; stabilization of intestinal microflora especially after severe gastrointestinal problems or the use of antibiotics [30,35]; relief of constipation [22]; reduction of serum cholesterol [36,37]; and inhibitory effects against mutagenicity [38]. Although many of these studies appear promising, much additional research is required to substantiate these claims.

The beneficial effects of the presence of bifidobacteria in the gastrointestinal tract are dependent on their viability and metabolic activity, aided by the presence of complex carbohydrates and other bifidogenic factors. To maximize the effectiveness of the bifidus-containing products, the bifidogenic factors are often included in the product itself. A recent review by Modler [39] lists several types of oligosaccharides and other bifidogenic factors, including some of dairy origin, as shown in the Table 11.3. In recent years, lactose has been one of the substrates used for production of bifidogenic factors such as lactulose, lactitol, or lactosucrose. Bifidogenic factors are also found in many natural sources including chicory, Jerusalem artichokes, onion, leek, and other plants. One such factor, inulin (a longer-chain oligosaccharide with a degree of polymerization higher than 30) has been available commercially for use in probiotic yogurts and other dairy products. In general, the bifidogenic

TABLE 11.3. Common Oligosaccharides and Other Bifidogenic Products Available Commercially.

Source	Product	Estimated Annual Production (t)
Lactose (milk)	Lactulose	20,000
	Lactosucrose	1,600
	Lactitol	n/a
Chicory, Jerusalem artichoke	Fructo-oligosaccharides	12,000
Starch	Malto- and isomalto-oligosaccharides	21,000
Soybean	Raffinose, stachyose	2,000

Source: Reference [25].

factors are mostly short-chain oligosaccharides (3–10 monosaccharide units) with unique functional properties, as they are not well digested by stomach acids and appear to stimulate the growth of bifidobacteria and lactobacillus, increase bioavailability of Ca and Mg, and prevent some stages in carcinogenesis [40,41].

The term "prebiotic" has been applied to products such as oligosaccharides, which promote the growth of beneficial organisms. Oligosaccharides have been recognized for their health benefits in Japan and since the early 1990s many products, especially drinks, have been developed and are being promoted for their oligosaccharide content. Products that contain both prebiotics and probiotics are sometimes referred to as "synbiotics." Synbiotic products such as the SymBalance yogurt (*Lac. reuteri, Lac. acidophilus, Lac. casei,* bifidobacteria, inulin) produced by Tonilait in Switzerland and Dutch Fysiq (*Lac. acidophilus* + Raftiline brand prebiotic) are now being marketed in Europe [42].

In North America, the 1970s and early 1980s were the period of "learning about yogurt," resulting in a large growth in the yogurt market. In the late 1980s and early 1990s, Europe has led the development of a new group of probiotic products. Countries such as France, which permit a bifidogenic health claim, have seen public awareness of bifidus and acidophilus increase to 80% and probiotics growing to 9% of the yogurt market by 1994 [23]. Recent FAO statistics [43] indicate that in Germany, the sales of probiotic products in 1996–97 have skyrocketed, reaching 5,927 tons compared to 1,925 tons a year earlier. These increases in consumption of new probiotic and synbiotic dairy products marketed by national and international companies indicate that the dairy industry will continue to play a leading role in this segment of the functional food market.

4. CASEIN-BASED BIOACTIVE PEPTIDES

Casein is the main protein component of milk, constituting about 80% of the total milk protein fraction. Until recently, the main physiological role of casein in the milk system was seen as the source of amino acids needed for the growth of the neonate. However, more recently, Holt [44] proposed the view that the main physiological importance of the casein micelle system appears to be the prevention of pathological calcification of the mammary gland. The inclusion of the calcium and phosphorus in the casein micelle structure appears to be in the form of "nanoclusters," allowing the retention and transport of these important but poorly soluble minerals to the recipient growing infant organism without the danger of calcium precipitation in the milk-producing tissues.

While no specific physiological property has been indicated for the total casein or the individual casein fractions (Table 11.4), the various peptides "hidden" in the casein amino acid sequence have been the subject of intensive studies in the recent past [45]. The most important casein-related bioactive peptides are casomorphins, possessing opioid-like activity; immunopeptides, providing immunostimulating activity; peptides with antihypertensive activity; and phosphopeptides having the ability to sequester calcium and possibly other minerals, thus acting as biocarriers [46]. Much research regarding the bioactive peptides is currently underway regarding their production by selective enzymatic hydrolysis [47] or specific activities that until now have been demonstrated primarily *in vitro* or, at best, in animal models. A recent comprehensive review of the subject of bioactive peptides [48] confirmed that most of the alleged physiological properties of the bioactive casein-based

TABLE 11.4. Main Casein and Whey Protein Fractions of Cow's Milk.

Fraction	Content (g/L)	Percent (w/w) of Total Milk Protein
Total casein	**26.0**	**80.0**
α_s-casein	13.0	39.0
β-casein	9.3	28.4
κ-casein	3.3	10.1
Total whey protein	**6.0**	**19.3**
β-lactoglobulin	3.2	10.0
α-lactalbumin	1.2	3.1
Serum albumin	0.3	1.2
Immunoglobulins	0.7	2.0
Other[a]	0.8	2.4

[a]Including lactoferrin, lysozyme and lactoperoxide.
Source: Adapted from Reference [98].

peptides remain to be proven in humans. Nevertheless, various industrial products are already being produced and marketed by several industrial processors. Table 11.5 lists several such products being offered by one large international dairy company.

Studies of the claimed effectiveness of the bioactive peptides involving human subjects are scarce. In one such study, [49] normotensive and slightly hypertensive volunteers were used to investigate the possible application of a hydrolyzate of casein as a hypertension-preventing food ingredient. A review on the subject of antihypertensive peptides from various sources [50] has indicated that while such peptides have been isolated from many plant or animal sources, their efficacy and safe use in humans as an alternative to drug medication still need to be investigated. Similarly, the ability of casein phosphopeptides (CPP) to bind calcium has been known for some time [51–53], but whether these peptides are effective enhancers of calcium metabolism (transport, absorption and/or utilization in bone mineralization) is not clear, and further studies with humans are required. Even some of the animal studies [54,55] could not demonstrate any improvement of the calcium metabolism resulting from the CPP-containing diet. Despite the need for more conclusive clinical trials, CPP products are being marketed in Australia as anticariogenic agents for use in foods and in products for personal hygiene [15].

TABLE 11.5. Examples of Commercially Available Physiologically Functional Dairy Products.

Product Class	Product	Claimed Properties
Bioactive peptides	Glutamine peptide	Maintain immune system Regulate protein turnover Glycogen replenishment
	Peptide FM	Inhibit dietary fat deposition Alter fat metabolism
	Casein phosphopeptides	Enhance Ca absorption Enhance Fe absorption Prevention of dental caries
Bioactive proteins	Lactoperoxidase	Promote beneficial intestinal flora Probiotic effects
	Lactoferrin	Regulate iron transport and absorption Promote beneficial intestinal flora
Bioactive minerals	Lactoval (natural milk calcium/mineral complex)	Enhance Ca absorption

Source: Based on technical literature of DMV International Co.

Several alternatives exist for delivery of the bioactive peptides to the consumer. Marshall [56] lists three common methods that can be relied upon in this regard: (a) regular meal digestion resulting in enzymatic hydrolysis of suitable protein sources included in the meal; (b) production of the bioactive peptides by bacteria in fermented foods, as demonstrated e.g., by the identification of casomorphins in milk incubated with various bacteria [57,58]; or (c) manufacture of functional food products containing industrially produced bioactive peptides.

The process technologies required to produce bioactive peptides are in most cases highly proprietary. In general, these processes are likely to be based on hydrolysis involving either enzymes and/or heat and/or acid/alkali conditions. The scarce publicly available information indicates that membrane separations combined with the use of specific enzymes can achieve the desired isolation of the specific peptides. Recently, immobilized glutamic acid specific endopeptidase was employed with α_s- or β-casein for experimental production of a novel calcium-binding CPP [59]. In their assessment of opportunities and limitations for widespread use of casein-derived bioactive peptides, Regester et al. [15] point out that successful large-scale production of these products will depend on the development of feasible technologies suitable for isolation and purification of the desired compounds from the mixture of various peptides likely to be produced in the hydrolysis step, as well as on overcoming the problem of low recovery from the raw material feedstock.

5. WHEY PROTEINS AS PHYSIOLOGICALLY FUNCTIONAL FOOD COMPONENTS

Approximately 20% of the total milk protein fraction consists of a heterogeneous group called whey proteins. In contrast to casein, the whey proteins, being insensitive to acid coagulation as well as to the action of chymosin, remain in both acid and rennet wheys resulting from manufacture of cheeses or industrial casein. The whey protein is a heterogeneous grouping of several dissimilar proteins (Table 11.4), many of which are now known to possess physiological functionality. For instance, the role of one of the more abundant whey proteins, α-lactalbumin, is as a co-enzyme active in synthesis of lactose, the milk sugar. Lactoferrin, lactoperoxidase or the various immunoglobulins (Ig) are examples of whey proteins having specific roles in the protection of the newborn calf, which does not receive the immunity *in utero*.

Use of whey proteins as specific ingredients in dairy or nondairy functional foods has been increasing steadily with improvements in the technological capabilities of the industry to produce commercially attractive whey protein concentrates (WPC), isolated total whey protein products or, most recently, enriched individual whey protein fractions. Until now, these products have been marketed as technologically functional or general nutritional ingredients. The high nutritional quality of whey proteins has been recognized for a long time [60]. Thus, whey protein is currently considered as one of the most desirable components in the diets of body-builders and athletes seeking to increase their muscle mass [61]. Extensive studies of specific physiological effects of the total—or individual—whey proteins as functional products in human nutrition are now in progress. One of these ongoing studies in Australia has concentrated on the notion that whey proteins—or at least some components of the whey protein group—may have unique physiological properties for cancer prevention. The research results available to date [62] have shown convincingly that whey protein-rich diets have a very significant effect ($p < 0.005$) on the decreased incidence of chemically induced colonic cancerous tumors in rats in comparison to other experimental diets containing casein, meat or soybean proteins. This effect was tentatively identified as possibly related to the concentration of glutathione, which was significantly ($p < 0.001$) stimulated by the whey protein diet. Anticarcinogenic effects of whey proteins were also reported by Bounous et al. [63].

More recently, studies with mice found strong immuno-enhancing effects of whey proteins, especially in combination with whey phospholipids. The serum IgM levels were more than doubled in mice fed diets based on whey protein and fresh whey cream [64]. Inclusion of total whey protein in experimental diets has been correlated with a stimulatory effect for the immune system [65]; an LDL-cholesterol lowering effect; and increased production of cholecystokinin involved in appetite suppression [66].

It is likely that at least some of these properties are linked to the individual protein species included in the total whey protein. Both of the two major whey proteins, α-lactalbumin and β-lactoglobulin, can be considered as having physiological properties. The uniqueness of α-lactalbumin as a calcium-binding protein has been known for some time [67,68]. This property may be the reason why the α-lactalbumin shows high renaturability and, as a result, can be considered as being highly resistant to thermal processing [69,70]. The lack of coagulative response upon heating of systems containing increased amounts of sufficiently purified α-lactalbumin may be important in development of UHT products with elevated whey protein content now being considered for industrial production. The possible role of α-lactalbumin in antitumor agent formulation is presently under consideration [71]. Similarly, one of the *in vivo* roles of the other major whey protein, β-lactoglobulin, appears to be binding of retinol and its transport into the small intestine [72]. The β-lactoglobulin can also bind fatty acids, as can the next most abundant whey protein, the bovine serum albumin. However, the role of bovine β-lactoglobulin as a physiologically active protein is somewhat controversial as, not being present in the human milk, it may be allergenic for certain humans. While the most widely publicized aspects of allergenicity of β-lactoglobulin are related to the production of hypoallergenic baby formulas [73], the allergenicity of certain adult consumers to this protein may need to be considered in the production and/or labeling of cheese made by the ultrafiltration technique which retains all the whey proteins in the final product.

Several minor whey proteins—in particular lactoferrin, lactoperoxidase, lysozyme, and immunoglobulins—have been under active investigation recently as antimicrobial proteins with numerous potential, and in some cases already fully commercial, applications in baby foods, chewing gum or mouthwash [74]. Lactoferrin in particular has been studied extensively for its role as an iron-binding protein, and its properties have been reviewed recently [75]. Although the commercial prospects of these minor proteins as functional food ingredients are potentially enormous, it must be remembered that the concentrations of these components in milk (or in the resulting whey) are low. Thus, a major limitation in industrial exploitation of the research findings currently lies in finding suitable extraction and/or separation technologies and especially viable applications of the resulting by-products. In addition, the bioactivity of the isolated whey proteins in humans is yet to be conclusively proven, including the dosages required for sustained effects.

In the case of immunoglobulins, their current utilization as functional food ingredients may be limited by the host specificity; however, much research is being conducted on in the area of induced specificity of bovine immunoglobulins produced by cows immunized against specific pathogens or viruses such as rotavirus. Marketing of two commercial products has been mentioned recently [15]. One of these products is a high-antibody-containing "immune milk" produced by cows immunized against various components of human intestinal microflora; the other is a dried modified colostrum powder. In both of these cases, the innovative technologies appear to be production-related, while the processing aspects must be controlled very carefully to avoid the loss of the biologically sensitive immunological properties.

In addition to the biological functionality of the individual protein fractions, some of the whey proteins are known to contain bioactive peptides with weak opioid or other biological activity as in the case of caseins. Examples of these include serorphin and albutensin from the serum albumin fraction; lactoferroxin from lactoferrin; or lactotensin from the β-lactoglobulin component [15]. In an investigation of enzymatic hydrolysis of α-lactalbumin or β-lactoglobulin by various enzymes (pepsin, trypsin and chymotrypsin), α-lactorphin produced from α-lactalbumin showed a definite but weak opioid activity whereas the effects of β-lactorphin, produced from β-lactoglobulin, were less clear [76]. Reports on industrial exploitation of these products are scarce.

Since many of the bioactive whey proteins are present in conventional milk or whey in small quantities, industrial production of these isolated compounds will result in large residual product streams requiring processing into additional products for which profitable uses must be found [77]. Traditional

TABLE 11.6. Composition of Industrially Produced α-Lactalbumin and β-Lactoglobulin Fractions.

	Percent Total Protein	
Product Component	α-Fraction (89.1% protein)	β-Fraction (89.7% protein)
α-Lactalbumin	70.6	13.8
β-Lactoglobulin	13.2	74.8
BSA + IGG[a]	10.4	4.6
Other proteins	5.8	6.8

[a]Bovine serum albumin and immunoglobulins.
Source: Reference [99].

cheese whey, the current source of most of the presently industrially available bioactive products, is considered a bothersome waste by traditional cheese-makers concentrating on the primary product of their efforts. Thus, it is likely that manufacturing of whey protein-based bioactive compounds will be carried out by few specialized processors such as the Dutch Borculo and DMV Companies, the Danish MD Foods, the Finnish Valio concern or some of the large cheese manufacturers in Australia. The present industrial approaches used to isolate the biologically active minor proteins from the milk or whey use specialized membrane technologies as the preferred tool [78]; however, the details of these highly confidential processes are not available. The two major whey proteins, α-lactalbumin and β-lactoglobulin, are being produced commercially as isolated protein fractions of relatively high purity (Table 11.6) using a variety of patented [79] or proprietary processes as that used by the Canadian Protose Separations company. Manufacture of total whey protein concentrates and isolates is widespread and many such products are available both as technological or nutritional ingredients and as highly prized items on the shelves of health stores catering to body-builders, competitive athletes, or others requiring special diets. Numerous processes are being used to produce these functional food products, including acid/base manipulation, ion exchange, electrodialysis or membrane techniques with resulting difference in the product properties. A recent advertising article [61] listed seven generations of such products differing in their properties as a result of different process technologies used (Table 11.7).

6. OTHER MILK-BASED BIOACTIVE COMPOUNDS

Although the protein fraction of milk attracts most of the present attention regarding the biologically active agents found in milk, there are other milk

TABLE 11.7. Classes of Whey Protein Preparations Marketed for Body Building Purposes.

Product Generation	Technological Characteristics	Content (%)	
		Protein	Lactose
1	Dried sweet whey	14	75
2	WPC[a] (low protein)	34	50
3	WPC (medium protein)	50–75	15–35
4	WPC (high protein)	80	6
5	Ion exchange treated	90–95	2
6	Hydrolyzed WPC	80–88	5
7	"Precision tailored" whey peptides	83–89	3

[a]Whey protein concentrate.
Source: Reference [61].

components with documented or presumed physiological significance. The case for calcium as a nutritionally important milk component involved in bone development and maintenance need not be restated here; however, other important effects of dietary calcium fit the contemporary notion of functional foods, including the role of calcium in blood pressure regulation [80]; the possible preventive effects in carcinogenesis [81]; or the suggested mediation of dental caries by calcium released into oral fluids from cheese [82,83]. Bioavailability of calcium from milk and dairy products is known to be excellent [1,84] and research is now aimed at increasing the low calcium content of some traditional dairy foods such as cottage cheese. An industrial food ingredient, Lactoval, produced by the Dutch DMV company is marketed as "label-friendly" natural milk calcium/mineral complex with a pleasing sensory profile and enhanced calcium absorption.

Cai [85] studied the bioavailability of calcium in a quark-like cheese product produced by using natural coagulants such as rhubarb extracts rich in calcium sequestrants. Due to the high content of oxalic acid in the rhubarb, the experimental quark had a significantly higher calcium content but the calcium bioavailability was drastically impaired. However, after pretreatment of the rhubarb juice to remove the undesirable oxalic acid, the resulting casein curd still had about 25% higher calcium content than a control quark, likely due to the citric and malic acids remaining in the rhubarb. The current image of milk as a rich source of calcium is probably the single most important nutraceutical attribute of the traditional dairy foods.

Lipid-based bioactive compounds of milk include mainly fatty acids. The importance of specific fatty acids for infant nutrition have been recognized for a long time by the manufacturers of infant formulas as well as researchers [86]. Most recent interests in functional foods and nutraceutical applications of milk-derived fatty acids include the potential of conjugated linoleic acid for inhibition of cancer and atherosclerosis and enhancement of immune system function [87]; the striking effects of butyric acid in elimination of cancerous cells in the colon [88]; and the regulatory involvement of membrane sphingolipids (e.g., sphingomyelin) in cell behavior [89]. Importantly and rather uncommonly, the latter research indicated that the amounts of sphingomyelin needed for effective suppression of colon carcinogenesis in experimental animals were not any greater than those found in common dairy products such as butter or cheese.

The single most abundant milk solids component, lactose, has been considered an enhancer of calcium absorption but the evidence is inconclusive [90]. In novel nutraceutical applications, lactose is important as a starting material for production of lactulose, used as a factor promoting probiotic growth (see Section 3) and added by some manufacturers to infant formulas and some other dairy foods produced in Japan [15]. Lacto-oligosaccharides are another class of probiotic growth promoters produced from lactose by enzymatic processes involving the reverse of the lactose hydrolysis reaction by the β-galactosidase enzymes [91]. Currently about 2000 tonnes of lacto-oligosaccharides are produced annually worldwide [15].

The enzymatic lactose hydrolysis by the β-galactosidase enzymes is an example of a modern industrial process aimed at producing a more physiologically acceptable milk for consumers experiencing the well-known problem termed alternatively "lactose intolerance," "lactose malabsorption" or "lactase deficiency." Lactose-free or lactose-reduced milk products have been available on the markets in many countries for some time and may be regarded as examples of modern dairy products manufactured to improve their physiological functionality. Some of the more advanced technological processes used in manufacture of these modified milk products and some whey beverages involve immobilized enzymes (e.g., the Finnish Valio process) or free soluble enzymes [92]. An experimental use of sonicated bacterial cultures [93] as an inexpensive enzyme source continues to be investigated. The main barrier to more widespread use of the lactose hydrolysis process is its high cost; however, from the standpoint of consumer needs, the production of lactose-free or lactose-modified dairy foods should be considered as one of the most important aims of the modern nutraceutically oriented dairy processors as the potential market worldwide is very significant.

7. CONCLUSIONS AND FUTURE PROSPECTS

Traditional milk and dairy products contain large amounts of components or precursors of agents of biological significance. While in some cases—such as calcium—their effects are well known and contribute to the positive image of dairy foods, many other physiologically active components of milk and milk products are now being discovered in intensive research efforts. As consumer interest in nutritional issues continues to grow, more definitive studies will become available, clearing up some of the uncertainties regarding the true effectiveness of these alleged bioactive agents. Clearly, if some of the anticipated effects suggested by the positive results of animal studies can be substantiated in clinical trials involving human subjects, this will be a major positive factor in marketing of dairy foods based on their health enhancement properties. Even now, "nutri-marketing" is becoming a major driving force in the international dairy industry as evidenced by a consultation organized by the IDF during the 1997 annual sessions. It appears that traditional dairy foods such as cheese, yogurt, ice cream, or even butter may be considered products with specific health benefits, if enough evidence will be forthcoming. Modifications of technologies—or developments of alternative processes—used to produce these foods will almost certainly occur as more knowledge regarding the specific desirable components of these products becomes available, as illustrated by the "new" class of probiotic yogurts now available in many countries. Whether these modified traditional products, which in some cases have somewhat different sensory properties due to technological needs, will be accepted by the consumer may depend on the strength of evidence regarding the health benefits, as well as the success of the manufacturer in adapting the technological process without major impairment of the traditional qualities. The nutri-marketing drive may be a major impetus for intensified product development efforts that will result in the emergence of truly novel dairy foods designed for maximum health benefits.

Some of the more significant changes resulting from increased public awareness of the functional foods concept may be expected in relation to whey protein. When the emerging health benefits of whey protein become generally accepted by the public, the natural presence of the whey protein in milk, ice cream, fermented dairy foods, and other products in which the complete milk protein fraction is retained, may become a strong marketing tool. Genetic engineering may be employed to produce milk with higher whey protein content or with higher content of only the most desirable whey protein components. Technological changes can be also foreseen to increase the whey protein content of these products by ultrafiltration of milk or the addition of an isolated whey protein fraction. However, as these products may have to be heat-treated, the limited heat stability of some of the whey protein components may have to be overcome, (e.g., by using only the heat-stable α-lactalbumin fraction [69] or by developing a heat-stable whey protein ingredient). The presence of whey protein in traditional cheese is known to result in difficulties during ripening, so either new ripening processes will need to be developed based on more precise knowledge of the biochemical events occurring during this complex process, or new whey protein-based cheeses may emerge in addition to the traditional ricotta. Yogurt drinks, popular in many countries, may be modified to be based on the whey protein-rich retentate of whey ultrafiltration [94]. Finally, whey protein products may be developed as freely available general nutritional supplements, much like the special whey protein preparations now used in the health food or medical food markets (products such as Ensure available for special dietary needs of hospital patients). Industrial whey protein concentrates have been marketed as industrial food ingredients for several decades but their success has been limited so far; with the heightened consumer awareness of their nutritional benefits, the WPCs may become major ingredients of choice in dairy as well as nondairy foods.

A major avenue for increasing the beneficial physiological effects of dairy products is likely to be "probiotic lines" of various traditional dairy foods. So far the success of probiotics has been limited to the fermented products, especially yogurt, probably due to the natural environment containing high counts of other dairy bacteria. However, since the probiotic bacterial cultures are usually added as a separate ingredient after the primary fermentation process has been completed, it is conceivable—as suggested by experimental research reports [95,96]—that other dairy products such as cheese, ice cream, or butter, will become equally suitable carriers of these healthful cultures if their sensitivity to environmental effects can be overcome. The limited commercial success of the A/B (acidophilus-bifidus) fluid milk products in certain markets (e.g., in Canada) indicates, however, that the consumer needs to be convinced of the added health benefits of these products, which are more expensive but sensorically identical to the regular milk (Jelen, personal experience).

Perhaps the most controversial direction in development of new functional dairy products will involve industrial production of the isolated physiologically active compounds such as peptides, specific proteins, enzymes, mineral mixtures, or other minor components of the milk systems. The difficulties of this approach have been noted in the discussion above; the high cost and other risks in embarking on such innovative ventures will have to be balanced by the more definitive proof of the efficacy of these preparations accompanied by major regulatory changes allowing health claims to be made. The need for sound science has never been greater but the rewards for positive results will be major. While the physiological attributes of traditional dairy foods will continue to increase in importance, the emergence of truly new physiologically functional dairy foods and nutraceuticals products of dairy origin remains a more distant goal.

8. REFERENCES

1. Flynn, A. and K. Cashman. 1997. "Nutritional aspects of minerals in bovine and human milks," Advanced Dairy Chemistry Vol. 3, Fox P. F., London, UK: Chapman & Hall. pp. 127–154.

2. Oste, R., M. Jagerstad and I. Andersson. 1997. "Vitamins in milk and milk products," Advanced Dairy Chemistry Vol. 3, Fox P. F., London, UK: Chapman & Hall. pp. 347–402.
3. Renner, E. 1991. Dictionary of milk and dairying. Munich: Volksvirtschaftlicher Verlag. p. 308.
4. Metchnikoff, E. 1908. The Prolongation of Life. New York, NY: G. Putnam & Sons.
5. Anon. 1993. "Demand outstrips supply for Gaio," Dairy Ind. Int. 58 (12):21.
6. Pearce, J. 1996. "Effects of milk and fermented dairy products on the blood cholesterol content and profile of mammals in relation to coronary heart disease," Int. Dairy J. 6:661–672.
7. IDF. 1991. "Cultured dairy products in human nutrition," Bulletin 255, Brussels, Belgium: IDF. 23 pp.
8. Jelen, P. 1993. "Pressure-driven membrane processes: principles and definitions," New Applications of Membrane Processes, Brussels, Belgium: IDF, Spec. Issue 9201. pp. 7–14.
9. Jelen, P. and A. Renz-Schauen. 1989. "Quark manufacturing innovations and their effects on quality, nutritive value and consumer acceptance," Food Technol. 43(3): 74–81.
10. Maubois, J. L. 1990. "Nouvelles applications des technologies à membrane dans l'industrie laitière," Proceedings, 23rd Int. Dairy Congress Montreal; Brussels, Belgium: IDF. pp. 1775–1790.
11. Jost, R. and P. Jelen. 1997. "Cross-flow microfiltration—an extension of membrane processing of milk and whey," Implications of Microfiltration on Hygiene and Identity of Dairy Products. Bulletin No. 320, Brussels, Belgium: IDF. pp. 9–15.
12. Kelly, P. M. and J. L. Tuohy. 1997. "The effectiveness of microfiltration for the removal of microorganisms," Implications of Microfiltration on Hygiene and Identity of Dairy Products. Bulletin No. 320, Brussels, Belgium: IDF. pp. 9–15.
13. Vilotte, J.-L., S. Soulier, M.-A. Persuy, L. Lepourry, S. Legrain, Ch. Printz, M.-G. Stinnakre, P. L'Huillier and J.-C. Mercier. 1997. "Application of transgenesis to modifying milk protein composition," Milk Composition, Production and Biotechnology, Welch, R. A. S., D. J. W. Burns, S. R. Davis, A. I. Popay and C. G. Prosser, New York, NY: CAB International. pp. 231–242.
14. Schanbacher, F. L. and M. D. Amstutz. 1997. "Direct transfection of the mammary gland: Opportunities for modification of mammary function and the production, composition and qualities of milk," Milk Composition, Production and Biotechnology, Welch, R. A. S., D. J. W. Burns, S. R. Davis, A. I. Popay and C. G. Prosser, New York, NY: CAB International. pp. 243–264.
15. Regester, G. O., G. W. Smithers, I. R. Mitchell, G. H. McIntosh and D. A. Dionysius, "Bioactive factors in milk: Natural and induced," Milk Composition, Production and Biotechnology, Welch, R. A. S., D. J. W. Burns, S. R. Davis, A. I. Popay and C. G. Prosser, New York, NY: CAB International. pp. 119–132.
16. Kurmann, J. A. and J. L. J. Rasic. 1991. "Health potential of products containing bifidobacteria," Therapeutic Properties of Fermented Milks, Robinson, R. K., Reading, UK: Elsevier Applied Science. pp. 137–144.
17. Dave, R. and N. P. Shah. 1997. "Viability of yoghurt and probiotic bacteria in yogurts made from commercial starter cultures," Int. Dairy J. 7:31–41.

18. Tamura, Z. 1983. "Nutrition of bifidobacteria," Bif. Microflora 2:3–16.
19. Vijayvendra, S. V. N. and R. C. Gupta. 1992. "Therapeutic importance of bifidobacteria and *Lactobacillus acidophilus* in fermented milks," Indian Dairyman 44:595–599.
20. Pettersson, L., W. Graf and U. Sewelin. 1983. "Survival of *Lactobacillus acidophilus* NCDO 1748 in the human gastrointestinal tract," Nutrition and the Intestinal Flora, Hallgren, B., Stockholm, Sweden: Almquist & Wiksell International.
21. Alm, L. 1991. "The therapeutical effects of various cultures," Therapeutical Properties of Fermented Milks, Robinson, R.K., London, UK: Elsevier Science Publishers. pp. 45–64.
22. Anon. 1995. Physiological Effects of *Bifidobacterium longum* BB536—*in Vitro* Tests and Administration to Humans and Animals. Tokyo, Japan: Morinaga Milk Industry. p. 14.
23. Hilliam, M. 1996. "Functional foods: the western consumer viewpoint," Nutrition Reviews 54(11):S189–194.
24. Sellars, R. L. 1991. "Acidophilus products," Therapeutic Properties of Fermented Milks, Robinson, R.K., London, UK: Elsevier Science Publishers. p. 84.
25. IDF. 1996. Oligosaccharides and Probiotic Bacteria. Bulletin 313, Brussels, Belgium: IDF. pp. 9–64.
26. McDonough, F. E., A. D. Hitchins and N. P. Wong. 1982. "Effects of yogurt and freeze-dried yogurt on growth stimulation of rats," J. Food Sci. 47:1463–5.
27. Hargrove, R. E. and J. A. Alford. 1978. "Growth rate and feed efficiency of rats fed yogurt and other fermented milks," J. Dairy Sci. 61:11–19.
28. Gorbach, S. L. 1997. Health Benefits of Probiotics, IFT Annual Meeting, Orlando, FL, Abstract 73–1.
29. Hughes, D. B. and D. G. Hoover. 1991. "Bifidobacteria: their potential use in American dairy products," Food Technology 45(4):74–83.
30. Klupsch, H. J. 1985. "Man and microflora," S. Afr. Dairy Tech. 17:153–156.
31. Hotta, M., Y. Sato, S. Iwata, N. Yamashita, K. Sunakawa, T. Oikawa, T. Tanaka, K. Watanabe, H. Takayama, M. Yajima, S. Sekiguchi, S. Arai, T. Sakurai and M. Mutai. 1987. "Clinical effects of *Bifidobacterium* preparations on pediatric intractable diarrhoea," Keio J. Med. 36:298–314.
32. Savage, D. C. 1977. "Interaction between the host and its microbes," Microbial Ecology of the Gut, Clarke, R. T. J. and T. Bauchop, London, New York: Academic Press. pp. 277–310.
33. Gilliland, S. E. 1979. "Beneficial interrelationships between certain microoganisms and humans: candidate microorganisms for use as dietary adjuncts," J. Food Protection 42:164–167.
34. Reddy, G. V., B. A. Friend, K. M. Shahani and R. E. Farmer. 1983. "Antitumor activity of yogurt components," J. Food Protection 46:8.
35. Alm, L., D. Humble, E. Ryd-Kjellen and G. Betterberg. 1983. Suppl. Näringsforskning, XV Symposium Swedish Nutrition Foundation. pp. 131–8.
36. Grunewald, K.K. 1982. "Serum cholesterol in rats fed skim milk fermented by *Lactobacillus acidophilus*," J. Food Sci. 47(6):2078–79.
37. Hepner, G., R. Fried, S. St. Jeor, L. Fusetti and R. Morin. 1979. "Hypocholesterolemic effect of yogurt and milk," Am. J. Clin. Nutr. 32:19–24.
38. Surono, I. S. and A. Hosono. 1996. "Antimutagenicity of milk cultured with lactic

acid bacteria from Dedih against mutagenic Terasi," Milchwissenschaft 51: 493–497.

39. Modler, W. H. 1994. "Bifidogenic factors—sources, metabolism and applications," Int. Dairy J. 4:383–407.
40. Roberfroid, M. B. 1997. "Prebiotics and synbiotics, concepts and overview of nutritional properties," IFT Annual Meeting, Orlando, FL, Abstract 73–2.
41. Oku, T. 1994. "Special physiological functions of newly developed mono- and oligosaccharides," Functional Foods, Goldberg, I., New York, NY: Chapman & Hall. pp. 202–218.
42. Young, J. N. 1997. "Developments in probiotics, prebiotics, and synbiotics: a European perspective." IFT Annual Meeting, Orlando, FL, Abstract 73–7.
43. Griffin, M. 1997. "Exceptional growth in probiotic products," Dairy Outlook 2: No 4. Rome, FAO.
44. Holt, C. 1997. "The milk salts and their interaction with casein," Advanced Dairy Chemistry, Vol. 3, Fox, P.F., London, UK: Chapman & Hall. pp. 233–256.
45. Meisel, H. and E. Schlimme. 1990. "Milk proteins: precursors of bioactive peptides," Trends in Food Sci. & Technol. 1(2):42–43.
46. West, D. W. 1986. "Structure and function of the phosphorylated residues of casein," J. Dairy Res. 53:333–352.
47. Pihlanto-Leppala, A., P. Antila, P. Mantsala and J. Hellman. 1994. "Opioid peptides by in-vitro proteolysis of bovine caseins," Int. Dairy J. 4:291–301.
48. Gaudichon, C. 1996. Bioactive peptides in milk. Proceedings, Seminar on Milk Proteins, Structure and Functions. Wadahl, Norway: Nat'l. Agric. Univ., Aas. pp. 1–5.
49. Sekiya, S., Y. Kobayashi, E. Kita, Y. Imamura and S. Toyama. 1992. J. Japanese Soc. Nutr. and Food Sci. 45:513–517 (abstract 00455866, Food Sci. & Technol. Abstracts, IFIS Publishing).
50. Ariyoshi, Y. 1993. "Angiotensin-converting enzyme inhibitors derived from food proteins," Trends in Food Sci. & Technol. 4:139–144.
51. Mellander, O. 1950. "The physiological importance of the casein phosphopeptide calcium salts. II. Peroral calcium dosage in infants. Some aspects of the pathogenesis of rickets," Acta Soc. Med. Ups. 55:247–255.
52. Meisel, H. and H. Frister. 1989. "Chemical characterization of bioactive peptides from in vivo digests of casein," J. Dairy Res. 56:343–349.
53. Berrocal, R., S. Chanton, M. A. Juillerat, B. Pavillard, J.-C. Scherz and R. Jost. 1989. "Tryptic phosphopeptides from whole casein. II. Physico-chemical properties related to solubilization of calcium," J. Dairy Res. 56:335–341.
54. Yuan, Y. V. and D. D. Kitts. 1991. "Confirmation of calcium absorption and femoral utilization in spontaneously hypertensive rats fed casein phosphopeptide diets," Nutr. Res. 11:1257–1272.
55. Pantako, T. O., M. Passos, T. Desrosiers and J. Amiot. 1994. "Effets des proteines laitiers sur l'absorption de Ca et P mesuree par les variations temporelles de leurs teneurs dans l'aorte et la veine porte chez le rat," Int. Dairy J. 4:37–58.
56. Marshall, W. E. 1994. "Amino acids, peptides, and proteins," Functional Foods, Goldberg, I., New York, NY: Chapman & Hall. pp. 242–260.
57. Hamel, V., G. Kielwein and H. Teschemacher. 1985. "β-Casomorphin immunoreactive material in cows' milk incubated with various bacteria species," J. Dairy Res. 52:139–148.

58. Matar, Ch. and J. Goulet. 1996. "β-Casomorphin from milk fermented by a mutant of *Lactobacillus helveticus,*" Int. Dairy J. 6:383–397.
59. Park, O. and J. C. Allen. 1997. Calcium-Binding of Casein Phosphopeptides Prepared with Immobilized Glutamic Acid Specific Endopeptidase. IFT Annual Sessions, Orlando, FL, Abstract 65–6.
60. Renner, E. 1983. Milk and Dairy Products in Human Nutrition. Munich: Volkswirtschaftlicher Verlag. p. 449.
61. Nettl, F. 1995. "The shocking truth about whey protein!" Muscle Media 2000, November 1995:72–77.
62. McIntosh, G. H., G. O. Regester, R. K. LeLeu, P. J. Royle and G. W. Smithers. 1995. "Dairy proteins protect against dimethylhydrazine-induced intestinal cancers in rats," J. Nutr. 125:809–816.
63. Bounous, G., G. Batist and P. Gold. 1991. "Whey proteins in cancer prevention," Cancer Letters 57:91–94.
64. Chinniah, T. B., M. Pedersen and R. Jimenez-Flores. 1997. "Effect of whey diets on serum immunoglobulin M levels in mice," J. Dairy Sci. 80 (Suppl. 1):134.
65. Bounous, G., P. A. L. Kongshavn and P. Gold. 1988. "The immunoenhancing property of dietary whey protein concentrate," Clin. Invest. Medicine 12:343–349.
66. Zhang, X. and A. Beynen. 1993. "Lowering effect of dietary milk-whey protein v. casein on plasma and liver cholesterol concentrations in rats," Brit. J. Nutr. 70: 139–146.
67. Hiraoka, Y. T. Segawa, K. Kuwajima, S. Sugai and N. Murai. 1980. "α-Lactalbumin: a calcium metalloprotein," Biochem. Biophys. Res. Commun. 95:1098–1106.
68. Bernal, V. and P. Jelen. 1984. "Effect of calcium binding on thermal denaturation of bovine α-lactalbumin," J. Dairy Sci. 67:2452–2454.
69. Peter, S., W. Rattray and P. Jelen. 1996. "Heat stability and sensory quality of protein-standardized 2% fat milk," Milchwissenschaft 51:611–616.
70. Rattray, W. and P. Jelen. 1997. "Thermal stability of skim milk/whey protein solution blends," Food Res. Int. 30:327–334.
71. Hakansson, A. B. Zhivotovsky, S. Orrenius, H. Sabharwal and C. Svanborg. 1995. Apoptosis Induced by a Human Milk Protein. Proc. U.S. Natl. Acad. Sci. 92: 8046–8068.
72. MacLeod, A., W. Fedio, L. Chu and L. Ozimek. 1996. "Binding of retinoic acid to β-lactoglobulin variants A and B: Effect of peptic and tryptic digestion on the protein-ligand complex," Milchwissenschaft 51:3–7.
73. Kuwata, T., T. Yajima and T. Kaneko. 1997. "Recent and future improvements of protein fraction in cow's milk-based infant formula," Milk Composition, Production and Biotechnology, Welch, R. A. S., D. J. W. Burns, S. R. Davis, A. I. Popay and C. G. Prosser, New York, NY: CAB International. pp. 215–230.
74. Burling, H. 1994. "Isolation of bioactive components from cheese whey," Scandinavian Dairy Inf. 3:54–56.
75. Hutchens, T. W., S. V. Rumball and B. Lonnerdal. 1994. "Lactoferrin: structure and function," Adv. Exp. Med. and Biol. 357:1–298.
76. Antilla, P., I. Paakkari, A. Jarvinen, M. J. Mattila, M. Laukkanen, A. Pihlanto-Leppala, P. Mantsala and J. Hellman. 1991. "Opioid peptides derived from in-vitro proteolysis of bovine whey proteins," Int. Dairy J. 1:215–229.
77. DeBoer, R. 1996. "Yogurt and other fermented dairy products," Advances of

Membrane Technology for Better Dairy Products. Bulletin 311, IDF, Brussels, Belgium. pp. 21–25.

78. Maubois, J. L., J. Leonil, S. Bouhallab and A. Garem. 1996. "Use of membrane processes in the manufacture of peptides and other nutritional preparations," Advances of Membrane Technology for Better Dairy Products. Bulletin 311, IDF, Brussels, Belgium. p. 28.
79. Pearce, R. J. 1988. Whey Protein Fractions. Patent application PCT/AU88/00141.
80. McCarron, D. A., C. D. Morris, H. J. Henry and J. L. Stanton. 1984. "Blood pressure and nutrient intake in the United States," Science 224:1392–1398.
81. Sorenson, W., M. L. Slattery and M. Ford. 1988. "Calcium and colon cancer: a review," Nutr. Cancer 11:135–145.
82. Patocka, G., J. A. Hargreaves, G. N. Jenkins and P. Jelen. 1991. "Effect of eating dairy products on plaque Ca and P," J. Dental Res. 70 (spec. issue): abstr. 1108.
83. Patocka, G. and Hargreaves, J. A. 1991. "Release and retention of calcium and phosphorus from various dairy products in the oral fluid," Int. Dairy J. 1:101–110.
84. Weaver, C. M. 1992. Calcium Bioavailability and Its Relation to Osteoporosis. Proc. Soc. Exp. Biol. Med. 200:157–160.
85. Cai, J. W. 1997. Utilization of Rhubarb in Manufacture of Quark Products and Investigation of Their Nutritive Value. M.Sc. Thesis, Edmonton: University of Alberta. p. 69.
86. Clandinin, M. T. 1995. "Infant nutrition: effects of lipid on later life," Current Opinion Lipidology 6:28–31.
87. Pariza, M. W. 1997. Conjugated Linoleic Acid: a Newly Recognized Nutrient. IFT Annual meeting, Orlando, FL, Abstract 15–3.
88. German, J. B. and L. C. Carter. 1997. Butyric Acid: a Nutrient Acting on the Cell Nucleus. IFT Annual meeting, Orlando, FL, abstr. 15–5.
89. Schmelz, E. M. and A. H. Merrill. 1997. Milk Sphingolipids: a New Category of Functional Food. IFT Annual meeting, Orlando, FL, Abstract 15–4.
90. Mustapha, A., S. R. Hertzler and D. A. Savaiano. 1997. "Lactose: nutritional significance," Advanced Dairy Chemistry Vol. 3, Fox, P. F., London, UK: Chapman & Hall. pp. 127–154.
91. Thelwall, L. A. W. 1997. "Lactose: chemical derivatives," Advanced Dairy Chemistry Vol. 3, Fox, P. F., London, UK: Chapman & Hall. pp. 39–76.
92. Modler, H. W., A. Gelda, M. Yaguchi and S. Gelda. 1993. "Production of fluid milk with a high degree of lactose hydrolysis," Lactose Hydrolysis Workshop. Bulletin 289, Brussels, Belgium: IDF. pp. 57–61.
93. Jelen, P. 1993. "Lactose hydrolysis using sonicated dairy cultures," Lactose Hydrolysis Workshop. Bulletin 289, Brussels, Belgium: IDF. pp. 54–56.
94. Jelen, P., M. Johnson, I. R. Mitchell, G. O. Regester and G. W. Smithers. 1996. "High protein whey drinks," Advances of Membrane Technology for Better Dairy Products. Bulletin 311, IDF, Brussels, Belgium. p. 25.
95. Modler, H. W., R. C. McKellar, H. D. Goff and D. A. Mackie. 1990. "Using ice cream as a mechanism to incorporate bifidobacteria and fructooligosaccharides into the human diet," Cultured Dairy Prod. J. 25(3):4–9.
96. Christiansen, P. S., D. Edelsten, J. R. Kristiansen and E. W. Nielsen. 1996. "Some properties of ice cream containing *Bifidobacterium bifidum* and *Lactobacillus acidophilus*," Milchwissenschaft 51:502–504.

97. Renner, E. and A. Renz-Schauen. 1992. Nutrition Composition Tables of Milk and Dairy Products. Giessen, Germany: Verlag B. Renner. pp. 1, 56, 314, 378, 422.
98. Walstra, P. and R. Jenness. 1984. Dairy Chemistry and Physics. New York, NY: J. Wiley and Sons. p. 107.
99. Rojas, S. A., H. D. Goff, V. Senaratne, D. G. Dalgleish and A. Flores. 1998. Gelation of commercial fractions of β-lactoglobulin and α-lactalbumin. Int. Dairy J. 7: 79–85.

CHAPTER 12

Functional Seafood Lipids and Proteins

F. SHAHIDI[1]

1. INTRODUCTION

THE popularity and image of seafoods have increased markedly in recent years. However, seafoods have served as a major source of animal protein and lipid since early civilization. Although seafood proteins are important by possessing a well-balanced amino acid composition, many species of fish remain underutilised because of a multitude of drawbacks, most of them relating to the small size, high bone content, unappealing shape, and look or fatty nature of the species. Therefore, production of novel protein preparations from such raw material has been attempted. These include protein concentrates/dispersions and hydrolyzates, among others. However, seafood lipids, which are rich in long-chain omega-3 polyunsaturated fatty acids (PUFA), have attracted much interest and are the main focus of attention. The interest in seafood lipids and their fatty acid constituents stems from observation of the diet of Greenland Eskimos [1] in which fish as well as seal meat and blubber were integral components. The incidence of cardiovascular disease (CVD) in Eskimos was considerably less than that of the Danish population, despite their high dietary fat intake.

The beneficial health effects of omega-3 PUFA have been attributed to their ability to lower serum triacylglycerol and cholesterol. In addition, omega-3 fatty acids are essential for normal growth and development and may also play a role in the prevention and treatment of hypertension, arthritis, other inflammatory and autoimmune disorders, and cancer [2,3].

[1]Department of Biochemistry, Memorial University of Newfoundland, St. John's, NF, A1B 3X9 Canada.

This chapter provides an account of novel uses of marine lipids and proteins in different applications. Issues related to the stability and stabilization of marine lipids, production of omega-3 concentrates, and formulation of other value-added products from underutilised fish species [4] are also discussed.

2. MARINE LIPIDS AND THEIR BENEFICIAL HEALTH EFFECTS

Marine lipids originate from the liver of lean white fish such as cod, the body of oily fish such as mackerel, and the blubber of marine mammals such as seal. These oils consist of saturated, monounsaturated and polyunsaturated fatty acids (PUFA). There are two classes of PUFA, namely, the omega-3 and the omega-6 families, which are differentiated from one another based on the location of the double bond from the terminal methyl group of the fatty acid molecule. Unlike saturated and monounsaturated fatty acids, which can be synthesized by all mammals, including humans, the PUFA cannot be easily synthesized in the body but must be provided through the diet. The omega-3 family of PUFA is descended from linolenic acid while its omega-6 counterparts are descended from linoleic acid. The unique feature that differentiates lipids of marine species from those of land animals is the presence of long-chain PUFA, namely, eicosapentaenoic acid (EPA; C20:5 ω3), docosahexaenoic acid (DHA; C22:6ω3) and, to a lesser extent, docosapentaenoic acid (DPA; C22:5 ω3) (see Table 12.1). These PUFA are formed in unicellular phytoplankton and multicellular sea algae and eventually pass through the food web to become incorporated into the body of fish and other higher marine species [5]. The high content of omega-3 fatty acids in marine lipids is suggested to be a consequence of cold temperature adaptation in which omega-3 PUFA remain liquid and oppose any tendency to crystallize [6].

Illingworth and Ullman [7] proposed that consumption of marine oils results in a decrease in plasma lipids by reduced synthesis of fatty acids and low-density lipoproteins (LDL). Nestel [8] suggested that the long-chain omega-3 PUFA have a direct effect on the heart muscle itself, increase blood flow, decrease arrhythmias, improve arterial compliance, decrease the size of the infarct, and reduce several cellular processes that comprise heart function. It has also been suggested that marine oils may retard artherogenesis through their effects on platelet function, platelet-endothelial interactions and inflammatory response. Most of these effects are mediated, at least in part, by alterations in eicosenoids formation in the human body [9].

The parents of the two PUFA families, namely, linoleic and linolenic acids (see above), are the precursors of long-chain PUFA (Table 12.1) which, in turn, produce a range of regulatory and biologically active substances, collectively known as eicosanoids (Table 12.2). In general, compounds derived from the omega-3 PUFA are less powerful than those derived from the omega-6 PUFA. Both the omega-3 and omega-6 pathways operate through the same set of en-

TABLE 12.1. Metabolism of Polyunsaturated Fatty Acids (PUFA).

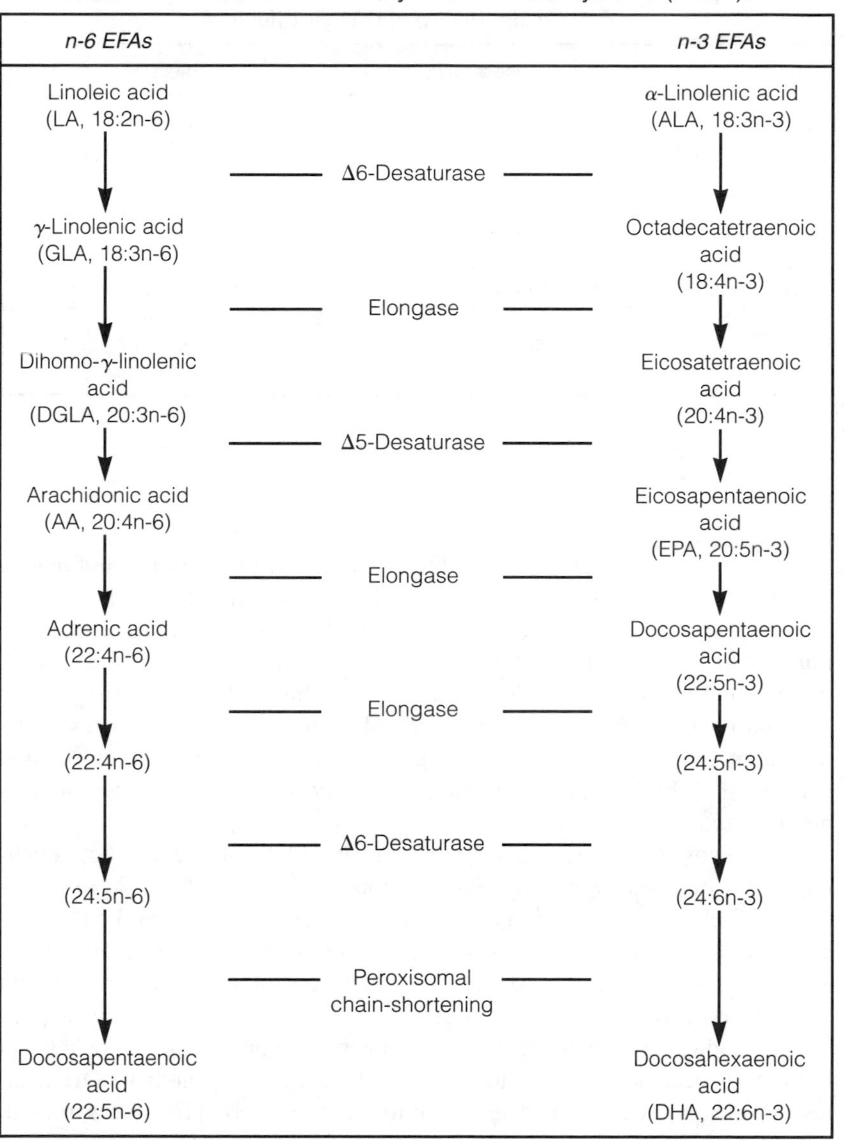

n-6 EFAs		*n-3 EFAs*
Linoleic acid (LA, 18:2n-6)		α-Linolenic acid (ALA, 18:3n-3)
↓	Δ6-Desaturase	↓
γ-Linolenic acid (GLA, 18:3n-6)		Octadecatetraenoic acid (18:4n-3)
↓	Elongase	↓
Dihomo-γ-linolenic acid (DGLA, 20:3n-6)		Eicosatetraenoic acid (20:4n-3)
↓	Δ5-Desaturase	↓
Arachidonic acid (AA, 20:4n-6)		Eicosapentaenoic acid (EPA, 20:5n-3)
↓	Elongase	↓
Adrenic acid (22:4n-6)		Docosapentaenoic acid (22:5n-3)
↓	Elongase	↓
(22:4n-6)		(24:5n-3)
↓	Δ6-Desaturase	↓
(24:5n-6)		(24:6n-3)
↓	Peroxisomal chain-shortening	↓
Docosapentaenoic acid (22:5n-6)		Docosahexaenoic acid (DHA, 22:6n-3)

zymes and may compete with each other. Consumption of high amounts of dietary marine oils leads to the production of the less powerful compounds.

Both arachidonic acid (AA) and EPA are precursors of eicosanoids [10], such as prostaglandins, thromboxanes and leukotrienes, all of which are oxygenated derivatives of C20 fatty acids (Table 12.2). Eicosanoids from

TABLE 12.2. Formation of Eicosanoids from ω-3 and ω-6 Polyunsaturated Fatty Acids (PUFA) and Their Effects.

PUFA	Eicosanoid	Effect
20:5 ω-3 Eicosapentaenoic acid (EPA)	Thrombaxane A_3 ($TBXA_3$)	Weak effect on platelet aggregation; Narrows blood vessels
	Prostacyclin I_3 (PGI_3)	Inhibits platelet aggregation
20:4 ω-6 Arachidonic acid (AA)	Thromboxane A_2 (TXA_2)	Strongly stimulates platelet aggregation; strongly narrows blood vessels
	Prostacyclin I_2 (PGI_2)	Inhibits platelet aggregation; relaxes blood vessels

these two fatty acids are different in structure and function [9] and have a broad spectrum of biological activity. Physiological effects of omega-3 fatty acids have been observed in the areas of (1) heart and circulatory, (2) immune response, and (3) cancer. The first group includes prevention or treatment of atherosclerosis [11,12], thrombosis [2], hypertriacylglycidemia [13], and high blood pressure [11]. The second area relates to the treatment of asthma, arthritis [14], migraine headache, psoriasis and nephritis [2]. Finally, the third category involves cancer of the breast [10], prostate and colon [14].

Since eicosanoids are ultimately derived from PUFA in the diet, both qualitative and quantitative changes in the supply of dietary PUFA have a profound effect on the production of eicosanoids. Therefore, omega-3 fatty acids are emerging as essential nutrients. As a structural component of brain, retina, testes, and sperm, DHA appears to be linked to proper tissue function and needs to be supplied in sufficient amounts during tissue development [15]. Recent studies have shown that DHA supplementation during pregnancy and lactation is necessary in order to prevent deficiency of the mother's DHA status in order to meet the high fetal requirement for DHA [16]. Carlson et al. [17] have shown that premature babies have lower levels of DHA in their tissues than full-term babies. Thus, supplementation of infant formula with marine oils/DHA is necessary in order to provide them with as much DHA as that available to their breast-fed counterparts. Feeding of infants with formula devoid of omega-3 fatty acids resulted in lack of deposition of DHA in their visual and neural tissues [18].

The Canadian Scientific Review Committee of Nutrition Recommendations [19] has suggested daily requirements for PUFA (omega-3 and omega-6) based on energy needs. Additional amounts of omega-3 and omega-6 fatty acids are recommended for lactating and pregnant women with increasing amounts from the first to the second trimester of pregnancy. The British Nutrition Foundation Task Force [20] on unsaturated fatty acids has recommended that 5% of total daily energy supply for humans originate from omega-3 fatty acids.

3. PROCESSING OF MARINE OILS

The basic processing steps for production of marine oils depend on the source of raw material used. Generally, however, they include heat processing or rendering to release the oil, degumming, alkali-refining, bleaching, and deodorization. Thus, processing of marine oils is similar to that of vegetable oils [21]. However, the quality of crude marine oils is less uniform than crude vegetable oils and proper handling of the raw material is of utmost importance. In addition, marine oils must be processed at the lowest possible temperature and under a blanket of nitrogen, when possible. Figure 12.1 provides a flow diagram to exhibit different processing steps involved in the production of marine oils.

4. OXIDATION OF MARINE OILS

Oils rich in PUFA are prone to oxidative deterioration and easily produce off-flavors and off-odors [22,23]. Therefore, inhibition of oxidation is a major criterion when marine oils are processed, stored or incorporated into food products.

Oxidation of marine oils proceeds via a free-radical chain mechanism involving initiation, propagation and termination steps. Peroxides are the primary products of oxidation, but these toxic compounds are unstable and degrade further to secondary products such as malonaldehyde and 4-hydroxynonenal that are also highly toxic. Secondary oxidation products are responsible for the development of off-flavor in stored seafoods and marine oils. Therefore, every attempt should be made to control deteriorative processes of oxidation in order to obtain the maximum benefit from their omega-3 components.

Methods that might be used to stabilize marine lipids include addition of antioxidants, microencapsulation and hydrogenation. However, hydrogenation negates the beneficial health effects of PUFA by producing saturated fatty acids as well as trans-isomers. Therefore, use of antioxidation and microencapsulation technology might be practised.

SOURCE OF MARINE LIPID

↓

heating/rendering

↓

2- or 3-phase separation

↓

CRUDE OIL

↓

refining

↓

REFINED OIL

↓

bleaching

↓

REFINED-BLEACHED OIL

↓

deodorization

(preferably at low t&p)

↓

REFINED-BLEACHED-DEODORIZED OIL

Figure 12.1 Process for production of crude, refined, refined-bleached, and refined-bleached-deodorized marine oils.

4.1. ANTIOXIDANTS

Synthetic antioxidants such as butylated hydroxyanisole (BHA), butylated hydroxytoluene (BHT), propyl gallate (PG), and *tert*-butylhydroquinone (TBHQ) as well as synthetic α-tocopherol may be incorporated into seafoods and/or marine oils in order to control their oxidative deterioration. However, the effectiveness of synthetic antioxidants other than TBHQ in the prevention of oxidation of marine oils is limited. In addition, synthetic antioxidants are regarded as suspects in cancer development when used at high concentrations in experimental animals. As a result, BHA has been removed from the GRAS (Generally Recognized As Safe) list by the U. S. Food and Drug Administration [24]. Furthermore, TBHQ has not been approved for use in Europe, Japan and Canada. Therefore, natural antioxidants may offer a practical solution to control oxidation of marine oils. Although antioxidants have traditionally been used to stabilize lipids, they may also augment body antioxidant defense systems for combatting cancer and degenerative diseases of aging. The natural antioxidants from dietary sources generally belong to the phenolic group of compounds, including tocopherols and flavonoids, as well as phospholipids and polyfunctional organic acids. Use of rosemary extract, plant tocopherols, oat oil, lecithin, and ascorbates, individually or in specific mixtures and combinations, may be encouraged in order to arrest oxidation.

Among the natural sources of antioxidants, green tea extracts might provide a practical and highly effective means for controlling oxidation and may also have the advantage of exerting beneficial health effects in the prevention of cancer. Thus, inclusion of green tea extracts in marine oils may afford products that are effective in the control and possible treatment of both CVD and cancer.

Recent studies in our laboratories have indicated that while ground green tea leaves and crude extracts from green tea are effective in inhibiting oxidation of cooked ground light muscles of mackerel (see Table 12.3), they may

TABLE 12.3. The Content 2-Thiobarbituric Acid Reactive Substances (milligram malonaldehyde equivalents/ kilogram sample) of Cooked Ground Light Muscles of Mackerel Treated with Different Antioxidants over a 7-day Storage Period at 4°C.[a]

Antioxidant (ppm)	Fresh	Stored
None	8.81	12.03
α-Tocopherol (296)	7.34	9.76
GGTL (1265)	4.09	4.25
GTE (1265)	4.03	5.58
EC (200)	5.81	6.53
EGC (211)	3.91	4.46
ECG (304	3.38	3.90
EGCG (316)	3.29	3.84

[a]Based on mole equivalents of 200 ppm epicatechin, EC. Other abbreviations are: GGTL, ground green tea leaves; GTE, green tea extract; EGC, epigallocatechin, ECG, epicatechin gallate; and EGCG, epigallocatechin gallate.

require complete dechlorophillization to be useful for incorporation into marine oils [25]. Meanwhile, the activity of individual catechins tested was in the order of epicatechin gallate (ECG) ≈ epigallocatechin gallate (EGCG) > epigallocatechin (EGC) » epicatechin (EC). However, ground green tea leaves protected the cooked fish meat against oxidation more effectively than individual catechins, perhaps due to the presence of other active components that might have acted synergistically with catechins. Further studies on the use of decholoriphillized green tea extracts (DGTE) and individual catechins revealed their efficacy in inhibiting oxidation of marine oils. These results, as reflected in the TBARS values of stored menhaden and seal blubber oils under Schaal oven conditions, are summarized in Table 12.4.

4.2. MICROENCAPSULATION

Oils rich in polyunsaturated fatty acids may be stabilized by their inclusion in microcapsules. In this process, the oil is entrapped in a wall material and is protected from oxygen, moisture and light [26]. The initial step in encapsulation of a food ingredient consists of selecting a suitable coating matter. Wall materials are basically film-forming substances that can be selected from a wide variety of natural or synthetic polymers, depending on the nature of the material to be coated and the desired characteristics of

TABLE 12.4. Percent Inhibition of Formation of 2-Thiobarbituric Acid Reactive Substances in Marine Oils as Affected by Antioxidants.

Antioxidant (ppm)	Menhaden Oil	Seal Blubber Oil
α-Tocopherol (200)	14.14	13.24
BHA (200)	25.28	22.97
BHT (200)	31.37	35.47
TBHQ (200)	51.80	56.25
DGTE (100)	25.25	22.97
DGTE (200)	32.91	32.91
DGTE (500)	41.44	41.81
DGTE(1000)	44.64	47.11
EC (200)	41.40	39.53
EGC (200)	46.46	40.50
ECG (200)	52.85	58.59
EGCG (200)	49.41	50.03

Abbreviations are: BHA, butylated hydroxyanisole; BHT, butylated hydroxytoluene; TBHQ, tert-butyl hydroquinone; DGTE, dechlorophillized green tea extract; EC, epicatechin; EGC, epigallocatechin; ECG, epicatechin gallate; and EGCG, epigallocatechin gallate.

the final microcapsules. Therefore, carbohydrates, both as such or modified, as well as proteins, may be used for this purpose. As an example, Taguchi et al. [27] have reported microencapsulation of sardine oil in egg white powder while Lin et al. [28] used gelatin and caseinate for microencapsulation of squid oil.

In a recent study [29], we used ß-cyclodextrin, Maltrin and corn syrup solids for microencapsulation of seal blubber oil. The efficacy of wall materials to prevent oxidation of the resultant coated products was in the order of ß-cyclodextrin >> corn syrup solids > Maltodextrin. It is possible that inclusion of alkyl chains of PUFA in the central cavity of ß-cyclodextrin provides better protection to the oil (Table 12.5).

4.3. OMEGA-3 CONCENTRATES

Omega-3 concentrates from marine oils may be produced in the form of the natural triacylglycerols or as modified triacylglycerols, as free fatty acids, or as the simple alkyl esters of these acids. Winterization or fractional crystallization may be employed to prepare concentrates with a total EPA, DHA and DPA content of up to 30%. Production of higher total concentration of the fatty acids is difficult because of the complexity of the combination of the fatty acids in triacylglycerol oils. However, these omega-3 concentrates might be prepared easily once they are transformed to free fatty acids or their simple alkyl esters. Urea complexation is one of the most promising methods for concentrating PUFA or their esters, as it allows handling of large quantities of material in simple equipment [30]. In this process, saturated and longer-chain monounsaturated fatty acids are complexed with urea as inclusion compounds while PUFA remain in the mixture and can be separated from it. In addition, lipase-assisted hydrolysis, alcoholysis and acidolysis may allow selective concentration of omega-3 fatty acids. The enzymes used for production of

TABLE 12.5. Changes in the Content (%) of Polyunsaturated Fatty Acids of Encapsulated (in β-cyclodextrin) Seal Blubber Oil upon Storage.

Fatty Acid	Initial	3 Weeks	7 Weeks
EPA	7.5	7.1 (3.3)	7.0 (3.0)
DPA	4.9	4.2 (2.1)	4.2 (2.1)
DHA	8.4	8.0 (3.8)	7.2 (3.0)
Total Polyunsaturates	24.7	23.3 (13.1)	22.2 (11.5)

Abbreviations are: EPA, eicosapentaenoic acid; DPA, docosapentaenoic acid; and DHA, docosahexaenoic acid. Values in parentheses are for unencapsulated oils.
Source: Adapted from Reference [29].

TABLE 12.6. Omega-3 Fatty Acids of Seal Blubber Oil Concentrates.

		Concentrate	
Fatty Acid	Original Oil	Enzymatic	Urea Complexation
EPA	9.1	12.2–17.1	24.6–27.7
DPA	5.0	6.9–8.4	5.0–9.3
DHA	10.0	15.4–26.6	38.9–46.1
Total Polyunsaturates	24.7	54.1	88.2

Abbreviations are: EPA, eicosapentaenoic acid; DPA, docosapentaenoic acid; and DHA, docosahexaenoic acid.

omega-3 concentrates may show selectivity for the position of acyl groups in the triacylglycerol molecule and also the degree of unsaturation of these acids. The degree and yield of concentration depend on the positional distribution of fatty acids in the triacylglycerol molecules.

Table 12.6 shows the degree of concentration of omega-3 fatty acids from seal blubber oil using enzyme-assisted hydrolysis and urea complexation procedures. The total content of omega-3 fatty acids from the enzymatic process, under optimum conditions, was approximately 54%; for the urea complexation process, it was 88%.

5. SEAFOOD PROTEINS

Seafood proteins possess excellent amino acid scores and digestibility characteristics. These constitute approximately 11–27% of seafoods and, like those of all other muscle foods, might be classified as sarcoplasmic, myofibrillar and stroma-type. In addition, non-protein nitrogen (NPN) compounds are present, to different extents, depending on the species under consideration. The dark muscles of fish generally contain a higher amount of NPN compounds than their light counterparts.

The sarcoplasmic proteins, mainly albumins, account for approximately 30% of the total muscle proteins; myoglobin and enzymes are also present. The content of sarcoplasmic proteins is generally higher in pelagic fish species than demersal fish. The dark muscles of some species contain less sarcoplasmic proteins than their white muscles [31]. However, the presence of large amounts of myoglobin, hemoglobin and cytochrome C in dark muscles may reverse this trend. Meanwhile, the presence of sarcoplasmic enzymes is responsible for deterioration of fish quality after death. These include glycolytic and hydrolytic enzymes, and their activity depends on the species of fish, type of muscle tissue, as well as seasonal and environmental factors.

The myofibrillar proteins in the muscles (approximately 60–70%) are composed of myosin, actin, tropomyosin and troponins C, I and T [31]. Myofibrillar proteins undergo changes during rigor mortis, resolution of rigor and long-term frozen storage. The texture of fish products and the gel-forming ability of fish mince and surimi may also be affected by these changes. The myofibrillar fraction of muscle proteins dictates the general functional properties of muscle tissues.

The residue after extraction of sacroplasmic and myofibrillar proteins is known as stroma, which is composed of collagen and elastin from the connective tissues. In general, fish muscles contain 0.2–2.2% collagen [32]. Although a higher content of collagen contributes to the toughness of the muscle, no such problems are encountered in fish. However, some species of squid may develop a tough and rubbery texture upon heat processing.

The non-protein nitrogen (NPN) compounds in muscle tissues are composed of free amino acids, amines, amine oxides, guanidines, nucleotides and their breakdown products, urea and quarternary ammonium salts [33]. The contribution of NPN compounds to the taste of seafoods is of paramount importance.

6. NOVEL FUNCTIONAL PROTEIN PREPARATIONS FROM UNDERUTILISED AQUATIC SPECIES

Novel functional protein preparations that might be produced from underutilised aquatic species include surimi, low-viscosity thermostable proteins and protein hydrolyzates, among others, as discussed below.

6.1. SURIMI

Surimi is mechanically deboned fish flesh that has been washed with water or very dilute salt solutions at 5–10°C and to which cryoprotectants have been added [34]. Removal of water-soluble sarcoplasmic proteins, including hemoproteins, enzymes and NPN compounds results in the production of a reasonably colorless and tasteless product. The yield of the process is 50–60% (see Figure 12.2). Surimi so produced may be used for the production of crab-leg analogues and other value-added food products. Colorants and flavorants may be added to surimi in order to form such products.

Factors that affect the surimi quality (gel-forming ability) and yield include storage technique, raw material quality and various processing factors. The process of surimi production from lean [34] and fatty [35] fish species has recently been reviewed and therefore will not be discussed here.

FISH

↓

heading and gutting

↓

deboning/mincing

↓

washing

↓

straining

↓

dewatering

↓

MYOFIBRILLAR PROTEINS

↓

adding cryoprotectants

↓

SURIMI

Figure 12.2 Flowsheet for preparation of surimi.

6.2. LOW-VISCOSITY THERMOSTABLE PROTEIN DISPERSIONS

Lack of solubility of myofibrillar proteins in water and their sensitivity to denaturation are among the reasons for the underutilization of proteins from low-cost fish. Under physiological conditions and in the presence of enzymes and low-molecular-weight components, myosin molecules interact with one another as well as with these other compounds [31,36]. Thus, improved processes for production of dispersion and soluble protein preparations are required.

The general process for production of protein dispersions from several species of fish, namely, capelin (*Mallotus villosus*), mackerel (*Scomber scombrus*), herring (*Clupea harengus*) and shark (*Isurus oxyrinchus*), is depicted in Figure 12.3. For capelin, mechanically deboned meat and other fish, light

FISH

↓

gutting and filleting

↓

mincing

↓

washing in cold water

↓

washing with sodium bicarbonate

↓

washing in cold water

↓

homogenization in cold water

↓

lowering of pH
using acetic acid
(if necessary)

↓

heating

↓

sieving

↓

spray drying
(if necessary)

↓

FUNCTIONAL PROTEIN DISPERSIONS/POWDERS

Figure 12.3 Flowsheet for preparation of functional protein dispersions from fish.

muscles were comminuted and used as raw material. The preparation of thermostable water dispersions of fish structural proteins, which may also be concentrated by suitable dehydration techniques, involves washing the comminuted muscle tissues to remove soluble components and lipids. Conformational changes in proteins enhance the entrapment of water in the gel matrices [37]. After a preliminary washing of the sample with water, solids are further washed with dilute saline and sodium bicarbonate solution followed by a subsequent wash with cold water. After removal of the water by straining, the washed meat is suspended in cold water, at up to 50% and homogenized. In some cases it is necessary to lower the pH to 3.0–3.5 in order to enhance gelation [38]. The pH-adjusted dispersion samples are then heated to 50°C. The acetic acid used for this purpose may also act as a preservative during storage of the product prior to its dehydration/concentration.

Table 12.7 summarizes the proximate composition of unwashed and washed fish meat before the final homogenization step in the production of thermostable protein products from capelin, herring, mackerel, and shark [39–43]. In all cases examined, the washed meat had a higher moisture and a lower lipid content and had a light color and a bland taste. The treatment also increased the mass of the sample by about 20% (w/w), presumably due to increased hydration of proteins.

The aqueous dispersions of washed meats from herring, mackerel and shark were highly viscous and their viscosity was both temperature- and concentration-dependent. As the temperature of the dispersions increased, their viscosity decreased, however, upon subsequent cooling the apparent viscosity of the dispersion was mostly recovered. In addition, the viscosity of the herring and mackerel dispersions was increased to >5 Pa•s when 2.4% pro-

TABLE 12.7. Proximate Composition (weight %) of Unwashed and Washed Fish Meat.

Species	Component	Unwashed	Washed
Capelin	Moisture	83.98 ± 0.20	93.19 ± 0.10
	Crude protein ($N \times 6.25$)	12.70 ± 0.31	4.51 ± 0.15
	Lipid	1.98 ± 0.01	1.13 ± 0.04
Herring	Moisture	72.40 ± 0.10	86.70 ± 2.30
	Crude protein ($N \times 6.25$)	17.40 ± 1.20	8.30 ± 0.20
	Lipid	8.10 ± 1.20	4.10 ± 0.10
Mackerel	Moisture	63.60 ± 0.30	82.20 ± 1.60
	Crude protein ($N \times 6.25$)	19.30 ± 0.20	9.60 ± 1.10
	Lipid	14.00 ± 0.50	5.30 ± 0.20
Shark	Moisture	79.80 ± 0.11	91.54 ± 0.16
	Crude protein ($N \times 6.25$)	18.25 ± 0.32	7.58 ± 0.51
	Lipid	1.03 ± 0.05	0.55 ± 0.01

teins were present. For capelin dispersions, heating of the samples to 80–100°C resulted in a permanent loss of viscosity. However, for herring, mackerel and shark dispersions, loss of viscosity was achieved only when a small amount of acetic acid was added to the washed samples prior to heat treatment. Thus, the solubility of protein dispersions, once formed, was ≥83% in all cases examined in our laboratory.

The dispersions with reduced apparent viscosity showed remarkable thermal stability. Thus, the proteins were stable when heated to 100°C for 30 min and even moderate concentrations of salt in the solution did not influence the solubility characteristics of such dispersions. Stable proteins are of interest in studying structure-function relationships and examining the possibilities of their use in biological applications [44]. Recently, Wu et al. [45] and Stanley et al. [46] have reported solubility of beef and chicken myofibrillar proteins in low ionic strength media, and Doi [47] has demonstrated that under controlled pH, ionic strength and heating, transparent gels may be obtained from globular protein that may have potential application in food preparations. Use of these dispersions is feasible as a protein supplement in extrusion cooking of cereal-based products and development of a functional powder by suitable dehydration of the dispersion.

The fish protein concentrates (powders) prepared from different species examined in our laboratory had a protein content of ≥85%. The amino acid composition of products so obtained was similar to that of the proteins present in the starting muscle tissues. However, the content of individual free amino acids in the products was much lower than those present in the starting materials as exemplified for capelin (see Table 12.7). Thus, the dispersions and powders so prepared had the advantage of being of equal nutritional value to their original fish proteins but having a bland taste. In addition, the washing process removed most of the hemoproteins from the original muscle tissues; products obtained in this way had a milky white colour. Use of such dispersions for fortification of cereal-based products is promising [48].

6.3. PROTEIN HYDROLYZATES

Freshly landed aquatic species such as male capelin may be mechanically deboned, similar to the procedure employed in surimi production. The comminuted raw materials are suspended in water and enzyme and added to the slurry [49]. The reaction may be allowed to proceed between 2 h and 1 week, depending on the activity of the enzyme employed as well as the process temperature and other factors. After separation of solids, the aqueous layer is clarified, the pH adjusted and the material dehydrated (Figure 12.4). The process may also include sterilization at different stages, if necessary.

Typical protein yield and proximate composition of hydrolyzates from capelin (Biocapelin) and shark (Bioshark) are given in Table 12.8. Although

FISH

↓

mincing

↓

adjustment of protein concentration

↓

pH adjustment

↓

enzymatic hydrolysis

↓

enzyme inactivation

↓

filtration

↓

decolorization

↓

filtration

↓

neutralization

↓

drying

(if necessary)

↓

PROTEIN HYDROLYZATE

Figure 12.4 Flowsheet for production of hydrolyzates.

TABLE 12.8. Typical Protein Recovery (%) and Composition of Hydrolyzates from Capelin (Biocapelin) and Shark (Bioshark).

Material	Protein Recovery	Composition (%)			
		Protein	Lipid	Moisture	Ash
Capelin	—	13.6–14.1	3.3–3.9	78.0–78.3	2.4–2.5
Biocapelin	51.6–70.6	65.9–73.3	0.2–0.4	5.3–6.3	14.9–20.6
Shark	—	17.9–18.6	1.0–1.1	79.6–80.0	0.8–0.9
Bioshark	58.0–72.4	77.4–78.0	0.2–0.3	7.4–8.2	13.4–14.3

many factors affect the yield of hydrolysis, the type of enzyme employed has a marked effect on this and also on the characteristics of the final product. The enzymes examined in our laboratory included papain, Alcalase, Neutrase and endogenous autolytic enzymes of each species. High yields of protein recovery by Alcalase and its low cost may provide an incentive for its use in commercial operations [50].

A close scrutiny of the results presented in Table 12.8 indicates that hydrolyzates generally possess a lower lipid content than their original protein source, on dry-weight basis. As hydrolysis proceeds, the elaborate membrane system of the muscle cells tends to round up and form insoluble vesicles, thus allowing the removal of membrane structural lipids. Consequently, protein hydrolyzates are expected to be more stable towards oxidative deterioration. In addition, hydrolyzates produced from capelin and seal meat had an ivory-white colour, which might have significance when formulating crab leg analogues and other fabricated products to which addition of colorants is generally desirable.

The amino acid composition of capelin protein hydrolyzate (Biocapelin) and shark protein hydrolyzate (Bioshark) produced by Alcalase-assisted hydrolysis was compared with that of their corresponding muscle tissues. Results indicated that the amino acid profiles for both species remained generally unchanged. However, sensitive amino acids such as methionine and tryptophan were slightly affected. Furthermore, the content of free amino acids in the hydrolysates was increased from 123 mg/100 g sample to 2,944 mg/100 g. Thus, the hydrolysates so prepared may be used for thermal generation of aroma when combined with sugars such as glucose [51].

The hydrolyzates prepared from capelin and shark had excellent solubility characteristics at pH values ranging from 2.0 to 10.4. While 90.4–98.6% of nitrogenous compounds of Biocapelin were soluble, corresponding values for Bioshark varied between 95.5 and 98.1%. The fat adsorption, moisture retention, emulsification properties, and whippability of the hydrolyzates were also excellent [23,43]. In addition, when capelin and shark protein hydrolyzates were added to meat model systems at 0.5–3.0% levels, an increase of up to 4.0% and 8.0%, respectively, in the cooking yield of processed meats was noticed [23,43]. Furthermore, Biocapelin inhibited oxidation of meat lipids by 17.7–60.4% as reflected in the content of 2-thiobarbituric acid reactive substances of the treated meat systems. The mechanism by which this antioxidant effect is exerted may be related to the action of hydrolyzed molecules as chelators of metal ions that could be released from hemoproteins during the heat processing of the meat. Furthermore, the phenolic nature of some amino acids such as tyrosine may allow their participation as free radical scavengers in the medium [52, 53].

7. CONCLUSIONS

Novel lipid and protein products may be prepared from underutilized aquatic species and their processing discards. These products may be used as pharmaceutical, food and specialty commodities. The beneficial health effects of seafood lipids and the nature of their proteins would provide the necessary incentive for consumers to modify their current dietary habits, particularly in the western world.

8. REFERENCES

1. Bang, H. O., J. Dyerberg and N. Hjorne. 1976. "The composition of food consumed by Greenland eskimos," Acta Med. Scand. 200:69–73.
2. Kinsella, J. E. 1986. "Food components with potential therapeutic benefits: The n-3 polyunsaturated fatty acids of fish oils," Food Technol. 40 (2):89–97.
3. Simopoulos, A. P. 1981. "Omega-3 fatty acids in health and disease and growth and development," Am. J. Clin. Nutr. 54:438–463.
4. Venugopal, V. and F. Shahidi. 1994. "Thermostable water dispersions of myofibrillar proteins from Atlantic mackerel (*Scomber scumbrus*)," J. Food Sci. 59: 265–268, 276.
5. Yongmanichai, W. and O. P. Ward. 1989. "Omega-3 fatty acids: Alternative sources of production," Prog. Biochem. 24:117–125.
6. Ackman, R. C. 1988. "The year of fish oil." Chemistry & Industry 3:139–145.
7. Illingworth, D. and D. Ullmann. 1990. "Effects of omega-3 fatty acids on risk factors for cardiovascular diseases," Omega-3 Fatty Acids in Health and Disease. R. S. Lees and Karel M., New York, NY: Marcel Dekker, Inc. pp. 39–69.
8. Nestel, P. J. 1990. "N-3 fatty acids, cardiac function and cardiovascular survival," Paper presented at the 2nd International Conference on the Health Effects of Omega-3 Polyunsaturated Fatty Acids in Seafoods. March 20–23, Washington, DC.
9. Fischer, S. 1989. "Dietary polyunsaturated fatty acids and eicosanoid formation in humans," Adv. Lipid Res. 23:169–198.

10. Branden, L. M. and K. K. Carroll. 1986. "Dietary polyunsaturated fats in relation to mammary carcinogenesis in rats," Lipids 21:285–288.
11. Dyerberg, J. 1986. "Linolenate-derived polyunsaturated fatty acids and prevention of atherosclerosis," J. Nutr. Rev. 44:125–134.
12. Mehta, J., L. M. Lopez, D. Lowton and T. Wargovich. 1988. "Dietary supplementation with omega-3 polyunsaturated fatty acids in patients with stable coronary disease: effects on indices of platelet and neurophil function and exercise performance," Am. J. Med. 84:45–52.
13. Phillipson, B. E., D. W. Rothrock, W. E. Conner, W. S. Harris and D. R. Illingworth. 1985. "Reduction of plasma lipids, lipoproteins and apoproteins by dietary fish oils in patients with hypertriglyceridemia," New Eng. J. Med. 312: 1210–1216.
14. Singh, G. and R. K. Chandra. 1988. "Biochemical and cellular effects of fish and fish oils," Prog. Food Nutr. Sci. 12:371–419.
15. Neuringer, M., G. J. Anderson and W.E. Conner. 1988. "The essentiality of n-3 fatty acids for the development and function of the retina and brain," Ann. Rev. Nutr. 8:817–821.
16. Al, M. D. M., G. Hornstra, Y. T. Schouw, M. E. E. W. Bulstra-Remakers and G. Huistes. 1990. "Biochemical EFA status of mothers and their neonates after normal pregnancy," Early Hum. Dev. 24:239–248.
17. Carlson, S. E., R. G. Rhodes and M. G. Ferguson. 1986. "Docosahexaenoic acid status of preterm infants at birth and following feeding with human milk or formula," Am. J. Clin. Nutr. 44:798–802.
18. Carlson, S. E., P. G. Rhodes, V .S. Rao and D. E. Goldgar. 1987. "Effect of fish oil supplementation on the n-3 fatty acid content of red blood cell membranes in preterm infants," Pediatr. Res. 21:507–511.
19. Canadian Scientific Review Committee, Nutrition Recommendation: Minister of National Health and Welfare, Ottawa, ON, 1990 (H49–42/1990E).
20. British Nutrition Foundation. 1992. Report of the Task Force on Unsaturated Fatty Acids, London, UK: Chapman & Hall.
21. Bimbo, A. P. and J. B. Crowther. 1991. "Fish oils: Processing beyond crude oil," Infofish Int. 6: 20–25.
22. Ke, P. J., R. G. Ackman and B. A. Linke. 1975. "Autoxidation of polyunsaturated fatty compounds in mackeral oil: Formation of 2,4,7-decatrianols," J. Am. Oil Chem. Soc. 52:349–353.
23. Shahidi, F., J. Synowiecki and J. Balejko. 1994. "Proteolytic hydrolysis of muscle proteins of harp seal (*Phoca groenlandica*)," J. Agric. Food Chem. 42:2634–2638.
24. Neito, S., A. Garrido, J. Sanhueza, L. A. Loyola, G. Morales, F. Leighten and A. Velenzuela. 1993. "Flavonoids as stablizers of fish oils: an alternative to synthetic antioxidants," J. Am. Oil Chem. Soc. 70:773–778.
25. Shahidi, F., U. N. Wanasundara, Y. He and V. K. S. Shukla. 1997. "Stabilization of marine lipids," Flavor and Lipid Chemistry of Seafood. ACS Symposium Series. Washington, DC: American Chemical Society. In press.
26. Shahidi, F. and X.-Q Han. 1993. "Encapsulation of food ingredients," CRC Crit. Rev. Food Sci. Nutr. 33:501–547.
27. Taguchi, K., K. Iwami, F. Ibuki and M. Kawabata. 1992. "Oxidative stability of sardine oil embedded in spray-dried egg white powder and its use in n-3 unsaturated fatty acid fortification of cookies," Biosci. Biotech. Biochem. 56:560–563.

28. Lin, C.-C., S.-Y. Lin and W. S. Hwang. 1995. "Microencapsulation of squid oil with hydrophillic macromolecules for oxidative and thermal stabilization," J. Food Sci. 60:36–39.
29. Wanasundara, U. N. and F. Shahidi. 1995. "Storage stability of microencapsulated seal blubber oil," J. Food Lipids. 2:73–86.
30. Shahidi, F., R. A. Amarowicz, J. Synowiecki and M. Naczk. 1993. "Extraction and concentration of omega-3 fatty acids of seal blubber," Developments in Food Engineering, Yano T., R. Matsuno, and K. Nakamura, London, UK: Blackie Academic and Professional. pp. 627–629.
31. Suzuki, T. 1981. Fish and Krill Processing Technology, London: Applied Science Publishers.
32. Sato, K., R. Yoshinaka, M. Sato and Y. Shimizu. 1986. "Collagen content in the muscle of fishes in association with their swimming movement and meat texture," Bull. Jpn. Soc. Sci. Fish. 52:1595–1598.
33. Ikeda, S. 1979. "Other organic components and inorganic components," Advances in Fish Science and Technology, Connell, J. J., Surrey: Fishing News Books. pp. 111–124.
34. Lee, C. M. 1994. "Surimi processing from lean fish," Seafoods: Chemistry, Processing Technology and Quality, Shahidi, F. and J. R. Botta, Glasgow: Blackie Academic and Professional. pp. 263–287.
35. Spencer, K. E. and M. A. Tung. 1994. "Surimi processing from fatty fish," Seafoods: Chemistry, Processing Technology and Quality, Shahidi F. and J. R. Botta, Glasgow: Blackie Academic and Professionals. pp. 288–319.
36. Nakagawa, T., F. Nagayama, H. Ozaki, S. Watabe and K. Hashimoto. 1989. "Effect of glycotytic enzymes on the gel forming ability of fish muscle," Nippon Suisan Gakkaishi.
37. Ziegler, G. R. and E. A. Foegeding. 1990. "The gelation of proteins," Advances in Food Research, Volume 34, Kinsella, J. E., New York, NY: Academic Press. pp. 203–298.
38. Freitheim, K., B. Egelandsdal, O. Harbitz and K. Samejima. 1985. "Slow lowering of pH induces gel formation of myosin," Food Chem. 18:169–177.
39. Shahidi, F. and V. Venugopal. 1993. "Production of functional proteins from underutilized fish species," Meat Focus International 2:443–445.
40. Shahidi, F. and V. Venugopal. 1994. "Solubilization and thermostability of water dispersions of muscle structural proteins of Atlantic herring (*Clupea harengus*)," J. Agric. Food Chem. 42:1440–1446.
41. Venugopal, V. and Shahidi, F. 1995. "Value added products from underutilized fish species," CRC Crit. Rev. Food Sci. Nutr. 35:431–435.
42. Shahidi, F. and Onodenalore, A. C. 1995. "Water dispersions of myofibrillar proteins from capelin (*Mallotus villosus*)," Food Chem. 53:51–54.
43. Onodenalore, A. C. and F. Shahidi. 1997. "Protein dispersions and hydrolyzates from shark (*Isurus oxyrinchus*)," J. Aquatic Food Prod. Technol. In press.
44. Nosoh, Y. and T. Sekiguchi. 1991. "Stability of proteins," Protein Stability and Stabilization through Protein Engineering, Sussex, UK: Ellis Horwood Ltd. pp. 101–123.
45. Wu, Y. J., M. T. Atallah and H. O. Hultin. 1992. "The proteins of washed minced fish muscle have significant solubility in water," J. Food Biochem. 15:209–218.
46. Stanley, D. W., A. P. Stone and H. O. Hultin. 1994. "Solubility of beef and

chicken myofibrillar proteins in low ionic strength media," J. Agric. Food Chem. 42:863.

47. Doi, E. 1993. "Gels and gelling of globular proteins," Trends Food Sci. Technol. 4:1.
48. Venugopal, V., S. N. Doke, P. M. Nair and F. Shahidi. 1994. "Protein powders and extruded products from shark muscle proteins," Meat Focus International 3:200–202.
49. Mohr, V. 1977. "Fish protein concentrate production by enzymatic hydrolysis," Biochemical Aspects of New Protein Food, Adler-Nissen, J., B. O. Eggum, L. Munck and H. S. Olsen. FEBS, Federation of European Biochemical Societies, 11th Meeting, Copenhagen, Vol. 44, pp. 259–269.
50. Shahidi, F., X.-Q. Han and J. Synowiecki. 1995. "Production and characteristics of protein hydrolyzates from capelin (*Mallotus villosus*)," Food Chem. 53: 285–293.
51. Ho, C.-T., C.-W. Chen, U. N. Wanasundara and F. Shahidi. 1997. "Natural antioxidants from tea," Natural Antioxidants: Chemistry, Health Effects and Applications, Shahidi, F., Champaign, IL: AOCS Press. pp. 213–223.
52. Shahidi, F. and R. Amarowicz. 1996. "Antioxidant activity of protein hydrolyzates from aquatic species," J. Am. Oil Chem. Soc. 73:1197–1199.
53. Amarowicz, R. and F. Shahidi. 1997. "Antioxidant activity of peptide fractions of capelin protein hydrolyzates," Food Chem. 58:355–359.

CHAPTER 13

Regulatory Aspects of Functional Products

A. M. STEPHEN[1]

1. INTRODUCTION

TRADITIONALLY, food products have been developed for taste, appearance, value, and convenience for the consumer. The development of products to confer a health benefit is a relatively new trend, and recognizes the growing acceptance of the role of diet in disease prevention and treatment. This change in motivation for product development has moved organizations and companies involved in formulating foods for health benefit into new areas of understanding, like health risk, risk/benefit analysis, evaluation of efficacy and toxicity, and health regulations. Legislation in relation to nutrient content and health to protect the consumer has not been encountered by many of these organizations before, and the regulations within this legislation are often viewed as barriers to product development and economic growth [1]. Many consumers, convinced of the benefits of certain products, also view regulations negatively, suggesting that such interference by government is detrimental to their pursuit of appropriate health choices [2]. On the other hand, health agencies have difficulty understanding why those developing new products are often reluctant to determine the active components in the natural product being developed or to evaluate their effectiveness in human trials. Those in the health profession view such levels of quality control and effectiveness as desirable for both developers and marketers of products and essential for consumers purchasing and consuming them. Differences in background and appreciation of the concerns of each side of this debate have led

[1]Division of Nutrition and Dietetics, College of Pharmacy and Nutrition, University of Saskatchewan, Saskatoon, SK, Canada.

to considerable discussion and even argument over the last few years in a number of countries. Fortunately, there is recognition by both sides that the status quo is unacceptable, and that dialogue is needed on how present regulations may be modified to address the growth of these products in the marketplace, and their place in health prevention and treatment. This chapter describes health regulations for natural products in some countries and attempts to outline how the field may be allowed to move forward. However, the area of regulation is constantly changing in many countries and it is difficult to describe even the present situation, far less attempt to forecast what may happen in the next few years.

2. WHAT TERMS SHOULD BE USED?

A number of different terms are used to describe the many natural products currently being developed for health benefit. These include *nutraceutical, functional food, pharmafood, designer food, vitafood, phytochemical,* and *foodaceutical.* Other terms, often considered separately, should also be included in discussions of regulatory issues like *medical foods, dietary supplements, herbal products,* and *botanicals.*

In North America, the terms *functional food* and *nutraceutical* have been used interchangeably, and a number of definitions of what is included under these all-encompassing headings have been advanced [3]. However, difficulties arise when it comes to regulation, in that some differentiation is required between those products that are sold and consumed as "foods," versus products where a particular component has been isolated from a food and is sold in the form of a tablet, capsule, powder, or other concentrated form. Clearly, products sold as foods are more self-limiting in terms of total daily consumption than a concentrate, where a dose higher than that suggested is far more likely. Hence, separation of these two types of products seems necessary. In Canada, the suggestion has been made by the Health Protection Branch of Health Canada that the terms *functional food* and *nutraceutical* be used separately to describe these two forms of presentation, with the following definitions:

> A functional food is similar in appearance to conventional foods, is consumed as part of a usual diet, and has demonstrated physiological benefits and/or reduces the risk of chronic disease beyond basic nutritional functions.
>
> A nutraceutical is a product produced from foods but sold in pills, powders, (potions) and other medicinal forms not generally associated with food and demonstrated to have a physiological benefit or provides protection against chronic disease [3].

Similarly, in the United Kingdom, the Ministry of Agriculture, Fisheries and Food (MAFF) has developed a definition of functional food as: "A food that has a component incorporated into it to give a specific medical or physiological benefit, other than a purely nutritional benefit" [4].

This definition was intended to help distinguish functional foods from products fortified with vitamins and minerals for nutritional benefit. While this distinction is not as clear in the Canadian definition, both terms indicate that a functional food is presented as a "food" and not as an isolated form, as a nutraceutical would be.

In Japan, where interest in functional foods has been growing since the early 1980s, these foods were defined as "Foods for Specified Health Use" (FOSHU) in 1991, with the introduction of a branch of the Ministry of Health and Welfare to deal specifically with their regulation [5].

FOSHU foods are those that:

- are expected to have a specific effect on health due to relevant constituents of foods
- are foods from which allergens have been removed, the effect of such addition or removal has been scientifically evaluated and permission has been granted to make claims regarding the specific beneficial effect on health to be expected from their consumption
- should not pose a health or hygiene risk [5]

Like the Canadian and United Kingdom proposals, FOSHU products are defined as "foods" consumed in the normal diet. The definitions proposed by Health Canada may be modified prior to being formalized, but the idea that there is a distinction between forms of presentation has been accepted by industry, health professionals and consumer groups in Canada.

For the purposes of discussion of health regulations, in this chapter the distinction between presentation as a food and a concentrated form or supplement is a useful one. The term *functional food* will be used for products in a food form, the term *nutraceutical* for a concentrated form. Both can be considered to be natural products with health benefit.

3. WHAT ARE THE REGULATIONS THAT AFFECT FUNCTIONAL FOOD AND NUTRACEUTICAL INDUSTRIES?

Generally, in discussions of regulations in regard to functional foods and nutraceuticals, the issue is the ability of those developing the products to say what their products does in relation to health, or in other words, whether or not they can "make a claim" about it. In order to understand the world situation in relation to these products, it is important to understand what is meant by a "claim," and also to understand the various items of information that already appear and that may appear in the future on a label or package. These are described below in a general sense, since countries have different regulations and also use terms somewhat differently.

3.1. INFORMATION ON THE PACKAGE

3.1.1. Ingredient List

For most countries, the ingredients in a food product must appear on the package, in descending order in terms of total content. Hence the first requirement of any food product is to know what is in it, in terms of food constituents.

3.1.2. Nutrient Information

Nutrient information is compulsory in some countries, like the United States, and voluntary in others. What constitutes the nutrient information (i.e., what nutrients *must* be listed and what nutrients *may* be listed) varies from country to country, generally depending on the scientific evaluation in each country of the importance for the consumer of each nutrient. Nutrient information appears usually in a box on the package, the layout of which is standardized in some countries, or more flexible in others. Nutrient information is given per serving in some countries and per 100 g in others, depending on what is most familiar to the consumer. Some countries give both. In some countries, the serving size is uniform and legislated; in others it is at the discretion of the manufacturer. Where the latter situation occurs, serving size can be altered to suggest desirable characteristics of the product and, as a result, there is a move in many countries to more regulated serving sizes, and/or expression per 100 g.

3.1.3. Nutrient Content Claims

Nutrient content claims on the package indicate the content of a particular nutrient that the manufacturer wants to promote, generally for health reasons, although the claim itself makes no connection with health. Examples of nutrient content claims would be "low fat," "cholesterol-free," "high fibre," "energy-reduced," "25% less fat," and "light." The criteria for the content of the nutrient in a food to comply with the nutrient claim are tightly regulated; they vary from country to country, and there has been considerable discussion about them in recent years. Some countries specify criteria for more than one nutrient to enable a claim for only one. For example, a product with a claim of "cholesterol-free" often has to have a low level of saturated fat as well, since saturated fat is considered a greater risk for coronary heart disease than is cholesterol. The aim of such a move is to ensure that the consumer does not buy a product that is cholesterol-free and high in saturated fat, assuming it is healthy. Some nutrient claims also must satisfy criteria "per 100 g" rather than simply "per serving," so that the serving size is not altered to enable the product to have the claim. In some countries, like Canada, the appearance of a nutrient claim on a package triggers the requirement for nutrient information, which otherwise is voluntary [6]. Hence all products with a claim of "low fat" or "fat-free" must present the nutrient content information.

As indicated above, nutrient content claims can indicate to the consumer that the product has a particular level of a nutrient, but they cannot relate that to any health issue; in other words, they cannot tell the consumer why they should care about this level of the nutrient. Consumers have to know why they would buy a product with "low fat" or "high fibre" on it.

3.1.4. Structure-Function Claims

Many nutrients are known to affect particular physiological or biochemical processes in the body. A "structure-function claim" is a claim on a package, which indicates that a nutrient plays a role in a particular biological process. These can also be described as "biological role claims" [6]. Examples of such claims would be to say that "high fibre promotes regularity" or that "iron is important for the functioning of red blood cells to carry oxygen" or that "calcium aids in the growth and maintenance of bones." None of these associations indicates a disease entity, and generally such claims cannot directly or indirectly refer to the treatment, mitigation or prevention of any disease, disorder, or abnormal physical state. One could *infer* from these claims that oversupply of a nutrient or a deficient intake could lead to a malfunction of the biological process described, but this is not stated in a "structure-function" claim. Many countries that at present do not allow "health" claims (i.e., where health or a disease entity is mentioned) do, however, allow "structure-function" claims. Generally, if a product contains a structure-function claim, this triggers the declaration of nutrient content information.

3.1.5. Health Claims

Health claims are statements that relate a nutrient, series of nutrients, food component or food product to the prevention or treatment of disease. The definition of health claim in the United States, as part of the Nutrition Labelling and Education Act (NLEA), is: "A health claim is any claim made on the label that either expressly or through implication (through the use of endorsements, written statements, symbols or vignettes), characterizes the relationship between any substance to a disease or health related condition" [7].

Claims relating to essential nutrient diseases are not included in this definition and are not considered health claims [7]. Health claims can relate to components of foods or foods themselves, and for purposes of clarification, it is useful to separate them into three types: (1) generic, (2) commodity, and (3) product-specific.

3.1.5.1. Generic Health Claims

Generic health claims are those that relate a nutrient, in the context of a total diet, to a particular disease or condition. Examples of generic health claims are those permitted in the United States under the NLEA such as: "Diets low in saturated fat and cholesterol and rich in fruits, vegetables and grain products that contain some types of fibre, particularly soluble fibre, may reduce the risk of heart disease, a disease associated with many factors" [8].

Generic claims do not apply to a specific product or food and thus the *products* on which they are placed cannot be said to be protective, only the nutrients in them. The basis for the claim to be permitted is the weight of scientific evidence demonstrating the beneficial effect of the nutrient in the prevention or treatment of the condition stated [7].

3.1.5.2. Commodity/Ingredient Health Claims

Commodity or ingredient claims describe claims for commodities or ingredients, like the statements recently permitted in the United States for oatmeal and oat bran: "Diets high in oat bran/oatmeal and low in saturated fat and cholesterol may reduce the risk of heart disease" [9].

Similar statements for psyllium are now being considered favourably by the Food and Drug Administration (FDA) [10]. Again, such claims are not product-specific, although it may be indicated that the commodity is present in the product [11]. However, it does not indicate in the claim that the *product* on which the claim is placed is protective [11]. Like the generic claims, the basis for allowing such claims is the weight of scientific evidence in support of the beneficial effect of the commodity or ingredient in the prevention or treatment of a condition.

3.1.5.3. Product-Specific Claims

A product-specific claim would be a claim that states that the product on which the claim is placed has a protective effect against a disease, that it either reduces the risk of the disease occurring or is useful in treating or reducing the symptoms of a pre-existing condition. Such claims can be made for food products in some countries, but in most cases in order to do so, the product must be evaluated under the guidelines for efficacy and toxicity specified for drugs [3]. For this type of claim, the product itself, rather than simply the ingredients or nutrients in it, have to be shown to have benefit.

4. FOODS VERSUS DRUGS

In most countries, an act of government regulates the sale and promotion of food and drugs. For some countries, the act is for both food and drugs, as in the Food and Drugs Act and Regulations in Canada or the Federal Food, Drug, and Cosmetic Act in the United States. In other countries there are separate acts for food and for drugs. For example, Sweden has a Food Act and an Act on Medicinal Products [12]. In the past, food and drugs were dealt with separately by different divisions or departments, sometimes within the same agency, branch or administrative unit of government as in Canada (Health Protection Branch, Health Canada), the United States (Food and Drug Administration), or in separate agencies as in the United Kingdom, where foods are regulated by the Ministry of Agriculture, Fisheries and Food (MAFF), often in conjunction with the Department of Health (DH), while drugs are regulated by the Medicines Control Agency (MCA). There was little apparent overlap, mainly because the definitions of *food* and *drug* were distinct when the acts of government were written and foods were not promoted on health grounds. The definitions of food and drug were distinct as in Canada:

Food: Any article manufactured, sold or represented for use as food or drink for man, chewing gum and any ingredient that may be mixed with food for any purpose whatsoever.

Drug: Any substance manufactured, sold or represented for use in a) the diagnosis, treatment, mitigation or prevention of disease or b) restoring correcting or modifying organic functions in man or animal [3].

These remain the definitions in Canada; hence there is no statement within the definition of a food that it can confer health benefits. If a company wants to indicate a health benefit, then the food must undergo evaluation as a drug, generally referred to as pursuing “the drug route” [3,12].

In recent years, with the growth of interest in foods and components of foods, natural products, herbal products, botanicals, and dietary supplements to promote health and reduce the risk or treat disease, the existing definitions of food and drug are being questioned. Many countries are dealing with this issue, and some have introduced separate categories for such products or indicated clearly under which department of government certain types of products must be regulated.

4.1. DIETARY SUPPLEMENTS

Definitions of the term *dietary supplements* vary. In many countries, these are thought of as purified nutrient preparations to “supplement” the diet, providing vitamins and minerals in amounts to ensure sufficient intake to prevent deficiency. However, what is now included under the term *supplement* has broadened in some countries, so that compounds other than vitamins and minerals are also included.

With the passing of the Dietary Supplement Health and Education Act

(DSHEA) in the United States in 1994, the term *dietary supplement* is now defined as:

- containing one or more nutrients, herbs, botanicals, or a concentrate, metabolite or constituent extract from the ingredients previously mentioned
- in the form of a supplement (meaning tablet, capsule or powder)
- is not represented as a food or sole item of a meal or the diet
- includes a similar new drug or biologic approved under previous legislation and not currently being investigated [13]

The DSHEA distinguishes dietary supplements from both foods and drugs and provides separate regulations for these preparations. Unlike the health claims now permitted for nutrients, which are strictly worded and where compliance with wording is mandatory, regulations for supplements are less rigid in terms of wording but can have no relationship with disease.

Unlike the U.S., most other countries have not created a special category for dietary supplements, and there are considerable differences in the way these products are regulated. In many countries, they continue to be regulated as foods; however, if a claim of medicinal purpose is assigned to a product, it is then regulated as a drug. There are many concerns worldwide about concentrated formulations where dosages above amounts recommended are easily achieved, and considerable discussion is presently occurring in how to regulate these products.

5. MEDICAL FOODS/FOODS FOR SPECIAL DIETARY USE

Many countries have separate regulations for foods specifically designed to be used for nutrition-related disorders. These come under two terms *medical foods* and *foods for special dietary use.* In the United States, medical foods are defined as "foods formulated to be consumed or administered under the supervision of a physician and which are intended for the specific dietary management of a disease or condition for which distinctive nutritional requirements, based on recognized scientific principle, are established by medical evaluation" [14].

These foods are formulated to aid in the dietary management of diseases or conditions that result in "distinctive nutritional requirements," which are different from the nutritional requirements of healthy people. These foods can be distinguished from "foods for special dietary use" [6,14], a term used in a number of countries, which are foods formulated to meet a special dietary need, such as a food allergy, but where the nutrients required are the same as for healthy people. These latter foods might have different ingredients or physical form of other foods, but not different nutrients. Medical foods are also given under the supervision of a physician, where the use of the food requires continued monitoring by a physician to ensure that the distinctive nutritional requirements of the patient are being met. In other words, they are not foods simply *recommended* by a physician [14].

Because of the very specific uses of medical foods, they are exempted from the nutrition labelling requirements of NLEA, although this should not compromise the standards of medical foods, either in content or in substantiation of their effects.

Because of the NLEA, the United States has had to address overlapping issues like dietary supplements and medical foods in more depth than other countries where claims are not permitted and where labelling is not mandatory. The distinction between *medical foods* and *foods for special dietary use* indicates the complexity of food and health issues, which many other countries are now considering or may have to consider in the future in the same way as the United States has done over the last decade.

6. THE PRESENT SITUATION

Because of the many different types of products that come under the umbrella of "natural products with health benefits," there is considerable confusion about what these products should be called, how they should be regulated, whether or not they raise safety concerns, and whether or not health claims should be permitted. These issues face governments, industry and academics around the world, particularly in the developed countries, where there is the strongest consumer interest. Some countries are viewed with envy by those in others, who see the regulatory environment in other countries as less rigid than their own. Many confuse the different types of health claims, implying that product-specific claims may be permitted when they are not, and many assume that if health claims are permitted in a country, then many companies are making those claims, when in reality they may not be. Finally, there appears to be an assumption that if health claims are permitted, then the level of proof for efficacy and safety is less than in those countries where no health claims are allowed. It is a common belief by industry that an inability to make health claims jeopardizes the success of a product and that this is a detriment to the growth of the entire field [1]. In order to address some of these concerns, it is important to know the situation in a number of key countries.

6.1. UNITED STATES

6.1.1. Foods

In 1984, the Kellogg Company, in conjunction with the National Cancer Institute, made a claim on their breakfast cereal All Bran, indicating that a high-fibre diet was protective against cancer. Although health claims of this kind were not permitted by law at that time, the claim was allowed to remain, and was followed by other claims on packages and in advertising in the United States through the 1980s [15,16]. Because of concern that consumers were being misled by the many unsubstantiated claims appearing, in 1990 the U.S. Congress passed the Nutrition Labelling and Education Act [17]. This act, which came into effect in 1994, regulates three components of information on food packages: nutrient information, nutrient claims, and health claims. Nutrient information is now in a uniform format, as "Nutrition Facts" on every package, and surveys of consumers indicate an increasing awareness of the label itself and the information it contains [18,19]. More importantly, purchases may have been affected by the information on the label, with trends toward healthier products [19,20]. With strictly controlled use of nutrient claims, the NLEA has also been very successful in ensuring uniform information on packaging when terms like *low fat, cholesterol–free, reduced,* and *lite* are used.

As for health claims, initially seven diet-disease health claims were permitted on packaging. The relationships permitted were:

- calcium and a reduced risk of osteoporosis
- sodium and an increased risk of hypertension
- dietary saturated fat and cholesterol and an increased risk of coronary heart disease
- dietary fat and an increased risk of cancer
- fibre-containing grain products, fruits, vegetables and a reduced risk of cancer
- fruits, vegetables and grain products that contain fibre, particularly soluble fibre, and a reduced risk of coronary heart disease
- fruits and vegetables and a reduced risk of cancer

For each of these claims, the wording is strictly controlled, as indicated earlier.

There is considerable debate about the use and usefulness of these claims. Estimates that a dozen food companies are using claims have been interpreted both as a large number [20], and a small number [21]. Others suggest that "few are visible in the marketplace" [22]. The general consensus is that they are little used by the food industry for a number of reasons. First, products that display health claims must contain certain nutrients within specified ranges, otherwise known as the "Jelly Bean Rule." The purpose here is not to allow a health claim for one nutrient when the product contains high levels or low levels of other nutrients of concern [23]. Second, the wording on the claims is onerous and unappealing. It would be unlikely to attract the attention of the target consumers, those who are interested in nutrition but are not so knowledgeable that they know the diet-disease link well already. For both these reasons, the food industry has not pursued rigorously the use of these generic health claims.

A different kind of health claim has recently been approved in the United States. In January 1997, the FDA authorized the use of health claims relating soluble fibre from oatmeal and oat bran and the risk of coronary heart disease [9]. This was the first time a specific commodity was identified as having beneficial effects that could be stated in claims on packaging. Although there has been some rewording of the permitted claims to ensure that it is soluble fibre from *oats* that is identified as the protective agent in a food, and that the soluble fibre must exist in whole oats, the claim stands and is now being used in products containing whole oats [11].

The claim for oatmeal and oat bran is likely to be followed by claims for other commodities. In fact, in May 1997, the FDA responded to a submission that a claim be permitted for products containing psyllium, another soluble dietary fibre source that lowers serum cholesterol [10]. Most recently, Kellogg has submitted a petition to allow a claim for wheat bran in relation to colon cancer [24]. However, both the oat and psyllium claims and others that follow are not product-specific, and are therefore open to use by a number of companies with a variety of products. Product-specific health claims for foods are not allowed in the United States, which is what many food companies wanted, as indicated by Silvergrade [19]. Thus, many food companies remain disappointed with the FDA's health claims policies; they had hoped that the FDA would authorize product-specific claims that could provide companies with a unique market advantage [20].

Those in other countries, particularly Canada, suggest that the health claims policies in the United States should be adopted in their country. What should be clear is that the claims presently permitted are generic, or for a commodity that can be incorporated into many different products. The claims for nutrients are used very seldom; it is yet unknown whether consumers are influenced by them but the evidence is not encouraging. If product-specific claims for foods are the goal, then adoption of the present US regulations would not achieve it.

6.1.2. Dietary Supplements

The situation for dietary supplements, or *nutraceuticals,* if this is the term being used for a broad range of concentrated formulations, is quite different. What is defined as a dietary supplement in the United States, under the new DSHEA, has been stated above. Statements can be made on labels about products classed as dietary supplements on the following issues:

- benefits related to classic nutrient deficiency disease and disclosing the prevalence of the disease
- description of the nutrient or dietary ingredient intended to affect the structure or function

- characterizes the mechanism of action
- describes general well-being from consumption of the nutrient or dietary ingredient [13].

In order to state one of these, the manufacturer must have substantiated that the label is truthful and not misleading. Labels cannot claim to diagnose, mitigate, treat, cure or prevent a disease. The label or advertisement must also state: "This statement has not been evaluated by the FDA. This product is not intended to diagnose, treat, cure or prevent any disease" [13].

Another important feature of the DSHEA is that pre-market clearance is not required for labelling or advertising, unlike most other regulations for health claims around the world. The passing of the DSHEA and the lack of requirement for pre-market clearance has led to a tremendous growth in promotion of dietary supplements of many kinds, with countless advertisements for them in U.S. magazines. It has become clear both to those frequently exposed to such advertisements and their scientific evaluation, and to the FDA, that many products are being promoted in relation to disease. "FDA has already received notifications for numerous statements that evidence an intent to cure, treat, mitigate, diagnose or prevent disease" [25]. Such statements are not authorized by the act, and "if the company continues to market the product, it risks regulatory action by the agency" [25]. As was clearly stated in 1994, a product that is intended for medicinal effects, that is, intended for use in the diagnosis, cure, mitigation, treatment, or prevention of disease, is a drug and not a food [13].

Examination of the *Federal Register* through 1996 and 1997 reveals that the Federal Trade Commission is acting on unsubstantiated claims. Products that have been advertised using statements where scientific proof is lacking are being requested to provide proof, withdraw sales or are being subjected to substantial fines [26–30]. Thus, concerns about the lack of pre-market clearance and a lack of resources to deal with fraudulent claims appear to be addressed. It will be important to monitor the success of the DSHEA regulations and their compliance to know if this approach to supplements, in the broad sense defined in this act, is a workable approach for other countries to follow.

6.1.3. Medical Foods

Medical foods as already defined are exempted from the requirements of the NLEA, but this only applies to a food if:

(1) It is a specially formulated and processed product (as opposed to a naturally occurring foodstuff used in its natural state for the partial or exclusive feeding of a patient by means of oral intake or enteral feeding by tube).

(2) It is intended for the *dietary* management of a patient who, because of therapeutic or chronic medical needs, has limited or impaired capacity to ingest, digest, absorb, or metabolize ordinary foodstuffs or certain nutrients, or who has other special medically determined nutrient requirements, the *dietary* management of which cannot be achieved by the modification of the normal diet alone.
(3) It provides nutritional support specifically modified for the management of the distinctive nutrient needs that result from the specific disease or condition, as determined by medical evaluation.
(4) It is intended to be used under medical supervision.
(5) It is intended only for a patient receiving active and ongoing medical supervision wherein the patient requires medical care on a recurring basis for, among other things, instructions on the use of the medical food.

As discussed earlier, these requirements of medical foods distinguish them from foods for special dietary use. The FDA has specifically addressed this confusion because of the many products that have appeared, apparently as medical foods and without the nutritional information required by NLEA. In addition, concerns have been expressed about reduced standards for such products because of the exemption, citing examples where formulations were incorrectly prepared, with serious repercussions. FDA has confirmed that standards of preparation and quality control, as well as evaluation of effects, are no less for medical foods, and because these products are intended for sick people rather than healthy, standards should, if anything, be stricter than for other foods [14].

6.1.4. Summarizing U.S. Regulations

In summary, in the United States health claims for foods permitted under the NLEA are generic, not product-specific. Products containing oats, and possibly psyllium and wheat bran later in 1997, are the only products to date where a *food* component can be mentioned. At present, functional foods would have to be regulated under these guidelines. Purified preparations or nutraceuticals may be considered as dietary supplements if they satisfy the criteria for that category. Claims can be made for supplements but only in relation to nutrient deficiency, structure function or general well-being. That is, dietary supplements cannot be said to be protective against or to treat a disease. Any purified products for which a disease is mentioned in a claim are considered drugs in the United States.

6.2. JAPAN

In Japan the interest in legislation is mainly concerned with functional foods, in other words, products sold as *foods*. This area has been developed in

Japan since the early 1980s in an attempt to address health problems in the growing elderly population [31]. Efforts were made by the Ministries of Agriculture and Health and Welfare to develop food components with potential health benefits, a concept in keeping with traditional oriental beliefs that food substances may play a role in the prevention and treatment of disease. In 1991, the Ministry of Health and Welfare introduced a system for licensing "Foods for Specified Health Use" (FOSHU), which are defined as described earlier. Functional foods for which a FOSHU licence is sought are submitted with evidence (1) of the ingredients and composition of the food, (2) of the health benefits of the food and (3) of its safety to the ministry in charge of their evaluation [5]. At present, 11 categories of functional ingredients exist in Japan as part of FOSHU:

- dietary fibre
- oligosaccharides
- sugar alcohols
- polyunsaturated fatty acids
- peptides and proteins
- glycosides, isoprenoides and vitamins
- alcohols and phenols
- cholines (lecithin)
- lactic acid bacteria
- minerals
- other

For each of these ingredients, the major potential health benefits have been identified. For example, under the oligosaccharide heading, benefits are likely to be: (a) low calories, (b) prevention of tooth decay, (c) intestinal control, and (d) bifidobacterium. For glycosides, isoprenoides and vitamins, categories include: (a) antioxidative effect, (b) intestinal control, (c) improvement of stomach, liver and kidney metabolism, (d) decrease in blood sugar and cholesterol, and (e) hypertensive effect.

An organized approval system through the ministry involves academics and the Health and Nutrition Research Laboratory. Before approval, the food must satisfy the following criteria.

(1) Contribute to the improvement of dietary habits and the maintenance and enhancement of health.
(2) The health benefits for the food or relative components should have a clear medical and nutritional basis.
(3) Appropriate consumption of the food or its constituents should be defined.
(4) The food and its constituents should be judged as safe.
(5) The test methods for the physiochemical properties of the constituents

and for the qualitative and quantitative determination of the constituents should be well defined.

(6) The composition of the product should not be significantly lower in nutritional components compared to those in similar foods.

(7) The food should be consumed in the usual way a food is consumed, and on a daily basis, not occasionally.

(8) The product should be in the form of an ordinary food, not in pill, capsule or other dosage form [5,31,32].

Once approved, the health benefits of the product may be stated on the label, but not in a misleading or exaggerated way. Manufacturers may not encourage overconsumption of the food, give advice that might deter the consumer from receiving medical care or defame competitors or their products [5,31,32].

The first two products were approved under this system in 1993 and about 20 products have been approved per year since. This is only a fraction of the functional foods sold in Japan. The reasons for the small number of submissions are thought to be the level of scientific information needed to show effectiveness and the rigour of the examination process [5,31,32].

Examples of FOSHU claims in Japan include:

- for Oligo cc, a carbonated beverage containing soybean oligosaccharides: This is suitable for those who are concerned about their GI conditions, as it increases intestinal bifidobacteria and helps maintain a good intestinal environment.
- for All Bran, containing wheat bran: All Bran is a food that helps regulate a GI condition, as it is made with wheat bran, which is rich in dietary fibre. Permits maintenance of a comfortable GI condition with a tasty food.
- Heme Iron Drink fe, a soft drink containing Heme iron: This is suitable for those who suffer from a mildly anemic condition that may require an iron supplement [31].

6.2.1. Summarizing Japanese Regulations

In summary, Japan has developed a process for approval of functional foods to enable health claims to be made. This process applies to products eaten as *foods* only. Approved claims, with examples shown above, appear to be modest and relate to health maintenance rather than disease prevention or treatment. Purified preparations or nutraceuticals for which a health effect is stated are regulated as drugs in Japan.

6.3. CANADA

6.3.1. Food and Drugs Act and Regulations

At present, there is no separate category in the Food and Drug Act in Canada for functional foods or nutraceuticals. While some "biological role claims" have been approved for foods through the Food Directorate, products seeking a relationship to a disorder or disease, whether eaten as food or prepared as a concentrate, can submit an application for approval as a drug through the Therapeutic Products Programme (previously Drugs Directorate) of the Health Protection Branch of Health Canada. If approved, the food can then make a claim of an action associated with a disease or disorder within certain limits. For example, chewing gum containing xylitol, which has proven anti-cariogenic activity, can claim to prevent cavities in Canada because it has gained approval through the Therapeutic Products Programme [3,32]. However, effects associated with a list of specific diseases, known as Schedule A, and containing such disorders as hypertension, diabetes, arteriosclerosis, cancer, arthritis, and obesity, cannot be advertised to the public. Hence an ability of either a food or a drug to lower cholesterol cannot be promoted as such to the public in Canada [32].

Recognizing the limitations of the Food and Drugs Act, and the growth of interest in functional foods and nutraceuticals, the Health Protection Branch has taken a number of initiatives to address concerns of many food and pharmaceutical companies, the agricultural community, health professionals and consumers about the present situation. In October of 1996, the Bureau of Nutritional Sciences at the Food Directorate of the Health Protection Branch issued a discussion paper on "Recommendations for Defining and Dealing with Functional Foods," which proposed the definitions for "functional foods" and "nutraceuticals" as outlined earlier [3]. Also included were different options for introducing a means to allow legitimate claims to be made about some natural products:

(1) Sell all functional foods as drugs (the present situation).
(2) Change the Food and Drugs Act (time-consuming and impractical). Opening of the Food and Drugs Act would lead to other changes in the act and would take years for approval.
(3) Invoke an exemption clause in the act: "exempting any food, drug, cosmetic or device from all or any of the provisions of this act."

The Bureau of Nutritional Sciences proposed this third option as their preferred route. The exemption would permit the sale of a functional food bearing a claim provided that the request to permit sale was accompanied by evidence to establish that the functional food was safe and had the beneficial physiological or disease risk reduction effect claimed [3].

Changes to or exemptions from the Food and Drugs Act would involve not only the Food Directorate, but also the Therapeutic Products Programme of Health Canada. In May 1997, these two directorates held a joint consultation with a number of stakeholder groups from across Canada to hear opinions and comments on issues of definition and risks and benefits of claims [33]. It is anticipated that the regulation for functional foods and nutraceuticals will change in Canada before the end of 1998.

6.3.2. Summarizing the Canadian Regulations

In Canada, no health claims can be made for foods, unless a submission is made through the Therapeutic Products Programme for the food to be regulated as a drug. There is no separate category for functional foods or nutraceuticals, although these terms have now been defined and consultations are taking place to consider amendment of the existing regulations to facilitate approval of functional foods. Purified preparations claimed to have benefit in the prevention or treatment of disease are considered drugs in Canada.

6.4. EUROPEAN UNION (EU)

6.4.1. Functional foods

The entire field of functional foods and nutraceuticals is rather fragmented in the EU, with each member country having its own direction at present. There is, for example, no legal definition of "food" in the EU, although there have been discussions about this for a number of years. This has led to a lack of an integrated policy on food legislation and there is therefore a need for a cohesive policy and harmonization among the 15 member states [32].

Most work to create a cohesive policy has been done in the area of functional foods (i.e., products eaten as foods). Purified preparations and supplements remain under the regulation of the member states; indeed, the term *nutraceutical* is not popular and little used [32]. Directives on foods with health effects appear to be following two lines—one as "foods for particular nutritional uses" (PARNUTS) and the other as functional foods, under an initiative called "Functional Food Science in Europe" coordinated through ILSI (International Life Science Institute) Europe [34]. PARNUTS is a directive involving nine separate categories of foods for special nutritional uses:

- infant formulae
- follow-up milk and other follow-up foods
- baby foods
- low-energy and energy-reduced foods intended for weight control
- dietary foods for special medical purposes

- low-sodium food, including low-sodium and sodium-free salts
- gluten-free foods
- food intended to meet the expenditure of intense muscular effort, especially for sportsmen
- foods for persons suffering from diabetes [32]

These foods, apart from those for athletes, would appear to come under the heading of foods for special dietary use or medical foods in other jurisdictions. To date, only the areas of infant foods and energy-reduced foods are being pursued [32].

The "Functional Food Science in Europe" strategy was initiated in order that "Europe should give a clear statement of its position with regard to functional foods in order to improve its industrial competitiveness in the context of a growing world market" [34]. The main goal of the project was to establish "a multidisciplinary discussion platform to reach consensus or concepts in functional food science and requirements for functional food applications" [35].

Six scientific areas have been identified for study:

- gastrointestinal functions
- behavioural and psychological functions
- conception and development
- modulation of lipid metabolism
- impact of food technology
- control of redox status

Following meetings and development of theme papers in 1997, a consensus is being developed and will be published by the end of 1998. While the emphasis in this initiative appears to be the scientific aspects of functional foods, it has been pointed out that "the principal area of interest relates to any food for which a health claim is made" and that researchers, industry and regulators need to work together so that the principles and criteria for substantiating claims can be assessed properly [36]. Presumably then the consensus document will provide guidance for evaluation of the scientific basis for claims. However, it would appear that this initiative is not intended to direct regulatory changes in the EU, indicating that it may remain up to each member to decide how functional foods and nutraceuticals or concentrates are regulated in their own country.

6.4.2. Summarizing the Situation in the EU

In summary, there are a number of initiatives in the EU about functional foods, but they appear to be largely focussed on the scientific issues. At present, regulation of functional foods and supplements/nutraceuticals/concentrates remains at the level of each member country. Regulations for concentrated formulations vary, although many countries consider them as foods. However, claims relating to a disease state are generally not permitted, and if such claims are made, products then come under the regulations for medicinal products or drugs.

6.5. THE WORLD IN SUMMARY

These four examples of different definitions, areas of emphasis and regulatory environment around the world point to the complexity and diversity of the field of natural products. There is at present little common ground and each country is choosing its own direction. However, with global trade and international research, this is highly undesirable. It would be of considerable benefit for industry if regulations were standardized and it would be more cost effective if criteria for evaluation of natural products were similar. While regulations do seem to be going in a number of directions that may converge at some later date, there is a growing willingness to evaluate natural products in a uniform way as the cost of carrying out the complex studies to provide evidence in support of products continues to increase. Moreover, whatever definitions, categorization and route of approval are used, the criteria for proof of beneficial effect do not seem to differ greatly. Each country has emphasized the need for detailed analysis and rigorous science in the evaluation of natural products.

7. EVALUATION OF FUNCTIONAL FOODS AND NUTRACEUTICALS: WHAT LEVEL OF PROOF FOR CLAIMS?

7.1. STEPS IN THE DEVELOPMENT OF A NATURAL PRODUCT

A list of six criteria that must be satisfied to promote a natural product for human use was developed for meetings on nutraceuticals and functional foods in 1995, and has proved useful in examining natural products:

- identification of a plant/crop with biological activity
- identification and characterization of the active principle(s) in the plant
- variation in content of the active principle(s)
- examination of biological activity and efficacy of a natural product or its active component(s)
- toxicity of natural product or active principle(s)
- assessment of natural product for use in human health and medicine [37,38]

7.1.1. Identification of a Plant/Crop with Biological Activity

This factor is almost redundant, since there appears to be an ever-increasing list of products with biological activity. However, further exploration of existing foods as well as new products should be encouraged. For example, in existing foods, there may be chemical entities not yet identified that have health benefits.

7.1.2. Identification and Characterization of the Active Principle(s) in the Plant

For functional foods and nutraceuticals, the active principle or principles is usually well known. Indeed, for many functional foods, the active principle is intentionally added to an existing food in order to confer the health benefit it exhibits. However, for many herbal products, the active principle, though often identified, is not always characterized. Many regard such analysis as unnecessary, citing the use of the product for centuries without knowledge of what brought about its beneficial effects. Several issues are confused here. First, knowledge of active principles and their quantification in products is for the purposes of claims. For example, in its response to concerns that herbal products would be banned under the Dietary Supplement Act as unapproved new drugs, FDA emphasized that their regulations in the act apply to labels and claims, not to sales [25]. In other words, it is only if claims are made about a product that it is necessary to know what it contains. The only situation in which attempts to restrict sales would occur is if there are safety concerns about the product [25].

The requirement of analysis for the active principle or principles is a universal regulation if claims are made, and seems logical. It is unacceptable anywhere to be told that a product of any kind has a particular action if it is uncertain whether or not it contains the necessary components to bring about that action. For example, if a headache medication is taken, it is assumed to contain the components necessary to cure the headache; if a high-fibre cereal is consumed for laxation, it is assumed it will contain high fibre. In both cases, this assumption can only be determined by knowing what helps the headache or colonic function and knowing that the amount required to bring about the effect is present in the product.

Functional foods, nutraceuticals and herbal products often contain complex organic compounds, the analysis of which may be difficult and expensive. Such expense does not preclude the need for analysis, but will have to be taken into account in the decision of whether or not to pursue a claim.

Sometimes, when isolated, the active principle or principles do not bring about the effect that occurs when present in the intact product, and often it is not clear exactly what the active principles are or how they interact. Sometimes the "active" principle is produced by a component in the product, not the component itself. Such is the case with bifidobacteria, which produce short-chain fatty acids, reduce pH, interact with other bacteria, or bring about some other action that is the true "protective" agent. In such cases, an analysis of a "marker" could be used to describe the level of the active principle. In this last case, counts of bifidobacteria would give an indication of the likely production of the real protective agent. Hence it is not always the principle itself that needs to be measured.

7.1.3. Variation in Content of the Active Principle(s)

Analysis of products must be ongoing, carried out at regular intervals on different batches of a product, whether a food or a concentrate. Using the examples given above, when a medication is taken for a headache, it is presumed to help the headache every time it is taken because it contains the same amount of active ingredient; if a cereal helps laxation when it is taken, it is expected that this will always happen, and that the same amount of fibre will be present in every serving to achieve this effect. Again, although often complicated, analytical analysis of the active principle or principles is a fundamental component of knowledge about a product.

7.1.4. Examination of Biological Activity and Efficacy of a Natural Product or Its Active Components

Efficacy or effectiveness of a functional food or nutraceutical can be assessed in a number of ways, using *in vitro* experiments, animal experiments and human studies. While all contribute to the knowledge about a product, in order to make a statement or claim about what a product might do in the human body to have an impact on health, the product has to be studied in humans. Thus, it is unacceptable to suggest that because a product has a certain action in the rat it will have the same action in the human body. That is not to say that animal studies are not valuable; because of access to body tissues in animal studies, more detailed mechanistic aspects of the action of a product can be studied than in human studies. However, these must be supplemented with human work.

Human studies can be carried out in a number of ways, with varying numbers of subjects, length of study periods, level of diet control, and varying detail in analytical methods. If a food is the product under study, then the only way to be able to say with certainty that the effect seen is due to the product under test, rather than another dietary change that might have occurred because of the product or by chance, is to control the rest of the diet consumed when the product is tested, or in other words, to carry out metabolically controlled diet studies. Very often the physiological or biochemical effects being observed are influenced by a number of dietary and lifestyle factors. Unless these factors are controlled, effects of the product may be masked by changes in the other factors. A good example of this is the effect of phytoestrogens from soy on markers of risk for breast cancer, like menstrual cycle length and level of certain reproductive hormones during the menstrual cycle. In 1994 Cassidy et al. [39] published a study where they carried out a diet-controlled human crossover experiment over several menstrual cycles, where half the study subjects ate a controlled western diet and the other half ate the same diet except that soy was added. Soy contains the phytoestrogens, diadzein and genistein, which are well defined chemically, and believed to have estrogenic effects. In Cassidy's experiment under controlled conditions, it was found that when soy was incorporated into the diet, the follicular phase of the menstrual cycle was 2–3 days longer, and levels of the hormones, progesterone, luteinizing hormone (LH), and follicle-stimulating hormone (FSH) were reduced [39]. The only difference between the periods to bring about these effects was the intake of soy. Without a controlled diet, it is unlikely that these effects would have been seen.

If a purified preparation or nutraceutical is being studied (not a food), diet-controlled studies may not be as critical since the product is being evaluated under a protocol similar to that of a drug. However, diet control remains the one way to ensure that no other dietary changes have brought about the effect seen. If diet is not controlled, the number of subjects needs to be higher than if diet is controlled; if the study is not a crossover diet, so that each subject receives each treatment, then again the number of subjects needs to be greater. Studies with diet control are thought to be the most expensive. However, the increased number of subjects required if there is no diet control balances this cost somewhat. In addition, the reliability and lack of ambiguity of the results far outweigh the additional cost, especially for submission for regulatory approval.

7.1.5. Toxicity of Natural Product or Active Principle(s)

It is sometimes suggested that because functional foods and nutraceuticals are natural products, there are no safety issues associated with them. This is not true. Whenever a product is introduced into the body with more of any component, nutrient or otherwise, than has been taken before, there are issues of concern. There are three main areas where problems may arise:

- from taking in more of the active principle than has been recommended
- from taking in more of other components in the product, either at the level of product recommended to be taken, or at higher levels
- from compounds used in the extraction and formulation of the product, and that may have not been removed entirely

It is therefore not only the active principle or principles that need to be considered in relation to toxicity. Contaminants or other compounds present in the food or preparation are often more of a concern than the active principle. Recent reports from a number of countries have identified contaminants as the agents bringing about illness as a result of taking certain preparations [40–43].

The ways in which any compound of concern can affect the human body are many. There can be numerous direct adverse effects on any tissue or organ. In addition, supplements or foods containing high levels of nutrients or other compounds can have effects on the presence of other nutrients in adequate amounts. This can occur as a result of:

- destruction of nutrients
- reduction of availability of nutrients
- interference with utilization of nutrients
- interference with digestion
- decrease in food intake [44]

Natural products can also interfere or interact with pharmacological therapeutic agents. Clearly, this must be known so that disease treatment is not compromised.

7.1.6. Assessment of Natural Product for Use in Human Health and Medicine

Simply because a product has an effect in the body does not guarantee that the product will have benefit against disease. While it would seem that in some cases this is true, for example, products that lower serum cholesterol levels are considered to be of benefit in reducing the risk for coronary heart disease; in other cases it has been found not to be true. The clearest example to date is the case of the antioxidant vitamins, particularly β-carotene. β-carotene is well defined chemically, its presence in foods is well documented, and there have been many experiments, both in animals and human subjects, to show that it has antioxidant properties [45,46]. There is also considerable observational evidence in populations that low β-carotene intakes or levels in the blood are associated with a higher risk of a variety of forms of cancer than in those with high intakes or serum levels [47,48]. However, since 1994, there have been a number of investigations, with two providing the strongest evidence, to suggest that when human subjects are supplemented with β-carotene for a number of years, no reduction in risk for cancer is observed. The ATBC (α-tocopherol β-carotene) study, published in 1994, demonstrated this lack of effect in a large sample of Finnish smokers who were supplemented, or not, for a period of 6 years [49]. In fact, there was a higher risk in those supplemented with β-carotene in one age group. More recently, the CARET [50,51] study results became available. This study had to be stopped because of increased risk in the supplemented group [50]. Hence, in spite of considerable evidence in experimental situations or from observational studies to indicate the β-carotene is protective against oxidative change, and hence cancer, when free-living subjects were given the vitamin over extended periods the protective effect was not seen. When the CARET findings were released, the director of the National Cancer Institute, Richard Klausner, addressed the issue of laboratory data suggesting a hypothesis that turned out not to bring about the desired effects when tested on a disease in the real world. Cautioning against assuming too much from experimental data, he said, "But such hypotheses cannot be presumed to be true because of hope or belief, no matter how fervently they are held" [52]. There are therefore few certainties in the area of protection against disease and there must always be an ability for opinions to change.

7.2. HOW MUCH EVIDENCE IS REQUIRED?

The question of how much evidence is required cannot be answered in abstract terms. In other words, each product has its own unique features that influence the amount and type of evidence needed to satisfy the factors outlined to gain some certainty that the product is safe, that it has the claimed benefits and that it contains a consistent concentration of the active principle. However, it is helpful to examine the evidence used by the FDA in the evaluation of oats for approval for a health claim and what is being used in evaluation of psyllium.

The preliminary requirements for a health claim under NLEA are that:

(1) The substances are associated with a disease for which the US population is at risk.
(2) The substances are a food.
(3) The substances are safe [9,10].

Both oats and psyllium were submitted as health claim petitions to the FDA to reduce the risk of coronary heart disease, which remains the number one cause of death in the United States. As for these substances being a food, oatmeal and oat bran are foods and have been used as ingredients in other foods. Psyllium husk is a concentrated source of soluble fibre derived from plants of the plantago genus, and has tentatively been considered as a food by FDA. As for safety, oatmeal and oat bran have a long history of safe use. For psyllium, there are some concerns about safety, including animal evidence of increased cell proliferation in the gastrointestinal tract, allergic reactions in some people and gastrointestinal obstruction. However, these have been evaluated in the context of the products being submitted, the likely level of consumption and using the results of a report from the Life Sciences Research

Office (LSRO) of FASEB (Federation of American Societies for Experimental Biology), which evaluated the safety of psyllium risk in 1993 [53]. Evaluation of effectiveness or safety by LSRO or similar organizations can be very useful for a company intending to submit a product for regulatory approval. For example, it can indicate the likelihood of success, and while it is not without cost, it would provide a company useful information and suggest areas where further evidence should be obtained before submission.

In the case of psyllium, LSRO suggested a safe level up to 25 g/d of psyllium, and the FDA "is not prepared to disagree with LSRO's conclusions on the safety of psyllium husk" [10].

In evaluating the scientific evidence for the effectiveness of both oats and psyllium on serum cholesterol levels, the FDA used human studies. Of the studies presented to them, they selected those studies that:

- presented data and adequate descriptions of the study design and methods
- were available in English
- included estimates, or enough information to estimate soluble dietary fibre intake
- included direct measurement of blood total cholesterol (TC) and other blood lipids related to CHD
- were conducted in persons who represented the general U.S. population (adults with TC $<$6.2 mmol/L) [9,10]

Studies were excluded that were in abstract form, conducted on special population groups, on groups with cholesterol $>$6.2 mmol/L (mean) or taking lipid-lowering medication, on children, or where there was a mixture of sources of soluble fibre.

In evaluating the studies, the FDA considered the reliability and accuracy of methods of nutrient intake and measurements of total dietary and soluble dietary fibre; information on the soluble-fibre content of the products containing oats or psyllium and the control food; estimates of intake of saturated fat and cholesterol; measurement of study endpoints; and general study design characteristics, such as randomization, controls, selection criteria for subjects, attrition rates, recall and interviewer bias, control of confounding factors (saturated fat and other nutrients, body weight maintenance), and statistical tests used and statistical power. The duration of the study periods was also considered, and it was considered highly desirable to have detailed information on nutrient intakes throughout the study, including accurate intakes of total and soluble dietary fibre [9,10].

For the oat proposal, the FDA examined 37 human studies presented in the submission. Of these, only 5 studies avoided problems with subject compliance, weight loss and appropriate controls; all of these studies showed a positive effect of lowering serum total and low-density lipoprotein (LDL) cholesterol with no adverse effects on CHD risk, such as lowering high-density lipoprotein (HDL) cholesterol. While other studies supported these findings, some design, subject or procedure issues excluded them from the most highly controlled group. Eleven studies did not show an effect of oats on serum lipids. In five of these, the lack of result was thought to be due to the oat source or oat processing; for the other six, as noted by FDA, "a lack of compliance and changes in dietary intakes by the subjects plagued a number of these studies" [9]. These problems could explain the lack of result and did not affect the conclusion that the claim that oats lowered cholesterol was valid [9].

For psyllium, 21 studies were submitted. Of these, 7 were given particular weight because they were well controlled, reported intakes of fat and cholesterol, and had appropriate sample size, placebo control, and blinding. Three of these studies were parallel and 4 were crossover designs. All were published between 1988 and 1996. All showed that psyllium, as part of a diet low in saturated fat, reduced blood cholesterol levels. It was on the basis of these 7 well-controlled studied that the FDA tentatively concluded that the relationship between psyllium and coronary heart disease is valid, and is proposing to authorize a health claim [10].

Examination of these two examples indicates that the most useful evidence in evaluating the relationship between a food and disease for the purposes of health claims are well-controlled human studies, conducted on a representative sample of the population of sufficient size, duration, with good diet control and analysis of foods, diet and endpoints. Studies with design or procedure deficiencies have not been used extensively in evaluation, and if inadequate studies are the only evidence for an aspect of evaluation, no conclusion can be drawn. Such is the situation regarding dose response with psyllium as there are questions of compliance surrounding the only available study [10].

If claims are to be proposed for functional foods or nutraceuticals, similar evidence is likely to be required. However, it is not the number of studies that is the important issue, but their scientific rigour and the ability to make unambiguous evaluations and conclusions from their results. It is unlikely that if regulations change to make health claims possible in countries where they are presently prohibited, the level of scientific evidence required to establish the validity of a claim will diminish in any way. These examples from FDA deliberations are described in detail in the *Federal Register.* Regulations and deliberations from other jurisdictions and other countries are not as freely available or available in English; however, the level of evidence required is likely to be similar. For organizations contemplating promotion of a food product or supplement of any kind through the use of a health claim, acquiring good scientific support for the disease relationship is clearly necessary and efforts must be made to carry out well-controlled studies before making a submission.

8. COSTS OF MAKING HEALTH CLAIMS

Three of the major costs in making claims are in the areas of chemical analysis, human studies and submission of the evidence to the regulatory authorities. As already outlined, inadequate chemical analysis or human experimental evidence will likely result in an unsuccessful submission. It is therefore imperative that there is adequate understanding of the level of science in analysis and human experimentation required. Analysis is relatively straightforward since there are only a small number of major types of analytical procedures appropriate for determining concentrations of chemical entities within products, like gas chromatography (GC) or high-pressure liquid chromatography (HPLC) or thin-layer chromatography (TLC). Many of the methods are time-consuming and hence costly, but it is unlikely that once the method is developed and validated, the results would be ambiguous.

With human studies, however, a considerable financial commitment can be incurred in a study for which the results are not useful, and that scenario must be avoided. All efforts should be made to determine that results will be meaningful and unambiguous before substantial costs are incurred. Less expensive alternatives may turn out to be a waste of money.

Since many functional foods and nutraceuticals are being developed by small and medium-sized companies and organizations, efforts should be made at a national level to enable controlled human studies to be done, and to make available funding directed to such initiatives. For example, if agricultural initiatives to develop functional products and nutraceuticals are in place, then agricultural funding agencies must consider the health aspects of that development to be within their mandate. This may require a change of the mandate or mission of some agencies in different parts of the world. Shared funding between industry and government may also be able to address the problem of high costs of trials; hence efforts should be made to promote joint ventures of this kind. Finally, those developing new products for health reasons must acquire a mind set that this development involves human testing, and that no claim will be conceivable without it. Embarking on the production of new products without recognizing the requirement of scientific proof of effect as a component of the overall development of a product is a recipe for failure. As indicated by Cave in his book on Medicinal Plants, "The methodology of research into medicinal plants must be rigorous. Often, simple technical errors undermine the value of research on natural products. There are many who believe that a little rapid research is sufficient to confirm the reputation of a plant, and then attempt to proceed from there toward lucrative industrial production" [54].

9. BURDEN OF PROOF

In most countries, the burden of proof to show an effect of a commodity or product on a physiological or biochemical process, or on a health condition, lies with the manufacturer. However, with the passing of the DSHEA, the burden of proof for dietary supplements, which under the definition in the act include herbal products and botanicals, was transferred to the FDA. Hence it is up to federal agencies, either the FDA or the Federal Trade Commission (FTC), to ensure that companies are complying with the act (i.e. that products are safe, that statements made are not misleading, and that supplements are not being promoted for a disease or disorder). Some groups such as the American Dietetic Association (ADA) have indicated that they believe that the burden of proof for liability and product safety should be on the manufacturer, not the government [55]. ADA suggested that it would be difficult for FDA "to take prompt action to protect the public from fraudulent claims made about a dietary supplement. Actual harm would have to occur to users before any action could be taken" and that "supplements should be subject to the labelling requirements specified for foods in the NLEA" [55].

As already indicated, the shift in the burden of proof has resulted in the promotion of a number of products without evaluation by the FDA, but with statements being made in relation to a disease [25]. However, this problem appears to be being addressed by the Federal Trade Commission. Although this is being done not only after "harm has occurred," it is clear that many consumers believe the prohibited statements, as witnessed by sales of the products being questioned. However, a climate of allowing claims without pre-clearance has led to a growth in statements that are hard to regulate, as on the Internet. For example, statements suggesting that shark cartilage "inhibits tumor growth and cancer" and melatonin "strengthens the body's immune system" are appearing, not only in the U.S. but also in countries where claims without pre-clearance are not permitted [56].

The issue of where burden of proof should lie remains one of considerable debate. As the authorities in each country deal with the regulatory issues facing them, the advantages and disadvantages of each approach will have to be evaluated in considerable depth.

10. ARE HEALTH CLAIMS NEEDED?

Many companies note that the lack of ability to make health claims is a major reason for reluctance to commit significant funds to rigorous human testing of efficacy and toxicity of products [1]. Product-specific claims are viewed as a means of recouping some of the financial outlay for such studies. However, the question should be addressed of whether health claims are really needed for a product to be successful in the marketplace. A number of indications and examples suggest that products can be successful and that companies can recover their research costs without the availability of claims or other forms of protection against competition.

The first factor to consider is the popularity and acceptability by the consumer of the type of product being promoted. Use of "alternative" solutions to the treatment or prevention of disease is growing rapidly in western countries like the U.S., Canada, Europe and Australia. For example, estimates from the U.S. indicate that the botanical industry has grown from nothing 20 years ago to $1.5 billion in sales per year and increasing at a rate of 15% per year [57]. There are estimated to be about 8000 natural health food stores, which in 1994 had about $553 million in sales. Other surveys suggest that over 40% of Americans take supplements [58]. In Europe, with a longer history of use of natural products, the market is thought to be about three times larger [57]. Surveys in several European countries show that consumers want natural products to help in the treatment and prevention of health problems. In the UK, a recent survey indicated that 40% of people believe that natural products are medicines, although health claims are restricted there [56]. In Germany alone in 1993, $1.9 billion was spent on plant-based allopathic medicines [57]. The Canadian market for herbal medicines was valued at $150 million in 1995, a 20% increase over 1994 [59]. A 1993 survey in Canada found that 20% of Canadians use some form of alternative medicine and at least 6% seek advice from health food stores.

Interest is not confined to herbal products, but is growing for foods as well. Consumer focus groups conducted in 1996 by the International Food Information Council (IFIC) in the United States indicated that consumers are interested in functional foods and are keen to learn more about them [60,61]. Specifically, participants said they would prefer to incorporate these components into their diets as foods rather than take them as supplements, a finding that has been confirmed in other surveys [62]. Respondents also indicated a preference for such products to be sold alongside regular food items, rather than in a separate section of a store [60,61].

These surveys and estimates of current interest in natural products indicate that the environment into which new products are introduced is an accepting and increasingly informed one. Consumers are able to find out more about natural products themselves. Further, sales of many of these products in countries where claims are not permitted indicate that health claims on packaging are not the only way to success. The situation in Japan is also indicative of this. While a considerable number of products, probably about 100, have now been licensed as FOSHU foods, this is a small number in comparison to the hundreds of functional products being successfully marketed in Japan. The population, accepting and knowledgeable about functional benefits, will buy products whether or not they have FOSHU status [31].

The situation is not that different in North America. Breakfast cereals and cookies fortified with vitamins and minerals and declaring their antioxidant content have sold well in the U.S., as have calcium-containing orange juice and mineral water, indicating that the companies producing these fortified or "functional" products are enjoying market success without product-specific claims [63].

Another example showing that health claims may not be necessary is that of olive oil. Until 1985, monounsaturated fatty acids, the main component of olive oil, were thought to be neutral in relation to coronary heart disease risk. In that year, and in the decade following, studies have shown that monounsaturated fatty acids are not neutral, but in fact lower serum total cholesterol levels. More importantly, they lower only LDL cholesterol, leaving HDL cholesterol unchanged, which is of greater benefit than the effect of polyunsaturated fatty acids, which lower both LDL and HDL cholesterol [64–66].

Since no product-specific health claims are permitted in the U.S. or elsewhere, these new findings could not be stated on labels. However, the findings have been reported at scientific meetings, in the literature, and from there to the popular press and media. The result has been a huge increase in sales of olive oil, such that olive oil by the litre is now commonplace, and supermarkets have difficulty keeping shelves stocked. There is a widespread promotion of the Mediterranean diet by numerous agencies and health professionals, and Italian food is the most commonly ordered ethnic food in the U.S. [63]. Without any ability to make a claim, the olive oil industry is benefitting through good research in the form of controlled human studies. The findings are sound, unambiguous and have been confirmed by a number of investigators worldwide.

Will health claims help? The examples above indicate that such claims are not always necessary, and that marketing success can be achieved without them if the science supporting their effects is rigorous and if the public is accepting of the type of product being sold. However, not all segments of society may obtain knowledge about products from outside sources. For them, a claim on the label may be useful. Evidence from the 1984 claim on All Bran by the Kellogg Company indicated that through the claim on the box, knowledge of the relationship between fibre and cancer increased, with the greatest change in those socioeconomic groups that do not read educational material [16]. There may, therefore, be an advantage to claims of packaging for those sectors.

Another potential advantage of an easier regulatory environment for health claims is that companies that perceive the present situation as constricting may be more inclined to initiate studies if a claim is a possible outcome. An increased knowledge of the contents of natural products and their effects in the body is a highly desirable goal.

11. CONCLUSION

There is no doubt that the increasing interest in natural products seen since the late 1980s will continue to grow into the next century. The recognition by consumers that they must take some responsibility for their own health has led to the explosion of interest in functional foods, nutraceuticals, dietary supplements, herbal products, and botanicals. Along with consumer interest, the food and pharmaceutical industries have seen the tremendous market potential for products with health benefit. However, the health of consumers is dependent on such products being safe, and having the effects they are said to have. It is the role of health agencies within the governments of all countries to ensure that the health of their population is not put at risk by the sale of unsafe products or the promotion of products for actions they do not have. Consumers should not be self-diagnosing illness or making decisions about medication for existing conditions without consulting health professionals; government health agencies are concerned that if this occurs, disorders may be treated inappropriately and ineffectively. Those developing and promoting products with health benefit must recognize the responsibility they take when they make a claim about a product in relation to health and disease. Because this is often not the case, government agencies have been compelled to institute regulations that limit what can and cannot be said on packaging and in advertising. There is a great need for dialogue between those developing products and government health agencies so that the potential benefit of new products and new scientific findings can be promoted to improve the health of the population, while at the same time limiting the sale and promotion of unsafe products and those making inappropriate claims. Most countries are working to create an environment of collaboration, drawing on each other's experiences to develop workable regulations. By the end of the decade, and hence the century, the confusion that presently surrounds the regulations on natural products will hopefully be much diminished.

12. REFERENCES

1. International Food Focus Limited. 1995. Nutraceuticals/Functioning Foods. An Exploratory Survey of Canada's Potential. Ottawa: Agriculture and Agri-Food Canada.
2. Rowland, D. W. 1997. "Foods or quasi-drugs?" Healthy Naturally, 28:14–17.
3. Scott, F. W., N. S. Lee, R. Mongeau, N. Hidiroglou, M. L'Abbé, A. Sarwar, R. Peace. 1996. "Recommendations for defining and dealing with functional foods. A discussion paper." Ottawa: Bureau of Nutritional Sciences, Food Directorate, Health Canada.
4. Cockbill, C. A. 1994. "Food law and functional foods." British Food J., 96(3):3–4.

5. Arai, S. 1996. "Studies on functional foods in Japan—state of the art." Biosci. Biotech. Biochem., 60:9–15.
6. Agriculture and Agri-Food Canada. 1997. Guide to Food Labelling and Advertising. Ottawa: Agriculture and Agri-Food Canada.
7. Department of Health and Human Services, Food and Drug Administration. 1993. "Food labelling: general requirements for health claims for foods," Federal Register, 58:2478–2536.
8. Department of Health and Human Services, Food and Drug Administration. 1993. "Food labelling: health claims and label statements: dietary fibre and cardiovascular disease." Federal Register, 58:2552–2605.
9. Department of Health and Human Services, Food and Drug Administration. 1996. "Food labelling: health claims; oats and coronary heart disease. proposed rule." Federal Register, 61:296–337.
10. Department of Health and Human Services, Food and Drug Administration. 1997. "Food labelling: health claims: soluble fibre from certain foods and coronary heart disease." Federal Register, 62:28234–28245.
11. Department of Health and Human Services, Food and Drug Administration. 1997. "Food labelling: health claims: soluble fibre from whole oats and risk of coronary heart disease." Federal Register, 62:15343–15344.
12. Swedish Nutrition Foundation. 1996. Health Claims in the Labelling and Marketing of Food Products. The Food Industry's Rules (Self-Regulating Programme). Lund, Sweden: Swedish Nutrition Foundation.
13. Department of Health and Human Services, Food and Drug Administration. 1994. "Food labelling; general requirements for health claims for dietary supplements. Final rule." Federal Register, 59(2):395–426.
14. Department of Health and Human Services, Food and Drug Administration. 1996. "Regulation of medical foods. Advance notice of proposed rulemaking." Federal Register, 61:60661–606711.
15. Ippolito, P. M. and A. D. Mathios. 1993. "New food labelling regulations and the flow of nutrition information to consumers." J. Pub. Policy and Marketing, 12:188–205.
16. Ippolito, P. M. and A. D. Mathios. 1989. Health Claims in Advertising and Labelling: A Study of the Cereal Markets. Washington, DC: Federal Trade Commission.
17. Department of Health and Human Services, Food and Drug Administration. 1993. "Food labelling: final rules." Federal Register, 58:2066–2941.
18. Ford, G. T., M. Mastak, A. Mitra and D. J. Ringold. 1996. "Can consumers interpret nutrition information in the presence of a health claim? A laboratory investigation." J. Pub. Policy and Marketing, 15:16–27.
19. Silverglade, B. A. 1996. "The nutrition labelling and education act—progress to date and challenges for the future." J. Pub. Policy and Marketing, 15:148–150.
20. Food Marketing Institute. 1995. Shopping for Health. Washington, DC: Food Marketing Institute.
21. Pappalardo, J. K. 1996. "Evaluating the NLEA: where's the beef?" J. Pub. Policy and Marketing, 15:153–156.
22. Petruccelli, P. J. 1996. "Consumer and marketing implications of information provision: the case of the nutrition labelling and education act of 1990." J. Pub. Policy and Marketing, 15:150–153.

23. Farley, D. 1993. "Look for 'LEGIT' health claims on foods." FDA Consumer, 27: 15–21.
24. Kellogg Canada Inc. 1997. Fibre Update: Wheat Bran in Colon Risk Reduction. Etobicoke, ON: Nutrition Communications, Kellogg Canada Inc.
25. Department of Health and Human Services, Food and Drug Administration. 1996. "Food labelling: dietary supplement; nutritional support statement; notification procedure. Proposed rule." Federal Register, 61:50771–50774.
26. Federal Trade Commission. 1996. "Home Shopping Network, Inc.; Home Shopping Club, Inc.; LISN Lifeway Health Products, Inc.: Proposed consent agreement with analysis to aid public comment." Federal Register, 61:38738–38741.
27. Federal Trade Commission. 1996. "Nutrition 21; Selene Systems, Inc.; Herbert H. Boynton: Analysis to aid public comment. Proposed consent agreement." Federal Register, 61:58562–58563.
28. Federal Trade Commission. 1997. "KCD Holdings, Inc., et al.; Interactive Medical Technologies, Ltd., et al.; William Pelzer, Jr.; and William E. Shell, M.D.: Analysis to aid public comment. Proposed consent agreements." Federal Register, 62:16587–16590.
29. Federal Trade Commission. 1997. "Universal Merchants, Inc., et al.; Prohibited trade practices, and affirmative corrective actions. Consent order." Federal Register, 62:15896.
30. Federal Trade Commission. 1997. "Amerifit, Inc.: analysis to aid public comment. Proposed consent agreement." Federal Register, 62:16584–16585.
31. Lapsley, K. G. 1996. Does the Process Work? Legislated Food Health Claims in Japan. Insight Communications.
32. Smith, B. L., M. Marcotte and G. Harrison. 1996. A Comparative Analysis of the Regulatory Framework Affecting Functional Food Development and Commercialization in Canada, Japan, the European Union and the United States of America. Ottawa, ON: Inter/sect Alliance Inc.
33. Health Canada. Food Directorate and Drugs/Medical Devices Programme. 1997. Discussion Document. Functional Foods and Nutraceuticals. Consultation Workshop. Ottawa: Health Canada.
34. International Life Sciences Institute (ILSI) Europe. 1997. Functional Food Science in Europe: State of the Art. A European Commission Concerted Action. Summary Report of a First Plenary Meeting. April 1996. Nice, Brussels: ILSI Europe.
35. Dance, B. 1997. "European concerted action programme on functional food science in Europe." First Plenary Meeting on Functional Food Science in Europe: State of the Art. Brussels: ILSI Europe, pp. 9–10.
36. Richardson, D. P. 1997. "Industry perspectives on foods with health claims." First Plenary Meeting on Functional Food Science in Europe: State of the Art. Brussels: ILSI Europe.
37. Stephen, A. M. 1996. "Nutraceuticals—the way forward." J. Nutraceut. Functional and Medical Foods, 1:103.
38. National Institute of Nutrition. 1996. "Nutraceuticals—towards consumer and market health." Rapport, 11 (Winter 1996):1, 4–5.
39. Cassidy, A., S. Bingham and K. D. R. Setchell. 1994. "Biological effects of a diet of soy protein rich in isoflavones on the menstrual cycle of premenopausal women." Amer. J. Clin. Nutr., 60:333–40.

40. Kew, J., C. Morris, A. Athie, R. Fysh, S. Jones and D. Brooks. 1993. "Arsenic and mercury intoxication due to indian ethnic remedies." BMJ, 306:507–8.
41. Shaw, D., I. House, S. Kolev and V. Murray. 1995. "Should herbal medicines be licensed?" Br. Med. J., 311:451–2.
42. Gertner, E., P. S. Marshall, D. Filandrionos, A. S. Potek and T. M. Smith. 1995. "Complications resulting from the use of Chinese herbal medications containing undeclared prescription drugs." Arthritis Rheu., 38:614–617.
43. Vanhaelen, M., R. Vanhaelen-Fastre, P. But and J. L. Vanderweighem. 1994. "Identification of Aristolochic acid in Chinese herbs." Lancet, 343:174.
44. Teutonico, R. A. 1987. "Impact of biotechnology on the nutritional quality of foods." Food Biotechnology, D. Knorr, ed., New York: Marcel Dekker Inc.
45. Burton, G. W. and K. U. Ingold. 1984. "β-Carotene: an unusual type of lipid antioxidant." Science, 224:569–73.
46. Krinsky, N. I. 1993. "Actions of carotenoids in biological systems." Ann. Rev. Nutr., 13:561–87.
47. Steinmetz, K. A. and J. D. Potter. 1991. "Vegetables, fruit, and cancer." Cancer Causes Control, 2:325–57, 427–42.
48. Block, G., B. Patterson and A. Subar. 1992. "Fruit, vegetables, and cancer prevention: a review of the epidemiology evidence." Nutr. Cancer, 18:1–19.
49. The Alpha-tocopherol, Beta Carotene Cancer Prevention Study Group. 1994. "The effect of vitamin E and beta carotene on the incidence of lung cancer and other cancers in male smokers." New Engl. J. Med., 330:1029–1035.
50. Omenn, G. S., G. E. Goodman, M. D. Thornquist, J. Balmes, M. R. Cullen, A. Glass, J. P. Keogh, F. L. Meykens, Jr., B. Valanis, J. H. Williams, Jr., S. Barnhart, and S. Hammar. 1996. "Effects of a combination of beta carotene and vitamin A on lung cancer and cardiovascular disease." New Engl. J. Med., 334:1150–55.
51. Omenn, G. S., G. E. Goodman, M. D. Thornquist, J. Balmes, M. R. Cullen and A. Glass. 1996. "Risk factors for lung cancer and for intervention effects in CARET, the beta-carotene and retinol efficacy trial." J. Nat. Cancer Inst., 88: 1550–1559.
52. Smigel, K. 1996. "Beta carotene fails to prevent cancer in two major studies: CARET intervention stopped." J. Nat. Cancer Inst., 88:145.
53. Life Sciences Research Office (LSRO), FASEB. 1993. The Evaluation of the Safety of Using Psyllium Seed Husk as a Food Ingredient. Bethesda, MD: FASEB.
54. Cave, A. 1986. "Methodology of research on medicinal plants." Advances in Medicinal Phytochemistry, D. Barton and W.D. Ollis, eds., London: John Libbey.
55. American Dietetic Association. 1993. "Labelling of dietary supplements stirs congressional debate." J. Amer. Diet. Assoc., 93(10):1110.
56. Bower, H. 1996. "Internet sees growth of unverified health claims." Br. Med. J., 313:381.
57. Marwick, C. 1995. "Growing use of medicinal botanicals forces assessment by drug regulators." J. Amer. Med. Assoc., 273:607–609.
58. Gannon, K. 1992. "Multivitamins are favored supplement among Americans." Drug Topics, 136:34.
59. Cottress, K. 1996. "Herbal products begin to attract the attention of brand-name drug companies." Can. Med. Assoc., 155(2):216–219.

60. Cooper, J. 1997. "Functional foods: fad or food of the future?" Can. Grocer, (March):14–16.
61. Schmidt, D. B. 1997. Communicating the Benefits of Functional Foods: Insights from U.S. Consumer and Health Professional Focus Groups, National Institute of Nutrition 1997 Annual General Meeting, Toronto.
62. Wrick, K. L., K. J. Briedman., J. K. Brewda and J. J. Carroll. 1993. "Consumer viewpoints on 'designer foods.'" Food Tech., (March):94–104.
63. Sloan, A. E. 1994. "Top ten trends to watch and work on." Food Tech., (July): 89–100.
64. Mattson, F. H. and S. M. Grundy. 1985. "Comparison of effects of dietary saturated, monounsaturated and polyunsaturated fatty acids on plasma lipids and lipoproteins in man." J. Lipid. Res., 26:194–202.
65. Baggio, G. 1988. "Olive-oil enriched diet: effect on serum lipoprotein levels and biliary cholesterol saturation." Amer. J. Clin. Nutr., 47:960–4.
66. Mensink, R. P. and M. B. Katan. 1989. "Effect of an enriched diet with monounsaturated or polyunsaturated fatty acids on levels of a low-density and high-density lipoprotein cholesterol in healthy women and men." New Engl. J. Med., 321: 436–441.

Index

About the Editor

G. (Joe) Mazza, Ph.D., is Senior Research Scientist and Head of the Food Research Program at the Agriculture and Agri-Food Canada, Pacific Agri-Food Research Centre, Summerland, British Columbia, Canada. He is also an Adjunct Professor in the Departments of Food Science at the University of Manitoba, Winnipeg, Manitoba, and University of British Columbia, Vancouver, British Columbia, Canada. Dr. Mazza was born in Pietrapertosa, Potenza, Italy, in 1946. He studied Agricultural Sciences at the University of Naples, Italy, and graduated with a B.Sc.A. degree in Food Science from the University of Manitoba in 1973. He received his Ph.D. degree from the University of Alberta, Edmonton, Alberta, and did postdoctoral studies at the Institut de Chimie, Université Louis Pasteur, Strausbourg, France.

Prior to joining the Research Branch of Agriculture and Agri-Food Canada, Dr. Mazza was a Food Scientist for Burns Foods Ltd., Winnipeg and Calgary, and at the Alberta Horticultural Research Center, Brooks, Alberta. Over the years he has served on a variety of national and international scientific and advisory committees involved in setting research priorities and identifying research needs for improved value-added processing, safety, and quality of plant products.

Dr. Mazza has published over 110 research papers, several critical reviews, and over 20 book chapters. He is a co-author of the CRC Press book *Anthocyanins in Fruits, Vegetables and Grains,* and the holder of several patents for food processes/products.

Dr. Mazza has also served as member of the editorial boards of the *Canadian Institute of Food Science and Technology Journal* and the *Journal of Food Quality,* and has reviewed several books and many research papers for journals and granting agencies. He is a member of the Canadian Institute of Food Science and Technology, the Institute of Food Technologists, the Potato Association of America, and the Groupe Polyphénols. He also serves on several regional, national, and international committees, including the Expert Committee on Plant Products of the Canada Committee on Food. One of Dr. Mazza's current major research interests concerns characterization, properties, and applications of phytochemicals in food/pharmaceutical products.

Dr. Mazza received the 1992 Public Service of Canada Merit Award for his outstanding research on behalf of the Canadian Potato Industry and was the 1994 recipient of the W.J. Eva Award of the Canadian Institute of Food Science and Technology for his contributions to food science in Canada through outstanding research and services.